ADVANCES IN HOST DEFENSE MECHANISMS
Volume 2

LYMPHOID CELLS

Advances in Host Defense Mechanisms
Volume 2

Lymphoid Cells

Editors

John I. Gallin, M.D.
Head, Bacterial Diseases Section
Laboratory of Clinical Investigation
National Institute of Allergy and Infectious
Diseases
National Institutes of Health
Bethesda, Maryland

Anthony S. Fauci, M.D.
Chief, Laboratory of Immunoregulation
National Institute of Allergy and Infectious
Diseases
National Institutes of Health
Bethesda, Maryland

Raven Press ■ New York

Raven Press, 1140 Avenue of the Americas, New York, New York 10036

The material contained in this volume was submitted as previously unpublished material, except in the instances in which credit has been given to the source from which some of the illustrative material was derived.

Great care has been taken to maintain the accuracy of the information contained in the volume. However, Raven Press cannot be held responsible for errors or for any consequences arising from the use of the information contained herein.

Materials appearing in this book prepared by individuals as part of their official duties as U.S. Government employees are not covered by the above-mentioned copyright.

Library of Congress Cataloging in Publication Data
Main entry under title:

Lymphoid cells.

(Advances in host defense mechanisms ; v. 2)
Includes bibliographical references and index.
1. Lymphocytes.   I. Gallin, John I.   II. Fauci,
Anthony S.   III. Series.   [DNLM: 1. Lymphocytes—
Immunology.   W1 AD636 / QW 568 L98603]
QR185.8.L9L98   1983   616.07′9   83-2848
ISBN 0-89004-729-4

Preface

The overlap between infectious diseases and immunology is best exemplified by an appreciation of the role of lymphoid cells and their products in host defense mechanisms. This critical relationship is the subject of this volume of the new series *Advances in Host Defense Mechanisms*. In early 1982, the first volume, devoted to the role of phagocytic cells in host defenses, met with considerable enthusiasm. This second volume presents the basic scientific foundation for the understanding and appreciation of the clinically relevant mechanisms of immune-mediated host defenses.

It is gratifying to have Dr. Robert A. Good provide the introductory chapter, Historic Perspectives. His contribution to this field is universally recognized, and his lifetime of commitment to this endeavor has played a major role in the feasibility of constructing such a volume.

One of the major areas of impact of immune function on host defenses is within the scope of the immunodeficiency diseases. These "experiments of nature" have allowed us to appreciate the role of various components of the immune response in providing the critical elements of host defenses against broad and specific categories of microorganisms. The chapter by Gelfand and Cohen, by analyzing certain of these immunodeficiency diseases with a focus on disorders of purine metabolism, provides a comprehensive and up-to-date review of several of the cellular metabolic processes involved in maintaining the integrity of the immune system. The multifaceted mechanisms available to the host in its defense against various types of microorganisms are presented in several chapters devoted to the distinct categories of organisms. Brunham and Holmes discuss the role of the lymphoid system in protection and recovery from bacterial infections.

Greenspan, Schwartz, and Doherty delineate the complex mechanisms of immune surveillance against viral infections and describe various components of the virus-host interaction, the different lymphocyte populations involved in host defense mechanisms, as well as the genetic restrictions in host defense against viral-infected cells. The latter point is of obvious importance in understanding the broader implications of genetic restrictions of immune reactivity. Mason and Kirkpatrick present a comprehensive review of the literature together with their own well-documented and extensive contributions to the area of immune-mediated host defense against mycotic and certain mycobacterial infections. They discuss cellular mechanisms, chemotherapy, and immunologic manipulations employed in the therapeutic approaches to these complex infectious diseases. Further insight into the complex mechanisms of host defense against mycobacterial infections is given by Bullock, who provides a most sophisticated approach toward these organisms in the cellular interactions which they elicit and upon which their containment depends.

v

The recent upsurge of interest and knowledge of the role of the immune system in host defenses against parasitic infections, particularly the protozoan infections, has been profound. The relevance of these disorders is clear, in that hundreds of millions of people as well as economically important domestic animals are infected with parasites. Only within the past few years have we come to a solid scientific base for understanding the role of specificity and nonspecificity of immune responses in host defenses against these multicellular organisms. The chapter by Allison and Eugui illustrates the multiplicity of immune responses elicited by protozoan parasitic infections and the various escape mechanisms from the infections. The authors review how parasite immunology has emerged from the stage of descriptive phenomenology to become one of the growing areas of biologic science that may lead to the control of these organisms.

Clearly, host defense mechanisms relate not only to infectious agents but to neoplastic transformation as well. In fact, keen insight into the subject of host defense mechanisms has evolved from an understanding of the similarity and overlap among mechanisms which the host employs in its defense against microbes and neoplastic cells. Herberman has been one of the major contributors in this area of immune-mediated host defense against neoplastic transformation. His chapter is a comprehensive discussion of the simplicity and complexity of these diverse mechanisms of host defense. The important impact of the nutritional status of the host on his ability to mount a specific immune response against microbial invaders is emphasized in the chapter by Keusch, Wilson, and Waksal on the relationship of nutrition and immune-mediated host defenses. The widespread malnutrition in certain parts of the world makes this aspect of host defense a globally important problem.

The science of immunology is rapidly expanding and becoming extraordinarily complex. Since immunology had its birth in the science of infectious diseases, it is appropriate that these irrevocably intertwined disciplines should continue to provide each other with complementary insights into their respective fields.

John I. Gallin
Anthony S. Fauci

Contents

Contributors

Anthony C. Allison: *Institute of Biological Sciences, Syntex Research, Palo Alto, California 94304*

Robert C. Brunham: *Department of Medicine and Medical Microbiology, University of Manitoba, Basic Medical Sciences Building, Winnipeg, Manitoba, Canada*

Ward E. Bullock, Jr.: *Division of Infectious Diseases, Department of Internal Medicine, University of Cincinnati College of Medicine, Cincinnati, Ohio 45267*

Amos Cohen: *Division of Immunology, Research Institute, Hospital for Sick Children, Toronto, Ontario, Canada*

P. C. Doherty: *The Wistar Institute of Anatomy and Biology, Philadelphia, Pennsylvania 19104*

Elsie M. Eugui: *Institute of Biological Sciences, Syntex Research, Palo Alto, California 94304*

Erwin W. Gelfand: *Division of Immunology, Research Institute, Hospital for Sick Children, Toronto, Ontario, Canada*

Robert A. Good: *Oklahoma Medical Research Foundation, Oklahoma City, Oklahoma 73104*

N. S. Greenspan: *858 Berick Drive, University City, Missouri 63132*

Ronald B. Herberman: *Laboratory of Immunodiagnosis, National Cancer Institute, National Institutes of Health, Bethesda, Maryland 20205*

King. K. Holmes: *Department of Medicine, University of Washington, and Division of Infectious Diseases, Seattle Public Health Hospital, Seattle, Washington 98114*

Gerald T. Keusch: *Division of Geographic Medicine, Department of Medicine, Tufts-New England Medical Center, Boston, Massachusetts 02111*

Charles H. Kirkpatrick: *The Conrad D. Stephenson Laboratory for Research in Immunology, Department of Medicine, National Jewish Hospital and Research Center/National Asthma Center, Denver, Colorado 80206*

Ulysses G. Mason: *The Conrad D. Stephenson Laboratory for Research in Immunology, Department of Medicine, National Jewish Hospital and Research Center/National Asthma Center, Denver, Colorado 80206*

D. H. Schwartz: *The Wistar Institute of Anatomy and Biology, Philadelphia, Pennsylvania 19104*

Samuel D. Waksal: *Division of Geographic Medicine, Department of Medicine, Tufts-New England Medical Center, Boston, Massachusetts 02111*

Carla S. Wilson: *Division of Geographic Medicine, Department of Medicine, Tufts-New England Medical Center, Boston, Massachusetts 02111*

Advances in Host Defense Mechanisms, Vol. 2,
edited by John I. Gallin and Anthony S. Fauci.
Raven Press, New York © 1983.

Historic Aspects of Cellular Immunology

Robert A. Good

Oklahoma Medical Research Foundation, Oklahoma City, Oklahoma 73104

When I began my work in cellular immunology in 1943, nothing was known of the cellular basis of immunity. It was widely held that macrophages were the antibody-producing cells because that had been the conclusion drawn by Sabin (222) from her work at the Rockefeller Institute. It was known from the studies of Tiselius and Kabat (250) that antibodies were contained in the electrophoretically defined gamma-globulin fraction, but nothing further was known of the chemistry of the antibody molecules. Complement was considered a single substance which complemented the functions of antibodies; and thymus, lymph nodes, and even spleen were organs whose functions seemed enigmatic. Lymphocytes were being aroused from a sleepy past by the studies of Dougherty and White (54) at Yale, who had concluded that lymphocyte dissolution under the influences of adrenal hormones might be the source of antibodies and gamma-globulin molecules in the circulating blood.

Today, in contrast, we have virtually complete chemical descriptions of antibodies reflecting immunoglobulins (Ig) of five distinct isotypes, plus four subclasses of IgG and two of IgA. The amino acid sequences of each of the Ig classes have been, or are soon to be, completed (49), and the basis of specificity of Ig for antigen has been linked firmly to variability of amino acid sequences in the so-called variable regions of kappa and lambda light chains and the heavy chains of each of the Ig isotypes and subclasses (160). Indeed, the gene sequences and the mechanisms of gene arrangement and rearrangement from germ line organization to the B cell differentiated form (153) are being progressively invoked to permit understanding of what has been called the essential miracle of immunology. The latter was defined by Medawar to be that a rabbit yet unborn should be able to make antibody to an antigen not yet synthesized.

Cellular immunology has developed apace. We now recognize that the thymus contains a central lymphoid organ site (239) where one class of lymphocytes, the T cells, are launched on a lineage of development which permits distinction of self from nonself, establishment of essentially permanent immunologic tolerance, and, early in life at least, production of large numbers of lymphocytes which seed to the periphery a self-perpetuating population of immunologically competent cells (111). The latter contribute to the development and functions of the antibody-producing cells. They are capable of exercising crucial immunologic functions and

1

contribute coordinate functions to maintain the integrity of the individual mammal in those seas of bacteria, viruses, fungi, and protozoa that have been selected as ecologic niches for mammals. We are coming to know the B lymphocytes, where their differentiation is initiated (204,205), how their total population and subpopulations are expanded and differentiated, and how their functions and differentiation are orchestrated by the T lymphocytes. We have dissected the different regions of lymph nodes, spleen, and other lymphoid aggregates (205,207) and defined and are rapidly expanding our knowledge of the crucial functions of the genes of the major histocompatibility complex (MHC) (110). We are learning the rules that govern the essential interactions of cells within the different lymphoid cell populations. We are also dissecting rapidly the mechanism whereby positive and negative influences of the lymphoid cells are exercised (74); we are learning the nature of crucial cell-cell interactions and are exploring the molecular nature of these interactions. Some scientists have been analyzing functions of lymphoid subpopulations in terms of surface determinants on their membranes and defining the chemical basis of surface-to-nuclear signals that control proliferation and differentiation of the T and B lymphocytes. We are even getting to know and to be able to identify precursors of plasma cells, such as pre-pre-B cells, pre-B cells, and B lymphocytes (135).

The knowledge at genetic, molecular, and cellular levels of immunologic development, although still rudimentary by some standards, is greater than for any other physiologically and pathologically important system (167). The development of our understanding is occurring so rapidly and with such precision that it is difficult for any modern-day immunologist to keep abreast of all aspects of the expanding understanding of immunologic function. Yet this entire explosion of immunologic knowledge has taken place during the lifetime of individuals who are still working productively in this exciting field. How did we get here? Can we visualize from the approaches that have taken us here the approaches that will be most useful in taking us where we shall be going in the future?

To accept the task of writing about immunologic development in historic perspective, any working immunologist would have to plead prejudice based on his personal involvement and realize that his account will suffer from, as well as have the advantage of, personal experience. Thus I accept my bias at the outset as I attempt herein to construct a picture of some of the extraordinary events in immunology which underlie the understanding of the immunologic systems and their organization and functions in 1983.

THE STORY OF THE PLASMA CELL

A beginning of modern immunology occurred in Denmark in the mid-1930s. Bing and Plum (19) had encountered an experiment of nature from a study of 11 cases of aplastic anemia. Three of these patients showed an exciting conjunction of high globulin levels and striking bone marrow plasmacytosis. The investigators, recognizing a thread of information that linked plasma cells to immunity, antibody-production, and protein synthesis which extended back to the earliest descriptions of the plasma cell, before 1900, drew an audacious conclusion. From their clinical investigations, they proposed that the plasma cells in their aplastic patients might actually be the cells that produced the globulin which was accummulating in the blood. This hypothesis, of course, was only a suggestion, but it struck a consonant note in Minneapolis, Minnesota, where Kolouch, then a medical graduate student with Downey, was interpreting another experiment of nature (138,139). Kolouch had followed to autopsy a patient with subacute bacterial endocarditis, at that time a regularly fatal disease. From study of the histology of bone marrow and spleen, Kolouch had become excited about the extraordinary accumulation of plasma cells in his patient. He already knew something of lymphocytes and mononuclear cells, because he had studied origins of the mononuclear cells in acute inflammation (140). He attempted in vain to learn from his teachers what the tremendous accumulations of plasma cells in the spleen and bone marrow of his patient might mean. However, both Downey, his teacher of hematology, and Clawson, his teacher of pathology, suggested that the plasma cells might have something to do with immunity. Downey thought that plasma cells had the morphologic appearance of secretory cells with their basophilic cytoplasma and distinctly eccentric nucleus (169), and Clawson had recognized many plasma cells in tissues of rats in which he had produced lesions pathologically like rheumatic fever by repeated infections with *Streptococcus viridans*. These discussions provoked Kolouch to prepare a heat-killed bacterial vaccine from the *S. viradans* organisms that had been grown from his patient. He repeatedly injected the vaccine intravenously into small rabbits. Kolouch reported in 1938 (139) that the repeated injections of *S. viridans* produced a rapidly developing plasmacytosis of the bone marrow in these rabbits. This was especially true if the rabbits signaled their immunity by developing anaphylactic shock. Kolouch reported his experiments and drew from them the conclusion that the plasma cells are responsible for producing the antibodies following antigenic challenge.

Kolouch, however, was removed from the scene of the embryonic field of cellular immunology for several years; after completing medical school, he had been almost forced to enter private medical practice to save his father's business after his father had had an attack of coronary vascular disease. Kolouch missed an opportunity to take a fellowship at Harvard with Menkin and practiced general medicine for several years. Upon returning to the academic scene at Minnesota, he joined the surgery department as a student of Wangensteen. In 1943, when I was beginning my research at Minnesota in Campbell's neurophysiology laboratories, Kolouch befriended me and urged me to help him with these experiments that were now somewhat tentative in his mind. He was wondering whether it was the complex physiologic consequences of anaphylaxis or whether it was the antibody production initiated by secondary exposure to the bacterial antigen that had generated the rapid development of plasma cells in his rabbits.

I had already become interested in lymphocytes and plasma cells which appeared in inflammatory exudates produced by virus infections of the central nervous system, and I thought I could suggest a simple experiment to help Kolouch. We compared experimentally passive anaphylaxis with active anaphylaxis and found that only the latter produced the extraordinary plasmacytosis that Kolouch had called attention to in his Master's thesis and initial publication. Thus we felt certain that we could link plasmacytosis to the secondary immune response to a bacterial vaccine (84). I subsequently carried out many experiments which showed that plasma cells were a reliable sign of allergic inflammation and that plasmacytosis was correlated to antibody production to several different kinds of antigens (85,86,88,141).

Kolouch's experiments also generated a response in Denmark. Stimulated by his studies, Bjorneboe and Gormsen (20) had launched experiments in which eight different types of heat-killed pneumococci were injected repeatedly into rabbits. This challenge produced extraordinary accumulations of plasma cells, massive antibody titers, and a huge peak of gamma-globulins in the blood. From their studies, these investigators concluded that plasma cells were the cells that made both antibody and gamma-globulins.

It was difficult for us few plasma cell hunters of the early 1940s because the experiments of Dougherty and White (55) and Dougherty et al. (53), as well as those of Ehrich and Harris (62), were being interpreted to indicate that lymphocytes were, indeed, responsible for antibody production. We on the other hand were impressed by the consistent association in our studies of plasmacytosis with immune responses, antibody production, and gamma-globulin levels and could show that plasmacytosis was even correlated with the rate of gamma-globulin accumulation in the blood (87). Thus we argued at every opportunity against the increasingly popular lymphocyte theory and for the plasma cell basis of antibody production.

Fagraeus (67), working in Sweden and separated from us not only by distance but by World War II, came forth with crucial experimental data. She had been stimulated to study plasma cells as antibody-producing cells after becoming impressed by myeloma cells. She recognized that in this disease, too, gamma-globulins often accumulate in the blood. Encouraged by Theorell, the virologist, Fagraeus (68) had also chosen to work with the secondary immune response, and after immunization of rabbits she challenged their tissues *in vitro* with an immunizing bacterial antigen. She compared the antibody produced by bits of lymphocyte-rich tissues, the Malpighian corpuscles of spleen, and bits of plasma cell-rich tissues, the red pulp of spleen. Her results were clear-cut and quite convincing: it was the plasma cell rich red pulp of spleen which, upon challenge with antigen *in vitro*, produced significant amounts of antibody. These findings provoked Ehrich to have a second look; with Drabkin and his student Forman (61), he completely switched his interpretation and now sided with the developing plasma-cell perspective. Harris and Harris (119), on the other hand, continued steadfastly to hold to the lymphocyte theory of antibody production on the basis of their analysis of proliferative responses of the lymphocytes to antigenic stimulation. There was much feeling in these disputes, particularly between the Harrises and Ehrich, who were former collaborators. There were also milder disputes between us plasma cell hunters at Minnesota and Dougherty, who did not like Kolouch's experiments but was more relaxed in his criticisms.

New methodology contributing to these analyses was introduced by Coons at Harvard who, with White of Scotland, Leduc, and Connally, had developed a new technology which permitted analysis of Ig as well as antibodies within cells. They used the technique developed by Coons that had permitted analysis of distribution of antigenic proteins in the tissues, namely immunofluorescence microscopy. In a spate of beautifully illustrated papers that they published in the *Journal of Experimental Medicine* (35,157,263), these investigators brought forward immunohistochemical testimony to support the view that it was plasma cells and their immediate round cell precursors that were the antibody- and gamma-globulin-producing cells.

I remember visiting Coons for the first time in his laboratories at Harvard in 1949. Stetson had taken me to see Coons following one of Cohn's seminars. In this particular seminar, Perutz, the Nobel Laureate-to-be, had described the crystallization of horse hemoglobin on which he had been working. During this visit, Coons listened critically to my analysis of the lymphocyte-plasma cell controversy and to my arguments that I felt permitted us to conclude that plasma cells and not lymphocytes were the antibody-producing cells. He advised me to publish all our data in the most critically edited journals and not to rely on publications in the *Proceedings of the Society for Experimental Biology and Medicine*. He also told me of the progress he was making in tracing antigens with his exciting new method. Two or three years later, he, White, Leduc, and Connally, using their new methods, came out with an impressive analysis of the questions I had raised with him.

THE CHALLENGE OF AGAMMAGLOBULINEMIA

Popper (214) has pointed out that the power of a scientific hypothesis is directly proportional to its refutability. In his book, he compared the lack of scientific power of explanatory but nonrefutable hypotheses, such as those of Marxism and Freudianism on the one hand with Einstein's theory of relativity on the other. The latter, he indicated, derived its great power because, had it been wrong, it could have been refuted by observations made at the first eclipse of the sun following its pronouncement.

The opportunity for complete refutation of the plasma cell theory of Ig and antibody production was provided by Bruton's discovery of the experiment of nature represented by a patient who could make neither antibody nor gamma-globulin. At the time, I was studying several patients with X-linked agammaglobulinemia who, as Bruton had shown, could make no antibody to antigenic challenge. We had already compared bone marrow and lymph nodes of immunologically normal volunteers and patients with rheumatic fever (87) and liver disease; we had linked quantitatively the bone marrow plasmacytosis with the slope of gamma-globulin accumulation in the blood in rheumatic fever and the abundant plasmacytosis in the liver with high gamma-globulin levels in patients with Kunkel's liver disease (146). The latter disease was called plasma cell hepatitis (91). We knew how many plasma cells could be expected in the marrow of normals (87) and in immunologically normal persons following antigenic stimulation by several routes. Thus as quickly as possible after Bruton's discovery of agammaglobulinemia, we checked plasma cell and antibody responses and established that patients with X-linked infantile agammaglobulinemia had no plasma cells in their bone marrow and did not respond by developing plasma cells in marrow after antigenic challenge by the intravenous route (89,90). Furthermore, these patients did not generate plasma cells in the medullary cords of the lymph node draining sites of antigenic stimulation in primary, secondary, or even tertiary immune responses after subcutaneous or intracutaneous injections of antigen.

Had the plasma cell theory of antibody and Ig production not been correct, our postulate of the cellular basis of antibody and Ig production would have been immediately refuted by study of these extraordinary patients who on the basis of a genetic abnormality could produce no gamma-globulin and no antibody. We also observed in these patients that germinal centers, which I called secondary follicles in those days, were also lacking and did not appear after antigenic challenge (90,106). By contrast, lymphocyte counts in the blood and lymphocyte populations in lymph nodes and spleens of such patients were normal. We also compared plasma cell accumulations in the lamina propria of the gastrointestinal tract and appendix of patients with agammaglobulinemia with those of immunologically normal children and adults (23). Our analyses showed that agammaglobulinemic patients had no plasma cells in these locations, but that immunologically intact persons, in contrast, had plenty of plasma cells at these sites. Finally, we compared chronic pathologic exudates, e.g., bronchiectatic lesions in normal and agammaglobulinemic patients, and established that plasma cells were regularly a prominent component in such exudates of immunologically vigorous persons. Plasma cells and certain nodular lymphoid accumulations regularly seen in immunologically normal persons and in most lymphoid tissues obtained at postmortem from persons with apparently normal immunologic vigor were lacking in the agammaglobulinemic patients. Our pathologic studies later revealed that the thymus was normal in these patients, as were circulating lymphocyte counts and lymphoid accumulations of the deep cortical regions of lymph nodes (88,106).

ORIGIN OF THE TWO CELL COMPONENT CONCEPT OF IMMUNE FUNCTIONS

These findings proved particularly provocative because we and others could show that agammaglobulinemic patients were susceptible especially to infections by certain high-grade encapsulated bacterial pathogens, e.g., *S. pneumoniae, S. pyogenes, Hemophilus influenzae,* and *Pseudomonas aeruginosa,* whereas other bacterial pathogens, such as *Bacillus tuberculosis,* atypical acid-fast organisms, fungi, and even certain viruses seemed to be resisted vigorously by these patients (23,88,106). We showed that although these patients with agammaglobulinemia lacked the ability to form antibodies after stimulation, they could normally develop delayed bacterial allergy and certain drug-induced allergies, e.g., allergy to 2-4,dinitrofluorobenzine. Their peripheral blood lymphocytes readily transferred specific delayed allergic reactions to nonsensitized immunocompetent donors, just as could the peripheral blood lymphocytes from normal donors (105). Thus from extensive study of these patients, we suggested the existence of two separate immunity systems. One related to antibody production and was based on plasma cell formation and germinal center lymphocyte development. The other seemed to be related to circulating blood lymphocytes (88,105,106). The latter system we later associated with a normal thymus morphology. At this early date, we concluded it was clearly associated with abundant lymphocyte populations in lymph nodes, spleen, and other lymphoid aggregates. This latter form of immunity system we linked to delayed-type hypersensitivity, resistance to infections with fungi, viruses, and facultative intracellular bacterial pathogens (88,98,106), and also to allograft rejection. Study of agammaglobulinemic patients particularly permitted new perspectives concerning the existence of two separate lymphoid systems representing distinct and separable mechanisms of the bodily defense. This conclusion also seemed to be consonant with findings we and others had been deriving from comparative investigations of the infections and immunologic responses in patients with multiple myeloma and Hodgkin disease (98,101,132).

Upon first coming to the Rockefeller Institute in 1949, I was seeking a source of C-reactive protein-containing body fluid to substitute for the streptococcal effusion fluid from which McCarty had crystallized the C-reactive protein. I found this valuable resource in patients with Hodgkin disease. These patients had been brought to my attention during 1949 and 1950 by Karnofsky at the Sloan-Kettering Institute in New York. I found chest fluids containing high concentrations of C-reactive protein in the Hodgkin disease patients and was even able to crystallize this protein from their effusions. I was stimulated by the fact that these patients seemed to be susceptible to tuberculosis, fungus infections, and certain viral infections and apparently not so susceptible to infection by pneumococcus, streptococcus, *H. influenzae*, or pseudomonas.

In striking contrast were the findings concerning infections in patients with multiple myeloma, whom I was also studying in order to help Kunkel obtain blood serum containing myeloma globulin. Myeloma patients, too, had many infections, but the organisms infecting them were different from those of patients with Hodgkin disease. In myeloma, pneumococcus, streptococcus, and *H. influenzae* caused the most trouble.

These two groups of patients, both with hematopoietic malignancy, proved also to be different from one another upon immunologic analyses. The patients with Hodgkin disease lacked delayed allergy to a battery of antigens (132,133,224) and rejected skin allografts poorly but could make antibodies very well to several antigens and had at least normal amounts of Ig in their blood and body fluids. In contrast, the myeloma patients, who could promptly reject skin allografts, possessed vigorous capacity to develop and express delayed allergies, but they did not make antibodies well and usually had lower than normal levels of Ig other than the pathologic Ig-spike that was often present in their blood (98,269).

On the basis of our investigations of these differences in susceptibility to different sets of infection and differences in ability to produce antibodies and to develop cell-mediated immunities, particularly from comparing the microbial universe to which each population of patients was susceptible, and also because of the relationship of these findings to the findings in patients with X-linked agammaglobulinemia, we drew the conclusion that there were two basically different kinds of cellular immunity (88,98,101). One of these cellular systems seemed to be based in antibody-producing plasma cells; the other could be related to the cell-mediated immunities like delayed allergy and homograft rejection, which we attributed to a separate population of lymphocytes. In several papers, I attempted to place these interpretations of the critical experiments of nature in the perspective of existing immunologic knowledge. Particularly in these communications, I was anxious to relate the findings of our clinical investigations with fundamental investigations of antibody production on the one hand and the analyses launched by Landsteiner and Chase (151) and Chase (30) of bacterial allergy or of cell-mediated immunity on the other. I also sought to link our findings in a sensible way to the fundamental studies of allograft immunity that had been carried out by Billingham et al. (17). Somewhat confusing in all this was the observation that one patient with agammaglobulinemia did not reject a skin allograft from an unrelated donor normally. However, subsequent experiments in our own and in other clinics showed that agammaglobulinemia patients, like myeloma patients, usually rejected skin allografts vigorously, despite their antibody deficiency (182).

ROLE OF THE THYMUS

Several investigators had sought to clarify the functions of the thymus by experiments based on thymectomy of adult animals; they drew the conclusion that the thymus does not exercise any important immunologic influence. Nonetheless, Fichtelius and Bryant (70) and several scientists whose work dates back to the studies of Beard (9) at the turn of the century had presented evidence that the thymus is an important if not crucial source of lymphoid cells for the blood, lymph, and lymphoid tissues. Indeed, it had been indicated that the thymus output of lymphocytes can provide in 1 day as many as five times the number of lymphocytes that at any one time are circulating in all the blood and lymph (24).

Metcalf (188) had also investigated the thymus as a potential source of noncellular factors that promote lymphocyte growth and differentiation. Our attention to the thymus as an important organ in immunology derived from interpretation of another provocative experiment of nature. A patient, whom Varco and I first studied in 1952, had a huge stromal-epithelial tumor of the thymus and a broadly based deficiency of immunologic function (165). The immunodeficiency included defects of delayed allergy, allograft rejection, low lymphocyte count, and hypogammaglobulinemia associated with profound deficiency in producing antibodies after primary, secondary, or tertiary exposure to antigen. From the information available, even though the findings in the patient represented a provocative constellation, it seemed impossible to ascertain the function of the thymus in immunity from study of him alone. Thus we turned to experimental animals and set about extirpating thymus in rabbits, mice, and rats at various times during life. Our studies had yielded only confirmation of earlier work, which indicated that the thymus extirpation did not exert readily measurable influences on immunologic function when this organ was removed from the body of rabbits during adult life or even from rabbits as young as 4 weeks of age (166).

In 1959, however, a close personal friend, Harold Wolfe of the University of Wisconsin, called to my attention the studies of Glick et al. (82), who had been removing the bursa of fabricius early in life in chickens and was profoundly influencing development of immunity. Because of the suggestions of the findings of Glick (81) and Mueller et al. (194), we began in early 1960 to remove the thymus from newly born rabbits and mice instead of from older animals. Because of a chance occurrence derived from a pedagogic responsibility, Glick, who was doing many experiments to ascertain the function of the bursa of fabricius, had discovered that extirpation of this organ in newly hatched chickens inhibited development of ability to produce antibody. He attempted to publish the observations made with his colleagues Chang and Jaap in a leading scientific journal, *Science*, but the experimental results were considered not to be of general interest. Thus they had published what proved to be a watershed paper in *Poultry Science* (182), a journal not read by most immunologists. This paper showed that extirpation of the bursa prior to 2 weeks of age inhibits development of ability to produce antibody. One fine immunologist, however, read *Poultry Science* regularly, and that was Harold Wolfe.

A great part of Wolfe's life work in immunology was contained in a long series of scientific papers published usually with one or more of his graduate students. These papers were each about an aspect concerning precipitin production in chickens. Wolfe and his colleagues used truly elegant immunologic techniques; the last of Wolfe's research prior to his death from stomach cancer in 1962 had been with his graduate students to confirm the discovery of Glick et al. (82). Wolfe told me of this adventure in 1959. The information he provided was especially revealing for me because Downey, my teacher of hematology, had repeatedly taught me that as early as 1911, Jolly had considered the bursa of fabricius to be the cloacal thymus (130). Thus we turned our efforts to influence immunity by thymic extirpation in rabbits, mice, and rats to the neonatal period (3,4,96,99,171–173). In each of these species, as well as later in hamsters, with Hard et al. (113), using thymectomy in the immediate newborn period, it was possible for us to prevent normal development of antibody-producing capacity to certain antigens, to prevent development of skin allograft and tumor allograft immunity, to inhibit development of capacity for delayed allergic responses, and to inhibit development of cells which initiate graft versus host responses.

The first of these experiments were done by Archer and Pierce in rabbits. Archer was a student from Australia who worked as a technician in my laboratory; Pierce was a surgical resident working with Varco and studying immunology with us in our laboratories in the Heart Hospital at the University of Minnesota. Sutherland, a freshman medical student, joined this group in 1961 (247), and another of the surgical trainees, McKneally, who also studied with Varco, later continued some of these studies (182,183). The experiments in mice addressed allograft immunity, tumor immunity, and antibody synthesis. The first experiments on the influence of neonatal thymectomy on allograft immunity in mice were carried out by John Kersey, who was a medical student transferring after 2 years of basic science at Dartmouth to the University of Minnesota Medical School. The experiments on development of tumor immunity were carried out by Augustin Dalmasso, a post-doctoral fellow, with my close friend and collaborator Carlos Martinez. Papermaster also carried out experiments with mice, chickens, and rats, but because of his interest in more fundamental issues, he was primarily responsible for launching our extensive phylogenetic inquiries (103).

Hard (113) later did experiments on neonatal thymectomy in hamsters. Once the perspective had turned to the role of the thymus in early development of lymphoid functions, the results regularly proved revealing and were well coordinated with each other. It was possible to show that removal of the thymus sufficiently early in life, with or without neonatal irradiation, interfered with lymphoid development, tumor and normal tissue allograft rejection, or development of cell populations that either could initiate or resist graft versus host reaction. Neonatal thymic extirpation also prevented the ability to produce antibodies to many antigens in each animal species studied (96,99). Thus from our analyses, thymus function was found to be essential to development of lymphoid tissues and to all recognized immunologic functions.

Our discoveries were first presented at the 1961 spring meeting of the American Association of Immunologists at the Federation of American Societies for Experimental Biology in Atlantic City (3). At this meeting, our formal presentation to the immunologists concerned deficient antibody production in neonatally thymectomized rabbits. However, in the discussion of that paper, I had also summarized our many additional observations on tumor immunity, allograft rejection, and antibody production in mice and rats which had been thymectomized as neonates. I insisted that the thymic influence on development of immunity represents a truly general case and thus was applicable to all species.

In apparently independent studies which derived impetus from the original observations of McEndy et al. in 1944 (181), who had inhibited leukemia development in AKR mice by neonatal thymectomy, Miller (192), at the Chester Beatty Institute in London, had launched studies of the influence of neonatal thymectomy in mice and had come to conclusions identical to ours. He presented his findings for the first time at a CIBA symposium in England in the summer of 1961, a few months after our presentation had been made to the American Association of Immunologists. Miller's initial paper, which was labeled *A Preliminary Communication*, appeared in *Lancet* in October, while our paper on neonatal thymectomy in mice with Martinez et al. (173), which was submitted prior to Miller's initial submission to *Lancet*, appeared in the following January issue of *Proceedings of the Society of Experimental Biology and Medicine*. Thus simultaneously and independently, the discovery of the crucial role played by the thymus in immunology was made in at least two places.

The time for the thymus had truly come. Parrott, working with Humphrey (208) in England, and Jancovic, who had initiated his experiments in Yugoslavia and extended them at Harvard at Byron Waksman's laboratory with Arnason et al. (5), were also conducting crucial studies of the influence of neonatal thymectomy on immunologic development respectively in mice and rats at approximately that same time.

THE THYMUS CONFERENCE

In October 1962, under support of the National Foundation–March of Dimes and also with NIH support, I had organized a symposium to consider the new work on the role of the thymus in immunobiology (99). All the principals in this scientific horse race were present, and each was clamoring for credit for his or her discoveries concerning thymus function. To relieve the tension, Fichtelius opened the conference by thanking the eager participants for leaving the thymus to him for so long (69).

It was at this meeting that Warner, who was a young scientist then, presented his work alleging that although the bursa may have been called the cloacal thymus by Jolly, it was now clear that the thymus and bursa of fabricius exercised different functions in chickens. Using hormonal approaches to bursectomy and thymectomy, the studies of Warner and Szenberg (262) linked hormonal bursectomy in developing chicks with inhibition of antibody production and hormonal thymectomy with inhibition of development of allograft immunity. However, the authors concluded erroneously that the bursa also controlled development of delayed-type allergy, while neither bursa nor thymus influenced development of ability of the lymphoid cells of spleen to mount a graft versus host reaction. This presentation, which electrified the conference, brought an intense and somewhat emotional challenge from me and some of my associates. This was because the findings did not fit in detail with the scheme we had been organizing concerning the grouping of immunity functions that had derived from study of the experiments of nature in our patients and our experimental work with mice, rats, and rabbits.

According to our way of sorting things out, it was antibodies, gamma-globulins, and all humoral immunities that should be grouped together with plasma cells. In contrast, the ability to develop delayed allergy, allograft rejection, and ability to initiate graft versus host reactions should be grouped together and linked to a lymphocyte population different from that of the plasma cell lineage, which we linked to production of conventional antibody.

Because of the confusion introduced by the experiments of Warner and Szenberg, I was determined to reinvestigate the influence of the bursa of Fabricius and thymus in chickens on development of the cellular immunity systems and immunologic functions. Raymond D. A. Peterson and Max Cooper, fellows in my laboratory, accepted this challenge; their collaborative experiments proved most crucial. Mary Ann South, another of my fellows, joined them later. Cooper coupled high-dose radiation with complete extirpation of either bursa or thymus, or both. The experiments were revealing. After irradiation of the newly hatched chick, thymectomy prevented development of the dense accumulations of lymphoid cells of one lymphoid population in spleen and lymph nodes. These manipulations reduced the numbers of circulating lymphocytes and prevented development of delayed allergy and capacity for allograft rejection. They also prevented development of ability to mount a graft versus host reaction. Irradiation plus bursectomy, on the other hand, prevented plasma cell and germinal center development in spleen and lymph nodes but left all the so-called cell-mediated immunities intact. Irradiation combined with both bursectomy and thymectomy inhibited all the lymphoid development and also inhibited development of all recognized immunity functions (42,43).

Van Alten, a young associate professor who later took a sabbatical leave with us, developed great operative skill and perfected operations that he carried out within the egg in late embryonization. He did these experiments with Cooper by operating on 17-day-old chick embryo and showed that this same grouping of immunologic functions and their linkage to thymus or to bursa of fabricius held as well when irradiation was not used in the experiments on the chicks (258).

Collaborative experiments with the scientists, led by Burmester at the regional poultry laboratories in East Lansing, and which were carried out also under the leadership of Peterson with Cooper et al. (37,41,213) and later with Dent et al. (50), showed that the bursa, like the thymus in Furth's experiments done many years before, could be the site of appearance of a virus-induced lymphoid malignancy. This malignancy, induced by the RPL-12 viruses, originated in a single bursal follicle and could be prevented by bursectomy in newly hatched chickens. This form of cancer was shown to be related to lymphoid cells that appeared in the bursa, later migrated to germinal centers, and became the plasma cells. Thus it involved what could be identified as a malignancy of the bursal-dependent B lymphocyte cell lineage. This finding, coupled with Furth's prevention of AKR leukemia by neonatal thymectomy and the later demonstration by Siegler and Rich (230) that the lymphoid tumors in AKR mice originated in the thymus and later metastasized to the periphery, were the experiments that launched our subsequent extensive efforts to dissect malignancies of the lymphoid tissues into those that originate in the thymus-dependent lymphoid system and those that originate in the thymus-independent lymphoid system, or what we called the bursal-dependent system (40,97).

This approach to classification of the lymphoid malignancies has been useful and has been highly developed by Lukes and Collins (164) as well as others, including ourselves (114,143). Until recently, it has been the most useful approach to classification of the malignancies of the lymphoid systems.

THE LOCAL IMMUNITY SYSTEMS
GALT, BALT, and MALT

Another revealing line of investigation was that launched in the 1930s with the discovery of coproantibodies. Later, Hanson (115), who himself lacked the local IgA system, recognized an extra immunochemically identifiable determinant on the IgA molecules present in milk. Tomasi (252,253), in an extensive and revealing series of studies, found that the IgA present in tears, saliva, intestinal juices, nasal secretions, and even in urine also presents this extra determinant. He named the extra determinant "secretory piece." With South, Hong, Cooper, and Wollheim, we studied the relationships of the secretory component to the IgA (235–237). We found that the secretory piece that we had dubbed "transport piece" is present in the saliva of all patients with agammaglobulinemia, even in the absence of IgA. It was not present on IgA in the plasma cells of the lamina propria and could be demonstrated in the epithelial cells of the intestinal lining or in epithelial salivary gland cells (235).

In attempting to define the bursal equivalent in rabbits, Cooper et al. (38,39) had extirpated the entire appendix, the sacculus rotundus, and each of the several Peyer patches. With this rather extensive surgery, we could inhibit the development of much of the Ig production in the rabbit.

Perey (211) did some rather ingenious surgical experiments in newborn rabbits which isolated the appendix and sacculus rotundus from the flow of gastrointestinal contents and thereby inhibited development of the extraordinary lymphoid tissue that normally was to be developed at these sites along the lower small bowel. It seemed likely that gastrointestinal contents, presumably but not certainly the bacterial flora, were stimulating the development of the extraordinary lymphoid accumulations which appear along the lower part of the small bowel in rabbits. It was Cebra et al. (29), however, who first carried out definitive experiments that showed that lymphoid cells generated in the subepithelial lymphoid aggregates of the Peyer patches can migrate especially to the lamina propria all along the small bowel, where they come to comprise a population of cells that may be stimulated to develop into IgA-producing plasma cells. In the lamina propria, in contradistinction to IgA-producing cells in spleen and lymph nodes, the plasma cells produce largely dimeric IgA. Later evidence revealed that it is the dimeric IgA produced by this local population of plasma cells in the submucosa that selectively combines with the transport or secretory piece at the antelumenal surface of the epithelial cells and then is transferred through the epithelial cells of the intestinal lining to the lumenal surface and then into the gut lumen or into the lumen of glands. This is surely a magnificant transport process of a specialized form of antibody across an epithelial membrane.

Thus a local immunity system was discovered which is generated by stimulation of lymphoid areas overlying a specialized epithelium (36) in the Peyer patches and similar lymphoid accumulations, e.g., in sacculus rotundus and appendix, that plays a special role in generating an army of plasma cells for the lamina propria of gut, glands, lungs, and breast. After maturation, these latter cells were shown to be able to be stimulated locally to produce a special Ig product that in turn can be coupled to a transport protein and transported across an epithelial barrier to the outside of the body (261). Henney and Waldman (120) discovered that a local immunity system also exists for cell-mediated immune functions when they showed that exposure to antigens locally via inhalation into the bronchial tree generated sensitized lymphocytes in the local secretions and local cellular immunity without stimulating development of systemic delayed allergy. With Müller-Schoop (195), we showed that the same situation exists for the bowel. Morphologically specialized sites overlying the domes of the Peyer patch follicles could permit penetration of whole bacterial antigens that provide the stimulation for formation of a special localized system of both T and B lymphocytes that ultimately generate the local T cell-mediated immunity and the local antibody system of the intestine. Perey (211) had called the specialized epithelial-lymphoid accumulations where both humoral and cellular immunities could be generated by exposure to antigens in the bowel, the gut-associated lymphoid tissues (GALT).

Bienenstock et al. (14) later showed that there were similar specialized epithelial sites where specialized lymphoid accumulations were generated along the bronchi. He then wrote about this bronchus-associated lymphoid tissue (BALT). He considered the BALT to be parallel for generation of local immunity functions in the lungs to the GALT of the Peyer patch type for the gut lymphoid system. Hanson and others (116) found that a mechanism parallel to enteroenteric cycle of cell traffic also could be viewed as a source for a local immunity system located in the salivary glands, lungs, and even in the breast. One thus could begin to think of enteroenteric, enteropulmonic, or pulmonoenteric generation of the cells responsible for local immunity. Indeed it became possible to visualize not only an enteromammaric system, but a mucosa-associated lymphoid tissue (MALT). This has now been studied. Elegant work of investigators led by Lamm (149,150) at New York University has shown that the migration of cells from Peyer patches to the lamina propria of the gut wall and even to the mammary gland is a reality. Indeed, from their analyses some cells stop off for a critical stage of development in mesenteric lymph nodes.

We now have evidence that the local immunity system arises in those nodular accumulations beneath specialized epithelium in gut and bronchi. Precursor cells then migrate to their definitive functional locations in the lamina propria of bowel, glands, and bronchi. The derivatives of these cells produce dimeric IgA molecules locally. The latter can be transported across the epithelium of the gut, glands, or bronchi by a process that involves combination with the transport peptide at the cell surface; transport through the cytoplasm of the epithelial cells while coupled to the secretory (or transport) peptide provide demeric IgA antibodies (attached to transport peptide) that protect the external parts of the body. The latter is an internal lining of the body, e.g., the gut and bronchial surfaces. Recent investigations continue to define this extraordinary local immunity function in impressive detail.

THE BEGINNINGS OF CELLULAR ENGINEERING

With progress in our understanding that the thymus plays a crucial role in the development of the lymphoid tissue and in particular in the development of a thymus-dependent lymphoid system, it seemed important to attempt to correct deficits produced in animals by neonatal thymectomy. One approach was thymus transplantation. With syngeneic donors or donors matched with recipient at the H-2 locus, sustained correction of the disastrous consequences of neonatal thymectomy was possible.

Later, we showed that transplantation of even tiny, wet membranes taken from the site of the epithelial region of the 11- to 12-day-old mouse embryo where the thymus was to develop, the thymus *Anlagen*, would correct the immunologic deficiencies that stemmed from neonatal thymectomy (16). The thymus precursor tissues developed into beautiful little thymuses following transplantation even from a H-2 identical allogeneic donor. If the transplants of the epithelial *Anlagen* of the thymus were made across major histocompatibility barriers, the bits of epithelial tissue were sometimes rejected in the neonatally thymectomized recipients; but they sometimes persisted for long periods. Indeed, they often persisted sufficiently long to permit the recipient to develop an impressively functional lymphoid system. Such recipients were often tolerant of tissues from the strain of mice from which the thymus transplant had been derived.

Experiments using transplantation of bone marrow, fetal liver, or thymus of syngeneic strains of mice where the lymphoid cells possessed a T6T6 marker chromosome permitted Ford et al. (117,118) and Ford and Micklem (72) to establish that traffic of cells from marrow to thymus and ultimately to the peripheral lymphoid tissue actually takes place. These observations established that traffic to the thymus, and residence in the thymus, was essential to development of functionally immunocompetent cells. It was also found from such studies that traffic from the thymus to the peripheral lymphoid tissue is unidirectional. The observations of Ford and Miklem (72) were confirmed and extended by Michlem et al. (190) and by Stutman et al. (242,246) in our laboratories. Davies et al. (48) showed that the lymphoid cells derived from the thymus contributed immunologically competent cells, a finding Stutman et al. (240,241) also confirmed. Stutman's studies, also employing sex chromosome markers, established further that precursors of lymphoid cells from bone marrow and fetal liver can traffic directly to the thymus to launch differentiation of the thymus-dependent lymphoid cell series. While initial experiments seemed to indicate that the yolk sac contains cells that can reconstruct the entire lymphoid system in lethally irradiated animals (240), Stutman's later studies (238) established that although bone marrow or fetal liver precursors traffic directly to the thymus, those from yolk sac are delayed in reaching the thymus.

The presumption from these investigations is that yolk sac cells must carry out a stage or several stages of differentiation at another site before being eligible for traffic to the thymus. Table 1 records stepwise the essential contributions and conditions of traffic to the thymus as described by Stutman (239) from a long series

TABLE 1. *Thymus cell differentiation*

Prethymus precursor acted on by thymic hormone
Traffic to thymus—bone marrow and fetal liver go direct
Yolk sac cells require additional step before thymus migration
H_2 identity preferred for thymus migration
H_2 preference for migration radiosensitive; intrathymic cell-cell interactions
Unidirectional migration from thymus
Short-lived postthymic precursor generated
Long-lived and short-lived effector cells generated
Defective differentiation—death in thymus
Steroid-resistant intrathymic medullary population, resident
Generation of competent T cells is a postthymic event

of experiments extending over a 10-year period. Traffic of cells to the thymus appears to be absolutely essential to full development of immunocompetence. Many lymphoid cells are generated and exported from the thymus by proliferation and differentiation of these cells within the thymus. Many cells are spawned in the thymus but are destroyed there. This process has been related to establishment of the repertoire of thymus-dependent lymphoid cell reactivity, development of immunocompetence, and to the creation of self-tolerance. It has also been linked to have the ability to recognize histocompatibility determinants on lymphoid cells with which the thymus-derived cells must be able to interact in collaborative function (239).

In addition to such profound influences as were achieved by transplantation of thymus or prethymic epithelial *Anlagen*, collaborative studies with Yunis et al. (268) showed it to be possible to achieve long-lasting, sustained immunocompetence in neonatally thymectomized mice if sufficiently large numbers of syngeneic peripheral lymphocytes from lymph nodes and/or spleen were injected parenterally into neonatally thymectomized recipients. The requirement that the cells be syngeneic or that they be from donors matched with the recipient at the major histocompatibility loci was absolute in these analyses (268). If such matching was not accomplished, the foreign lymphocytes would regularly initiate lethal graft versus host disease in the neonatally thymectomized mice, which were inordinately susceptible to graft versus host reaction. Thus it was possible to correct immunologic defects consequent to neonatal thymectomy in mice by transplantation of thymus from a very young donor, transplantation of even very small tissue *Anlagen* in which thymus was destined to develop (16), or transplantation of sufficiently large numbers of peripheral fully or partially differentiated lymphoid cells where donor and recipient were syngeneic or allogeneic but matched with one another at the major histocompatibility loci.

THE DIGEORGE SYNDROME

With the establishment of the separate roles for the thymus and bursa of Fabricius as being essential to the development of two separate systems of lymphoid cells, and with the recognition that X-linked agammaglobulinemia is the equivalent of an irradiated, bursectomized chicken, it seemed essential to find a clinical condition equivalent to the chicken that had been thymectomized following irradiation in the newly hatched period. No sooner had Cooper et al. (40,42,43) and Warner and Szenberg (262) presented their findings differentiating the origins of two separate lymphoid systems, than DiGeorge (52) and co-workers in Philadelphia described a complex set of developmental anomalies; in human infants, one component was failure of thymic development and consequent absence of the thymus-dependent lymphoid tissues. Peterson et al. (212) could then write confidently about the pathogenesis of the immunodeficiency diseases.

DiGeorge syndrome was usually associated with hypoparathyroidism expressed as neonatal tetany plus failure of development of the thymus and thymus-dependent lymphoid tissue. In addition, these children regularly suffered from congenital cardiac abnormalities or abnormalities of the development of the large vessels representing the outflow tract from the heart. They also had peculiar ears and a strange downward bow to the mouth.

THYMUS TRANSPLANTATION

With the recognition by DiGeorge that survival of these athymic patients was often limited by susceptibility to infection due to failure to develop thymus-dependent immunocompetence, it was natural to consider the possibility of correcting this clinical immunologic anomaly by transplantation of thymus or thymic *Anlagen*, as had been so successful in the neonatally thymectomized mouse. This feat of cellular engineering was first accomplished by the endocrinologist Cleveland in collaboration with Fogel, Brown, and Kay of England (33). They transplanted an allogeneic thymus from an aborted first trimester fetus to a child with DiGeorge syndrome. The transplant corrected the immunodeficiency and led to repopulation of the thymus-dependent lymphoid tissue. This first immunologic reconstitution has now been sustained through many years. Almost immediately, lasting reconstitution of this immunodeficiency was also achieved by embryonic thymus transplantation of DiGeorge syndrome by August et al. (6) in Boston and subsequently by several others, including ourselves (15). These achievements revealed the practical value of a penetrating analysis of lymphoid tissue development that had so recently focused on the role of the thymus in the body economy. Thus the value of experiments of nature in the clinic to provide both crucial questions of fundamental nature to be taken to the laboratory and also to provide a valuable testing ground for the usefulness of the developing understanding of lymphoid development was revealed.

BONE MARROW TRANSPLANTATION

Another example of analysis in clinical perspective of lymphoid tissue development was provided by discovery of patients in Switzerland who had a disease originally called lymphocytopthisis by Glanzmann and Riniker (80). This disease I later dubbed Swiss-type agammaglobulinemia, and, more recently we have called it severe combined immunodeficiency disease (SCID). This form of primary immunodeficiency was especially well studied pathologically by Tobler and Cottier (251) and clinically and immunologically by Hitzig et al. (121) in Switzerland. Several different genetic variations of this form of immunodeficiency exist in which neither the thymus-dependent nor thymus-independent lymphoid systems have developed (104). With the new understanding of the processes underlying development of the two lymphoid systems from precursors in bone marrow or fetal liver, it seemed reasonable to postulate that SCID might be correctable if a transplant of lymphoid stem cells from either bone marrow or fetal liver could be provided. Initial efforts to make such corrections failed because they induced graft versus host disease when donor and recipient were not suitably matched at the MHC (122,123).

To use bone marrow from sibling donors matched with the recipient at the major histocompatibility region of chromosome 6 seemed the logical next step. In 1968 we accomplished full correction of SCID using marrow from a sibling donor matched with the recipient male child at the C-B and D loci of the MHC (73). In this initial instance, donor and recipient were mismatched at the A locus of the major histocompatibility region and also according to major blood groups. The recipient was of blood group A and the donor of blood group O. This transplant corrected the immunodeficiency and reconstituted both the thymus-dependent lymphoid system and thymus-independent plasma cell system. However, a graft versus host reaction ensued, which led to potentially fatal aplastic anemia. With a subsequent marrow transplant from the same donor, the aplastic anemia was corrected, the recipient's blood group was switched from the genetic A to the donor's O blood group, and a sustained full correction of the SCID was accomplished (93,94,100). This correction of an inborn error of metabolism by a feat of cellular engineering that corrected two fatal diseases, SCID and immunologically based aplastic anemia or pancytopenia, has already lasted more than 14 years.

This approach, based on using a matched sibling donor, was also employed by Bach et al. (7) almost simultaneously with our initial achievement to permit partial correction of the immunologic abnormalities in the Wiskott-Aldrich syndrome. Subsequently, several different forms of SCID have been repeatedly corrected by bone marrow transplantation or by an alternative fetal liver transplantation (189,199). Sustained correction of SCID has been accomplished with fetal liver transplantation most reproducibly, however, if thymus is also given from the same fetal donor. The basis for this discrepancy between stem cells given as bone marrow and those given as fetal liver is not clear but may relate to recent observations which show that bone marrow transplants induce hormonal functions of the recipient's thymus, while fetal liver transplants do not (126). The latter is an exciting new lead which requires further and more direct analysis. Thus with SCID, these clinical experiments of nature again served as a testing ground for emerging concepts of lymphoid development. The interpretations and observations also illustrate the power of continued interaction of the emerging science of cellular immunology with the questions and challenges from the clinic. On the basis of recent advances it now is regularly possible to achieve correction of SCID when matched sibling donors are not available (92).

IT TAKES TWO TO TANGO

Another development that first came to attention at the international conference on the thymus in 1962 was a discovery by Claman. He and co-workers (32) observed that bone marrow cells developed much more efficiently as antibody-producing cells *in vitro* if they were cultured together with cells from the thymus. This discovery was later followed by a series of most important contributions led by those of Miller and Mitchell (193), which established that a crucial interaction of the thymus-derived cells and cells of the plasma cell lineage was necessary to achieve most efficient antibody production *in vitro*. Thus the concept of helper lymphoctyes from the thymus-dependent lineage and of a dual signal for B cell differentiation to antibody-producing cells was born (34). This line of investigation has culminated in recognition of B cell growth and differentiation factors produced by thymus-derived cells that are essential for B cell development. Only recently have these factors that are implicated in B cell development been defined chemically. The molecular basis of their influence is still being elucidated (196,266,267).

GERSHON'S SUPPRESSOR LYMPHOCYTES

Following Claman's discovery that thymus-dependent cells can act as helpers for the development of plasma cell precursors, Gershon and Kondo (76–78) showed that the negative controls responsible for down-regulation, like those responsible for up-regulation, of antibody synthesis represent a most important function of the thymus-derived lymphoid cell populations. Earlier, the cellular transfer of immunologic tolerance was demonstrated in our own work (175,177,229), but these observations did not initiate from us sufficient consideration of the possibility that a suppressor cellular mechanism attributable to lymphocytes might explain the passive transfer of some forms of immunologic tolerance. Gershon and his associates carried out experiments in which they clearly demonstrated that for both antibody production and cell-mediated immunities following immunization, lymphoid cell populations can inhibit immune responses as well as participate in their facilitation (76,77). These seminal experiments opened the door to a set of experimental analyses which by now have established beyond doubt that in a well-modulated immunologic system, suppressor cells of thymic origin may act specifically to suppress responses to the stimulating antigen (74,78).

We now write and speak confidently of antigen-specific suppression of both B and T cell functions by antigen-specific suppressor T cells (74), Ig class-specific (137,259) suppression of B lymphocyte development, and even nonspecific suppression of both T and B cell development and function by suppressor T cells (79). Indeed, we have from Waldman and his co-workers (260) evidence that some forms of primary or secondary immunodeficiency diseases of man can be based on T suppressor cell influences or even inhibition of the immune responses by macrophage suppressors. The network of T helper and suppressor lymphocytes, their interactions, and the existence of countersuppressor circuits (75) has been elaborately developed and is currently the basis of extensive experimental study. It seems certain already that clinically significant immunologic disturbances are based on perturbations of these functions and that one may be able to manipulate immunologic functions by the pharmacologic control of the functions of these several classes of suppressor cells.

THE NETWORK CONCEPT OF JERNE

These suppressor cell circuits are not the only control mechanisms. Some of the earliest observations in modern immunology recognized that antibodies can inhibit antibody responses to antigens (200). It was Uhr and Baumann (257), however, who showed in reproducible systems that downward regulation of immunity responses can be exercised by circulating antibody, particularly of the IgG class. Since the original papers were published, much study of the negative regulatory influences of antibodies has appeared.

On a backdrop of extensive study of rheumatoid factors, antiidiotype antibodies (147,203), and Najjar's (197) autologous antiantibodies, Jerne (129) postulated that idiotypes and anti-idiotype antibodies exercise a dominant control of both positive and negative regulatory components of specific immunity. He urged immunologists to think of network interactions to better understand immunologic controls. Now positive and negative control of immunologic functions are being attributed to antiidiotype antibodies as well as to autoantiidiotypic antibodies (63). Such antibodies have been shown to exist, and are currently the subject of extensive investigations as we strive to understand the extraordinary regulation that exists for immunity functions. Thus through the operation of specific helper and suppressor T cells, countersuppressor T cells, isotype-specific suppressor T cells, nonspecific suppressor T cells, suppressor macrophages, accessory or nonspecific helper monocyte-macrophage populations, negative feedback influences of antibodies, influences of circulating immune complexes on cellular differentiation, existence of idiotypes on T and B cells, antiidiotypic antibodies, and autoantiidiotype antibodies, we seek to explain the myriad of immunologic regulations that are readily apparent as immunologic processes are studied. It seems now that the immunologic systems can be considered to spend more of their energy talking to themselves than to reacting to potentially destructive foreign organisms, internally derived mutant cells, or virus-infected host cells. This is probably an absolute requirement for any complex system of cells and molecules such as comprise the immunological systems, that are vital to the body and yet may also be most harmful.

THE ENDOCRINE FUNCTION OF THE THYMUS

From the earliest days after the discovery that the thymus plays a vital role in immunologic development, evidence began to appear which indicated that thymic hormones exist and that part of thymic function might be attributable to the action of these hormones. Levey et al. (158) and Osoba and Miller (202) showed that thymuses housed in cell-impenetrable millipore chambers exert reproducible influences on immunologic development. Indeed, in some neonatally thymectomized female mice (201), partial restoration of immunologic function was achieved when the mice became pregnant. These experiments were interpreted to indicate that thymic function could be explained in part by indirect actions attributable to thymic hormones.

Stutman et al. (243,244) produced functional stromal-epithelial thymomas by injecting chemical carcinogens directly into the thymus. In these experiments, it was shown that the rather infrequent functional stromal-epithelial thymomas which were generated were active in restoring immunologic functions of neonatally thymectomized mice. The activity of these stromal-epithelial thymomas, however, required that immunoincompetent postthymic precursor cells be present in the peripheral lymphoid system. Like thymuses in millipore chambers, the stromal-epithelial thymomas exerted an influence even when housed in cell-impenetrable chambers (245). Postthymic precursor cells, which subsequently have been extensively defined and studied by Stutman (239), were found to be short-lived cells that possess markers characteristic of thymus-derived elements. These cells proved to be dependent on thymus; if the thymus had been removed in mice, they gradually disappeared from the lymphoid tissues and were entirely gone within a period of 6 weeks to 2 months. Following elimination of the postthymic precursors from the lymphoid tissues, neither the functional stromal thymomas nor thymic epithelium in millipore chambers could restore immunologic function in neonatally thymectomized mice (245).

Metcalf and his colleagues (188) had long been contending that they could extract a growth factor from the thymus that influenced culture of lymphocytes *in vitro* and also exercised an influence on activities of developing lymphoid cells *in vivo*. Later Goldstein, Slater, and White (83), working with relatively crude fractions of thymus that they called fraction V, demonstrated interesting influences on lymphocyte development both *in vivo* and *in vitro* which seemed attributable thymic hormones. The chemistry of these putative thymic hormones has developed rapidly. A. Goldstein has purified and with his colleagues sequenced several molecules that they contend are thymic hormones (163). They have even cloned the genes for thymosin α_1 and β_4 of this series and synthesized active molecules by introducing the responsible genes into coliform bacteria.

Schlessinger and G. Goldstein (225) have purified chemically from aqueous extracts of thymus and sequenced a molecule comprising 49 amino acids which they put forth as a thymic hormone. This molecule proved to have an active site residing between the 32nd and 36th amino acid sequences. This component can be readily synthesized and has proved to have impressive biologic functions (226) comprising some thymopoitin-like actions.

Bach et al. (8) purified from pig serum a putative thymic hormone which is a small molecule: a nonapeptide. This molecule requires zinc for its activity; when the nonapeptide is synthesized in the absence of zinc, it is inactive, whereas it is active as a zinc-containing peptide when synthesized in the presence of zinc (45). Receptors for FTS or thymulin, as the zinc-containing functional molecule is now called, have been found on T cells and T cell lines (45). Evidence has also been presented that thymulin is synthesized by the thymus epithelial cells and that some of these cells possess vacuoles containing zinc.

Thus in 1983, an apparent embarrassment of riches exists with respect to thymus hormones. Which of the molecules described, if any, is a true thymic hormone has not yet been resolved. What thymus-derived factors are in actuality synthesized by thymus epithelial cells, which, if any, are the hormones that exert long-range influences on precursor cells before the latter enter the thymus, which operate while cells are present in the thymus, and which act on the cells that have been differentiated in the thymus and have already left this organ as committed cells will have to be worked out in the future.

The experiments of Komuro and Boyse (142) showed that precursor cells could be induced by thymosin fraction V to express at their surface differentiation antigens which define the thymocyte surface phenotype (22,198). The process involved in this developmental step in thymus cell differentiation in the mouse, as well as an initial step in differentiation of human thymus-dependent lymphocytes, was shown to involve transcription and translation but not cell division. This differentiative step occurred quickly after exposure to the thymic extracts and was completed within 90 min. For mouse precursor cells, antigens coded for in the TL-a locus, Thy-1, and Lyt-1, 2, and 3 loci were all expressed after exposure of the precursor cells to thymic hormones.

LYMPHOCYTE SUBPOPULATIONS

Evidence that T lymphocytes develop into different subpopulations specialized for certain functions was first presented from analysis of the surface antigenic phenotype when Kisielow et al. (136) showed that the population of mouse post-thymic lymphocytes capable of exerting either helper or suppressor functions could be differentiated from one another by analysis of the surface phenotype for the Thy-1 and Lyt antigens expressed on their surface. This initial observation was extended and elaborately developed by Cantor and Boyse (27,28). Thus the concept of distinct subsets of postthymic lymphocytes which exercise specialized functions and can be distinguished phenotypically by cell surface expression of differentiation antigenic markers was born. The observation has been of crucial historic importance and has provided a point of departure for much of modern immunobiology.

Subsequently, Evans et al. (64,65) developed heteroantisera that were capable of distinguishing the cells that express the suppressor cytotoxic phenotype in man from those that express the helper function. A collaborative interaction between Kung and Goldstein of Ortho laboratories and Reinherz of Schlossman's group at Harvard (219) resulted in development of an extensive set of monoclonal antibodies which have permitted recognition and definition of early stages of thymocyte development, the common thymocytes, late thymocytes, and, ultimately, the specialized subsets of postthymic T lymphocytes for humans. Thus two major subpopulations of T lymphocytes that subserve helper-inducer functions on the one hand or suppressor-cytotoxic function on the other can be identified (219). Some of these reagents have been commercialized and thus have been extensively used by many investigators to define lymphocyte subpopulation disturbances in human disease and the nature of malignancies of the T cell series. Evans and co-workers (66,152), as well as a number of other investigators, have also been developing monoclonal antibodies which can be used to distinguish subpopulations of human T lymphocytes. Some of these also have been marketed and are proving useful in analyzing human disease.

B lymphocyte subpopulations in the plasma cell series can be identified at different stages of differentiation and as pre-B cells containing small amounts of cytoplasmic Ig, B lymphocytes with IgM, IgM and IgD, IgG, IgA, or IgE, at their surface. These surface immunoglobulins function as Ig receptors for specific antigens. Indeed, monoclonal antibodies to recognize both prepre-B cells and pre-B cells of mouse have been forthcoming and are already providing new ways for analyzing B cell development. Particularly important is that the antigens recognized by these antisera are present on what appear to be early stages of B cell differentiation of human B cells as well (134).

Thus both B and T cell subpopulations exist that subserve distinct and separate functions and that are interactive with each other. It seems from these and the many evidences of cell-cell interaction that the two major cellular immunity systems represent highly integrated systems of cells that have distinguishable functional properties and which are occupied in interacting with, modulating, and controlling each other. It is the urgent business of modern clinical immunology to analyze the subpopulations in pathology and, in the light of disturbances that occur in these cellular subpopulations and their functions with circadian time, stages of life, and with physiologic stress. How much of the new information about the fascinating lymphocyte populations and subpopulations and their interactions is of particular value and how much of this new information will turn out to be "brownian movement" going nowhere remains to be seen. It is hoped that through these analyses of cell populations will come cellular and molecular manipulations that can relieve suffering or be life-saving as has already been the case from earlier analyses of development and interaction of the components of the lymphoid system.

DISSECTING LYMPHOID MALIGNANCIES

It seems certain that these new means of describing and defining the stages of differentiation of the normal lymphocytes of the T and B cell series can be applied to the analysis, classification, and, ultimately, the improvement of treatment of human malignant diseases of the lymphoid systems (10,71,143,144,145,159,187). At present, it is useful to consider malignancies of the hematopoietic cells to represent uncontrolled proliferation of cells generally combined with uncoupled differentiation (223). As such, the malignant proliferations of the lymphoid systems are being defined by monoclonal antibodies which recognize surface phenotypes of the lymphoid cancers. These antibodies, and the cell surface antigen phenotypes they permit one to describe, should improve analysis of the relationship of lymphoid cancers to the normal lymphoid cells which have undergone the malignant change. Indeed, some of the malignancies of the lymphoid system seem to be deviant cell clones where differentiation is frozen at one or another level of development of the lymphoid cells. On the other hand, the malignant clone may be deviated at an early stage of differentiation and an entire developmental lineage may derive by differentiation from the cells of this malignant clone (M. D. Cooper, personal communication). It even seems possible that for some of them, the oncogene expression that is responsible for the malignant nature of the cells may be intimately related to the components involved in normal development and function of the cells as immunocompetent elements, e.g., to the expression of the Ig genes (44).

It is also hoped that detailed analysis of the cell surfaces of the malignant cells may permit immunologically directed chemotherapy, focused immunotoxic therapy, or true immunotherapy that will add to the armamentarium for treatment of lymphoid cancers.

GENETICS AND IMMUNITY

Consideration of historic underpinnings of modern cellular immunology must take cognizance of the extraordinary contributions made by the surging fields of genetics and molecular biology. The latter is currently in day-to-day and almost moment-to-moment interaction with the developing discipline of modern cellular immunobiology. Genetic considerations have been vital to modern immunology in many ways. The greatest impact of genetics on immunology has come through the following three developments:

1. Discovery and analysis of the role of the MHC on the body economy have subserved the understanding of transplantation immunity, the vigor of antibody responses, and the cooperation and interaction of cells. All these clearly are functions of genetic determinants.
2. The replacement of instructional theories of antibody production by selective theories, especially clonal selection, has been of immense importance in the development of cellular immunology.
3. The movement and rearrangement of genes which subserve the establishment of specificity toward antigen of the light and heavy Ig chains and of the multichain Ig molecules is the most recent and perhaps one of the most important of all genetic advances. The best interpretation at present is that this system of rearrangements accounts for the massive heterogeneity of antibody molecules that is essential to their capacity to recognize antigens.

ROLE OF THE MHC IN THE BODY ECONOMY

The history of the crucial contributions of analysis of the major histocompatibility system to modern cellular immunology began long ago with the keeping and inbreeding of Japanese waltzing mice as a biologic curiosity. Japanese waltzing mice had a genetically determined anomaly of the inner ear which contributed to their peculiar behavior. Inbreeding of these animals was extensively carried out about the turn of the century. Loeb (162) in Philadelphia first used these Japanese waltzing mice to study tumor immunity. He showed that he could transfer a tumor that arose in the waltzing mice to other animals of the same strain but not to unrelated strains. Jensen (127) later showed in experiments in another strain of pen-bred white mice, which was by present standards only partially inbred, that he could carry a spontaneous alveolar cancer by transplantation within this stock for many generations but could not transfer this tumor to other stocks of mice. Tyzzer (255) and Little and Tyzzer (161) also made extensive use of the inbred Japanese waltzing mice and showed that transplantable carcinomas were permitted from animal to animal within but not outside the strain. The genetics clearly involved dominant genes. Haldane (112) later linked tumor rejection to rejection of normal blood cells and developed the concepts of alloantigens to explain this relationship.

Perhaps the most important contributions to early immunogenetics and transplantation immunity in the mouse were made by Gorer, Snell, and Medawar. Gorer's (107–109) contribution showed that in the mouse, blood group and tumor immunogenetics were dominated by a genetic system which he called H-2. The author showed that this same genetic system also determined susceptibility genes that controlled tumor transplantation. He also demonstrated that tumor rejection frequently was an immunologic process.

With Snell (234), Gorer compared tumor and normal tissue rejection and linked tumor and tissue transplant immunity to the H-2 system. This set the stage for elucidation of the basic rules of transplantation immunity (234). These contributions, together with those of Medawar, established clearly that most allogeneic tissue transplantation rejection is based on an immunologic process. In brilliant experiments, Medawar (184–186) linked tissue transplantation rejection, which he had shown to be immunologic in several species, to the H-2 system in the mouse. He made critical observations which distinguished transplantation immunity from ordinary antibody production; with his colleagues Billingham and Brent (18), he discovered immunologic tolerance. The experimental lines of investigations of immunologic tolerance that were pursued by Medawar and his associates were based historically on the interpretation of two natural experiments—one in cattle, the other in mice.

IMMUNOLOGIC TOLERANCE

Prior to Medawar's experiments, Burnet and Fenner (26) had postulated that exposure to antigen early in development would render an animal forever tolerant to that antigen. His postulate was based on Owen's (206) earlier discovery that fraternal twin cattle often have two blood types—their own and that of their fraternal twin. This phenomenon was attributable to exchange of hematopoietic precursors through a synchorious placenta during development. Traub (256) had discovered that mice infected with lymphocytic choriomeningitis virus during embryonation could not reject immunologically the infecting virus. By contrast, the same virus could be readily eliminated from the body if infection occurred after the immunity systems had matured. Based on these observations, Burnet and Fenner (26) postulated that immunologic tolerance could be induced by exposure of a host to any antigen during a crucial stage of development. Billingham and his colleagues (18), however, successfully carried out certain critical experiments. They injected lymphoid cells from the prospective donor mouse strain into the prospective recipient strain in late embryonic life or in the neonatal period and induced long-lasting immunologic tolerance. These findings led to experiments showing that the phenomenon holds not only for mice but also for rats (264) and that it could be induced not only by lymphoid cells but by injection of simple protein antigens (31). Smith and Bridges (232), working in my laboratories, showed that tolerance induced with simple protein antigens is antigen dose dependent and is of finite duration. This finding implied that replication of the cells used in the experiments by Medawar's group was crucial to the long-sustained tolerant state.

Soon after the publication of the work by Billingham, Brent, and Medawar, my associates and I tried, and failed, to confirm their experiments, using strains of mice where donor and recipient differed from one another across the strongest histocompatibility barriers. We finally succeeded in inducing tolerance only when we chose mouse strains that were matched or partly matched with one another at the MHC (H-2) (102,168,170,173,174,176,229). It then became clear to us that Billingham, Brent, and Medawar also had chosen strains of mice that were partly matched at the major histocompatibility region (MHR).

Once we had chosen such a matching of donor and recipient, we could induce tolerance regularly and could perform many dramatic experiments, including transplantation across allogeneic barriers of functioning pituitary and adrenal glands, functional ovaries, and other organs and tissues without rejection. We could even passively transfer the tolerant state. Our experiments convinced us, at that juncture, that to have a degree of matching, especially with respect to the MHC, could pave the way for impressive achievements in clinical organ or tissue transplantation (102).

THE MAJOR HISTOCOMPATABILITY SYSTEM OF MAN: HLA

Dausset and Nenna (47) and Miescher and Fauconnet (191) discovered leukoagglutinins which were sometimes associated with clinical agranulocytosis. Dausset's antigen was the antigen Mac (46), which was the first antigen discovered that was coded for in the major histocompatibility region of chromosome 6 of man. Payne (210) and Van Rood (221) then employed serum from grand multiparae or post-transfusion patients as a source of the agglutinating antibodies. Van Rood's work led him to propose that there exists in man a complexity of highly polymorphic systems of antigens that could be recognized by the leukoagglutinins (220). Terasaki et al. (249) introduced the cytotoxicity analysis as a more reproducible means of analyzing for the antibodies, which recognize antigens of the MHR. His work set the stage for Gorer's student, Amos (1), to utilize in cooperative international workshops the talents of many outstanding contributors, including Dausset, Payne, Cepellini, Bodmer, Van Rood, Walford, Bach, Svegaard, Kiesmeyer-Nielsen, and many others, to analyze the MHR located on the 6th chromosome of humans. These investigations showed that the HLA system is dramatically like the H-2 system located on the 17th chromosome of the mouse which Gorer had discovered. It controls a major proportion of the antigens involved in transplantation immunology and also many important interactions of lymphoid cell populations.

The HLA system functions as a super-gene complex which has multiple loci, each of which is highly polymorphic (21). These systems in mouse and man have been shown to control genetically cell-mediated transplantation immunity, immunity for certain tumors, mixed leukocyte culture responses, susceptibility to virus infection, and antibody-producing capacity, and even to influence such functions as sex preference in mice (265). Of greatest importance to the development of modern immunology was the finding that a major control of the vigor of the antibody response is also linked to this genetic system. This linkage was discovered independently by Benacerraf (11) and McDevitt and Chinitz (180). It was worked out both jointly (13) and independently by these two scientists and their colleagues.

Benacerraf et al. (12) had discovered earlier that the vigor of antibody response in guinea pigs is genetically determined. McDevitt, desiring to study genetic control of immune responses, was a postdoctoral fellow in Humphrey's laboratory at Mill Hill. Because Humphrey did not take the concept of genetic control of immunity seriously, McDevitt left to join Michael Sela at the Weizmann Institute in Israel to carry out initial experiments that not only showed genetic control of immunity but linked immunity inextricably to the H-2 system in mice. The latter finding was confirmed for mice by Benacerraf.

Both groups of investigators continued their experiments, showing that the influence of genetics on immune responses in mice is largely determined by the H-2 complex. Furthermore, they found the controlling genes to be located in the H-2 region on the 17th chromosome on the right-hand side of the K locus and to the left-hand side of the D locus.

This newly defined region was then dubbed the Ir region or immune response region. Following these important discoveries, these investigators and their colleagues, as well as many others, have made contributions which establish that cooperation of T lymphocytes with B lymphocytes in mouse and man and between T cells and both B cells and macrophages often involve restrictions of interaction that are controlled genetically at the MHR. The rules and regulations that govern immunity function operate on both the afferent and efferent limbs of immunity and involve helper and suppressor functions in many different systems. They involve delayed allergies, defense against virus-infected cells, cytotoxicity of T lymphocytes for foreign allogeneic cells, and cytotoxicity for foreign and host tumor target cells.

Thus investigations that have established the value of the inbred mouse as a critical teacher of immunology have been greatly extended by the discovery that tissue and tumor transplantation immunities are linked to immunogenetics of red cells and leukocytes in the mouse. Man and all other species that have been critically studied to date have a similar system of linked genetic loci that determine the rules of transplantation immunology and tumor immunology and that also control the vigor of antibody production, determine capacity for cooperation and interaction of T cells with B cells, underly the effectiveness of helper and suppressor T cell functions, and influence or control most of the important cell-cell interactions that subserve cellular immunology. These determinants inherited in this region of chromosome 6 also determine levels of complement and certain complement components in man.

SELECTION VERSUS INSTRUCTION AS THE
BASIS OF IMMUNE RESPONSES

Brilliant postulates by Pauling (209) concerning the nature of forces involved in protein-protein interaction and extrapolation of these processes to immunology as a basis for the influences of antigens on antibody production had convinced most but not all immunologists of the 1940s that antibodies are formed by a process that involved an action of antigens to form a protein template. The product of the latter was then supposed to be replicated as antibody by the protein-synthesizing machinery of the cells. Jerne, Burnet, and Talmage, however, did not accept Pauling's concepts. It was Jerne (128) who first proposed that antigen-selected cells are favored in producing their protein product as the antigen provides a stimulus to immunologically competent cells to induce the latter to express a genetically determined biosynthetic process. Talmage (248), made similar postulates and began to carry out both calculations and experiments to analyze the influence of combination of antibody with antigen at the surface of cells that might provoke the cells to multiply and develop as antibody-producing cells. About this same time, Burnet (25) formulated his now universally accepted theory of clonal selection as the basis for antibody production. His postulate gave central position to selective stimulation by specific antigen to cells capable of becoming antibody-producing cells.

Furthermore, he postulated that antigen stimulates such cells not only to divide but also to differentiate to the antibody-producing cells. This stimulation was visualized as generating an expanding clone of immunologically competent cells which could act as specific effector cells in immunity. He reasoned that cells of these clones not only produce the antibody, but some members of the clone are reserved in a poised state of so-called memory cells capable of responding quickly by rapid proliferation and differentiation upon recontact with the antigen. These exciting postulates concerning clonal selection stimulated many experiments from all corners of the western immunologic world. They also provided reasonable postulates to explain autoimmunities. Even the Nobel Laureate Lederberg (156) was enticed to offer rather extensive advice and comments on immunologic experimentation because of the stimulus afforded by this new paradigm in immunology, which brought molecular genetics, of which Lederberg was a recognized leader, onto the stage of the developing science of cellular immunology. Since efforts to refute these new ideas were not productive, and since the postulates themselves proved immensely productive, few scientists since the early 1960s have taken instructional theories of antibody production seriously, and modern genetics has had a major stake in modern cellular immunology.

THE ANTIBODY MOLECULES AND THEIR JUMPING GENES

As stated above, in the early 1940s, we knew nothing about antibody molecules except that they were globulins and migrated with the gamma-globulins upon electrophoretic fraction (2). This all began to change when scientists, including Kunkel et al. (148), Putnam (217), and Deutsch et al. (51), began to take advantage of chemical and immunologic studies of the uniformities in the myeloma proteins and used serum from patients with multiple myeloma as a source for purification of highly uniform immunoglobulins. Large amounts of a single species of antibody could be obtained in pure form from myeloma sera. This was because myeloma, as a form of plasma cell cancer, represents a monoclonal expansion of the antibody-producing cell factories, and large amounts of myeloma proteins accumulate in serum of these patients. Kunkel and his associates (148,231) compared myeloma proteins to one another and to normal gamma-globulins immunochemically. In these studies, the authors showed that the myeloma proteins had clear relationships to one another and also to normal gamma-globulins. In these earliest studies, we also found significant immunochemical differences to exist between the individual myeloma proteins. These investigations took an important turn when Porter (215), who worked with initially purified antibody from rabbits, and Edelman (59), using myeloma proteins, began studies which identified a multiple chain structure to the characteristic of the immunoglobulins. These investigations ultimately culminated in the development by Edelman et al. (60) of a strategy for achieving the full sequencing of IgG.

Putnam (218), who over the years has been a most consistent contributor in this field, then worked out the amino acid sequence of several of the major immunoglobulin peptide chains. From Putnam's work and that of his associates, as well as others, we now have full or nearly full amino acid sequences for representative heavy chains of each of the Ig classes and the two major light chains, as well. Furthermore from work by many scientists, we now have amino acid sequences for the critical regions of numerous myeloma proteins, particularly those that exhibit antibody activity. It became clear from these studies that for each of the Ig isotypes, and for the heavy and light chains that make up the Ig molecules, there are both variable terminal regions and a constant portion comprised of several separate domains. In the variable regions of the Ig heavy and light chains which determine specificity of the peptide for antigen, the amino acid sequences of different myeloma proteins are highly variable. Indeed, in some regions in this part of the molecule, extreme variability was noted. The latter have been called the hypervariable regions by Kabat and Wu (131). By contrast, each of the Ig chains possesses constant regions which are similar from one myeloma protein to the others. The amino acid sequences of the myeloma proteins of mice derived from the myelomas that were produced by Potter (216) showed that the myeloma proteins and thus the antibodies of this species are molecularly akin to the myeloma proteins and antibodies of humans. These findings set the stage for one of the most dramatic and important developments in modern cellular immunology.

Reflecting on the striking differences between the constant and variable regions of the Ig molecules, and attempting at the same time to elucidate the basis for the apparently unlimited heterogeneity of antibody molecules, Dreyer and his colleague Bennett at Cal Tech (56) proposed that many different antibody specificities could be explained by different combinations of light and heavy chains. These investigators also noted the great differences between constant and variable regions present on each of the several Ig chains. They reasoned that the genes responsible for one part, the variable regions, of each of the light and heavy chains has undergone rapid evolutionary change to account for the variability of these Ig components. In contrast, the genetic components responsible for the other part of the Ig chain, the constant regions, must have been highly conserved in evolution. The authors drew from these observations the conclusion that there must be many different genes which code for the variable regions of the Ig chains and few, or but a single genetic determinant, separate from that responsible for the variable portions of the molecule that codes for the constant region. This was a revolutionary concept. It implied two genes for a single peptide chain and also required that there be a method for splicing of the two separate genetic components to make a single effective sequence of base pairs which could act as the genetic determinant for the whole peptide chain. Needless to say, this new perspective was not popular at first. Nonetheless, it provided a new way to explain the great heterogeneity of antibodies while at the same time explaining the conservation of the protein structure that subserves other functions of the antibody molecule. Included among the latter are those that relate to distribution of immunoglobulins and antibodies in the circulation extracellular fluids and external secretions of the body, the attachment of immunoglobulins to cells, their transfer across the placenta, their capacity to activate the complement amplification system, and their capacity to involve certain effector cells in cyto-toxicity.

In 1972, the Dreyer-Bennett postulate began to receive experimental support when Leder with his colleagues (154), working with the molecular biology of mouse myeloma, prepared a DNA probe for one constant region gene. They showed that there were, as predicted by Dreyer and Bennett, only a few copies of the gene for the light chain constant region per cell. Hozumi and Tonegawa (125) then provided the first experimental demonstration that a difference in arrangement of DNA sequence exists between embryonic mouse cells and differentiated mouse myeloma cells. This extraordinary discovery that implied rearrangement of Ig light chain genes was based on use of a powerful new method to analyze relationships of the components of the DNA within the cells.

This method was made possible by the discovery and use of restriction endo-nucleases (233). Subsequently, using recombinant DNA technology and a method for cloning of genes in bacteriophage that Leder and his associates (153) had developed for studying the coding for globin molecules, and a new method for rapidly sequencing DNA (179), Tonegawa and his colleagues (254) showed by direct analysis that the coding for the constant and variable portions of the lambda light chains of the mouse are located far apart in the embryonic mouse cells, while in mouse plasma cells, they form virtually a continuous coding sequence.

More complex genetic rearrangements were then revealed by Leder and his colleagues (155,227,228) for kappa light chains and, in even more elaborate form, for heavy chain genes by Hood and his associates (57,58). These fantastic new discoveries about the way genes responsible for antibodies are deployed in the germ line and rearranged in the differentiated cells utilized the rapidly developing and powerful tools of modern molecular biology. The methods used included restriction endonuclease technology, recombinant DNA technology, gene cloning and amplification of the cloned genes in bacteria or bacteriophages, rapid DNA sequencing, and, in its more recent detail, a gene-machine developed by Hood and his associates at Cal Tech.

The discoveries have provided understanding of the genetic basis for literally billions of different possible specificities for antibody molecules (153). Thus recombination of determinants of the V regions, with different joining (J) sequences, different diversity (D) regions (special for the heavy chains), and even slight shifting of the coding sequences at the point where V regions are joined to J regions (178) are all involved in determining the variability of the variable and hypervariable parts of the Ig molecules. Thus the capability to generate a massive number of specificities of the Ig molecules is ascertained. The number of possible antibodies which can be generated by the genetic rearrangements already understood could be as large as 10 to 20 billion.

In a broader perspective, these discoveries of the bases for antibody diversity could yield genetic mechanisms to account for generation of diversities in any other system. Indeed, it seems certain that such recombinant developmental genetic processes will be found to underlie other developmental processes which require a high degree of diversity. For example, such mechanisms could account for diversity of T cell specificities, even if the latter are independent of the bases for specificity involved in the Ig molecules. Most important for the development of understanding of this aspect of immunity have been (a) the experiments of nature represented by multiple myeloma, (b) the bold postulates which addressed the perplexing issue of antibody diversity and the paradox of constant and variable regions of the Ig peptide chains, and (c) application of the surging new technology of molecular biology and molecular genetics to immunologic issues. The conjunction and interaction of these processes and events have brought molecular biologists to the center of the stage of immunology.

The involvement of the molecular biologists in immunology should ensure continued rapid and progressively fundamental analysis of immunologic processes which surely will be translated into new approaches that can be of great practical significance. We should soon learn from these approaches, for example, how to cope definitively with the several immunodeficiency diseases and perhaps also with leukemias, lymphomas, myelomas, autoimmunities, and allergies. Perhaps we can even cope with the processes involved in aging of the immunologic systems and thus with some of the diseases of aging.

In the historic perspective, we can see that an extraordinary new science of cellular immunology has developed in a short time. This development has already provided the means of treating effectively a number of otherwise lethal diseases. This is only a beginning. One cannot help being optimistic and thus feeling certain that the future of this rapidly developing and exciting field holds great promise for permitting development of ever more effective approaches to diagnosis, analysis, understanding, prevention, and treatment for currently unsolved problems in human disease (95).

ACKNOWLEDGMENTS

The original work reported here was aided by Public Health Service grants AI-19495 and NS-18851 and by the March of Dimes, Birth Defects Foundations 1-789.

REFERENCES

1. Amos, D. B. (1981): The era of the immunogeneticist. *J. Immunol.*, 127:1727.
2. Archer, O. K., Papermaster, B. W., and Good, R. A. (1964): Thymectomy in rabbit and mice: Consideration of time of lymphoid in peripheralization. In: *Thymus in Immunobiology*, edited by R. A. Good and A. E. Gabrielsen, p. 431. Harper & Row, New York.
3. Archer, O. K., and Pierce, J. C. (1961): Role of the thymus in development of the immune response. *Fed. Proc.*, 20:26.
4. Archer, O. K., Pierce, J. C., Papermaster, B. W., and Good, R. A. (1962): Reduced antibody response in thymectomized rabbits. *Nature*, 195:191.
5. Arnason, B. G., Jankovic, B. D., Waksman, B. H., and Wennersten, C. (1962): Role of the thymus in immune reactions in rats. II. Suppressive effect of thymectomy at birth on reactions of delayed (cellular) hypersensitivity and the circulating small lymphocyte. *J. Exp. Med.*, 116:177.
6. August, C. S., Rosen, F. S., Filler, R. M., Janeway, C. A., Markowski, B., and Kay, H. E. M. (1968): Implantation of a foetal thymus restoring immunological competence in a patient with aplasia (DiGeorge's syndrome). *Lancet*, 2:1210.
7. Bach, F. H., Albertine, R. J., Joo, P., Anderson, J. L. Y., and Bortin, M. M. (1968): Bone marrow transplantation in a patient with the Wiskott-Aldrich syndrome. *Lancet*, 1:1364.
8. Bach, J. F., Dardenne, M., Pleau, J. M., and Rosa, J. (1977): Biochemical characterization of a serum thymic factor. *Nature*, 266:55.
9. Beard, J. (1900): The source of leucocytes and the true function of the thymus. *Anat. Anz.*, 18:515.
10. Beck, J. D., Haghbin, M., Wollner, N., Mertelsmann, R., Garrett, T., Koziner, B., Clarkson, B., Miller, D., Good, R. A., and Gupta, S. (1980): Subpopulations of human T lymphocytes. VI. Analysis of cell markers in acute lymphoblastic leukemia with special reference to Fc receptor expression on E-rosette forming blasts. *Cancer*, 46:45.
11. Benacerraf, B. (1973): The genetic control of specific immune responses. *Harvey Lect.*, 67:109.
12. Benacerraf, B., Green, I., and Paul, W. E. (1967): The immune response of guinea pigs to hapten-poly-L-lysin conjugates as an example of the genetic control of the recognition of antigen citing. *Cold Spring Harbor Symp. Quant. Biol.*, 32:569.
13. Benacerraf, B., and McDevitt, H. O. (1972): Histocompatability linked immune response genes. *Science*, 175:273.
14. Bienenstock, J., Rudzik, O., Clancy, R. L., and Perey, D. Y. E. (1974): Bronchial lymphoid tissue. In: *The Immunoglobulin A System: Advances in Experimental Medicine and Biology*, edited by J. Mestecky and A. R. Lawton, III, vol. 45, p. 47. Plenum Press, New York.
15. Biggar, W. D., Park, B. H., and Good, R. A. (1973): Immunologic reconstitution. *Annu. Rev. Med.*, 24:135.
16. Biggar, W. D., Stutman, O., and Good, R. A. (1972): Morphological and functional studies of fetal thymus transplants in mice. *J. Exp. Med.*, 135:793.

17. Billingham, R. E., Brent, L., and Medawar, P. B. (1953): Actively acquired tolerance of foreign cells. *Nature*, 172:603.
18. Billingham, R. E., Brent, L., and Medawar, P. B. (1955): Acquired tolerance of skin homografts. *Ann. NY Acad. Sci.*, 59:409.
19. Bing, J., and Plum, P. (1937): Serum proteins in leucopenia. *Acta Med. Scand.*, 92:415.
20. Bjoerneboe, M., and Gormsen, H. (1943): Experimental studies on the role of plasma cells as antibody producers. *Acta Pathol. Microbiol. Scand.*, 20:649.
21. Bodmer, W. F. (1978): HLA—A super supergene. *Harvey Lect.*, 72:91.
22. Boyse, E. A., and Old, L. J. (1978): The immunogenetics of differentiation in the mouse. *Harvey Lect.*, 71:23.
23. Bridges, R. A., Condie, R. M., Zak, S. J., and Good, R. A. (1959): The morphologic basis of antibody formation. Development during the neonatal period. *J. Lab. Clin. Med.*, 53:331.
24. Bryant, B. J. (1972): Renewal and fate in the mammalian thymus: Mechanisms and inferences of thymocytokinetics. *Eur. J. Immunol.*, 2:38.
25. Burnet, F. M. (1959): *The Clonal Selection Theory of Acquired Immunity.* Cambridge University Press, Cambridge.
26. Burnet, F. M., and Fenner, F. (1949): *The Production of Antibodies.* Macmillan, New York.
27. Cantor, H., and Boyse, E. A. (1975): Functional subclasses of T lymphocytes bearing different Ly antigens. I. The generation of functionally distinct T cell subclasses is a differentiative process independent of antigens. *J. Exp. Med.*, 141:1376.
28. Cantor, H., and Boyse, E. A. (1975): Functional subclasses of T lymphocytes bearing different Ly antigens. II. Cooperation between subclasses of Lyt cells in the generation of killer activity. *J. Exp. Med.*, 141:1390.
29. Cebra, J. J., Craig, S. W., and Jones, P. O. (1973): Cell types contributing to the biosynthesis of IgA. In: *The Immunoglobulin A System*, edited by J. Mestecky and A. R. Lawton, III, p. 23. Plenum Press, New York.
30. Chase, M. W. (1943): Production of local skin reactivity by passive transfer of antiprotein sera. *Proc. Soc. Exp. Biol. Med.*, 52:238.
31. Cinader, B., and Dubert, J. M. (1955): Acquired immune tolerance to human albumin and the response to subsequent injections of diazo albumin. *Br. J. Exp. Pathol.*, 36:515.
32. Claman, M. N., Chaperon, E. A., and Triplett, R. F. (1966): Thymus marrow cell combination; synergism in antibody production. *Proc. Soc. Exp. Biol. Med.*, 122:1167.
33. Cleveland, W. W., Fogel, B. J., Brown, W. T., and Kay, H. E. M. (1968): Foetal thymic transplant in a case of DiGeorge's syndrome. *Lancet*, 2:1211.
34. Cohn, M. (1971): The take home lesson. *Ann. NY Acad. Sci.*, 190:529.
35. Coons, A. H., Leduc, E. H., and Connolly, J. M. (1955): Studies on antibody production. I. A method for the histochemical demonstration of specific antibody and its application to a study of the hyperimmune rabbit. *J. Exp. Med.*, 102:49.
36. Cooper, M. D., Kincade, P. W., Dale, E., Bockman, D. I., and Lawton, A. R. (1974): Origin, distribution and differentiation of IgA-producing cells. *The Immunoglobulin A System*, edited by J. Mestecky and A. R. Lawton, III, p. 13. Plenum, New York.
37. Cooper, M. D., Payne, L. M., Dent, P. B., Burmester, B. R., and Good, R. A. (1968): The pathogenesis of avian lymphoid leukosis. I. Histogenesis. *J. Natl. Cancer Inst.*, 41:373.
38. Cooper, M. D., Perey, D. Y., McKneally, M. F., Gabrielsen, A. E., Sutherland, D. E. R., and Good, R. A. (1966): A mammalian equivalent of the avian bursa of fabricius. *Lancet*, 1:1388.
39. Cooper, M. D., Perey, D. Y., Gabrielsen, A. E., Sutherland, D. E. R., McKneally, M. F., and Good, R. A. (1968): Production of an antibody deficiency syndrome in rabbits by neonatal removal of organized intestinal lymphoid tissues. *Int. Arch. Allergy Appl. Immunol.*, 33:65.
40. Cooper, M. D., Perey, D. Y., Peterson, R. D. A., Gabrielsen, A. E., and Good, R. A. (1968): The two component concept of the lymphoid system. In: *Immunologic Deficiency Diseases in Man*, edited by R. A. Good and D. Bergsma, vol. IV, no. 1, p. 7. Birth Defects Original Article Series, The National Foundation Press, New York.
41. Cooper, M. D., Peterson, R. D. A., Gabrielsen, A. E., and Good, R. A. (1966): Lymphoid malignancy and development, differentiation and function of the lymphoreticular system. *Cancer Res.*, 26:1165.
42. Cooper, M. D., Peterson, R. D. A., and Good, R. A. (1965): Delineation of the thymic and bursal lymphoid systems in the chicken. *Nature*, 205:143.

43. Cooper, M. D., Peterson, R. D. A., South, M. A., and Good, R. A. (1966): The functions of the thymus system and the bursa system in the chicken. *J. Exp. Med.*, 123:75.

44. Croce, C. M. (1982): Mouse-human hybridomas to study the genetics of human immunoglobulins. In: *Regulation and Manipulation of Immune Responses*, The Oji Symposium on Immunology, p. 27.

45. Dardenne, M., Pleau, J. M., Lefrancier, P., and Bach, J. F. (1981): Role du zinc et d'autres metavox dans Lactivite biologique du FTS (Thymuline). *CR Acad. Sci. (D) (Paris)*, 292:793.

46. Dausset, J. (1954): Leuko-agglutinin IV leukoagglutinins and blood transfusion. *Vox Sang.*, 4:190.

47. Dausset, J., and Nenna, A. (1952): Pressance d'une leuko-agglutinine dans le serum d'un cas d'agranulocytose chronique. *CR Soc. Biol. (Paris)*, 146:597.

48. Davies, A. J. S., Leuchars, E., Wallis, V., and Koller, P. C. (1966): The mitotic response of thymus-derived cells to antigenic stimulus. *Transplantation*, 4:438.

49. Debuire, B., and Putnam, F. W. (1982): Structural studies of human IgD. In: *Protides of the Biological Fluids*, edited by H. Peeters, p. 41. Pergamon Press, Oxford.

50. Dent, P. B., Cooper, M. D., Payne, L. N., Good, R. A., and Burmester, B. R. (1967): Characterization of avian lymphoid leukosis as a malignancy of the bursal lymphoid system. In: *Perspectives in Virology V*, edited by M. Pollard, p. 251. Academic Press, New York.

51. Deutsch, H. F. Morton, J. I., and Kratochvil, C. H. (1956): Antigenic identity of hyperglobulinemia serum components with proteins of normal serum. *J. Biol. Chem.*, 222:39.

52. DiGeorge, A. M. (1968): Congenital absence of the thymus and its immunologic consequences: Concurrence with congenital hypoparathyroidism. In: *Immunologic Deficiency Diseases in Man*, edited by R. A. Good and D. Bergsma, p. 116. The National Foundation Press, New York.

53. Dougherty, T. F., Chase, J. H., and White, A. (1945): Pituitary-adrenal cortical control of antibody release from lymphocytes. An explanation of the anamnestic response. *Proc. Soc. Exp. Biol. Med.*, 58:135.

54. Dougherty, T. F., and White, A. (1945): Regulation of functional alterations in lymphoid tissue induced by adrenal cortical secretion. *Am. J. Anat.*, 77:81.

55. Dougherty, T. F., and White, A. (1943): Effect of pituitary adrenotropic hormone on lymphoid tissue. *Proc. Soc. Exp. Biol. Med.*, 53:132.

56. Dreyer, W. J., and Bennett, C. J. (1965): The molecular basis of antibody formation: A paradox. *Biochemistry*, 54:864.

57. Early, P. W., Davis, M. M., Kaback, D. B., Davidson, N., and Hood, L. (1979): Immunoglobulin heavy chain gene organization in mice: Analysis of a myeloma genomic clone containing variable and alpha constant regions. *Proc. Natl. Acad. Sci. USA*, 76(2):857.

58. Early, P. W., Huang, H. V., Davis, M. M., Calame, C., and Hood, L. (1980): An immunoglobulin heavy chain variable region is generated from three segments of DNA: V_H, D and J_H. *Cell*, 19:981.

59. Edelman, G. M. (1959): Dissociation of γ-globulin. *J. Am. Chem. Soc.*, 81:3155.

60. Edelman, G. M., Cunningham, A., Gall, W. E., Gottlick, P. D., Rutishauser, V., and Wandal, M. J. (1969): The covalent structure of an entire gamma G immunoglobulin molecule. *Proc. Natl. Acad. Sci. USA*, 63:78.

61. Ehrich, W. E., Drabkin, D. L., and Forman, C. (1949): Nucleic acids and the production of antibody by plasma cells. *J. Exp. Med.*, 90:157.

62. Ehrich, W. E., and Harris, T. N. (1945): Site of antibody formation. *Science*, 101:23.

63. Eichmann, K., Brown, D. G., Feizi, T., and Krause, R. M. (1970): The emergence of antibodies with either identical or unrelated individual antigenic specificity during repeated immunizations with streptococcal vaccines. *J. Exp. Med.*, 131:1169.

64. Evans, R. L., Breard, J. M., Lazarus, M., Schlossman, S. F., and Chess, L. (1977): Detection, isolation and functional characterization of two human T-cell subclasses bearing unique differentiation antigens. *J. Exp. Med.*, 145:221.

65. Evans, R. L., Lazarus, H., Penta, A. C., and Schlossman, S. F. (1978): Two functionally distinct subpopulations of human T cells that collaborate in the generation of cytotoxic cells responsible for cell-mediated lympholysis. *J. Immunol.*, 129:1413.

66. Evans, R. L., Wall, D. W., Platsoucas, C. D., Siegal, F. P., Fikrig, S. M., Testa, C. M., and Good, R. A. (1981): Thymus-dependent membrane antigens in man: Inhibition of cell-mediated lympholysis by monoclonal antibodies to the T_{H2} antigen. *Proc. Natl. Acad. Sci. USA*, 78:544.

67. Fagraeus, A. (1947): Plasmacellular reaction and its relation to formation of antibodies in vitro. *Nature*, 159:499.

68. Fagraeus, A. (1948): Antibody production in relationship to development of plasma cells. *Acta Med. Scand. [Suppl.]*, 130:7.
69. Fichtelius, K. E. (1962): Chairman's remarks at the International Conference on the Role of Thymus in Immobiology. *Unpublished.*
70. Fichtelius, K. E., and Bryant, B. J. (1964): On the fate of thymocytes. In: *The Thymus in Immunobiology*, edited by R. A. Good and A. Gabrielsen, p. 274. Harper & Row, New York.
71. Filippa, D. A., Lieberman, P. H., Erlandson, R. A., Koziner, B., Siegal, F. P., Turnbull, A., Zimring, A., and Good, R. A. (1978): A study of malignant lymphomas using light and ultramicroscopic, cytochemical and immunologic technics. Correlation with clinical features. *Am. J. Med.*, 64:259.
72. Ford, C. F., and Micklem, H. S. (1963): The thymus and lymph nodes in radiation chimeras. *Lancet*, 1:359.
73. Gatti, R. A., Meuwissen, J. H., Allen, H. D., Hong, R., and Good, R. A. (1968): Immunological reconstitution of sex-linked lymphopenic immunological deficiency. *Lancet*, 2:1366.
74. Gershon, R. K. (1980): Suppressor T cells; a miniposition paper celebrating a new decade. In: *Immunology 80*, edited by M. Fourgereau and J. Dausset, p. 175. Academic Press, New York.
75. Gershon, R. K., Eardley, D. D., Durum, S., Green, D. R., Shen, F. W., Yamauchi, K., Cantor, H., and Murphy, D. B. (1981): Contrasuppression: A novel immunoregulatory activity. *J. Exp. Med.*, 153:1533.
76. Gershon, R. K., and Kondo, K. (1971): Antigenic competition between heterologous erythrocytes. I. Thymic dependency. *J. Immunol.*, 106:1524.
77. Gershon, R. K., and Kondo, K. (1970): Cell interactions in the induction of tolerance: The role of thymic lymphocytes. *Immunology*, 18:723.
78. Gershon, R. K., and Kondo, K. (1972): Infectious immunological tolerance. *Immunology*, 21:903.
79. Gershon, R. K., Maurer, P. H., and Merryman, C. F. (1973): A cellular basis for genetically controlled immunologic unresponsiveness in mice: Tolerance induction in T cells. *Proc. Natl. Acad. Sci. USA*, 70:250.
80. Glanzmann, E., and Rinniker, P. (1950): Essentielle Lymphocytophthise ein neues Krankheitsbild aus dem Sauglingspathologie. *Ann. Paediatr. (Basel)*, 175:1.
81. Glick, B. (1964): The bursa of fabricius and the development of immunologic competence. In: *The Thymus in Immunobiology*, edited by R. A. Good and A. E. Gabrielsen, p. 343. Harper & Row, New York.
82. Glick, B., Chang, T. S., and Jaap, R. G. (1956): The bursa of Fabricius and antibody production. *Poult. Sci.*, 35:224.
83. Goldstein, A. L., Slater, F. D., and White, A. (1966): Preparation, assay and partial purification of a thymic lymphocytopoietic factor (thymosin). *Proc. Natl. Acad. Sci. USA*, 56:1010.
84. Good, R. A. (1948): Effect of passive sensitization and anaphylactic shock on rabbit bone marrow. *Proc. Soc. Exp. Biol. Med.*, 67:203.
85. Good, R. A. (1947): The morphologic mechanisms of hyperergic inflammation in the brain; with special reference to the significance of local plasma cell formation. Doctoral dissertation, University of Minnesota, Minneapolis.
86. Good, R. A. (1950): Experimental brain inflammation, a morphological study. *J. Neuropathol. Exp. Neurol.*, 9:78.
87. Good, R. A., and Campbell, B. (1950): Relationship of bone marrow plasmacytosis to the changes in serum gamma globulin in rheumatic fever. *Am. J. Med.*, 9:330.
88. Good, R. A. (1957): Morphological basis of the immune response and hypersensitivity. In: *Host-Parasite Relationships in Living Cells*, edited by H. M. Felton, p. 78. Charles C Thomas, Springfield, Ill.
89. Good, R. A. (1954): Absence of plasma cells from bone marrow and lymph nodes following antigenic stimulation in patients with aggamaglobulinemia. *Rev. Hematol.*, 9:502.
90. Good, R. A. (1955): Studies on agammaglobulinemia. II. Failure of plasma cell formation in the bone marrow and lymph nodes of patients with agammaglobulinemia. *J. Lab. Clin. Med.*, 46:167.
91. Good, R. A. (1956): Plasma cell hepatitis and extreme hypergammaglobulinemia in adolescent females. *J. Dis. Child.*, 92:508.
92. Good, R. A. (1982): Immunologic reconstitution, achievements and potential. *Hosp. Pract.*, 17:115.
93. Good, R. A. (1969): Immunologic reconstitution: The achievement and its meaning. *Hosp. Pract.*, 4:41.
94. Good, R. A. (1970): Progress toward a cellular engineering. *JAMA*, 214:1289.

95. Good, R. A. (1981): Anticipating the exciting future of immunology. In: *Basic Research and Clinical Medicine*, edited by S. P. Bralow, p. 125. Hemisphere Publishing, New York.

96. Good, R. A., Dalmasso, A. P., Martinez, C., Archer, O. K., Pierce, J. C., and Papermaster, B. W. (1962): The role of thymus in development of immunological capacity in rabbits and mice. *J. Exp. Med.*, 116:773.

97. Good, R. A., and Finstad, J. (1968): The association of lymphoid malignancy and immunologic functions. In: *The International Conference on Leukemia-Lymphoma*, edited by C. J. D. Zarafonetis, p. 175. Lea & Febiger, Philadelphia.

98. Good, R. A., Finstad, J., and Gatti, R. A. (1970): Bulwarks of the bodily defense. In: *Infectious Agents and Host Reactions*, edited by S. Mudd, p. 76. Saunders, Philadelphia.

99. Good, R. A., and Gabrielsen, A. E. (1964): *The Thymus in Immunobiology*. Harper & Row, New York.

100. Good, R. A., Gatti, R. A., Hong, R., and Meuwissen, J. H. (1969): Successful marrow transplantation for correction of immunological deficit in lymphopenic agammaglobulinemia and treatment of immunologically induced pancytopenia. *Exp. Hematol.*, 19:4.

101. Good, R. A., Kelly, W. D., Rotstein, J., and Varco, R. L. (1962): Immunological deficiency diseases. Agammaglobulinemia, Hodgkin's disease and sarcoidosis. In: *Progress in Allergy, Vol. 6*, edited by P. Kallos and B. H. Waksman, p. 187. Karger, Basel.

102. Good, R. A., Martinez, C., and Gabrielsen, N. E. (1964): Progress toward transplantation of tissues in man. In: *Advances in Pediatrics, Vol. 13*, edited by S. Z. Levine, p. 93. Yearbook Medical Publishers, New York.

103. Good, R. A., and Papermaster, B. W. (1964): Ontogeny and phylogeny of adaptive immunity. *Adv. Immunol.*, 4:1.

104. Good, R. A., Peterson, R. D. A., Perey, D. Y., Finstad, J., and Cooper, M. D. (1968): The immunological deficiency diseases of man: Consideration of some questions asked by these patients with an attempt at classification. In: *Immunologic Deficiency Diseases in Man*, edited by D. Bergsma and R. A. Good, p. 17. The National Foundation, New York.

105. Good, R. A., Varco, R. L., Aust, J. B., and Zak, S. J. (1957): Transplantation studies in patients with agammaglobulinemia. *Ann. NY Acad. Sci.*, 64:882.

106. Good, R. A., and Zak, S. J. (1956): Disturbances in gamma globulin synthesis as "experiments of nature". *Pediatrics*, 18:109.

107. Gorer, P. A. (1936): The detection of antigenic differences in mouse erythrocytes by the employment of immune sera. *Br. J. Exp. Biol.*, 17:42.

108. Gorer, P. A. (1937): The genetic and antigenic basis of tumor transplantation. *J. Pathol. Bacteriol.*, 44:691.

109. Gorer, P. A. (1938): The antigenic basis of tumor transplantation. *J. Pathol. Bacteriol.*, 47:231.

110. Gotze, D. (1977): *The Major Histocompatability System in Man and Animals*. Springer-Verlag, Berlin.

111. Greaves, M. F., Owen, J. J. T., and Raff, M. C. (1973): *T & B Lymphocytes*. American Elsevier, New York.

112. Haldane, J. B. S. (1933): The genetics of cancer. *Nature*, 132:265.

113. Hard, R. C., Martinez, C., and Good, R. A. (1964): Intestinal crypt lesions in neonatally thymectomized hamsters. *Nature*, 204:455.

114. Hansen, J. A., and Good, R. A. (1974): Malignant disease of the lymphoid system in immunologic perspective. *Hum. Pathol.*, 5:567.

115. Hanson, L. A. (1961): Comparative immunological studies of the immune globulins of human milk and of blood serum. *Int. Arch. Allergy Appl. Immunol.*, 18:241.

116. Hanson, L. A., Ahlstedt, S., Carlsson, B., Kaijser, B., Larson, P., Mattsby, I., Baltzer, A., Akerlund, S., Svanberg, C. E., and Svennerholm, A. M. (1977): Secretory IgA antibodies to enterobacterial virulence antigens: Their induction and possible relevance. In: *Secretory Immunity and Infection, Advances in Experimental Medicine and Biology*, Vol. 107, edited by J. R. McGhee, J. Mestecky, and J. L. Babb, p. 165. Plenum Press, New York.

117. Harris, J. E., and Ford, C. E. (1963): Role of the thymus: Migration of cells from thymic grafts to lymph nodes in mice. *Lancet*, 1:389.

118. Harris, J. E., and Ford, C. E. (1964): Cellular traffic of the thymus: Experiments with chromosome markers. Evidence that the thymus plays an instructional part. *Nature*, 201:884.

119. Harris, S., and Harris, T. N. (1954): Studies on the transfer of lymph node cells into the donor and collection of its lymph node cells. *J. Exp. Med.*, 100:269.

120. Henney, C. S., and Waldman, R. H. (1970): Cell-mediated immunity shown by lymphocytes from the respiratory tract. *Science*, 169:696.

121. Hitzig, W. H., Biro, Z., Bosch, H., and Huser, H. J. (1958): Agammaglobulinamie und alymphocytose mit schwund des lymphatischen. *Helv. Paediatr. Acta.*, 13:551.

122. Hong, R., Gatti, R. A., and Good, R. A. (1968): Hazards and potential benefits of blood transfusion in immunological deficiency. *Lancet*, 2:388.

123. Hong, R., Kay, H. E. M., Cooper, M. D., Meuwissen, H., Allen, M. J. G., and Good, R. A. (1968): Immunological restitution in lymphopenic immunologic deficiency syndrome. *Lancet*, 1:503.

124. Hopper, J. E., and Nisonoff, A. (1971): Individual antigenic specificity of immunoglobulin. In: *Advances in Immunology, Vol. 57*, edited by F. J. Dixon and H. J. Kunkel, p. 113. Academic Press, New York.

125. Hozumi, N., and Tonegawa, S. (1976): Evidence for somatic rearrangement of immunoglobulin genes coding for variable and constant regions. *Proc. Natl. Acad. Sci. USA*, 73:3628.

126. Iwata, T., Incefy, G. S., Cunningham-Rundles, C., Smithwick, E., Geller, N., O'Reilly, R., and Good, R. A. (1981): Circulating thymic hormone activity in patients with primary and secondary immunodeficiency diseases. *Am. J. Med.*, 71:385.

127. Jensen, C. O. (1903): Experimentelle untersuchungen uber krebs bei mausen. *Zentralbl. Bakteriol. Parasitenk. Infect.*, 34:28.

128. Jerne, N. K. (1955): The natural selection theory of antibody formation. *Proc. Natl. Acad. Sci. USA*, 41:849.

129. Jerne, N. K. (1974): Towards a network theory of the immune system. *Ann. Immunol. (Paris)*, 125C:373.

130. Jolly, J. (1911): Sur la function hematopoietique de la burse de fabricius. *Comple. Rend. Soc. Biol.*, 70:498.

131. Kabat, E. A., and Wu, T. T. (1971): Attempts to locate complementarity-determining residues in the variable positions of light and heavy chains. *Ann. NY Acad. Sci.*, 69:2659.

132. Kelly, W. D., Good, R. A., and Varco, R. L. (1958): Anergy and skin homograft survival in Hodgkin disease. *Surg. Gynecol. Obstet.*, 107:565.

133. Kelly, W. D., Lamb, D. L., Varco, R. L., and Good, R. A. (1960): An investigation of Hodgkin's disease with respect to the problem of homotransplantation. *Ann. NY Acad. Sci.*, 87:187.

134. Kincade, P. W., Lee, G., Watanabe, T., Sun, L., and Scheid, M. P. (1981): Antigens displayed on murine B lymphocyte precursors. *J. Immunol.*, 127:2262.

135. Kincade, P. W. (1981): Formation of B lymphocytes in fetal and adult life. In: *Advances in Immunology, Vol. 31*, edited by F. Dixon and H. G. Kunkel, p. 177. Academic Press, New York.

136. Kisielow, P., Hirst, J. A., Shiku, H., Beverley, P. C. L., Hoffmann, M. K., Boyse, E. A., and Oettgen, H. F. (1975): Ly antigens as markers for functionally distinct subpopulations of thymus-derived lymphocytes of the mouse. *Nature*, 253(5488):219.

137. Kishimoto, T. (1982): IgE class-specific suppressor T cells and regulation of the IgE response. *Prog. Allergy*, 32:265.

138. Kolouch, F. (1938): The bone marrow plasma cell. Doctoral dissertation, University of Minnesota, Minneapolis.

139. Kolouch, F. (1938): Origin of bone marrow plasma cell associated with allergic and immune states of rabbits. *Proc. Soc. Exp. Biol. Med.*, 39:147.

140. Kolouch, F. (1939): The lymphocyte in acute inflammation. *Am. J. Pathol.*, 15:413.

141. Kolouch, F., Good, R. A., and Campbell, B. (1947): The reticulo-endothelial origin of the bone marrow plasma cells in hypersensitive states. *J. Lab. Clin. Med.*, 32:749.

142. Komuro, K., and Boyse, E. A. (1973): *In vitro* demonstration of thymic hormone in the mouse by conversion of precursor cells into lymphocytes. *Lancet*, 1:740.

143. Koziner, B., Filippa, D. A., Mertelsmann, R., Gupta, S., Clarkson, B., Good, R. A., and Siegal, F. P. (1977): Characterization of malignant lymphomas in leukemic phase by multiple differentiation markers of mononuclear cells. Correlation with clinical features and conventional morphology. *Am. J. Med.*, 63:556.

144. Koziner, B., Kempin, S., Passe, S., Gee, T., Good, R. A., and Clarkson, B. D. (1980): Characterization of B-cell leukemias: A tentative immunomorphological scheme. *Blood*, 56:815.

145. Koziner, B., Mertelsmann, R., Filippa, D. A., Good, R. A., and Clarkson, B. D. (1978): Adult lymphoid neoplasias of T- and null-cell types. In: *Differentiation of Normal and Neoplastic Hematopoietic Cells*, edited by B. Clarkson, P. A. Marks, and J. E. Till, Cold Spring Harbor

Conferences on Cell Proliferation, Vol. 5, p. 843. Cold Spring Harbor Laboratory, Cold Spring Harbor, New York.

146. Kunkel, H. G., Ahrens, E. H., Jr., Eisenmenger, W. J., Bongiovanni, A. M., and Slater, R. J. (1951): Extreme hypergammaglobulinemia in young women with liver disease. *J. Clin. Invest.*, 30:654.

147. Kunkel, H., Mannik, M., and Williams, R. C. (1963): Individual antigenic specificity of isolated antibodies. *Science*, 140:1218.

148. Kunkel, H. G., Slater, R. J., and Good, R. A. (1951): Relation between certain myeloma proteins and normal gamma globulins. *Proc. Soc. Exp. Biol. Med.*, 76:190.

149. Lamm, M. E. (1976): Cellular aspects of immunoglobulin A. In: *Advances in Immunology, Vol. 22*, edited by F. J. Dixon and H. G. Kunkel, p. 223. Academic Press, New York.

150. Lamm, M. E., Weisz-Carrington, P., Roux, M. E., McWilliams, M., and Phillips-Quagliata, J. M. (1978): Development of the IgA system in the mammary gland. In: *Secretory Immunity and Infection, Advances in Experimental Medicine and Biology*, Vol. 107, edited by J. R. McGhee, J. Mestecky and J. L. Babb. p. 35. Plenum Press, New York.

151. Landsteiner, K., and Chase, M. W. (1942): Experiments on transfer of cutaneous sensitivity to simple compounds. *Proc. Soc. Exp. Biol. Med.*, 49:688.

152. Ledbetter, J. A., Evans, R. L., Lipinski, M., Cunningham-Rundles, C., Good, R. A., and Herzenberg, L. A. (1981): Evolutionary conservation of surface molecules that distinguish T lymphocyte helper/inducer and cytotoxic/suppressor subpopulations in mouse and man. *J. Exp. Med.*, 153:310.

153. Leder, P. (1982): Genetics of antibody diversity. *Sci. Am.*, 246:102.

154. Leder, P., Honjo, T., Packman, S., Swan, D., Nau, M., and Norman, B. (1974): The organization and diversity of immunoglobulin genes. *Proc. Natl. Acad. Sci. USA*, 71:3659.

155. Leder, P., Max, E. E., and Seidman, J. G. (1980): The organization of immunoglobulin genes and the origin of their diversity. In: *Immunology 80*, edited by M. Fourgereau and J. Dausset, pp. 34–50. Academic Press, New York.

156. Lederberg, J. (1959): Genes and antibodies. *Science*, 129:1649.

157. Leduc, E. H., Coons, A. H., and Connolly, J. M. (1955): Studies on antibody production. II. The primary and secondary responses in the popliteal lymph node of the rabbit. *J. Exp. Med.*, 102:61.

158. Levey, R. H., Trainin, N., and Law, L. W. (1963): Evidence for function of thymic tissue in diffusion chambers implanted in neonatally thymectomized mice. Preliminary report. *J. Natl. Cancer Inst.*, 31:199.

159. Lieberman, P. H., and Good, R. A. (1981): In *Diseases of the Hematopoietic System*. Proc. 45th Annual Anatomic Pathology Slide Seminar of the American Society of Clinical Pathologists, 1979. Educational Products Division, Chicago.

160. Litman, G. W., and Good, R. A. (eds.) (1978): *Comprehensive Immunology 5: Immunoglobulins*. Plenum, New York.

161. Little, C. C., and Tyzzer, E. E. (1916): Further experimental studies on the inheritance of susceptibility to a transplantable tumor, carcinoma (J.W.A.) of the Japanese waltzing mouse. *J. Med. Res.*, 33:393.

162. Loeb, L. (1908): Ueber die Entstehung eines Sarkoms nach Transplantation eines Adenocarcins einer Japanischen Maus. *Z. Krebsforsch.*, 7:80.

163. Low, T. L. K., and Goldstein, A. L. (1979): Thymosin and other thymic hormones and their synthetic analogues. *Semin. Immunopathol.*, 2:169.

164. Lukes, R. J., and Collins, R. D. (1974): Immunologic characterization of human malignant lymphomas. *Cancer*, 34:1488.

165. MacLean, L. D., Zak, S. J., Varco, R. L., and Good, R. A. (1965): Thymic tumor and acquired agammaglobulinemia—a clinical and experimental study of the immune response. *Surgery*, 40:1010.

166. MacLean, L. D., Zak, S. J., Varco, R. L., and Good, R. A. (1957): The role of the thymus in antibody production: An experimental study of the immune response in thymectomized rabbits. *Transplant. Bull.*, 4:21.

167. Makinodan, T. (1977): Retrospect and prospect in biology of aging. In: *Comprehensive Immunology*, edited by T. Markinodan and E. Yunis, p. 1, Plenum, New York.

168. Mariani, T., Martinez, C., Smith, J. M., and Good, R. A. (1960): Age factor and induction of immunological tolerance to male skin isografts in female mice subsequent to the neonatal period. *Ann. NY, Acad. Sci.*, 87:93.

169. von Marschalko, T. (1895): Ueber die sogenannten plasmazellen, ein Beitrag Zur Kenntnis der Herkunft der erzundlichen Infiltrationzellen. *Arch. Dermatol. Syph.*, 30:241.

170. Martinez, C., Aust, J. B., and Good, R. A. (1956): Acquired tolerance to ovarian homografts in castrated mice. *Transplant. Bull.*, 3:128.

171. Martinez, C., Dalmasso, A., and Good, R. A. (1962): Acceptance of tumor homografts by thymectomized mice. *Nature*, 194:1289.

172. Martinez, C., Dalmasso, A. P., and Good, R. A. (1964): Homotransplantation of normal and neoplastic tissue in thymectomized mice. In: *Thymus in Immunobiology*, edited by R. A. Good and A. E. Gabrielsen, p. 465. Harper & Row, New York.

173. Martinez, C., Kersey, J., Papermaster, B. W., and Good, R. A. (1962): Skin homograft survival in thymectomized mice. *Proc. Soc. Exp. Biol. Med.*, 109:193.

174. Martinez, C., Shapiro, F., and Good, R. A. (1960): Essential duration of parabiosis and development of tolerance to skin homografts in mice. *Proc. Soc. Exp. Biol. Med.*, 104:256.

175. Martinez, C., Shapiro, F., and Good, R. A. (1961): Transfer of tolerance induced by parabiosis to isologous newborn mice. *Proc. Soc. Exp. Biol. Med.*, 107:553.

176. Martinez, C., Smith, J. M., and Good, R. A. (1958): Acquired tolerance to homologous transplantation of endocrine glands in inbred strains of mice. *Br. J. Exp. Pathol.*, 39:574.

177. Martinez, C., Smith, J. M., Shapiro, F., and Good, R. A. (1959): Transfer of acquired immunological tolerance of skin homografts in mice joined in parabiosis. *Proc. Soc. Exp. Biol. Med.*, 102:413.

178. Max, E. E., Seidman, J. G., and Leder, P. (1979): Sequences of five potential recombination sites encoded close to an immunoglobulin K constant region gene. *Proc. Natl. Acad. Sci.*, 76:3450.

179. Maxam, A. M., and Gilbert, W. (1977): A new method for sequencing DNA. *Proc. Natl. Acad. Sci. USA*, 74:560.

180. McDevitt, H. O., and Chinitz, A. (1969): Genetic control of the antibody response: Relationship between immune response and histocompatibility H-2 type. *Science*, 163:1207.

181. McEndy, D. P., Boon, M. C., and Furth, J. (1944): On the role of thymus, spleen and gonads in the development of leukemia in high leukemia stock of mice. *Cancer Res.*, 4:377.

182. McKneally, M. F., and Good, R. A. (1971): The central lymphoid tissues of rabbits. I. Functional studies in newborn animals. *Surgery*, 69:166.

183. McKneally, M. F., Sutherland, D. E. R., and Good, R. A. (1971): The central lymphoid tissues of rabbits. II. Functional and morphologic studies in adult animals. *Surgery*, 69:345.

184. Medawar, P. B. (1944): The behaviour and fate of skin autografts and skin homografts in rabbits. *J. Anat.*, 78:176.

185. Medawar, P. B. (1945): Experimental study of skin grafts. *Br. Med. Bull.*, 3:79.

186. Medawar, P. B. (1958): The homograft reaction. *Proc. R. Soc. Lond. [Biol.]*, 149:145.

187. Mertelsmann, R., Filippa, D. A., Koziner, B., Grossbard, E., Beck, J., Moore, M. A. S., Lieberman, P. H., Clarkson, B. D., Gupta, S., and Good, R. A. (1979): Correlation of biochemical and immunological markers with conventional morphology and clinical features in 120 patients with malignant lymphomas. In: *Function and Structure of the Immune System*, edited by W. Muller-Ruchholtz and H. K. Muller-Hermelink, p. 553. Plenum, New York.

188. Metcalf, D. (1966): The nature and regulation of lymphopoiesis in the normal and neoplastic thymus. In: *The Thymus: Experimental and Clinical Studies*. Ciba Foundation Symposium, edited by G. E. W. Wolstenholme and R. Porter, p. 242. Little, Brown, and Company.

189. Meuwissen, J. H., Gatti, R. A., Terasaki, P. I., Hong, R., and Good, R. A. (1969): Treatment of lymphopenic hypogammaglobulinemia and bone marrow aplasia by transplantation of allogeneic marrow: Crucial role of histocompatibility matching. *N. Engl. J. Med.*, 281:691.

190. Micklem, H. S., Clarke, C. M., Evans, E. P., and Ford, C. E. (1968): Fate of chromosome-marked mouse bone marrow cells transfused into normal syngeneic recipients. *Transplant*, 6:299.

191. Miescher, P., and Fauconnet, M. (1954): Misé en evidence de differents groupes leukocytaires chez l'homme. *Schweiz. Med. Wochenschr.*, 84:597.

192. Miller, J. F. A. P. (1961): The immunological function of the thymus. *Lancet*, 2:748.

193. Miller, J. F. A. P., and Mitchell, G. F. (1968): Cell-cell interactions in immune response I. Hemolysin-forming cells in neonatally thymectomized mice reconstituted with thymus or thoracic duct lymphocytes. *J. Exp. Med.*, 128:801.

194. Mueller, A. P., Wolfe, H. R., and Meier, R. K. (1960): Precipitin production in chickens 21: Antibody production in bursectomized chickens and in chickens injected with 19-nortestosterone on 5th day of incubation. *J. Immunol.*, 85:172.

195. Müller-Schoop, J. W., and Good, R. A. (1975): Functional studies of Peyer's patches: Evidence for their participation in intestinal immune responses. *J. Immunol.*, 114:1757.

196. Muraguchi, A., Kashara, T., Oppenheim, J. J., and Fauci, A. S. (1983): B cell growth factor and T cell growth factor produced by mitogen-stimulated normal human peripheral blood T lymphocytes are distinct molecules. *J. Exp. Med. (in press).*

197. Najjar, V. A. (1963): Some aspects of antibody-antigen reactions and theoretical consideration of the immunologic response. *Physiol. Rev.*, 43:243.

198. Old, L., and Boyse, E. A. (1973): Current enigmas in cancer research. *Harvey Lect.*, 67:273.

199. O'Reilly, R. J., Pahwa, R., Dupont, B., and Good, R. A. (1978): Severe combined immunodeficiency: Transplantation approaches for patients lacking an HLA genotypically identical sibling. *Transplant. Proc.*, 10:187.

200. Osborn, J. J., Dancis, J., and Julin, J. F. (1952): Studies of the immunology of the newborn infant. I. Age and antibody production. *Pediatrics*, 9:736.

201. Osoba, D. (1964): Immune reactivity in mice thymectomized soon after birth: Normal response after pregnancy. *Science*, 147:298.

202. Osoba, D., and Miller, J. F. A. P. (1963): Evidence for a humoral thymus factor responsible for the maturation of immunological faculty. *Nature*, 199:653.

203. Oudin, J., and Michel, M. (1963): A new allotype form of rabbit serum gamma globulins apparently associated with antibody function and specificity. *CR Acad. Sci. (Paris)*, 257:805.

204. Owen, J. J. T. (1980): B cell development. In: *Immunology 80*, edited by M. Fourgereau and J. Dausset, p. 303. Academic Press, New York.

205. Owen, J. J. T., Raff, M. C., and Cooper, M. D. (1976): Studies on the generation of B lymphocytes in the mouse embryo. *Eur. J. Immunol.*, 5(7):468.

206. Owen, R. D. (1945): Immunogenetic consequences of vascular anastomoses between bovine twins. *Science*, 102:400.

207. Parrot, D. M. V., and De Sousa, M. (1971): Thymus-dependent and thymus-independent populations: Origin, migratory patterns and lifespan. *Clin. Exp. Immunol.*, 8:663.

208. Parrot, D. M. V., and East, J. (1962): The role of the thymus in neonatal life. *Nature*, 195:347.

209. Pauling, L. (1940): A theory of the structure and process of formation of antibodies. *J. Am. Chem. Soc.*, 62:2643.

210. Payne, R. (1957): Leukoaggluttinins in human serum. *Arch. Intern. Med.*, 99:587.

211. Perey, D. Y. E., and Good, R. A. (1968): Experimental arrest and induction of lymphoid development in intestinal lymphoepithelial tissues of rabbits. *Lab. Invest.*, 18:15.

212. Peterson, R. D. A., Cooper, M. D., and Good, R. A. (1965): The pathogenesis of immunologic deficiency diseases. *Am. J. Med.*, 38:579.

213. Peterson, R. D. A., Purchase, H. G., Burmester, B. R., Cooper, M. D., and Good, R. A. (1966): Relationships among visceral lymphomatosis, the bursa of Fabricius and the bursa-dependent lymphoid tissue of the chicken. *J. Natl. Cancer Inst.*, 36:585.

214. Popper, K. R. (1963): *Conjectures and Refutations.* Routledge and Kegan Paul, London.

215. Porter, R. R. (1959): The hydrolysis of rabbit gamma globulin and antibodies with crystalline papain. *Biochem. J.*, 73:119.

216. Potter, M. (1973): The developmental history of the neoplastic plasma cell in mice. A brief review of recent developments. *Semin. Hematol.*, 10:19.

217. Putnam, F. W. (1955): Abnormal human serum globulins. *Science*, 122:275.

218. Putnam, F. W., Florent, G., Paul, C., Shinoda, T., and Shimizu, A. (1973): Complete amino acid sequence of the Mu heavy chain of a human IgM immunoglobulin. *Science*, 182:287.

219. Reinherz, E. L., Kung, P. C., Goldstein, G., and Schlossman, S. F. (1979): Separation of functional subsets of human T cells by a monoclonal antibody. *Proc. Natl. Acad. Sci. USA*, 76:4061.

220. Van Rood, J. J. (1962): Leukocyte grouping, a method and its application. Doctoral dissertation, Drukkerij Pasmans, Den Haag.

221. Van Rood, J. J., Ernisse, J. G., and van Leeuwen, A. (1958): Leukocyte antibodies in sera from pregnant women. *Nature*, 181:1735.

222. Sabin, F. (1939): Cellular reactions to a dye-protein with a concept of the mechanism of antibody formation. *J. Exp. Med.*, 70:67.

223. Sachs, L. (1974): Regulation of membrane changes, differentiation and malignancy in carcinogenesis. In: *Harvey Lectures, 1972–1973* (series 68). Academic Press, New York.

224. Schier, W. W. (1954): Cutaneous anergy and Hodgkin's disease. *N. Engl. J. Med.*, 250:353.

225. Schlesinger, D. H., and Goldstein, G. (1975): The amino acid sequence of thymopoietin II. *Cell*, 5:361.
226. Schlesinger, D. H., Goldstein, G., Scheid, M. P., and Boyse, E. A. (1975): Chemical synthesis of a peptide fragment of thymopoietin II that induces selective T-cell differentiation. *Cell*, 5:367.
227. Seidman, J. G., and Leder, P. (1978): The arrangement and rearrangement of antibody genes. *Nature*, 276:790.
228. Seidman, J. G., Leder, A., Nau, M., Norman, B., and Leder, P. (1978): Antibody diversity. *Science*, 202(4363):11.
229. Shapiro, F., Martinez, C., Smith, J. M., and Good, R. A. (1961): Tolerance of skin homografts induced in adult mice by multiple injections of homologous spleen cells. *Proc. Soc. Exp. Biol. Med.*, 106:472.
230. Siegler, R., and Rich, M. A. (1963): Unilateral histogenesis of AKR thymic lymphoma. *Cancer Res.*, 23:1669.
231. Slater, R. J., Ward, S. M., and Kunkel, H. G. (1955): Immunological relationships among the myeloma proteins. *J. Exp. Med.*, 101:85.
232. Smith, R. T., and Bridges, R. A. (1958): Immunological unresponsiveness in rabbits produced by neonatal injection of defined antigens. *J. Exp. Med.*, 108:227.
233. Smith, H. O., and Wilcox, K. W. (1970): A restriction enzyme from hemophilus influenzae. I. Purification and general properties. *J. Mol. Biol.*, 51:379.
234. Snell, G. D. (1958): Histocompatibility genes of the mouse. II. Production and analysis of isogenic resistant lines. *J. Natl. Cancer Inst.*, 21:843.
235. South, M. A., Cooper, M. D., Wollheim, F. A., and Good, R. A. (1968): The IgA system. II. The clinical significance of IgA deficiency: Studies in patients with agammaglobulinemia and ataxia-telangiectasia. *Am. J. Med.*, 44:168.
236. South, M. A., Cooper, M. D., Wollheim, F. A., Hong, R., and Good, R. A. (1966): The IgA system. I. Studies of the transport and immunochemistry of IgA in the saliva. *J. Exp. Med.*, 123:615.
237. South, M. A., Warwick, W. J., Wollheim, F. A., and Good, R. A. (1967): The IgA system. III. IgA levels in the serum and saliva of pediatric patients. Evidence for a local immunological system. *J. Pediatr.*, 71:645.
238. Stutman, O. (1976): Migration of yolk sac cells to thymus grafts: Requirement of prior sojourn in bone marrow (or liver?). *Ann. Immunol. (Paris)*, 127C:943.
239. Stutman, O. (1978): Intrathymic and extrathymic T cell maturation. *Immunol. Rev.*, 142:138.
240. Stutman, O., and Good, R. A. (1971): Immunocompetence of embryonic hemopoietic cells after traffic to thymus. *Transplant. Proc.*, 3:923.
241. Stutman, O., and Good, R. A. (1971): Immunocompetence of cells derived from hemopoietic liver after traffic to thymus. In: *Morphological and Functional Aspects of Immunology*, edited by K. A. Lindahl-Kiessling, A. Alan, and M. G. Hanna, p. 129. Plenum, New York.
242. Stutman, O., and Good, R. A. (1969): Traffic of hemopoietic cells to the thymus: Influence of histocompatibility differences. *Exp. Hematol.*, 19:12.
243. Stutman, O., Yunis, E. J., and Good, R. A. (1968): Carcinogen-induced tumors of the thymus. I. Restoration of neonatally thymectomized mice with a functional thymoma. *J. Natl. Cancer Inst.*, 41:1431.
244. Stutman, O., Yunis, E. J., and Good, R. A. (1969): Carcinogen-induced tumors of the thymus. II. Lung colonies as a means of separating different cell types of a functional thymoma. *J. Natl. Cancer Inst.*, 42:783.
245. Stutman, O., Yunis, E. J., and Good, R. A. (1969): Carcinogen-induced tumors of the thymus. III. Restoration of neonatally thymectomized mice with thymomas in cell-impermeable chambers. *J. Natl. Cancer Inst.*, 43:499.
246. Stutman, O., Yunis, E. J., and Good, R. A. (1970): Studies on thymus functions. II. Cooperative effect of newborn and embryonic hemopoietic liver cells with thymus function. *J. Exp. Med.*, 132:601.
247. Sutherland, D. E. R., Archer, O. K., Peterson, R. D. A., Eckert, E., and Good, R. A. (1965): Development of "autoimmune processes" in rabbits subjected to neonatal removal of central lymphoid tissue. *Lancet*, 1:130.
248. Talmage, D. W. (1959): Immunological specificity. *Science*, 129:1643.
249. Terasaki, P. I., Vredevoe, D. L., and McClelland, J. D. (1965): Serotyping for homotransplan-

tation: IV use of cyogenically stored cells for purification of antisera. In: *Histocompatibility Testing*, pp. 265–270. Munksgaard, Copenhagen.

250. Tiselius, A., and Kabat, E. A. (1939): An electrophoretic study of immune sera and purified antibody preparations. *J. Exp. Med.*, 69:119.

251. Tobler, R., and Cottier, H. (1958): Familare lymphopenie mit agammaglobulinamie und schwerer moniliasis. *Helv. Paediatr. Acta*, 13:1333.

252. Tomasi, T. B. (1965): Studies on the immunoglobulin A proteins of serum and nonvascular fluids. Doctoral dissertation, Rockefeller University, New York.

253. Tomasi, T., Jr., and Bienenstock, J. (1968): Secretory immunoglobulins. In: *Advances in Immunology, Vol. 9*, edited by F. J. Dixon and H. G. Kunkel, p. 1. Academic Press, New York.

254. Tonegawa, S., Maxam, A. M., Tizard, R., Bernard, O., and Gilbert, W. (1978): Sequence of a mouse germ-line gene for a variable region of an immunoglobulin light chain. *Proc. Natl. Acad. Sci. USA*, 75(3):1485.

255. Tyzzer, E. E. (1909): A study of inheritance in mice with reference to their susceptibility to transplantable tumors. *J. Med. Res.*, 21:519.

256. Traub, E. (1939): Epidemiology of lymphocytic choriomenengitis in a mouse stock observed for four years. *J. Exp. Med.*, 69:801.

257. Uhr, J. W., and Baumann, J. B. (1961): Antibody formation. I. The suppression of antibody formation by passively administered antibody. *J. Exp. Med.*, 113(2):935.

258. Van Alten, P. J., Cain, W. A., Good, R. A., and Cooper, M. D. (1968): Gamma globulin production and antibody synthesis in chickens bursectomized as embryos. *Nature*, 217:358.

259. Waldmann, T. A., Broder, S., Krakauer, R., Diurm, M., Meade, B., and Doldman, M. D. (1976): Defect in IgA secretion and IgA specific suppressor cells in patients with selective IgA deficiency. *Trans. Assoc. Am. Physicians*, 89:215.

260. Waldmann, T. A., Broder, S., Krakawer, R., MacDermott, R. P., Durm, M., Goldman, C., and Meade, B. (1976): The role of suppressor cells in the pathogenesis of common variable hypogammaglobulinemia and the immunodeficiency associated with multiple myeloma. *Fed. Proc.*, 35:3067.

261. Walker, W. A., Isselbacher, K. J., and Block, K. (1974): The role of immunization in controlling antigen uptake from the small intestine. In: *The Immunoglobulin A System*, edited by J. Mistecky and A. R. Lawton, III, p. 295. Plenum, New York.

262. Warner, N. L., and Szenberg, A. (1964): Immunologic studies on hormonally bursectomized and surgically thymectomized chickens: Dissociation of immunologic responsiveness. In: *The Thymus in Immunobiology*, edited by R. A. Good and A. E. Gabrielsen, p. 395. Harper & Row, New York.

263. White, R. G., Coons, A. H., and Connolly, J. M. (1955): Studies on antibody production. III. The alum granuloma. *J. Exp. Med.*, 102:73.

264. Woodruff, M. A. F., and Simpson, L. O. (1955): Induction of tolerance to skin homografts in rats by injection of cells from the prospective donor soon after birth. *Br. J. Exp. Pathol.*, 36:494.

265. Yamazaki, K., Boyse, E. A., Mike, V., Thaler, H. T., Mathieson, B. J., Abbott, J., Boyse, J., Zayas, J. A., and Thomas, L. (1976): Control of mating preferences in mice by genes in the major histocompatibility complex. *J. Exp. Med.*, 144(2):1324.

266. Yoshizaki, K., Nakagawa, T., Kaieda, T., Muraguchi, A., Yamamura, Y., and Kishimoto, T. (1982): Induction or proliferation and Ig production in human B leukemic cells by anti-immunoglobulins and T cell factors. *J. Immunol.*, 128:1296.

267. Yoshizaki, K., Nakagawa, T., Fekunaga, K., Kajeda, T., Maruyana, S., Kishimoto, S., Yamamura, Y., and Kishomoto, T. (1983): Characterization of human B cell growth factor BCGF from a cloned T cell on mitogen-stimulated T cells. *J. Immunol. (in press)*.

268. Yunis, E. J., Hilgard, H. R., Martinez, C., and Good, R. A. (1965): Studies on immunologic reconstitution of thymectomized mice. *J. Exp. Med.*, 121:607.

269. Zinneman, H. H., and Hall, W. H. (1954): Recurrent pneumonia in multiple myeloma and some observations on immunological response. *Ann. Intern. Med.*, 41:1152.

Advances in Host Defense Mechanisms, Vol. 2,
edited by John I. Gallin and Anthony S. Fauci.
Raven Press, New York © 1983.

Disorders of Purine Metabolism and Immunodeficiency

Erwin W. Gelfand and Amos Cohen

Division of Immunology, Research Institute, Hospital for Sick Children, Toronto, Canada

The study of immunodeficiency has contributed significantly to the advancement of immunology and to our understanding of normal host resistance to infection. Since the discovery of hypogammaglobulinemia in the early 1950s, a large and increasing number of deficiency states has been described. The primary immunodeficiency diseases fall into one of three major categories: defects within the B-cell system, isolated disorders of T-cell or cell-mediated immunity, and combined T- and B-cell immunodeficiency. Attempts at simple classification are complicated by the significant interplay between the T- and B-cell systems and the application of new and sophisticated technology to the study of these patients, revealing alternative mechanisms which result in similar disease states.

The human lymphoid system is comprised of discrete subsets of T- and B-lymphocytes. In addition to the functional integrity of these cells, it is the balance between effector and regulatory subsets of cells that ultimately determines or governs the actual immune response. The divergence of T- and B-cells into functionally distinct subpopulations of cells represents the culmination of a complex sequence of events. The rapid advances in cell marker analysis, generation of monoclonal antibodies, and *in vitro* assays have provided the necessary initial probes for the identification of the discrete stages of lymphocyte ontogeny. Many of the immunodeficiency diseases now can be identified as primary disorders of lymphocyte differentiation. For example, severe combined immunodeficiency disease (SCID) is comprised of a heterogeneous group of diseases, in which the combined absence of cell-mediated and humoral immunity can be traced in some patients to a failure of normal T-cell differentiation and a consequent failure of B-cell maturation. Several phenotypes of SCID have been identified on the basis of the stage of maturation at which T-cell development is arrested (46,50). Similarly, congenital agammaglobulinemia may actually reflect a heterogeneous group of patients with arrests of B-cell maturation at different stages of development (99).

If one group of the immunodeficiency diseases can be viewed within the framework of lymphocyte differentiation, then the second group may be considered to reflect abnormalities or imbalances among the immunoregulatory subsets. Since terminal differentiation of B-cells to immunoglobulin-secreting plasma cells is regulated by T-cells, the presence of an abnormal suppressor cell (36) or an excess of normal suppressor cells (106) can be implicated in the pathogenesis of some forms of hypogammaglobulinemia. Such suppressor cells may play a role in the hypogammaglobulinemia following infectious mononucleosis (125) or dilantin therapy (38). Alternatively, agammaglobulinemia may result from the absence of T-helper cells (107).

The association of profound immunodeficiency with the deficiency of a specific enzyme of purine metabolism comprises the third group and has been of particular interest in our laboratories. In these disorders, we find abnormalities of differentiation and immunoregulation. Observations from patients with a rare inherited disease and the studies they have evoked have important implications for our understanding of the biochemical control of lymphocyte differentiation and the role this biochemical pathway plays in the regulation of immune function. In this chapter, we focus on purine metabolism and lymphocyte function since they represent the clearest examples of the contributions of the study of immunodeficiency disease to the expansion of knowledge of the normal immune system.

PURINE METABOLISM: AN OVERVIEW

Purine metabolites are linked to many aspects of intermediary metabolism as substrates, cofactors, and regulatory molecules. In addition to their common roles in the biosynthesis of nucleic acids, proteins, lipids, and carbohydrates, purine compounds have specialized regulatory roles in hormonal actions, neurotransmission, and immune regulation. Most human cells have alternative pathways for purine nucleotide biosynthesis, *de novo* purine biosynthesis and purine salvage.

The *de novo* pathway of purine biosynthesis builds the purine ring on the ribose-5-phosphate moiety from common substrates, such as glutamine, glycine, formate, aspartate, and bicarbonate (Fig. 1). The end product of *de novo* purine biosynthesis is inosine monophosphate, from which all other purine nucleotides are made through interconversions and phosphorylation. *De novo* purine biosynthesis is tightly regulated by various purine nucleotides. The targets of end product inhibition are the first two enzymes in this pathway, phosphoribosylpyrophosphate synthetase and glutamine phosphoribosylpyrophosphate amidotransferase (4,43,65,139,140).

Purine nucleotides also can be synthesized through the purine salvage pathway (Fig. 1). The enzymes of this metabolic pathway are ubiquitous in man; their role is to reutilize preformed purine bases and purine nucleosides for nucleotide and nucleic acid synthesis. The purine phosphoribosyltransferases hypoxanthine guanine phosphoribosyltransferase (HGPRT) and adenine phosphoribosyltransferase (APRT) catalyze the transfer of the ribose-5-phosphate moiety to the purine bases hypoxanthine, guanine, and adenine to form the corresponding nucleosides inosine monophosphate (IMP), guanosine monophosphate (GMP), and adenosine monophosphate (AMP). Nucleoside kinases catalyze the phosphorylation of nucleosides to produce nucleoside monophosphate. Adenosine and 2′-deoxyadenosine are phosphorylated by adenosine kinase. 2′-Deoxyadenosine and 2′-deoxyguanosine also can be phosphorylated by deoxycytidine kinase. There is no phosphorylation of guanosine or inosine in human tissues.

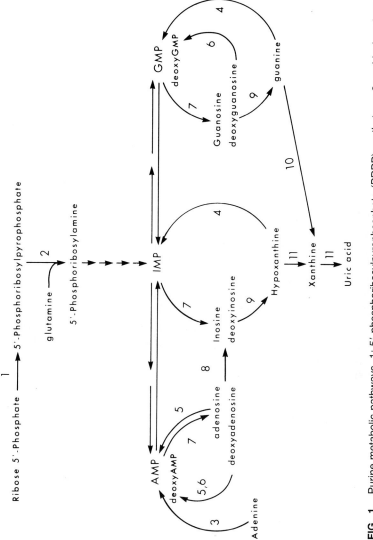

FIG. 1. Purine metabolic pathways. 1: 5'-phosphoribosylpyrophosphate (PRPP) synthetase; 2: amidophosphoribosyl transferase; 3: adenine phosphoribosyl transferase (APRT); 4: hypoxanthine-guanine phosphoribosyl transferase (HGPRT); 5: adenosine kinase; 6: deoxycytidine kinase; 7: 5'-nucleotidase; 8: adenosine deaminase (ADA); 9: purine nucleoside phosphorylase (PNP); 10: guanase; 11: xanthine oxidase.

The balance between purine salvage and the *de novo* pathways largely depends on the availability of purine salvage substrates. For example, the addition of purine bases to cultured mammalian cells results in inhibition of *de novo* purine synthesis (5,108). Inhibition of *de novo* synthesis results from the accumulation of products formed through the salvage pathway (5,108). Evidence that the majority of purine nucleotides are produced through the purine salvage pathway comes from observations made in children deficient in HGPRT and in purine nucleoside phosphorylase (PNP), who are unable to salvage hypoxanthine and guanine (Fig. 1). As a result, the nonutilized purines are excreted in their urine (23,81), but higher amounts of purines are excreted than the equivalent uric acid excretion in normal children. These differences in purine excretion are an estimate of the amounts normally salvaged by these enzymes. The purine salvage pathway may serve two physiologic roles: (a) to enable purines synthesized in one tissue to be made available to other tissues, and (b) to allow intracellular reutilization of purines produced by nucleic acid and nucleotide turnover. The relative importance of these two roles is not known.

Purine nucleotides that are not reutilized by the salvage pathway are subjected to a common purine degradation pathway (Fig. 1). Several enzymes can catalyze the dephosphorylation of nucleotides. Specific 5'-phosphomonoesterase (or 5'-nucleotidase) and nonspecific phosphatases hydrolyze AMP, IMP, and GMP to their corresponding nucleosides. Most of the activity of 5'-nucleotidase is localized on the outside surface of the plasma membrane (ecto-5'-nucleotidase). Deoxynucleoside monophosphates, on the other hand, are hydrolyzed by a specific cytoplasmic enzyme, endo-5'-nucleotidase. Inosine, deoxyinosine, guanosine, and deoxyguanosine are converted to the corresponding purine base and ribose-1-phosphate or deoxyribose-1-phosphate by PNP. Adenosine and deoxyadenosine are first deaminated to inosine or deoxyinosine by adenosine deaminase (ADA) and subsequently are converted to hypoxanthine by PNP. PNP is the only major enzyme in mammalian cells that converts purine nucleosides to the corresponding purine bases; there is no adenosine phosphorylase in mammalian cells. Guanine is deaminated to xanthine by guanine deaminase. Finally, hypoxanthine and xanthine are oxidized to uric acid by xanthine oxidase. All the enzymes that catalyze the degradation of purine nucleotides to the purine bases guanine and hypoxanthine are ubiquitous in mammalian tissues, whereas the final common pathway of purine degradation which produces uric acid is located mainly in the liver and small intestinal mucosa (135).

Another major source of adenosine production is 5'-adenosylhomocysteine, a product of methyltransferase reactions, which is degraded further to adenosine and homocysteine by 5'-adenosylhomocysteine hydrolase (Fig. 2).

PURINE ENZYME ACTIVITIES IN LYMPHOCYTE DIFFERENTIATION

In the course of differentiation, lymphocytes undergo morphologic, surface membrane, and biochemical changes. Although the role of these changes is not clear,

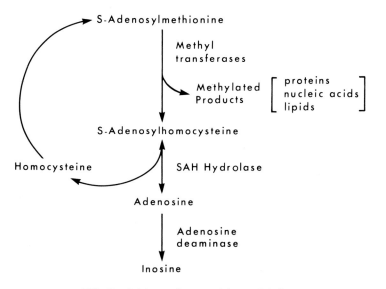

FIG. 2. 5-Adenosylhomocysteine metabolism.

they do provide tools for identification and classification of lymphocyte populations in normal and disease states. Activities of several purine enzymes change markedly during T-cell differentiation.

Adenosine Deaminase (ADA)

Thymocytes have the highest activity of ADA when compared to other tissues (1,66). As T-cell differentiation proceeds, ADA activity decreases. Mature medullary thymocytes have lower activities than immature cortical thymocytes, and T-cells from peripheral blood have decreased activity (9,21).

Purine Nucleoside Phosphorylase (PNP)

PNP is the next in sequence to ADA in the purine degradation pathway (Fig. 1). PNP activities are inversely related to activities of ADA during T-lymphocyte differentiation. PNP activity is low in immature cortical thymocytes and increases in the more mature medullary thymocytes (10). Peripheral blood T-lymphocytes have activities similar to those of B-cell lines (126).

Deoxycytidine Kinase

Thymocytes have the highest level of deoxycytidine kinase, an enzyme that catalyzes the phosphorylation of deoxycytidine, deoxyguanosine, and deoxyadenosine (16,27,79,93). B- and T-cells from peripheral blood or lymph nodes have comparable but lower levels of deoxycytidine kinase than immature T-cells (27).

Ecto-5′-Nucleotidase

The activity of this ectoenzyme increases markedly during T-cell differentiation. Thymocytes have a low activity, which increases in mature T-cells from peripheral blood and lymph nodes (27,41). Thymic-derived factors, known to stimulate T-cell differentiation, can also increase the activity of 5′-nucleotidase in cultured human thymocytes (29). Peripheral blood B-lymphocytes have high levels of activity (27,41). On the other hand, chronic lymphocytic leukemic cells, which may represent the clonal expansion of an immature B-cell population, have low activities (24,102). 5′-Nucleotidase may be associated with the differentiation of both B- and T-lymphocytes.

Terminal Deoxynucleotidyl Transferase

Terminal deoxynucleotidyl transferase (TdT) catalyzes the polymerization of DNA in the absence of a template (13). It is present only in immature lymphocytes (8,56). Intrathymic T-lymphocytes as well as prethymic precursor cells in the bone marrow contain high levels of TdT, whereas postthymic peripheral blood T- or B-cells have no TdT activity (8,56). TdT activity in leukemic cells correlates with ADA: T-leukemic cells contain high activity, null leukemic cells intermediate activity, and B-leukemic cells low activity of both ADA and TdT (33).

SIGNIFICANCE OF PURINE METABOLISM
IN T-LYMPHOCYTE DIFFERENTIATION

The thymus provides an essential microenvironment for the differentiation of T-lymphocytes. It has been suggested that thymus is involved in the selection of lymphocyte populations, with the ability to recognize self major histocompatibility antigens (145). There is evidence that in addition to cell differentiation and cell division, the majority of lymphocytes die within the thymus (90,112,137). This combination of massive cell death together with cell division and cell differentiation in the same microenvironment poses certain metabolic difficulties. Dying cells can release large amounts of the degradation products of DNA and RNA, including purine and pyrimidine ribonucleosides, deoxyribonucleosides, and bases. This is of special relevance in the thymus, since it is a tissue containing a low number of macrophages, the natural scavengers of dying cells (11).

Extracellular purine and pyrimidines may supply the salvage substrates for RNA and DNA synthesis and thus enhance cell division in situations where *de novo* synthesis is rate limiting. However, imbalances in the amounts of these extracellular purine nucleosides can lead to cell death (57,58,130). Intrathymic T-cells have an unusually high capacity for salvaging both purine and pyrimidine deoxynucleosides (27,35); these metabolic aspects may have significant effects on the differentiation of intrathymic T-lymphocytes. On one hand, the abundance of purine salvage substrates which can be used for DNA synthesis would permit rapid cell division.

These substrates may also play a regulatory role in this process, causing thymocyte death due to the cytotoxic effects of the accumulation of certain purine nucleosides. The end result is dependent on two factors. The first is the balance between the levels of different nucleosides in the cell microenvironment. For example, extracellular deoxyguanosine alone is cytotoxic, whereas deoxyguanosine in the presence of deoxycytidine supports cell division (58). The second reflects the profile of purine enzyme activities of a particular cell or intrathymic cell population. For instance, high activity of ADA could protect cells from adenosine or deoxyadenosine toxicity, and a subpopulation of thymocytes with low activity could be killed by extracellular adenosine or deoxyadenosine.

INHERITED ENZYME DEFICIENCIES

The genetic deficiency of three enzymes in the purine degradation pathway can result in a life-threatening immunodeficiency disease. ADA deficiency can result in one form of SCID, a uniformly fatal inherited disorder characterized by a failure of normal development of cell-mediated and humoral immunity. In contrast, PNP deficiency results in a selective deficiency of particular aspects of T-cell immunity. Transcobalamin II deficiency leads to deficiency of humoral immunity alone.

Clinical Syndromes

ADA Deficiency

The association of the deficiency of ADA with profound immunodeficiency has been reported in more than 30 families and 50 patients (reviewed in ref. 69). In 85 to 90% of the ADA-deficient patients, the clinical picture and laboratory findings are those of early onset of symptoms, lymphopenia, and no detectable evidence for cell-mediated or humoral immunity. In this group, the patients present within the first few months of life with recurrent infections, diarrhea, and failure to thrive. Fungal, protozoal, and viral infections pose the major problems. All show delayed growth and development and an absence of lymphoid tissue. Absolute lymphocyte counts generally are less than 500 and often less than 200/mm^3; indeed, lymphocytes may not be detectable in peripheral blood or bone marrow. Correspondingly, few E-rosetting T-cells can be identified, and *in vitro* lymphocyte proliferative responses to lectins or allogeneic cells are at background levels. Similarly, agammaglobulinemia is the rule, and specific antibody responses are absent.

In perhaps 10 to 15% of the patients, the disease may present in a somewhat different manner. The onset of symptoms may be delayed beyond 6 to 12 months of life. They may initially have normal levels of serum immunoglobulins. Although specific antibody formation often is impaired, some patients have responded with specific responses to herpes virus, adenovirus, and allogeneic cells (53). Lymphopenia is common and cell-mediated immunity often absent or grossly abnormal; again, some exceptions are described. The majority of the patients in this group suffer immunologic attrition with progressive fall-off in immune function.

In several patients with ADA deficiency, prethymic precursor T-cells can be identified. Their maturation could be induced *in vitro* following contact with cultured thymic epithelium but only if a source of ADA is provided (114). This suggests that for T-cell maturation, ADA is required, even for the earliest stages of differentiation. In additional studies, corformycin, a potent inhibitor of ADA, has been shown to impair the maturation of precursor T-cells but not the maturation of B-cell precursors into immunoglobulin-secreting cells (6).

In five patients with ADA-deficient SCID, thymus histology was reported to differ from that seen in SCID with normal ADA activity (71). Although these differences may not be as clearcut as originally suggested (68), ADA-deficient SCID thymus may not be embryonal in type but mimic the picture of extreme thymic involution with the preservation of some Hassall corpuscles.

In any rare autosomal recessive disease, it is not surprising to find some degree of genetic heterogeneity. Nonetheless, the findings of normal lymphocyte function in several patients with complete deficiency of ADA in red cell lysates was surprising. Subsequent studies have indicated 25 to 50% of normal activity in the lymphocytes, a level of activity sufficient *in vivo* to almost totally prevent the accumulation of potentially toxic metabolites (105). These cases indicate the pitfalls in attempting to correlate red cell enzyme activities with specific abnormalities of lymphocyte function.

PNP Deficiency

Complete deficiency in the activity of the next enzyme in the reaction sequence, PNP, was reported in 1975 in a child presenting with an isolated deficiency of T-cell immunity (54). More than 10 patients have now been evaluated (reviewed in ref. 3). Many of the patients had a history of chronic and recurrent infections with bacterial as well as viral agents, including cytomegalovirus and toxoplasmosis. The onset of infections has been generally later than in SCID. Surprisingly, many of the patients have tolerated live virus immunization, Bacillus Calmette-Guérin (BCG), or blood transfusions without incident early in life; some have developed progressive vaccinia or fatal varicella infections.

Most of the patients were lymphopenic at the time of presentation or developed a progressive decrease in lymphocyte numbers. All patients failed to respond to delayed hypersensitivity skin testing. E-rosetting T-cells were always reduced, not only in absolute numbers (given the lymphopenia) but as a percentage of the mononuclear cell fraction after gradient centrifugation. In parallel, lymphocyte proliferative responses were markedly depressed, despite the addition of normal numbers of T-cells to the cultures.

In contrast to the T-cell deficiencies described, B-cell immunity was intact and even hyperresponsive in some. Although circulating numbers of B-cells were reduced, immunoglobulin levels were normal or high, and specific antibody responses were elicited to a variety of antigens. Monoclonal gammopathy also has been observed.

Overall, it appears that these patients have normal B-cell immunity but lack selective aspects of T-cell immunity. Thus, despite the profound circulating lymphopenia and absence of lymphocytes in the paracortex of the lymph node, they are capable of generating T-dependent specific antibodies *in vivo* and *in vitro* (47). The T-cells present appear incapable of proliferating in response to lectins, antigens, or allogeneic cells. Furthermore, all stages of precursor T-cell differentiation appear intact (47), and the thymus appears reasonably normal (2). Several of the patients have developed autoimmune hemolytic anemia, autoantibodies, or monoclonal immunoglobulins. These findings, coupled with the heightened antibody responsiveness, suggest that these patients may have a significant abnormality in immunoregulation.

Transcobalamin II Deficiency

Congenital transcobalamin II deficiency is a rare condition which can affect the immune system. Deficiency of this carrier protein has known effects on the hematopoietic system. Recently, it has been shown to be vital for the normal proliferation and function of B-lymphocytes. In the patient best studied, failure to thrive, diarrhea, and recurrent infections were associated with a progressive anemia and pancytopenia (70). The presence of macrocytes and hypersegmented neutrophils suggested a diagnosis of pernicious anemia. Agammaglobulinemia also was observed, although circulating B-cell numbers were normal. All aspects of cell-mediated immunity were normal. Following institution of vitamin B_{12} therapy, immunoglobulin levels rose to normal, plasma cells appeared, and specific antibodies were elicited. Surprisingly, specific antibodies to diphtheria and tetanus appeared without reimmunization and boosted rapidly on reimmunization. It appears that the B-cells could become primed in the vitamin B_{12}-deficient phase but not secrete antibodies. Following institution of vitamin B_{12} therapy, clonal expansion and specific antibody synthesis became possible.

Biochemical Bases of the Diseases

ADA Deficiency

In general, a deficiency of an enzyme activity can change cellular metabolism as a result of the absence of a product of the enzymatic reaction or, alternatively, secondary to an excessive accumulation of its substrate(s). In ADA deficiency, it is generally believed that the failure of normal lymphocyte development and function is the result of the accumulation of ADA substrates adenosine and 2'-deoxyadenosine. The lack of ADA products is probably not causally related to the immune deficiency, since inosine and 2'-deoxyinosine can either be salvaged to their corresponding nucleotides by HGPRT or degraded to uric acid by xanthine oxidase (Fig. 1). Deficiency of either one of these enzymes does not result in immune deficiency in man (75,141).

The ADA substrates adenosine and 2'-deoxyadenosine accumulate in excessive amounts in the serum and urine of these patients (34,117). Both are cytotoxic to lymphocytes and to other cultured mammalian cells (55,57,77,83,94,101,119,130). Several possible mechanisms have been postulated to explain adenosine- and deoxyadenosine-induced toxicity. Among these are: pyrimidine starvation (55,57,129), increased intracellular cyclic AMP levels (138), inhibition of methylation reactions (61,62,78), and inhibition of ribonucleotide reductase (82,93,119,130).

Pyrimidine starvation.

In the presence of inhibitors of ADA, adenosine at micromolar concentrations is cytotoxic to a variety of cultured cells, including lymphocytes (55,57,129). The toxicity of low adenosine concentrations is relieved by the simultaneous addition of uridine (55,57,129). In addition, it has been shown that adenosine can cause depletion of intracellular pyrimidine nucleotides (55).

The molecular mechanism of adenosine toxicity has been studied in detail in S49 mouse lymphoma cells (25,57,129). Adenosine toxicity is dependent on the transport and phosphorylation of adenosine. Mutants deficient in adenosine transport or in adenosine kinase activity are resistant to adenosine toxicity (57,130). The toxicity is associated with depletion of intracellular phosphoribosylpyrophosphate, resulting in inhibition of *de novo* pyrimidine biosynthesis (57). Lymphoid cells, incubated in the presence of adenosine, excrete orotic acid, an intermediary metabolite in pyrimidine biosynthesis (57). Phosphoribosylpyrophosphate depletion may be caused by feedback inhibition of phosphoribosylpyrophosphate synthetase due to the excessive accumulation of adenine nucleotides resulting from adenosine phosphorylation (57,101). Although the occurrence of pyrimidine starvation as a result of ADA inhibition is well documented in cultured cells, it is unlikely that ADA-deficient children suffer from pyrimidine starvation, since there is no excessive orotic acid in the urine of these patients (57).

Cyclic AMP accumulation.

Adenosine can cause elevation of intracellular cyclic AMP levels by binding to surface membrane receptors, resulting in stimulation of adenylate cyclase activity in various cell types, including T-lymphocytes (25,138). Adenosine-induced elevation of cyclic AMP levels can cause inhibition of cell-mediated cytotoxicity by T-lymphocytes (138) and transient inhibition of proliferation of mouse thymocytes (111). The cytotoxicity of adenosine to mouse T-lymphoma cells is independent of cyclic AMP metabolism, however, since mutants unresponsive to cyclic AMP are still sensitive to adenosine toxicity (26). Although elevation of extracellular adenosine may contribute to the immune dysfunction of ADA-deficient patients, it is unlikely that an elevation in cyclic AMP is responsible for the marked reduction of lymphocyte numbers and abnormal function in these patients.

Inhibition of ribonucleotide reductase.

2'-Deoxyadenosine in the presence of inhibitors of ADA is cytotoxic to various cultured mammalian cells (83,93,119,130). In order to exert its toxicity, deoxy-

to low concentrations of deoxyguanosine and accumulate large amounts of deoxy-GTP. A double mutant, deficient in both PNP and deoxycytidine kinase, does not accumulate deoxy-GTP and is less sensitive to deoxyguanosine toxicity (131). Another mutant, resistant to deoxyguanosine toxicity, involves the enzyme ribonucleotide reductase, which became resistant to deoxy-GTP inhibition (42). These studies imply that deoxyguanosine cytotoxicity to these T-lymphoma cells is a result of the accumulation of deoxy-GTP, which leads to the inhibition of ribonucleotide reductase, depletion of deoxy-CTP pools, and inhibition of DNA synthesis (88).

Thymocytes are significantly more sensitive to deoxyguanosine toxicity than any other human cell type tested (27,47). The exquisite sensitivity of thymocytes is accompanied by an increased capability of these cells to accumulate deoxy-GTP (27). Inhibition of ribonucleotide reductase by deoxy-GTP in thymocytes is the only proposed explanation for the selective T-cell deficiency associated with PNP deficiency.

Transcobalamin II Deficiency

Transcobalamin II is a β-globulin which transports the absorbed vitamin B_{12} to the tissues (59). Interestingly, methylcobalamin is a cofactor in the remethylation of homocysteine to methionine (136). The involvement of cobalamin in homocysteine methylation may suggest a common biochemical mechanism, linking the hypogammaglobulinemia seen in both ADA and transcobalamin II deficiencies. It is possible that immunoglobulin production requires S-adenosylmethionine-mediated methylation. In ADA deficiency, these reactions may be inhibited by the accumulation of S-adenosylhomocysteine, whereas in transcobalamin II deficiency, these methylation reactions are absent secondary to the deficiency in methionine production.

SECONDARY ENZYME DEFICIENCIES

The enzyme 5'-nucleotidase is present on the plasma membrane of both T- and B-cells; and, as discussed earlier, the level of activity may be related in both cases to the stage of differentiation of the lymphocytes (29,49). Depending on the technique and laboratory, mature B-cells have up to threefold higher levels of activity than mature T-cells (41,121). There are several conditions in which lymphocyte 5'-nucleotidase activity is significantly reduced or absent.

Cord Blood Lymphocytes

Cord blood mononuclear cells have significantly less 5'-nucleotidase activity than mononuclear cells isolated from normal adults. This appears to be due to lower activities on both B- and T-lymphocytes (109).

T-Cell Acute Lymphoblastic Leukemia

Most T-cell acute lymphoblastic leukemia (T-ALL) cells are thought to be derived from an early stage of maturation corresponding to the intrathymic stage of differentiation (113). T-ALL cells have significantly lower 5'-nucleotidase levels than do mature T-cells (103).

Chronic Lymphocytic Leukemia

The B-lymphocytes from most patients with chronic lymphocytic leukemia have low levels of 5'-nucleotidase activity (82,102). These cells may be arrested at an early stage of development, since they express low concentrations of surface IgM and can be induced to differentiate in the presence of the phorbol ester tetradeca-noylphorbol acetate (97).

Hypogammaglobulinemia

A deficiency of 5'-nucleotidase activity has been reported in a number of patients with hypogammaglobulinemia, including those with congenital X-linked agam-maglobulinemia, common variable immunodeficiency, and some with a selective deficiency of serum IgA (40,41,73,109,121). These findings have been confirmed by histochemical staining as well as by assay for enzyme activity (89,104). There is no evidence for a cause and effect relationship between lymphocyte 5'-nucleo-tidase deficiency and the hypogammaglobulinemic state. There is no obvious disorder of purine nucleotide degradation or increased sensitivity to deoxyadenosine or deoxyguanosine *(unpublished observations)*. Nevertheless, in many of these patients, circulating T-cells (as well as B-cells) can be shown to have reduced levels of enzyme activity (40,121). Whether this deficiency is a marker indicating a maturational block of lymphocyte development or reflects an imbalance in the proportions of lymphocyte subsets is unclear. The demonstration of an abnormal T-suppressor cell or increase in suppressor T-cell numbers in many of these patients may provide a clue to the findings (36). Unfortunately, we have been unable to demonstrate any correlation between the presence of suppressor T-cells and 5'-nucleotidase deficiency in our patients.

The deficiency of 5'-nucleotidase in congenital X-linked agammaglobulinemia also has been utilized to detect the heterozygote state. Lymphoblastoid cell lines established from presumed carriers were characterized by low ecto-5'-nucleotidase activity and a reduced percentage of surface immunoglobulin-bearing cells (122).

Familial Reticuloendotheliosis

Familial reticuloendotheliosis (Omenn's Syndrome) with eosinophilia was originally described by Omenn in 1965 (98). Since then, a number of reports have documented a variable degree of impairment of humoral or cell-mediated immunity, including combined immunodeficiency, in this syndrome (7,20,28,95). The characteristics of the syndrome include frequent infections, eosinophilia, hepato(spleno)megaly, morbilliform rash, high IgE levels, and a lymphocyte-depleted thymus without Hassall corpuscles. In three patients we have studied, there has been a selective absence of B- and T-cell ecto-5'-nucleotidase activity despite activity in other cells (granulocytes, bone marrow) and in fibroblast cell lines established from the patients (28,52). In addition, levels in the parents are normal, as are endonucleotidase activities, and there are no derangements in nucleoside metabolism.

It appears that the association of this syndrome with the absence of lymphocyte ecto-5'-nucleotidase is not causally related but may reflect some abnormality of lymphocyte differentiation. The delineation of this syndrome in one infant with combined immunodeficiency, in one with cartilage-hair hypoplasia, and a lympho-proliferative syndrome in the third may suggest a common pathogenetic event being expressed in a susceptible host.

NUCLEOSIDE-MEDIATED MODULATION OF IMMUNE FUNCTION

In Vivo Administration of Inhibitors of ADA

Induction of T-Cell Deficiency

The development of specific inhibitors of ADA permitted the utilization of animal models to study the relationship of nucleoside metabolism to lymphocyte function *in vivo*. ADA activity in mouse tissues can be virtually abolished by the *in vivo* administration of a potent and specific inhibitor, deoxycoformycin. Following daily intraperitoneal injections of the drug (1.0 mg/kg), Burridge et al. (15) showed that although ADA activity was reduced by more than 90%, the drug did not impair the response of mouse thymocytes to stimulation with concanavalin A (con-A) or spleen cells to allogeneic cells. In contrast, following continuous intraperitoneal infusion of the drug, immunodeficiency resulted in parallel to the inhibition of ADA. The immunodeficiency was indicated by a reduction in T- and B-cell mitogenic responses, impairment of delayed hypersensitivity reactions, a decrease in both *in vivo* and *in vitro* antibody production, prolongation of skin allografts, and lymphopenia. Histologic examination of the tissues revealed lymphocyte depletion in the thymus, lymph nodes, and spleen (120).

Inhibition of Graft Rejection

Animals treated with another inhibitor of ADA, Erythro-9-[2-Hydroxyl-3-Nonyl] Adenine Hydrochloride (EHNA), have been shown to be sufficiently immunosuppressed to prevent skin allograft rejection (84). In Balb/c mice rendered diabetic with stretozocin and treated with daily intraperitoneal injections of EHNA, intrasplenic transplantation of pancreatic islets from DBA/2 animals restored glucose homeostasis and prolonged graft survival in 60% of recipients (86). These studies suggest that inhibitors of ADA can modify the host's immune response and may be of potential benefit as an immunosuppressive agent for organ allografting.

Inhibition of Suppressor T-Cell Function

The generation of antibody responses *in vivo* or *in vitro* requires the cooperation of both B- and T-cells, and the height of the response reflects the balance between

T-helper and T-suppressor cells. The differentiation of B-cells to an antibody-secreting stage and the activation of antigen-specific T-suppressor cells requires proliferation; antigen-induced activation of T-helper cells does not (36). We examined the effects of deoxyguanosine on *in vitro* plaque-forming cell responses. In the presence of as little as 2.5 μM deoxyguanosine, there was a failure of expression of T-suppressor cell activity, suggesting that this population of T-cells is more sensitive to the drug than helper T-cells (48).

In another system, Hayward (60) studied the suppression of plasma cell differentiation using newborn T-cells and pokeweed mitogen. Suppressor cells are induced by pokeweed mitogen and, in parallel, the percentage of OKT 8$^+$ cells rises. This increase can be prevented by the addition of 50 μM deoxyguanosine to the cultures; this concentration of drug also prevents suppression of plasma cell differentiation.

In *in vivo* studies in mice, we monitored the generation of T-suppressor cells capable of abrogating a primary IgM response. Following daily intraperitoneal injections of deoxyguanosine, the selective inhibition of T-suppressor cell activity was observed in both primary recipients of the drug and those receiving spleen cells from treated animals (37).

Using a mouse malaria model, Lelchuk et al. (80) have shown T-cell-mediated suppression of the contact sensitivity response to oxazolone in infected mice. Daily treatment with 2-deoxyguanosine did not affect the response in normals but largely abrogated the suppression in mice infected with *Plasmodium berghei*. However, treatment with deoxyguanosine did not affect the parasitemia during infection or alter the survival pattern of the treated animals.

In Vitro Modulation of Immune Function

T-Cell Differentiation

Studies in ADA-deficient patients have indicated the role of ADA in the earliest stages of T-cell differentiation (110,114). Inhibition of ADA also appears to affect precursor T-cell development but does not impair the maturation of precursor B-cells into immunoglobulin-secreting cells (6).

E-Rosette Formation

Mononuclear cell surface markers were tested in the presence of EHNA. Only E-rosette formation was significantly inhibited and sIg and C3-rosette formation was unchanged (85).

Lymphocyte Proliferation

A number of studies have assayed the effects of the addition of different nucleosides on lymphocyte proliferation. Deoxyguanosine is a potent inhibitor of lymphocyte proliferation (48,91,96); the more immature the T-cell, the lower the concentration of drug required (27,48). Adenosine and deoxyadenosine are also potent inhibitors, particularly in the presence of inhibitors of ADA (17,18,48, 67,91,117). The proposed mechanism for this lymphotoxicity may be through the inhibition of ribonucleotide reductase, as discussed above. On the basis of their studies, Uberti et al. (127) proposed that adenosine and deoxyadenosine inhibit lymphocyte proliferation at some point before DNA synthesis begins (128). This implies that the purine nucleosides inhibit thymidine uptake by interfering with early events following lectin binding and not by inhibiting DNA synthesis directly. Support for interference with events in the mitogen recognition phase rather than direct DNA inhibition has come from studies assessing T-cell growth factor (TCGF) production. In the presence of deoxyadenosine and 2-deoxycoformycin, con-A-induced production of TCGF was markedly inhibited (124).

Inhibition of Lymphocyte-Mediated Cytolysis

The *in vitro* destruction of tumor cells by specifically sensitized mouse lymphocytes may be inhibited by adenosine (138). This inhibition was markedly potentiated in the presence of an inhibitor of ADA and was accompanied by a rapid elevation in lymphocyte cyclic AMP. Since adenosine receptors and stimulation of lymphocyte adenylate cyclase are now well described (25,51,138), the adenosine-mediated inhibition of cytolysis may not be related to nucleoside metabolism. More recently, however, the same group has shown that 3-deazaadenosine can inhibit lymphocyte-mediated cytolysis (143,144). The mechanism is not through elevation of cyclic AMP but rather through elevation of adenosylhomocysteine and/or deazaadeno-sylhomocysteine and consequent inhibition of 5-adenosylmethionine-utilizing methyltransferases.

Inhibition of Lymphocyte Capping

Capping of B-lymphocyte surface Ig receptors results from the rapid redistribution of the receptors to one pole of the cell. This is a highly organized contractile process which may also involve methyltransferase reactions. Treatment of murine or human B-cells with adenosine and an inhibitor of ADA, or with 3-deazaadenosine, resulted in the inhibition of Ig capping (14). Anti-Thy-1 antigen or membrane sites reactive with antilymphocyte antibodies were not affected, confirming their noninvolvement with the contractile process.

Inhibition of Human Monocyte Chemotaxis

A requirement for 5-adenosylmethionine-mediated methylation has also been shown for monocyte chemotaxis. Methylation was inhibited in monocytes by treating the cells with substances that resulted in increased levels of 5-adenosylhomocysteine. Treatment of isolated monocytes with adenosine plus an ADA inhibitor resulted in a marked increase in 5-adenosylhomocysteine and inhibition of monocyte chemotaxis; monocyte phagocytosis was unimpaired (100).

USE OF PURINE ENZYMES AND ANALOGS IN DIAGNOSIS AND CHEMOTHERAPY OF LEUKEMIA

The selective lymphopenia associated with ADA and PNP deficiencies stimulated interest in utilizing purine enzymes and analogs in the diagnosis and treatment of lymphoid leukemia. Measurements of ADA and TdT activities have proved useful in the classification of ALLs (32). T-ALL cells have the highest levels of both ADA and TdT, whereas non-T-non-B-cells have intermediate levels and B-cells have the lowest activities of both enzymes (32).

The availability of a potent inhibitor of ADA, 2'-deoxycoformycin, prompted clinical trials testing its efficacy as an antileukemic agent. In phase I clinical trials, marked lymphopenia was observed, accompanied in some cases with other cytotoxic effects (12,92,118). The administration of deoxycoformycin to patients has revealed metabolic and toxic phenomena which are not present in ADA-deficient patients. Thus deoxycoformycin administration was associated with central nervous system toxicity, hemolytic anemia, and reduction of ATP levels (92,115). These phenomena may be associated with direct side effects of deoxycoformycin, which is phosphorylated to the monophosphate level and can inhibit not only ADA but also adenylate deaminase (45,133). Because of its toxicity, the use of this drug may be limited; in addition the response of leukemic cells is highly variable (92).

No comparable potent inhibitor of PNP is available. A relatively weak PNP inhibitor, 8-aminoguanosine, has been shown to potentiate deoxyguanosine cytotoxicity toward T-lymphoblasts (74). However, the high concentrations (100 μM) required for effective inhibition exclude its potential use in chemotherapy. Deoxyguanosine at micromolar concentrations is selectively cytotoxic toward T-ALL cells *in vitro* (30). Preliminary trials with deoxyguanosine *in vivo* showed that it is rapidly cleared by the PNP activity present in the red blood cells *(unpublished observations)*. Therefore, it is necessary to use deoxyguanosine analogs which are resistant to cleavage by PNP. One such analog is arabinosylguanine, which is resistant to PNP cleavage but still can be phosphorylated to the triphosphate arabinosyl-GTP (30). Arabinosylguanine proved to be 100-fold more toxic than deoxyguanosine toward T-ALL cells, whereas it is essentially nontoxic to B-lymphoblasts (30). Future studies are required to test its effectiveness as an antileukemic and immunosuppressive agent.

CONCLUSIONS

The discovery of the association of immunodeficiency with inherited disorders of purine metabolism has sparked new interest in the effects of purine nucleosides on lymphocyte function. The implications for these findings are far-reaching and have undoubtedly contributed to a new understanding of the biochemical ontogeny of T- and B-cells and modulation of specific lymphocyte functions. In addition, this initial insight will be applied to other aspects of diagnosis, classification, and, hopefully, treatment of some of the immunodeficiency diseases, lymphoid leukemias, and perhaps autoimmune states.

Many aspects remain to be clarified. We are only beginning to understand the biochemical pathogenesis of the immunodeficiency states accompanying the inherited enzyme deficiencies and are somewhat naive about the remarkable tissue-specific and, in some cases, function- or lymphocyte-subset-specific consequences of the diseases. There are many hypotheses and perhaps many explanations. Nevertheless, the interdisciplinary approaches of the last 5 to 10 years have contributed enormously to the expansion of knowledge of the critical role of purine metabolism in lymphocyte ontogeny, lymphocyte function, immunodeficiency, and the potential for pharmacologic manipulation of normal and malignant cells.

ACKNOWLEDGMENTS

This work was supported by grants from the Medical Research Council of Canada, The National Cancer Institute of Canada, and the Ontario Cancer Treatment and Research Foundation. Dr. Cohen is the recipient of a scholarship from the National Cancer Institute.

REFERENCES

1. Adams, A., and Harkness, R. A. (1976): Adenosine deaminase activity in thymus and other human tissues. *Clin. Exp. Immunol.*, 26:647–649.
2. Ammann, A. J., Wara, D. W., and Allen, T. (1978): Immunotherapy and immunopathologic studies in a patient with nucleoside phosphorylase deficiency. *Clin. Immunol. Immunopathol.*, 10:262–269.
3. Ammann, A. J. (1979): Immunological aberrations in purine nucleoside phosphorylase deficiencies. In: *Enzyme Defects and Immune Dysfunction*, pp. 55–69. Elsevier, Amsterdam.
4. Bagnara, A. S., Brox, L. W., and Henderson, J. F. (1974): Kinetics of amidophosphoribosyltransferase in intact cells. *Biochim. Biophys. Acta*, 350:171–182.
5. Bagnara, A. S., Letter, A. A., and Henderson, J. F. (1974): Multiple mechanisms of regulation of purine biosynthesis de novo. *Biochim. Biophys. Acta*, 374:259–270.
6. Ballet, J. J., Insel, R., Merler, E., and Rosen, F. S. (1976): Inhibition of maturation of human precursor lymphocytes by coformycin, an inhibitor of the enzyme adenosine deaminase. *J. Exp. Med.*, 143:1271–1276.
7. Barth, R. F., Vegara, G. G., Khurana, S. K., Lawman, J. T., and Beckwith, J. B. (1972): Rapidly fatal familial histiocytosis associated with eosinophilia and primary immunologial deficiency. *Lancet*, 2:503–506.
8. Barton, R., Goldschneider, I., and Bollum, F. J. (1976): The distribution of terminal deoxynucleotidyl transferase (TdT) among subsets of thymocytes in the rat. *J. Immunol.*, 116:462–468.
9. Barton, R., Martiniuk, F., Hirschhorn, F., and Goldschneider, I. (1979): The distribution of adenosine deaminase among lymphocyte populations in the rat. *J. Immunol.*, 122:216–220.
10. Barton, R., Martiniuk, F., Hirschhorn, R., and Goldschneider, I. (1980): Inverse relationship between adenosine deaminase and purine nucleoside phosphorylase in rat lymphocyte populations. *Cell. Immunol.*, 49:208–214.
11. Beller, D. I., and Unanue, E. R. (1980): Ia antigens and antigen-presenting function of thymic macrophages. *J. Immunol.*, 124:1433–1440.
12. Benjamin, R. S., Plunkett, W., Keating, M. J., Fenn, L. G., Hug, V., Nelson, J. A., Bodey, G. P., and Freireich, E. J. (1980): Phase I and biochemical pharmacological studies of deoxycoformycin. *Proc. Annu. Assoc. Cancer Res.*, 21:337.
13. Bollum, F. J. (1974): Terminal deoxynucleotidyl transferase. In: *The Enzymes, Vol. 10*, edited by P. D. Boyer, pp. 145–177. Academic Press, New York.
14. Braun, J., Rosen, F. S., and Unanue, E. R. (1980): Capping and adenosine metabolism. Genetic and pharmacologic studies. *J. Exp. Med.*, 151:174–183.
15. Burridge, P. W., Paetkau, V., and Henderson, J. F. (1977): Studies of the relationship between adenosine deaminase and immune function. *J. Immunol.*, 119:675–678.

16. Carson, D. A., Kaye, J., and Seegmiller, J. E. (1977): Lymphocyte specific toxicity in adenosine deaminase deficiency and purine nucleoside phosphorylase deficiency: Possible role of nucleoside kinase(s). *Proc. Natl. Acad. Sci. USA*, 74:5677–5681.

17. Carson, D. A., Kaye, J., and Seegmiller, J. (1978): Differential sensitivity of human leukemic T cell lines and B cell lines to growth inhibition of deoxyadenosine. *J. Immunol.*, 121:1726–1731.

18. Carson, D. A., Kaye, J., Matsumoto, S., Seegmiller, J. E., and Thompson, L. (1979): Biochemical basis for the enhanced toxicity of deoxyribonucleosides toward malignant human T cell lines. *Proc. Natl. Acad. Sci. USA*, 76:2430–2433.

19. Carson, D. A., Kaye, J., and Wasson, D. B. (1981): The potential importance of soluble deoxynucleotidase activity in mediating deoxyadenosine toxicity in human lymphoblasts. *J. Immunol.*, 126:348–352.

20. Cederbaum, S. D., Niwayama, G., Stiehm, E. R., Neerhout, R. C., Ammann, A. J., and Berman, W. (1974): Combined immunodeficiency presenting as the Letterer-Siwe syndrome. *J. Pediatr.*, 85:466–471.

21. Chechik, B. E., Schroder, W. P., and Minowada, J. (1981): An immunomorphological study of adenosine deaminase distribution in human thymus tissue, normal lymphocytes, and hematopoietic cell lines. *J. Immunol.*, 126:1003–1007.

22. Chen, S. H., Ochs, H. D., Scott, C. R., Giblett, E. R., and Tingle, A. J. (1978): Adenosine deaminase deficiency. Disappearance of adenine deoxynucleotides from a patient's erythrocytes after successful marrow transplantation. *J. Clin. Invest.*, 62:1386–1389.

23. Cohen, A., Doyle, D., Martin, D. W., Jr., and Ammann, A. J. (1976): Abnormal purine metabolism and purine overproduction in a patient deficient in purine nucleoside phosphorylase. *N. Engl. J. Med.*, 295:1449–1454.

24. Cohen, A., Hirschhorn, R., Horowitz, S. D., Rubinstein, A., Polmar, S. H., Hong, R., and Martin, D. W., Jr. (1978): Deoxyadenosine triphosphate as a potentially toxic metabolite in adenosine deaminase deficiency. *Proc. Natl. Acad. Sci. USA*, 75:472–476.

25. Cohen, A., Gudas, L. J., Ullman, B., and Martin, D. W., Jr. (1979): Nucleotide metabolism in cultured T-cells and in cells of patients deficient in adenosine deaminase and purine nucleoside phosphorylase. In: *Enzyme Defects and Immune Dysfunction*, pp. 101–114. Elsevier, Amsterdam.

26. Cohen, A., Ullman, B., and Martin, D. W., Jr. (1979): Characterization of a mutant mouse lymphoma cell with deficient transport of purine and pyrimidine nucleosides. *J. Biol. Chem.*, 254:112–117.

27. Cohen, A., Lee, J. W. W., Dosch, H.-M., and Gelfand, E. W. (1980): The expression of deoxyguanosine toxicity in T lymphocytes at different stages of maturation. *J. Immunol.*, 125:1578–1582.

28. Cohen, A., Mansour, A., Dosch, H.-M., and Gelfand, E. W. (1980): Absence of lymphocyte ecto 5'-nucleotidase in familial reticuloendotheliosis and combined immunodeficiency. *Clin. Immunol. Immunopathol.*, 15:245–250.

29. Cohen, A., Dosch, H.-M., and Gelfand, E. W. (1981): Induction of ecto 5'nucleotidase activity in human thymocytes. *Clin. Immunol. Immunopathol.*, 18:287–289.

30. Cohen, A., Lee, J. W. W., and Gelfand, E. W. (1983): Selective toxicity of deoxyguanosine and arabinosyl guanine for T-leukemic cells. *Blood (in press)*.

31. Coleman, M. S., Donofrio, J., and Hutton, J. J. (1977): Abnormal concentrations of deoxynucleotides in adenosine-deaminase (ADA) deficiency and severe combined immunodeficiency disease (SCID). *Blood*, 50:292–297.

32. Coleman, M. S., Donofrio, J., Hutton, J. J., Hahn, L., Daoud, A., Lampkin, B., and Dyminski, J. (1978): Identification and quantitation of adenine deoxynucleotides in erythrocytes of a patient with adenosine deaminase deficiency and severe combined immunodeficiency. *J. Biol. Chem.*, 253:1619–1626.

33. Coleman, M. S., Greenwood, M. F., Hutton, J. J., Holland, P., Lampkin, B., Krill, C., and Kastelic, J. E. (1978): Adenosine deaminase, terminal deoxynucleotidyl transferase (TdT), and cell surface markers in childhood acute leukemia. *Blood*, 52:1125–1131.

34. Donofrio, J., Coleman, M. S., and Hutton, J. J. (1978): Overproduction of adenine deoxynucleosides and deoxynucleotides in adenosine deaminase deficiency with severe combined immunodeficiency disease. *J. Clin. Invest.*, 62:884–887.

35. Donofrio, J. C., Meier, J., and Hutton, J. J. (1979): Nucleotide metabolism and nucleic acid synthesis in mouse thymocytes. *Cell. Immunol.*, 42:79–89.

36. Dosch, H.-M., and Gelfand, E. W. (1979): Specific in vitro IgM responses of human B-cells: A complex regulatory network modulated by antigen. *Immunol. Rev.*, 45:243–274.

37. Dosch, H.-M., Mansour, A., Cohen, A., Shore, A., and Gelfand, E. W. (1980): Inhibition of suppressor T-cell development following deoxyguanosine administration. *Nature*, 285:494–496.

38. Dosch, H.-M., Jason, J., and Gelfand, E. W. (1982): Transient antibody deficiency and abnormal T-suppressor cells induced by diphenylhydantoin. *N. Engl. J. Med.*, 306:406–409.

39. Durham, J. P., and Ives, D. H. (1969): Deoxycytidine kinase. I. Distribution in normal and neoplastic tissues and interrelationships of deoxycytidine and 1-beta-D-arabinofuranosylcytosine phosphorylation. *Mol. Pharmacol.*, 5:358–375.

40. Edwards, N. L., Magilavy, D. B., Cassidy, J. T., and Fox, I. H. (1978): Lymphocyte ecto-5′-nucleotidase deficiency in agammaglobulinemia. *Science*, 201:628–630.

41. Edwards, N. L., Gelfand, E. W., Burk, L., Dosch, H.-M., and Fox, I. H. (1979): Distribution of 5′-nucleotidase in human lymphoid tissues. *Proc. Natl. Acad. Sci. USA*, 76:3474–3476.

42. Eriksson, S., Gudas, L. J., Ullman, B., Clift, S. M., and Martin, D. W., Jr. (1981): DeoxyATP-resistant ribonucleotide reductase of mutant mouse lymphoma cells. *J. Biol. Chem.*, 256:10184–10188.

43. Fox, I., and Kelley, W. N. (1971): Human erythrocyte phosphoribosylpyrophosphate synthetase: Conformational changes and regulation. *Fed. Proc.*, 30:1255–1258.

44. Fox, R. M., Piddington, S. K., Tripp, E. H., and Tattersall, M. H. N. (1981): Ecto-adenosine triphosphatase deficiency in cultured human T and null leukemic lymphocytes. *J. Clin. Invest.*, 68:544–552.

45. Frieden, C., Gilbert, H. R., Miller, W. H., and Miller, R. L. (1979): Adenylate deaminase: Potent inhibition by 2′-deoxycoformycin 5′-phosphate. *Biochem. Biophys. Res. Commun.*, 91:278–283.

46. Gelfand, E. W., and Dosch, H.-M. (1982): Review. Differentiation of precursor T lymphocytes in man and delineation of the selective abnormalities in severe combined immune deficiency disease. *Clin. Immunol. Immunopathol.*, 25:303–315.

47. Gelfand, E. W., Dosch, H.-M., Biggar, W. D., and Fox, I. H. (1978): Partial purine nucleoside phosphorylase deficiency: Studies of lymphocyte function. *J. Clin. Invest.*, 61:1071–1080.

48. Gelfand, E. W., Lee, J. W. W., and Dosch, H.-M. (1979): Selective toxicity of purine deoxynucleosides for human lymphocyte growth and function. *Proc. Natl. Acad. Sci. USA*, 76:1998–2002.

49. Gelfand, E. W., Dosch, H.-M., Cohen, A., and McClure, P. D. (1980): Post-transplant immunodeficiency: Secondary to thymic epithelial cell dysfunction? In: *Biology of Bone Marrow Transplantation*, edited by R. P. Gale and C. F. Fox, pp. 97–117. Academic Press, New York.

50. Gelfand, E. W., Dosch, H.-M., Shore, A., Limatibul, S., and Lee, J. W. W. (1980): The role of the thymus in human T-cell differentiation. In: *The Biological Basis for Immunodeficiency Disease*, edited by E. W. Gelfand, and H.-M. Dosch, pp. 39–56. Raven Press, New York.

51. Gelfand, E. W., Cheung, R., Hastings, D., and Dosch, H.-M. (1980): Characterization of lithium effects on two aspects of T-cell formation. In: *Effects of Lithium on Granulopoiesis and Immune Functions*, edited by A. H. Rossof and W. H. Robinson, vol. 127, pp. 429–446. Plenum Press, New York.

52. Gelfand, E. W., Rao, C. P., McCurdy, D., Sigal, N. H., and Cohen, A. (1982): Familial reticuloendotheliosis—A primary or secondary disease? *Pediatr. Res.*, 16:222.

53. Giblett, E. R., Anderson, J. E., Cohen, F., Pollara, B., and Meuwissen, H. J. (1972): Adenosine-deaminase deficiency in two patients with severely impaired cellular immunity. *Lancet*, 2:1067–1069.

54. Giblett, E. R., Ammann, A. J., Wara, D. W., Sandman, R., and Diamond, L. K. (1975): Nucleoside-phosphorylase deficiency in a child with severely defective T-cell immunity and normal B-cell immunity. *Lancet*, 1:1010–1013.

55. Green, H., and Chan, T. S. (1973): Pyrimidine starvation induced by adenosine in fibroblasts and lymphoid cells: Role of adenosine deaminase. *Science*, 182:836–837.

56. Gregoire, K. E., Goldschneider, I., Barton, R. W., and Bollum, F. J. (1979): Ontogeny of terminal deoxynucleotidyl transferase-positive cells in lymphohemopoietic tissues of rat and mouse. *J. Immunol.*, 123:1347–1352.

57. Gudas, L. J., Cohen, A., Ullman, B., and Martin, D. W., Jr. (1978): Analysis of adenosine-mediated pyrimidine starvation using cultured wild type and mutant mouse T-lymphoma cells. *Somatic Cell Genet.*, 4:201–219.

58. Gudas, L. J., Ullman, B., Cohen, A., and Martin, D. W., Jr. (1979): Deoxyguanosine toxicity

in a mouse T-lymphoma: Relationship to purine nucleoside phosphorylase-associated immune dysfunction. *Cell*, 14:531–538.

59. Hall, C. A., and Finkler, A. E. (1965): The dynamics of transcobalamin II. A vitamin B12 binding protein in plasma. *J. Lab. Clin. Med.*, 65:459–468.

60. Hayward, A. R. (1981): Development of lymphocyte responses and interactions in the human fetus and newborn. *Immunol. Rev.*, 57:39–60.

61. Hershfield, M. S. (1979): Apparent suicide inactivation of human lymphoblast S-adenosylhomocysteine hydrolase by 2'-deoxyadenosine and adenine arabinoside. *J. Biol. Chem.*, 254:22–25.

62. Hershfield, M. S., and Kredich, N. M. (1978): A mechanism for adenosine cytotoxicity in adenosine deaminase (ADA) deficiency. *Clin. Res.*, 26:329A.

63. Hershfield, M. S., Kredich, N. M., Ownby, D. R., and Buckley, R. (1979): In vitro inactivation of erythryocyte S-adenosylhomocysteine hydrolase by 2'-deoxyadenosine in adenosine deaminase-deficient patients. *J. Clin. Invest.*, 63:807–811.

64. Hershfield, M. S., and Kredich, N. M. (1980): Resistance of an adenosine kinase-deficient human lymphoplastoid cell line to effects of deoxyadenosine on growth, S-adenosyl-homocysteine hydrolase inactivation, and ATP accumulation. *Proc. Natl. Acad. Sci. USA*, 77:292–296.

65. Hershko, A., and Mager, J. (1969): Relation of the synthesis of 5'-phosphoribosyl-1-pyrophosphate in infant red blood cells and in cell free preparations. *Biochem. Biophys. Acta*, 184:64–76.

66. Hirschhorn, R., Martiniuk, F., and Rosen, F. S. (1978): Adenosine deaminase activity in normal tissues and tissues from a child with severe combined immunodeficiency and adenosine deaminase deficiency. *Clin. Immunol. Immunopathol.*, 9:287–292.

67. Hirschhorn, R., Bajaj, S., Borkowsky, W., Kowalski, A., Hong, R., Rubinstein, A., and Papageorgiou, P. (1979): Differential inhibition of adenosine deaminase deficient peripheral blood lymphocytes and lymphoid line cells by deoxyadenosine and adenosine. *Cell. Immunol.*, 42:18–423.

68. Hirschhorn, R., Vawter, G. F., Kirkpatrick, J. A., and Rosen, F. S. (1979): Adenosine deaminase deficiency: Frequency and comparative pathology in autosomally recessive severe combined immunodeficiency. *Clin. Immunol. Immunopathol.*, 14:107–120.

69. Hirschorn, R. (1979): Clinical delineation of adenosine deaminase deficiency. In: *Enzyme Defects and Immune Dysfunction*, pp. 35–49. Elsevier, Amsterdam.

70. Hitzig, W. H., and Kenny, A. B. (1975): The role of vitamin B12 and its transport globulins in the production of antibodies. *Clin. Exp. Immunol.*, 20:105–111.

71. Huber, J., and Kersey, J. (1975): Pathological features. In: *Combined Immunodeficiency Disease and Adenosine Deaminase Deficiency: A Molecular Defect*, edited by H. J. Meuwissen, R. J. Pickering, B. Pollara, and I. H. Porter, pp. 279–288. Academic Press, New York.

72. Ives, D. H., and Durham, J. P. (1970): Deoxycytidine kinase II. Purification and general properties of the calf thymus enzymes. *J. Biol. Chem.*, 245:2276–2284.

73. Johnson, S. M., Asherson, G. L., Watts, R. W. E., North, M. E., Allsop, J., and Webster, A. D. B. (1977): Lymphocyte purine 5'-nucleotidase deficiency in primary hypogammaglobulinemia. *Lancet*, 1:168–170.

74. Kazmers, I. S., Mitchell, B. S., Daddona, P. E., Worting, L. L., Townsend, L. B., and Kelley, W. N. (1981): Inhibition of purine nucleoside phosphorylase by 8-aminoguanosine: Selective toxicity for T lymphoblasts. *Science*, 214:1137–1139.

75. Kelley, W. N., and Wyngaarden, J. B. (1972): The Lesch-Nyhan syndrome. In: *The Metabolic Basis of Inherited Disease*, edited by J. B. Stanbury, J. B. Wyngaarden, and D. S. Fredrickson, pp. 969–991. McGraw-Hill, New York.

76. Kerr, S. J. (1972): Competing methyltransferase systems. *J. Biol. Chem.*, 247:4248–4252.

77. Klenow, H. (1959): On the effect of some adenine derivatives on the incorporation in vitro of isotopically labelled compounds into nucleic acids of Ehrlich ascites tumor cells. *Biochem. Biophys. Acta*, 35:412–421.

78. Kredich, N. M., and Martin, D. W., Jr. (1977): Role of S-adenosylhomocysteine in adenosine-mediated toxicity in cultured mouse lymphoma cells. *Cell*, 12:931–938.

79. Krenitsky, T. A., Tuttle, J. V., Koszalka, G. W., Chen, I. S., Beacham, L., Rideaut, J. L., and Elion, G. B. (1976): Deoxycytidine kinase from calf thymus. *J. Biol. Chem.*, 251:4055–4061.

80. Lelchuk, R., Sprott, V. M. A., and Playfair, J. H. L. (1981): Differential involvement of non-specific suppressor T cells in two lethal murine malaria infections. *Clin. Exp. Immunol.*, 45:43–438.

81. Lesch, M., and Nyhan, W. L. (1964): A familial disorder of uric acid metabolism and central nervous system function. *Am. J. Med.*, 36:561–570.

82. Lopes, J., Zucker-Franklin, D., and Silber, R. (1973): Heterogeneity of 5'--nucleotidase activity in lymphocytes in chronic lymphocytic leukemia. *J. Clin. Invest.*, 52:1297–1300.

83. Lowe, J. K., Gwans, B., and Brox, L. (1977): Deoxyadenosine metabolism and toxicity in cultured LS178Y cells. *Cancer Res.*, 37:3013–3017.

84. Lum, C. T., Sutherland, D. E. R., Foker, J. E., and Najarian, J. S. (1977): Low-toxicity immunosuppression by specific inhibition of adenosine deaminase (ADA): Prolongation of mouse skin grafts with erythro-9-(2-hydroxy-3-nonyl) adenine hydrochloride (EHNA). *Surg. Forum*, 28:320–322.

85. Lum, C. T., Schmidtke, J. R., Sutherland, D. E. R., and Najarian, J. S. (1978): Inhibition of human T-cell rosette formation by adenosine deaminase inhibitor erythro-9-(2-hydroxy-3-nonyl) adenine hydrochloride (EHNA). *Clin. Immunol. Immunopathol.*, 10:258–261.

86. Lum, C. T., Sutherland, D. E. R., Eckhardt, J., Matas, A. J., and Najarian, J. S. (1979): Effect of an adenosine deaminase inhibitor on survival of mouse pancreatic islet allografts. *Transplantation*, 27:355–357.

87. Majias, E., Mitchell, B. S., Cassidy, J. (1979): Deoxyribonucleoside triphosphate pools in immunodeficiency states. *Clin. Res.*, 27:331A.

88. Martin, D. W., Jr., and Gelfand, E. W. (1981): Biochemistry of diseases of immunodevelopment. *Ann. Rev. Biochem.*, 50:845–877.

89. Matamoros, N., Horwitz, D. A., Newton, C., Asherson, G. L., and Webster, A. D. B. (1979): Histochemical studies for 5'-nucleotidase and alpha-naphthyl (non-specific) esterase in lymphocytes from patients with primary immunoglobulin deficiencies. *Clin. Exp. Immunol.*, 36:102–106.

90. Matsuyama, M., Wiadrowski, N. N., and Metcalf, M. N. (1966): Autoradiographic analysis of lymphopoiesis and lymphocyte migration in mice bearing multiple thymus grafts. *J. Exp. Med.*, 123:559–576.

91. Mitchell, B. S., Mejias, E., Daddona, P. E., and Kelley, W. N. (1978): Purinogenic immunodeficiency diseases: Selective toxicity of deoxyribonucleosides for T cells. *Proc. Natl. Acad. Sci. USA*, 75:5011–5014.

92. Mitchell, B. S., Kaller, C. A., and Heyn, R. (1980): Inhibition of adenosine deaminase activity results in cytotoxicity to T lymphoblasts in vivo. *Blood*, 56:556–559.

93. Monparler, R. L., and Fischer, G. A. (1968): Mammalian deoxynucleoside kinases; purification properties and kinetic studies with cytosine arabinoside. *J. Biol. Chem.*, 243:298–344.

94. Morris, N. R., Reichard, P., and Fischer, G. A. (1963): Studies concerning the inhibition of cellular reproduction by deoxyribonucleosides. II. Inhibition of the synthesis of deoxycytidine by thymidine, deoxyadenosine and deoxyguanosine. *Biochem. Biophys. Acta*, 68:93–99.

95. Ochs, H. D., Davis, S. D., Mickelson, E., Lerner, K. G., and Wedgwood, R. J. (1974): Combined immunodeficiency and reticuloendotheliosis with eosinophilia. *J. Pediatr.*, 85:463–465.

96. Ochs, U. H., Chen, S. H., Ochs, H. D., Osborne, W. R., and Scott, C. R. (1979): Purine nucleoside phosphorylase deficiency: A molecular model for selective loss of T cell functions. *J. Immunol.*, 22:2424–2429.

97. Okamura, J., Letarte, M., Stein, L. D., Sigal, N. H., and Gelfand, E. W. (1982): Modulation of chronic lymphocytic leukemia cells by phorbol ester: Increase in Ia expression, IgM secretion, and MLR stimulatory capacity. *J. Immunol.*, 128:2276–2280.

98. Omenn, G. S. (1965): Familial reticuloendotheliosis with eosinophilia. *N. Engl. J. Med.*, 273:427–432.

99. Pearl, E. R., Vogler, L. B., Okos, A. J., Crist, W. M., Lawton, A. R., and Cooper, M. D. (1978): B lymphocyte precursors in human bone marrow: An analysis of normal individuals and patients with antibody deficiency states. *J. Immunol.*, 120:1169–1175.

100. Pike, M. C., Kredich, N. M., and Snyderman, R. (1978): Requirement of S-adenosyl-L-methionine mediated methylation for human monocyte chemotaxis. *Proc. Natl. Acad. Sci.*, 75:3928–3932.

101. Planet, G., and Fox, I. H. (1976): Inhibition of phosphoribosylpyrophosphate synthesis by purine nucleosides in human erythrocytes. *J. Biol. Chem.*, 251:5839–5844.

102. Quagliata, F., Faig, D., and Conklyn, M. (1974): Studies on the lymphocyte 5'-nucleotidase in chronic lymphocyte leukemia, infectious mononucleosis, normal subpopulations, and phytohemagglutinin-stimulated cells. *Cancer Res.*, 34:3197–3202.

103. Reaman, G. H., Levin, N., Muchmore, A., Holiman, B. J., and Poplack, D. G. (1979): Diminished lymphoblast 5'-nucleotidase activity in acute lymphoblastic leukemia with T-cell characteristics. *N. Engl. J. Med.*, 300:1374–1377.

104. Recker, D. P., Edwards, N. L., and Fox, I. H. (1980): Histochemical evaluation of lymphocytes in hypogammaglobulinemia. Decreased number of 5'-nucleotidase-positive cells. *J. Lab. Clin. Med.*, 95:175–179.

105. Reem, G. H., Borkowsky, W., and Hirschhorn, R. (1979): Purine and phosphoribosylpyrophosphate metabolism of lymphocytes and erythrocytes of an adenosine deaminase deficient immunocompetent child. *Pediatr. Res.*, 13:649–653.

106. Reinherz, E. L., Cooper, M. D., Schlossman, S. F., and Rosen, F. S. (1981): Abnormalities of T cell maturation and regulation in human beings with immunodeficiency disorders. *J. Clin. Invest.*, 68:699–705.

107. Reinherz, E. L., Geha, R., Wohl, M. E., Morimoto, C., Rosen, F. S., and Schlossman, S. F. (1981): Immunodeficiency associated with loss of T4 inducer T-cell function. *N. Engl. J. Med.*, 304:811–816.

108. Rosenbloom, F. M., Henderson, J. F., Caldwell, I. C., Kelley, W. N., and Seegmiller, J. E. (1968): Biochemical basis of accelerated purine biosynthesis de novo in human fibroblasts lacking hypoxanthine-guanine phosphoribosyltransferase. *J. Biol. Chem.*, 243:1166–1173.

109. Rowe, M., De Gast, G. C., Platts-Mills, T. A. E., Asherson, G. L., Webster, A. D. B., and Johnson, S. M. (1980): Lymphocyte 5'-nucleotidase in primary hypogammaglobulinemia and cord blood. *Clin. Exp. Immunol.*, 39:337–343.

110. Rubinstein, A., Hirschorn, R., Sicklick, M., and Murphy, R. A. (1979): In vivo and in vitro effects of thymosin and adenosine deaminase on adenosine-deaminase-deficient lymphocytes. *N. Engl. J. Med.*, 300:387–392.

111. Sandberg, G., and Fredholm, B. B. (1981): Regulation of thymocyte proliferation: Effects of L-alanine, adenosine and cyclic AMP in vitro. *Thymus*, 3:63–75.

112. Scollay, R. G., Butcher, E. C., and Weissman, I. L. (1980): Thymus cell migration quantitative aspects of cellular traffic from the thymus to the periphery in mice. *Eur. J. Immunol.*, 10:210–218.

113. Shore, A., Dosch, H.-M., and Gelfand, E. W. (1979): Expression and modulation of C3 receptors during early T-cell ontogeny. *Cell. Immunol.*, 45:157–166.

114. Shore, A., Dosch, H.-M., Gelfand, E. W. (1981): Role of adenosine deaminase in the early stages of precursor T-cell maturation. *Clin. Exp. Immunol.*, 44:152–155.

115. Siaw, M. F. E., Mitchell, B. S., Kaller, C. A., Coleman, M. S., and Hutton, J. J. (1980): ATP depletion as a consequence of adenosine deaminase inhibition in man. *Proc. Natl. Acad. Sci. USA*, 77:6157–6161.

116. Siegenbeek van Heukelom, L. H., Akerman, J. W. N., Staal, G. E. J., De Bruyn, C. H. M. M., Stoop, J. W., Zegers, B. J. M., DeBree, P. K., and Wadman, S. K. (1977): A patient with purine nucleoside phosphorylase deficiency: Enzymological and metabolic aspects. *Clin. Chim. Acta*, 74:271–279.

117. Simmonds, H. A., Panayi, G. S., and Corrigall, V. (1978): A role of purine metabolism in the immune response: Adenosine deaminase activity and deoxyadenosine catabolism. *Lancet*, 1:60–63.

118. Smyth, J. F., Poine, R. M., Jackman, A. L., Harrap, K. R., Chassin, M. M., Adamson, R. H., and Johns, D. G. (1980): The clinical pharmacology of the adenosine deaminase inhibitor 2'deoxyformycin. *Cancer Chemother. Pharmacol.*, 5:93–101.

119. Tattersal, M. G. N., Ganeshagwu, K., and Hoffbramal, A. V. (1975): The effect of external deoxyribonucleosides on deoxyribonucleoside triphosphate concentrations in human lymphocytes. *Biochem. Pharmacol.*, 24:1495–1498.

120. Tedde, A., Balis, M. E., Ikehara, S., Pahwa, R., Good, R. A., and Trotta, P. P. (1980): Animal model for immune dysfunction associated with adenosine deaminase deficiency. *Proc. Natl. Acad. Sci. USA*, 77:4899–4903.

121. Thompson, L. F., Boss, G. R., Spiegelberg, H. L., Jansen, I. V., O'Connor, R. D., Waldmann, T. A., Hamburger, R. N., and Seegmiller, J. E. (1979): Ecto-5'-nucleotidase activity in T and B

lymphocytes from normal subjects and patients with congenital x-linked agammaglobulinemia. *J. Immunol.*, 123:2475–2478.

122. Thompson, L. F., Boss, G. R., Spiegelberg, H. L., Bianchinda, A., and Seegmiller, J. E. (1980): Ecto-5'-nucleotidase activity in lymphoblastoid cell lines derived from heterozygotes for congenital X-linked agamma-globulinemia. *J. Immunol.*, 125:190–193.

123. Thomson, M. J., Garland, M. R., and Richards, J. F. (1971): Metabolic effects of nucleosides in rat thymus cells in vitro. *J. Cell. Physiol.*, 77:17–30.

124. Thuillier, L., Garreau, F., and Cartier, P. (1981): Inability of immunocompetent thymocytes to produce T-cell growth factor under adenosine deaminase deficiency conditions. *Cell. Immunol.*, 63:81–90.

125. Tosato, G., Magrath, I., Koski, I., Dooley, N., and Blaese, M. (1979): Activation of suppressor T cells during Epstein-Barr-virus-induced infectious mononucleosis. *N. Engl. J. Med.*, 301:1133–1137.

126. Tritsch, G. L., and Minowada, J. (1978): Differences in purine metabolizing enzyme activity in human leukemic T-cell, B-cell, and null cell lines. *J. Natl. Cancer Institute*, 60:1301–1304.

127. Uberti, J., Lightbody, J. J., Wolf, J. W., Anderson, J. A., Reid, R. H., and Johnson, R. M. (1978): The effect of adenosine on mitogenesis of ADA-deficient lymphocytes. *Clin. Immunol. Immunopathol.*, 10:446–458.

128. Uberti, J., Lightbody, J. J., and Johnson, R. M. (1979): The effect of nucleosides and deoxycoformycin on adenosine and deoxyadenosine inhibition of lymphocyte activation. *J. Immunol.*, 123:189–193.

129. Ullman, B., Cohen, A., and Martin, D. W., Jr. (1976): Characterization of a cell culture model for the study of adenosine deaminase and purine nucleoside phosphorylase-deficient immunologic disease. *Cell*, 9:205–211.

130. Ullman, B., Gudas, L. J., Cohen, A., and Martin, D. W., Jr. (1978): Deoxyadenosine metabolism and cytotoxicity in cultured mouse T-lymphoma cells: A model for immunodeficiency disease. *Cell*, 14:365–376.

131. Ullman, B., Gudas, L. J., Clift, S. M., and Martin, D. W., Jr. (1979): Isolation and characterization of purine-nucleoside phosphorylase-deficient T-lymphoma cells and secondary mutants with altered nucleotide reductase: Genetic model for immunodeficiency disease. *Proc. Natl. Acad. Sci. USA*, 76:1074–1078.

132. Ullman, B., Levinson, B. B., Hershfield, M. S., and Martin, D. W., Jr. (1981): A biochemical genetic study of the role of specific nucleoside kinases in deoxyadenosine phosphorylation by culture human cells. *J. Biol. Chem.*, 256:848–852.

133. Venner, P. M., and Glazer, R. I. (1979): The metabolism of 2'-deoxycoformycin by L1210 cells in vivo. *Biochem. Pharmacol.*, 28:3239–3242.

134. Wortmann, R. L., Mitchell, B. S., Edwards, N. L., and Fox, I. H. (1979): Biochemical basis for differential deoxyadenosine toxicity to T and B lymphoblasts: Role for 5'-nucleotidase. *Proc. Natl. Acad. Sci. USA*, 76:2434–2437.

135. Watts, R. W. E., Watts, J. E. M., and Seegmiller, J. E. (1965): Xanthine oxidase activity in human tissues and its inhibition by allopurinol. *J. Lab. Clin. Med.*, 66:688–697.

136. Weissbach, H., and Taylor, R. (1966): Role of vitamin B12 in methionine biosynthesis. *Fed. Proc.*, 25:1649–1653.

137. Weissman, I. L. (1967): Thymus cell migration. *J. Exp. Med.*, 126:291–304.

138. Wolberg, G., Zimmerman, T. P., and Hiemstra, K. (1975): Adenosine inhibition of lymphocyte-mediated cytolysis: Possible role of cyclic adenosine monophosphate. *Science*, 187:957–959.

139. Wong, P. C. L., and Murray, A. W. (1969): 5'-Phosphoribosyl pyrophosphate synthetase from Ehrlich ascites tumor cells. *Biochemistry*, 8:1608–1614.

140. Wyngaarden, J. B., and Ashton, D. M. (1959): The regulation of activity of phosphoribosylpyrophosphate amidotransferase by purine ribonucleotides: A potential feedback control of purine biosynthesis. *J. Biol. Chem.*, 234:1492–1496.

141. Wyngaarden, J. B. (1972): Xanthinuria. In: *The Metabolic Basis of Inherited Disease*, edited by J. B. Stansbury, J. B. Wyngaarden, and D. S. Fredrickson, pp. 992–1002. McGraw-Hill, New York.

142. Xeros, N. (1962): Deoxyriboside control and synchronization of mitosis. *Nature*, 194:682–683.

143. Zimmerman, T. P., Wolberg, G., and Duncan, G. S. (1978): Inhibition of lymphocyte-mediated cytolysis by 3-deazaadenosine: Evidence for a methylation reaction essential to cytolysis. *Proc. Natl. Acad. Sci. USA*, 75:6220–6224.

144. Zimmerman, T. S., Schmitgas, C. J., Wolberg, G., Deeprose, R. D., Duncan, G. S., Cuatrecasas, P., and Elion, G. B. (1980): Modulation of cyclic AMP metabolism by s-adenosylhomocysteine and S-3-deazaadenosylhomocystein in mouse lymphocytes. *Proc. Natl. Acad. Sci. USA*, 77:5639–5643.
145. Zinkernagel, R. M., and Doherty, P. C. (1979): MHC-restricted cytotoxic T cells: Studies on the biological role of polymorphic major transplantation antigens determining T-cell restriction specificity. *Adv. Immunol.*, 27:52–74.

Advances in Host Defense Mechanisms, Vol. 2,
edited by John I. Gallin and Anthony S. Fauci.
Raven Press, New York © 1983.

Immune Mechanisms Involved in Bacterial Infections

Robert C. Brunham and *King K. Holmes

*Department of Medicine and Medical Microbiology, University of Manitoba,
Basic Medical Sciences Building, Winnipeg, Manitoba, Canada; and
*Department of Medicine, University of Washington, and
Division of Infectious Diseases,
Seattle Public Health Hospital, Seattle, Washington 98114*

Bacteria are complex pathogenic agents which present a variety of antigenic stimuli to the infected host. Elucidation of the mechanisms of acquired resistance is of fundamental importance in understanding the pathogenesis of bacterial infections and in the development of immunotherapy and immunoprophylaxis.

In most if not all instances of bacterial infection, both a humoral and a cellular host immune response are elicited (23,44,67,111,126). Acquired resistance to bacterial infection represents a complex interplay between several components of the immune system. Normal activity of T-lymphocytes and of the immunoglobulin products of B-lymphocytes is required for host resistance to a number of bacterial infections. One or the other aspect of the immune response characteristically predominates for certain types of host-parasite relationships and has been conveniently characterized as purulent or granulomatous responses in an excellent recent review of the role of cell-mediated immunity in bacterial infections (49a). For example, pyogenic organisms (such as *Neisseria gonorrheae, Hemophilus influenzae,* and group A and B streptococci), which multiply extracellularly, appear to be effectively dealt with by a humoral immune response in concert with polymorphonuclear leukocytes. Organisms that are able to successfully parasitize host mononuclear phagocytes, such as *Mycobacterium tuberculosis, Salmonella typhi,* and *Brucella abortus,* elicit a more prominent cellular immune response.

The immune response to bacteria represents a means by which the host is able to focus the inflammatory response to eliminate the parasite with minimal damage to host tissue. For many infections, however, the immune response produces tissue injury and the clinical manifestations of inflammatory disease. Host hyperreactivity to specific bacterial antigens may contribute to tissue damage. For example, subjects with acute rheumatic fever show increased cellular immune responses to streptococcal antigens when compared to subjects with uncomplicated streptococcal infection (100), and subjects with *Chlamydia trachomatis*-associated Reiter syndrome have increased lymphocyte transformation responses to chlamydial antigens when compared with subjects who have uncomplicated chlamydial urethritis (D. Martin, K. Holmes, and T. Kuo, *unpublished data*). In some instances, bacteria may elicit immunocompetent cells and/or antibody which are cross-reactive to host cell constitutents. For example, in acute rheumatic fever, antistreptococcal antibodies cross-react with heart and subthalamic neuronal tissue (44,56). Bacterial antigens present in blood may complex with antibacterial antibody, resulting in immune complex disease. Leprosy-associated erythema nodosum (15,125), glomerulonephritis associated with endocarditis (10,73) or infected shunts (51), and poststreptococcal glomerulonephritis (120,132) all represent such diseases.

In many acute bacterial infections, suppression (59,60,108) of immune function occurs. Anergy, widely appreciated as a feature of some acute viral infections, may also occur during acute bacterial meningitis (1,48), pneumonia (91,113), and chronic mycobacterial disease. Impairment of mitogen and microbial antigen-induced *in vitro* lymphocyte proliferation also occurs during such infections. The basis of depressed lymphocyte function during acute or chronic bacterial disease is not fully defined, and further studies of immunoregulation during bacterial infection are clearly needed.

Multiple interactions between host and bacterial pathogen occur which can be helpful or harmful. This chapter concerns mechanisms by which immune reactions protect the host against bacterial infection or which play a role in the immuno-pathogenesis of specific infections. It selectively emphasizes recent advances to illustrate well-established concepts. Data from human infections are emphasized, except where animal data illustrate principles that appear most applicable to human disease.

HUMORAL MECHANISMS OF IMMUNE RESISTANCE TO BACTERIAL INFECTION

Induction and Kinetics of the Humoral Immune Response

The humoral immune response to infection at nonmucosal sites is induced within lymph nodes if the antigen is present in tissue or within the spleen if present mainly in blood (76). Bacteria arrive at lymphatic tissue either free or within macrophages and usually remain localized within the lymphoid system. The immune response generated within local lymphatic tissue disseminates to the rest of the body. Elegant studies by Hall et al. (50) have defined the role of lymph nodes in the development and dissemination of the immune response following local antigenic challenge. Antigenic stimulation of lymph node tissue results in the trapping of antigen-specific lymphocytes within such lymph nodes (52). Cell traffic in efferent lymphatics markedly decreases during the initial 24 to 48 hr following antigenic stimulation and then increases. Removal of efferent lymph flow prevents the systemic deployment of the humoral immune response and its development elsewhere in the body. Transfer of lymphoid cells from efferent lymphatics to an unprimed and unchallenged recipient results in the development of a humoral immune response in the recipient.

During acute bacterial infection in man, the appearance of peripheral blood lymphocytes changes (91,113). The number of large and medium-sized lymphocytes and plasma cells increases (27). Although the total lymphocyte number remains unchanged, the number of B-lymphocytes substantially increases, while the number of T-lymphocytes remains normal or decreases. However, "activated" T-lymphocytes appear in markedly increased numbers (113).

Disruption or destruction of lymphatic tissue interferes with the development of an effective and appropriate immune response. After radical mastectomy with removal of regional lymph nodes, women are at increased risk for severe and disseminating bacterial infection of that extremity. After splenectomy, humans are inordinately susceptible to severe and overwhelming bacterial sepsis, usually due to pyogenic organisms (54). Such subjects are less responsive to vaccination and require increased amounts of opsonizing antibody for phagocytic clearance of antigens following hematogenous particulate challenge.

The humoral immune reponse involves the development of antibody of changing isotype [immunoglobulin (Ig) heavy chain class] and idiotype (antigenic specificity). Early after antigenic challenge, antibody of the IgM class predominates. *In vitro*, human B-lymphocytes release polyclonal IgM following stimulation by a variety of microbial products, including lipopolysaccharide of gram-negative bacteria, purified protein derivative of *M. tuberculosis*, and protein A of *Staphylococcus aureus* (33). It is speculated that this polyclonal IgM response occurs *in vivo* and represents an early "primitive" immune response requiring little cellular collaboration and which serves to contain the bacterial pathogen until more specific immunoglobulin and effector T-cell deployment occurs.

IgM antibody is restricted intravascularly by its size and usually is of low affinity but is a potent activator of complement. Phagocytes do not have surface receptors for the Fc portion of IgM, and immune enhanced phagocytosis proceeds as a result of complement binding to phagocyte C3b receptors. With continued antigenic exposure or following reexposure, IgG and IgA antibody are the major isotypes of Ig produced. Antibody of these classes can diffuse outside the vascular compartment. IgG molecules can effectively engage with phagocyte Fc receptors and can activate the complement sequence after binding to bacterial antigen. IgG antibody generally has higher affinity for the immunizing antigen than does IgM antibody (30). The function of serum IgA antibody is not clearly understood.

Although specific antibody is produced following antigenic challenge, this accounts for only half or less of the incremental increase in serum Ig that follows intense exposure (60). The specificity and mechanism of induction for the remaining "nonspecific" Ig is unknown. It has been hypothesized that the excess Ig may represent autoantiidiotypic Ig, which regulates the immune response; "bystander" B-cells are nonspecifically acted upon by mitogenic helper factors released by antigen-activated T-helper cells; or, as described above, bacterial products may directly stimulate a polyclonal IgM response. Bacteria serve as mitogens of human B-lymphocytes *in vitro*, perhaps related to their ability to nonspecifically bind to IgD, which forms part of the surface antigen receptors of B-lymphocytes (9,37).

Several mechanisms may account for the excess Ig synthesis that occurs following antigenic challenge.

Experiments of Nature

The relative importance of T- or B-cell activity in specific infections can be inferred from observations of the pattern of infectious morbidity among individuals with congenital or acquired defects in the immune system. Deficiency of serum Ig (e.g., Bruton agammaglobulinemia, multiple myeloma) predisposes to infection with pyogenic bacteria, such as *Streptococcus pneumoniae* and *H. influenzae*. In Bruton aggamaglobulinemia, this susceptibility is effectively reduced by parenteral therapy with gammaglobulin (103). The effect of congenital defects in T-cell function on the patterns of infectious morbidity is described later.

Animal Models

In rodent models of experimental infections with *Str. pneumoniae* (17), group A and B streptococci (68,69), and *H. influenzae* (89), specific antibody provides protection. Although convincingly showing the protective role of serum antibody, these experiments have not excluded a role for cell-mediated immunity, since the response to infection of naive recipients of immune spleen cells has not been assessed. It is likely that even in those situations where antibody is of paramount importance, T-lymphocytes have an important role in host defense through helper function influencing cells of the B-lymphocyte series and through enhancing the phagocytic activities of mononuclear phagocytes.

Serotherapy

Prior to the discovery and widespread use of antibacterial agents, immunotherapy represented a major therapeutic approach to bacterial infection. Immune serum benefited subjects with pneumonia due to *Str. pneumoniae* or meningitis due to *N. meningitides* or *H. influenzae*. Early in this century, Flexner (36) observed that antimeningococcal serum significantly reduced mortality in meningococcal meningitis (see Table 1). Similarly, Finland (35) showed the efficacy of type-specific antisera in pneumococcal pneumonia (Table 2). Mortality was approximately halved

TABLE 1. *Effect of antimeningococcal antiserum on mortality in patients with meningococcal meningitis[a]*

Group	No. of cases	Mortality (%)	p
Serum treated	176	30	<0.0001
Not serum treated	74	85	

[a]From ref. 36.

TABLE 2. *Effect of specific antiserum on deaths from pneumonia caused by types 1, 2, 5, and 7 Str. pneumoniae*[a]

Pneumococcal pneumonia	Serum treated		Not serum treated		
	N	% Mortality	N	% Mortality	p
Bacteremic	296	37	330	79	<0.0001
Nonbacteremic	557	9	645	19	<0.0001

[a]From ref. 35.

among patients with either bacteremic or nonbacteremic disease and was further reduced if therapy was initiated within 3 days of the onset of disease.

Mechanisms for Antibacterial Activity of Serum Antibody

Antibody to surface structures of the bacterial pathogen appears to be most critical in host defense against many bacterial infections. Extracellular survival of pyogenic bacteria depends on subversion of host phagocytosis (129). Such bacteria often possess antiphagocytic factors. Capsular polysaccharides of *Str. pneumoniae, H. influenzae, N. meningitidis*, group B streptococci, and some strains of *Staph. aureus* reduce the efficiency of phagocytosis. Surface protein moieties, such as pili of *N. gonorrheae* and "M" fimbriae of *Str. pyogenes*, also serve as antiphagocytic structures. Antibody directed to these particular bacterial molecules enhances phagocytosis, and the development of such antibodies is correlated with development of specific immunity.

Opsonization

Since phagocytosis is the primary mechanism by which the host rids itself of invasive bacterial pathogens, it is primarily phagocytosis which the humoral immune response serves to amplify. Antibody of either the IgM or IgG class, by coating bacteria, neutralizes antiphagocytic surface structures. Host polymorphonuclear or mononuclear phagocytes possess Fc receptors which fix the Fc portion of IgG antibody only after the antibody has engaged antigen. IgG-Fc receptor interaction then elicits immune phagocytosis of the engaged antigen by either polymorphonuclear or mononuclear phagocytes. Host phagocytes also possess membrane receptors for the cleaved third component of complement, C3b. IgG and IgM molecules, when engaged with antigen, activate complement, depositing C3b on the parasite surface. This further augments binding of bacteria to host phogocytes via C3b receptors (immune adherence). Other activated components of complement recruit additional phagocytes by the chemoattractant activity of C5a.

Many bacteria also directly activate the alternate complement pathway (34). The particular activating structures are unknown. Those unusual bacterial species having capsular sialic acid, such as type III group B streptococcus, groups B and C *N.*

meningitidis, and type K1 *Escherichia coli*, are poor activators of the alternate complement pathway and are especially pathogenic for humans. Antibody to capsular material in these and other bacterial species augments alternate complement pathway activity and C3b immune adherence without participation of the immunoglobulin Fc fragment. The molecular basis for this is not presently understood.

Phagolysosomal Fusion

Antibody coating of bacteria promotes more efficient phagolysosomal fusion. This may be critical for certain bacterial pathogens, such as *S. aureus*, which are otherwise able to survive within unfused host phagosomes (72). Other bacterial pathogens, such as *M. tuberculosis* (7), *C. psittaci* (40,130), and *C. trachomatis* (70) also inhibit fusion of the phagosome with the lysosome. Specific antibody in these instances promotes phagolysosomal fusion. The mechanism by which some bacteria are able to prevent phagolysosomal fusion and how specific antibody reverses this effect are unknown. Antibody may neutralize a surface component of the bacterial cell which inhibits fusion, or antibody may inactivate the bacterial cell and prevent the secretion of an inhibitory factor.

Bacteriolysis

Although opsonization is the prime function of serum antibody for most pyogenic bacteria, for systemic neisserial infection, induced bactericidal antibody is the prime function of the humoral immune response. Systemic neisserial infections appear unique in this regard. Goldschneider et al. (45,46) showed that bactericidal serum antibody against a colonizing strain of *N. meningiditis* is associated with protection against disease caused by that strain. Of 54 military recruits who developed systemic meningococcal disease during prospective study, only three had bactericidal antibody to the infecting strain in the predisease serum; of 550 controls who did not develop systemic meningococcal disease, 444 had bactericidal antibody against the homologous colonizing strain. The evidence for a protective role of bactericidal antibody in gonococcal injection is more indirect. Strains of *N. gonorrheae* isolated from patients with disseminated gonococcal disease are more resistant to the IgM-mediated, complement-dependent bactericidal activity of normal human serum than are many strains associated with local mucosal infection (107). The unique susceptibility of patients with deficiencies in the terminal components of the complement sequence (C5-8) to disseminated neisserial disease further supports the role of bactericidal antibody in limiting gonococcal and meningococcal bacteremia (71).

Toxin Neutralization

Some bacterial pathogens, such as *Corynebacterium diphtheriae, Clostridium tetani, and Cl. botulinum*, produce disease predominantly or exclusively through the elaboration of exotoxins. Exotoxin is passively adsorbed as the organism replicates on mucosal surfaces or in wounds. Other bacteria are both invasive and toxin producing. *Pseudomonas aeruginosa* represents an invasive bacterial pathogen which produces a toxin, exotoxin A, which causes many of the manifestations of disease (97,98). Similarly, *Staph. aureus* and group A streptococci are invasive, pyogenic bacteria which produce important exotoxins. In cases of toxin-mediated disease, neutralization of toxin activity is of particular importance for immunity and host survival. For example, among patients with *P. aeruginosa* bacteremia, survival correlates with the presence of antibody to exotoxin A in acute phase serum. Antiexotoxin A becomes even more important among bacteremic patients who lack intact host defense mechanisms. Humoral antitoxin completely prevents the clinical effects of toxins of *Cl. tetani, Cl. botulinum, or C. diphtheriae.*

T-Lymphocyte Activity Augments Effects of Antibody on Phagocytosis by Monocytes

Although T-lymphocyte activity plays a background role in infections with all the agents described above, such activity clearly is present. Ig synthesis in response to many of these bacterial antigens is T-lymphocyte dependent; i.e., many bacterial antigens are T-dependent antigens. In addition, augmentation of host mononuclear phagocyte function occurs during infection even with pyogenic organisms. Delayed type hypersensitivity (114) and enhanced activity of the reticuloendothelial system (122) have been described among patients with pneumococcal pneumonia. Such activity would benefit the host by enhancement of the phagocytic and bactericidal activity of recruited mononuclear phagocytes. For instance, upon immune activation, mononuclear phagocytes acquire the ability to phagocytose bacteria which have bound C3b to their surface. In the nonactivated state, mononuclear phagocytes are unable to engulf particles coated with C3b, even though adherence to the phagocyte occurs (13).

Mucosal Antibody

Serum antibody may not only protect against systemic bacterial infection but is, in some instances, correlated with alterations of bacterial host interactions occurring at mucosal surfaces. For example, immunization with pertussis vaccine prevents respiratory infection with *Bordetella pertussis*, and immunization with capsular antigens of *N. meningiditis* or *Str. pneumoniae* suppresses the carrier state. However, ever since the observations of Besredka (12) of bacterial dysenteric infection, it has been suspected that local immune responses may occur independently of systemic immune responses (14). Studies of cholera have supported this concept.

Cholera as a Prototype Mucosal Pathogen

In endemic areas, cholera induces solid immunity (88). Reinfection with the homologous serotype rarely occurs. Although a reciprocal relationship exists between age-specific attack rates and the age-specific prevalence of serum vibriocidal antibody in areas of high endemicity (see Fig. 1), serum antibody is not well

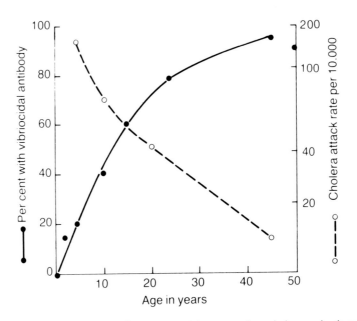

FIG. 1. Serum vibriocidal antibodies are an epiphenomen. In a cholera endemic area, a reciprocal relationship exists between the prevalence of serum bactericidal antibody to *V. cholera* and age-specific attack rates. (Data from ref. 88.)

correlated with immunity in individual patients with experimental cholera. Experimental infection with *Vibrio cholera* confers solid immunity lasting at least 12 months, but serum antibody, whether measured by bactericidal or other assays, does not correlate with resistance. For example, Cash et al. (25) fed *V. cholera* to 51 subjects with vibriocidal serum antibody titers ≥1:20; 20 were convalescent from experimental cholera infection, and 31 had never had a known attack of cholera. Symptomatic cholera did not occur in any of the convalescent subjects, but did occur in 77% of those who had no history of cholera. These and other investigators have concluded that serum antibodies do not mediate immunity to *V. cholera* but are convenient markers of the immune state in the general population.

Since cholera is a disease strictly limited to the epithelial surface of the small intestine and mediated by a locally active toxin, it is not surprising that the relevant immune mechanism can be induced and expressed locally within the gastrointestinal tract. Burrows and Ward (21) identified antibody to *V. cholera* in feces of experimentally infected animals. This coproantibody occurred independently of serum antibody. Freter et al. (39) detected specific antibody to *V. cholera* in duodenal fluid obtained from humans convalescent from the disease. In animal studies, specific secretory IgA (sIgA) was protective against experimental *V. cholera* infection (41). In humans, it is still not established whether sIgA mediates recovery or resistance to cholera.

Secretory Immune System

The nature and cellular basis of local mucosal immunity have been the subject of extensive recent investigation. Tomasi et al. (116) characterized the unique qualitites of the predominant mucosal Ig, sIgA. In contradistinction to serum IgA, which is dimeric, sIgA on secretory surfaces is predominantly polymeric, contains secretory component, and exists in two allotypic forms, IgA1 and IgA2, in nearly equal amounts (14,115). As the IgA molecule is transferred from submucosal plasma cells across the mucosal epithelial cell to the mucosal surface, secretory component is added in the epithelial cell, making the IgA molecule resistant to proteolytic enzymes found within or on secretory surfaces.

Much of the sIgA found on mucosal surfaces is synthesized locally in plasma cells located beneath the mucosal epithelium. Recent information from experiments in rats, however, has revealed an enterohepatic circulation for IgA (94). The liver efficiently removes IgA from the circulation via hepatocyte secretory component receptors and excretes it as sIgA into bile and into the gut lumen. Some of the sIgA in the gut may be derived from bile and some secreted directly into the lumen from plasma cells in the lamina propria. Whether other mucosal sites, such as salivary or lacrimal glands or the genital tract, can actively transport IgA from the circulation has not been studied. Active export of IgA from serum at various mucosal sites could be one mechanism by which the sIgA antibody response is dispersed over the mucosal surfaces of the body. Serum IgA, when complexed with antigen, is also selectively transported into bile actively by the liver (105). The removal of IgA immune complexes by liver potentially represents a mechanism for disposal of antigen which circumvents the inflammatory consequences of the activation of complement and phagocytosis.

Antibacterial activity of sIgA.

There are several possible mechanisms for the antibacterial activity of sIgA. sIgA does not activate complement by the classic pathway, and not all components of the complement cascade are found on mucosal surfaces. The opsonic activity of sIgA has varied in different experiments. Impure preparations of sIgA may account for some of these disparate findings. By an undefined mechanism, IgA does enhance monocyte-mediated, antibody-dependent antibacterial activity *in vitro* (74), and this may be a major function of sIgA in those situations where mononuclear phagocytes are present, such as in lung alveoli and colostrum.

The most likely mechanism for the antibacterial activity of sIgA is inhibition of bacterial adherence to epithelial surfaces, the first step in the initiation of most infections. Nonadherent bacteria are removed by peristaltic, flushing, or ciliary activity present at all mucosal surfaces. Early studies by Freter et al. (38,39) demonstrated that immune serum inhibited attachment of *V. cholera* to intestinal epithelium without affecting the growth rate of the organism (Table 3). Subsequent studies showed that specific sIgA obtained from mice following enteral immuni-

TABLE 3. *Immune serum to* V. cholera *inhibits intestinal epithelial attachment but not the growth rate of* V. cholera[a]

Serum	Growth ($\log_{10}$ per 90 min) of *V. cholera* in intestinal loops in the presence of antiserum	Percent *V. cholera* adherent to intestinal epithelium
V. cholera antiserum	2	1.0
Control serum	1.9	32.5

[a]See refs. 38 and 39.

zation with *V. cholera* had similar activity. The antibacterial effect of sIgA was dependent on intact metabolic activities of mucosal cells, suggesting that only in cooperation with an unidentified mucosal cell could sIgA exert antibacterial activity (41). Experiments in infant mice challenged enterally with *V. cholera* suggest that IgA is more effective than IgG or IgM in inhibiting attachment of bacteria to epithelial surfaces (110). Further studies by Williams and Gibbons (128) demonstrated that sIgA isolated from parotid fluid specifically prevented the adherence of bacteria to epithelial cells. sIgA functions in this way to clear bacteria in a noninflammatory fashion.

B-cells of the secretory immune system.

Studies of gut-associated lymphatic tissue in the mouse have shown that the cellular basis of sIgA Ig production begins with antigen processing and presentation in highly organized lymphatic collections, called Peyer patches (26). Within Peyer patches are found unique T-lymphocytes which function as helper cells specifically for IgA-secreting B-lymphocytes and which are not found in spleen or peripheral lymph nodes (3,32). Once stimulated by antigen, IgA-specific B-lymphocytes migrate from Peyer patches via mesenteric lymph nodes to the thoracic duct and disseminate widely throughout the body (96). They are found in the peripheral blood of humans and produce IgA predominantly of the polymeric type found in external secretions (66). B-lymphocytes producing IgA antibody to enterically presented antigens are found within colostrum, indicating that such lymphocytes have migrated from the gut to the mammary gland in an enteromammary mucosal IgA B-cell cycle (115). B-lymphocytes derived from any mucosal site appear to be able to home to other distant surfaces, such as salivary and lacrimal glands and the genitourinary tract (82,124). Mestecky et al. (87) found that sIgA to *Str. mutans* appeared both in saliva and in lacrimal fluid of human subjects orally immunized with this organism. Antigen stimulation at any mucosal site thus serves to clonally expand and augment the sIgA response at that site, as well as at other mucosal sites (55,87). A system for dissemination of sIgA-producing cells to multiple mucosal sites certainly would enhance host protection, since many infections, such as *C. trachomatis* and *N. gonorrheae*, commonly affect multiple mucosal sites.

The distribution of IgA-specific B-lymphocytes to some mucosal surfaces may be hormonally determined (82). As seen in Table 4, during the follicular (proestrus) phase of the menstrual cycle of mice, more mensenteric lymph node cells home to the cervix and vagina than do peripheral lymph node cells. Such homing was not seen in the luteal (or metestrus) phase of the menstrual cycle. During late pregnancy and with lactation, mesenteric lymph node cells also preferentially home to the breast.

"Homing" may not precisely describe this phenomenon; as pointed out by Elson et al. (32), the circulating IgA-producing B-cells may lodge and terminally differentiate only in sites where there is sufficient IgA T-cell help. This might be a function of the presence of (a) T-cells with helper function for IgA-secreting B-cells, or (b) antigen at the site, which could lead to local activation of helper T-cells by the mechanisms described below. It remains to be shown, however, that the lamina propria of the intestine or of other mucosal sites contains specific IgA T-cell helper activity; thus far, such helper cells have been found only in Peyer patches.

Expanding knowledge of the secretory immune system will lead to improved understanding of the pathogenesis and mechanism of immunity in many bacterial infections and may lead to improved strategies for administration of bacterial vaccines.

Examples of mucosal antibody response in bacterial infection in humans.

C. trachomatis and N. gonorrheae: Specific sIgA responses are evoked in men with gonococcal urethritis and in women with gonococcal cervicitis. Tramont (117) observed that among women with gonococcal infection, genital secretions containing mainly sIgA effectively inhibited adherence of the homologous strain of *N. gonorrheae* to epithelial cells. Women who had cervicovaginal sIgA antibody to *N. gonorrheae* had asymptomatic cervical infection, whereas those who lacked

TABLE 4. *Homing of radiolabeled mesenteric lymph node cells (MLN), peripheral lymph node cells (PLN) to genital tissue, and mammary glands in the mouse is preferential[a]*

Recipient tissue	Donor cells injected	No. of radiolabeled cells per 10³ high power fields (HPF) on microscopic examination of histologic sections of tissue	Homing index[b]
Proestrual cervix and vagina	MLN	15.7	7.9
	PLN	2.0	
Mammary glands[c]	MLN	26.8	2.8
	PLN	9.6	

[a]From ref. 82.
[b]Mean no. of labeled cells per 10³ HPF in MLN recipients

Mean no. of labeled cells per 10³ HPF in PLN recipients.
[c]Examined on the 19th day of pregnancy.

cervicovaginal sIgA antibody had pelvic inflammatory disease; their cervicovaginal secretions did not inhibit gonococcal attachment to epithelial cells. It is speculated but unproved that when gonococcal infection occurs in the absence of sIgA, the risk of gonococcal salpingitis may be increased.

Among women with *C. trachomatis* infection of the cervix, there is a reciprocal relationship between the presence or absence of cervical sIgA antibody to *C. trachomatis* and the numbers of organisms isolated from the cervix (see Fig. 2) (R. Brunham, *unpublished*). Furthermore, the greater numbers of organisms recovered from the cervix, the greater the frequency of clinical cervicitis. In this infection, sIgA antibody may inhibit replication of *C. trachomatis* and consequently limit the extent of local inflammation. It remains possible, however, that in genital infection with *N. gonorrheae* and *C. trachomatis* sIgA may only reflect other more important immune responses.

H. influenzae type b: Many bacterial agents produce systemic invasion following infection of mucosal surfaces. The mucosal antibody response to one such agent, *H. influenzae* type b, recently has been studied. Pichichero et al. (95) demonstrated that 17 of 18 children with invasive disease due to this organism developed a mucosal IgA antibody response. The mucosal antibody response tended to be detected sooner than the serum antibody response. The authors noted, as have others, that infants mounted a poor serum antibody response to this infection. Six of seven children less than 1 year of age failed to develop serum antibody to capsular polysaccharide of *H. influenzae* type b. Remarkably, however, all seven infants developed an early and persistent mucosal immune response to this antigen. This result is consistent with the ontogeny of the secretory and humoral antibody systems: adult levels of sIgA (detected in saliva) are obtained between 1 and 8 months of age, sooner than adult levels of serum Ig. Pichichero's observation may suggest alternate methods for immunoprophylaxis of *H. influenzae* disease, since it is in infants < 18 months of age that parenteral polysaccharide vaccine has failed to induce adequate protective immunity or serum antibody.

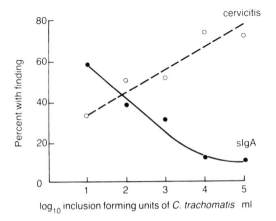

FIG. 2. Among women who have cervical infection with *C. trachomatis*, a reciprocal relationship exists between the quantity of organism recovered in culture and the proportion of women with sIgA antibody to *C. trachomatis*. A direct relationship also exists between the quantity of organism recovered in culture and the proportion of women with clinically apparent cervicitis.

Immunopathology Resulting From the Humoral Immune Response

Antibody-mediated immunopathologic consequences of bacterial infection can be caused by immune complex disease, cross-reactive antibody formation, and autoantibody formation.

Immune Complex Disease

Immune complexes normally are formed during many infections; they become pathogenic when they are of intermediate size and cannot be cleared from the circulation by the mononuclear phagocyte system and are able to activate mediator systems (127). Genetic factors appear to be involved in determining the type and size of immune complexes formed after antigenic stimulation and may be involved in the susceptibility to immune complex disease. Immune complexes frequently deposit in organs with specialized vasculature, such as the kidneys, skin, joints, and choroid plexus, which thus are the target organs of immune complex disease (112).

The immunopathologic sequelae of infection with *Str. pyogenes* include erythema nodosum, acute rheumatic fever, and acute poststreptococcal glomerulonephritis. The latter frequently is associated with infection by nephritogenic group A streptococcal strains, which form a unique protein that can be detected in the glomeruli of patients with glomerulonephritis (121). Immune complexes are detectable in the acute phase serum of about 75% of subjects with poststreptococcal glomerulonephritis and appear responsible for this condition (120). Other bacterial infections in which immune complexes have been demonstrated and in which such complexes are thought to behave pathologically are shown in Table 5.

TABLE 5. *Examples of bacterial infections in which pathologic immune complexes have been demonstrated*[a,b]

Disease or bacteria	Manifestation of immune complex injury
Bacterial endocarditis	Glomerulonephritis
	Janeway spots
	Osler nodes
Infected ventriculoatrial shunts	Glomerulonephritis
Intraabdominal abscess	Glomerulonephritis
Syphilis (congenital and secondary)	Glomerulonephritis
Lepromatous leprosy (following therapy)	Erythema nodosum leprosum
Disseminated gonococcal infection	Tenosynovitis
	Cutaneous lesions
Systemic meningococcal infection	Tenosynovitis
	Cutaneous lesions

[a]From ref. 112.
[b]The role of immune complexes is not established in some of these conditions.

Cross-Reactive Antibody Formation

Cross-reactive antibody formation occurs when both the bacterial pathogen and host cell share common antigenic determinants. It has been best described with *Str. pyogenes* infection. Antibodies to cell wall or cell membrane constituents of the organism and which cross-react with host cardiac smooth muscle cells, with glycoproteins of heart valves, or with subthalamic neuronal cells are thought to be involved in the pathogenesis of acute carditis and chorea in acute rheumatic fever (44,56).

Autoantibody Formation

Autoantibody formation occurs when infection produces antibodies to host cell antigens which are not shared by the bacterial parasite. Autoantibodies have been demonstrated in some bacterial infections. The antibody detected in the VDRL test in syphilis may be an autoantibody to lipid-containing antigens of mitochondria-rich tissues. These antibodies, if harmless, are of diagnostic importance. However, the Donath-Landsteiner antibody produced in some patients with syphilis reacts with blood group P substance and may cause hemolysis. These autoantibodies are not known to be cross-reactive antibodies to *T. pallidum*. The cold hemagglutinins to blood group I antigen occurring during *M. pneumoniae* infection also may cause hemolysis (44).

Reiter Syndrome

For some disorders occurring with or following bacterial infection, an immunopathologic basis is postulated but not yet proved. For example, following enteric infection with *Salmonella, Yersina,* or *Campylobacter species*, or following urethral infection with *C. trachomatis*, recurrent arthritis, characteristic mucocutaneous lesions, uveitis, conjunctivitis, and urethritis may develop. The major histocompatibility antigen, HLA-B27, is associated with this disorder. The fact that these infections all involve mucosal surfaces suggests that in some way the secretory immune system may be involved.

CELLULAR MECHANISMS OF IMMUNE RESISTANCE TO BACTERIAL INFECTION

The previous section described reactions of serum and mucosal antibody with bacterial pathogens. This section concerns cellular or cell-mediated immune (CMI) reactions to bacterial infections. These reactions are mediated by T-lymphocytes independent of antibody. In addition, new information suggests that killer (K) lymphocytes may cooperate with antibody in response to bacterial infection.

Immune Granulomas—Pathologic Hallmark of CMI Antibacterial Reactions

Certain bacterial infections are characterized histologically by a host granulomatous reaction and/or by multiplication of bacteria within host mononuclear phagocytes and are dealt with primarily by a CMI reaction rather than by a humoral immune reaction (118). An example of such a granulomatous host reaction is seen in Fig. 3 resulting from a *C. trachomatis* (lymphogranuloma venereum L2 serotype) infection of rectal mucosa (99). Such immune granuloma formation appears to be the basic characteristic of the host response to infection by intracellular pathogens. Immune granulomas differ from foreign body granulomas in having a rapid rate of turnover of recruited blood monocytes. Immune granuloma formation is closely correlated with delayed type hypersensitivity; both are dependent on the activity of T-lymphocytes. The select group of obligate and facultative intracellular bacterial pathogens which induce a predominantly CMI reaction is listed in Table 6.

Evidence supporting an important or exclusive role for CMI for these infections in humans is in many cases scant. A delayed type mononuclear cell inflammatory response is elicited by intradermal inoculation of the bacterial antigen in many of these infections, and exposure of peripheral blood leukocytes to relevant bacterial antigen *in vitro* results in production of macrophage migration inhibition factor (MIF), lymphocyte transformation, or other *in vitro* correlates of a cellular immune response. For example, recovery from typhoid fever has been correlated with the *in vitro* production of leukocyte MIF but not with the development of serum antibody (8,53).

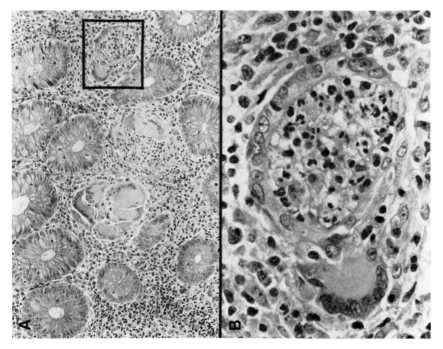

FIG. 3. Submucosal giant cell formation in a homosexual male with rectal infection by a lymphogranuloma venereum immunotype of *C. trachomatis. Enlarged inset*, giant cell abutting a crypt abscess. (From ref. 99, with permission of the author and publisher.)

TABLE 6. *Obligate and facultative intracellular bacterial pathogens[a]*

Mycobacterium tuberculosis, other atypical mycobacteria
Mycobacterium leprae
Salmonella typhi
Listeria monocytogenes
Brucella species
Francisella tularensis
Rickettsia species
Chlamydia trachomatis
Chlamydia psittaci
Bartonella bacilliformes
Treponema pallidum
Calymmatobacterium granulomatis
Legionella pneumophila

[a]Evidence that certain of these agents (e.g., *T. pallidum, C. granulomatis*) are intracellular pathogens is indirect and based primarily on histopathologic studies.

Experiments of Nature

Acquired or congenital defects in T-lymphocyte-derived function most often give rise to infection with viruses or fungi. Less frequently, deficiencies in T-lymphocyte function (e.g., DiGeorge syndrome, Hodgkin disease) have been associated with bacterial infection with such agents as *M. tuberculosis* and other atypical mycobacteria, *Nocardia asteroides, Listeria monocytogenes, B. abortus,* and *Salmonella* species (47).

Animal Models

Experiments in animals have provided detailed information concerning the induction, mechanisms, and regulation of cellular antibacterial responses. The results of these experiments are described below and are expected to apply in principle to humans.

General Mechanisms of Effector T-Cell Responses

In general, the reactions encompassed by CMI are characteristically associated with effector-target cell interactions involved in (a) acquired microbial resistance, particularly that associated with intracellular infections, (b) transplantation immunity, and (c) tumor rejection. CMI reactions may be relatively more important than antibody-mediated mechanisms in limiting early spread of bacteria within the host (11,134).

Two general classes of acquired T-lymphocyte-mediated immune reactions are recognized. T-lymphocytes directly cytotoxic to virus-infected cells, to tumors, or to foreign tissue constitute one type of effector T-cells: the cytotoxic T-lymphocyte (TCTL). T-lymphocytes actively secreting regulatory molecules which recruit and activate mononuclear phagocytes forming immune granulomas constitute the second type of effector T-cell: the delayed hypersensitivity T-lymphocyte (TDTH). Cy-totoxic T-lymphocytes have not been studied in bacterial infections, but since bacteria are not known to induce neoantigens on infected host cells, such TCTL response may not be important. Bacteria which can subvert and survive within host mononuclear phagocytes are the target for the TDTH response (77). Bacteria which infect mononuclear phagocytes appear to induce a prominent TDTH response (84,126).

Cell-to-Cell Interaction in the Induction of TDTH Response

The induction of a TDTH response requires the presentation of bacterial antigen to T-lymphocytes in an immunogenic form by macrophages in association with the macrophage cell surface antigens (Ia antigens) specified by the H-2I region of the mouse major histocompatibility complex (the analogous region in the human is HLA-D) (104,119). Such induced T-lymphocytes, if transferred to a new host, are restricted in their future recognition of an identical antigen by the specificity of the Ia molecule on the macrophages of the new host. This restricted induction is apparent in adoptive transfer experiemnts, where immune T-lymphocytes cooperate most effectively in recipients whose H-2I region gene products match those of the T-lymphocyte donor (135). Similar results have also been found in the rat (57,58). As in helper T-lymphocyte interactions with B-lymphocytes, this restriction is limited to the I-A subregion of the H-2 complex. *In vitro* experiments by Ziegler and Unanue (133) confirm that lymphokine production by T-cells immune to *L. monocytogenes* is also I-A restricted.

Upon induction, TDTH cells disseminate widely throughout the host. Antibac-terial effector TDTH cells for listerial immunity are short lived, nonrecirculating, and preferentially recruited into sites of inflammation (61–63,85,86,93). The surface Ly phenotype of such cells in mice is Ly $1+2+3+$ and differs from T-cells, which help B-lymphocyte production of antibody, which are Ly $1+2-3-$ (61).

Mechanisms of TDTH Activity

Upon activation of TDTH lymphocytes by the relevant bacterial antigens, a variety of biologically active mediators are secreted. Factors which attract, immobilize, and activate mononuclear phagocytes have been identified (64,101). These lym-phocyte-derived factors, or lymphokines, are thought to mediate the dramatic al-teration of behavior and physiologic function of monocytes observed *in vivo* during a CMI reaction (see Fig. 4). Mononuclear phagocytes differ from polymorphonu-clear phagocytes in their responsiveness to T-cell-derived immunologic signals. It is the recruited monocyte rather than the *in situ* macrophage which provides the key antibacterial effect (92). Such stimulated monocytes undergo a marked increase in the secretion of proteases active at neutral pH and in the secretion of reactive metabolites of oxygen, such as superoxide, hydrogen peroxide, hydroxyl radical, and singlet oxygen (90). This burst in oxygen metabolism may underly the bac-tericidal activity of activated mononuclear phagocytes. Activated mononuclear phagocytes also have altered endocytic activity. Fc receptor phagocytosis proceeds more rapidly, and C3b receptors no longer mediate simply adherence but also immune phagocytosis (6,13,28).

Characteristics of the TDTH Response *In Vivo*

Mackaness (78,79,81) and associates have described the *in vivo* characteristics and activity of the TDTH system. The unique characteristics of acquired cellular resistance are (a) a consistent association with delayed type hypersensitivity (DTH), (b) a nonspecific *expression* of acquired resistance despite an immunologically specific *induction*, (c) a change in the physiologic and antibacterial activity of host mononuclear phagocytes, (d) the passive transfer of specific resistance only with immune T-lymphocytes and not with serum antibody, and (e) the efficient induction TDTH by challenge with living and not with killed bacteria.

Many of the bacterial granulomatous diseases of man are associated with DTH. As studied by use of Rebuck skin windows, DTH to purified protein derivative (PPD) in individuals with active tuberculosis is characterized by the delayed recruitment of mononuclear cells (5) (Fig. 5). The development of DTH in the host also correlates with the onset of the antibacterial process in experimental listeriosis, salmonellosis, brucellosis, mycobacteriosis, and tularemia (102,126). The skin test response elicited by intradermal injection of the microbial antigen recapitulates the antibacterial process occurring at deeper parenchymal sites of bacteria deposition (80).

As described above, the immunologic induction of TDTH requires a specific interaction of microbial antigen with host T-lymphocytes. The expression of TDTH response through enhanced antibacterial activity of host macrophages is antigenically unrestricted. Mackaness (79) observed that mice infected with *B. abortus* become resistant to challenge with *L. monocytogenes* at the onset of the brucella antibacterial response. Intracellular bacterial pathogens thus are able to induce enhanced activity of host macrophages following stimulation by immune T-lymphocytes; such activated macrophages are nonspecifically bactericidal for unrelated bacterial pathogens (31).

The ability to transfer antibacterial resistance to naive recipients with immune spleen cells but not with immune serum is the *sine qua non* of a solely cell-mediated antibacterial process. Such has been convincingly shown for many experimental infections, including *L. monocytogenes* (78) and *Francisella tularensis* (65). We have found that mice develop acquired resistance to experimental infection with the lymphogranuloma venereum biotype of *C. trachomatis* (Fig. 6). This resistance

FIG. 4. Mononuclear cells obtained from peritoneal cavity of **(A)** normal mice and **(B)** mice infected with *M. bovis* (BCG) and adhered to glass for 15 min. Mononuclear cells obtained from mice with BCG infection undergo more rapid spreading than do mononuclear cells obtained from uninfected mice, a sign of macrophage activation. (From ref. 47, with permission of the publisher.)

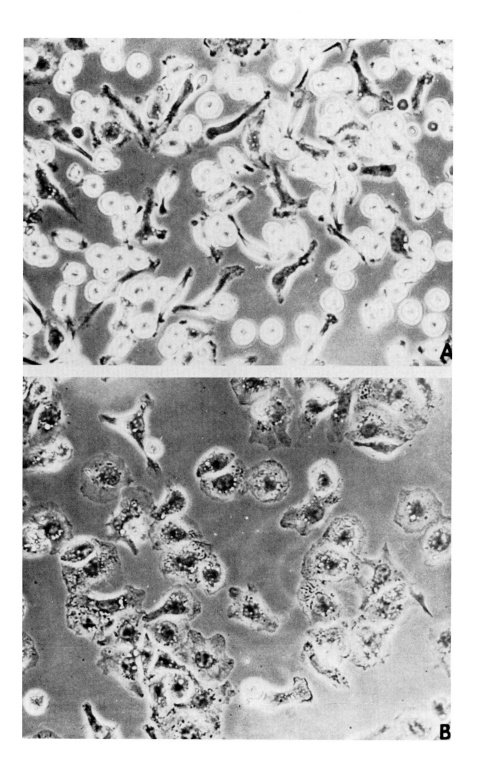

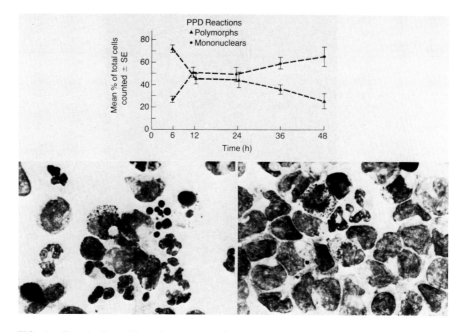

FIG. 5. Examination of the inflammatory cell recruitment into Rebuck skin windows following intradermal inoculation with PPD. *Upper panel,* early influx of polymorphonuclear inflammatory cells and the later influx and predominance of mononuclear inflammatory cells. *Lower panels,* examples of the inflammatory cell population as seen at 24 hr **(left)** and 48 hr **(right)**. (From ref. 5, with permission of the author and publisher.)

is transferable with immune spleen cells but not with immune serum (see Fig. 7) (19).

The acquired resistance to bacteria which induce a protective CMI reaction appears to be critically dependent on immunizing with live rather than dead organisms. This dependence on immunization with living bacteria further differentiates the CMI process from the humoral immune process. Table 7 illustrates that living organisms are more immunogenic than dead organisms for the induction of resistance to *F. tularensis* in the rat (65). This same phenomenon has been seen in humans vaccinated with *F. tularensis*. As summarized in Table 8, vaccination with a live attenuated strain of *F. tularensis* also was more immunogenic than vaccination with a dead vaccine strain in human subjects who were subsequently challenged with virulent *F. tularensis* by aerosol (29,106).

The basis for the requirement of living organisms for the induction of cell-mediated antibacterial immunity is not understood. It is speculated that parasitization of host macrophages by live organisms may allow the presentation of bacterial antigens to host T-lymphocytes in a fashion which most efficiently induces TDTH cells. In any case, these observations have great implications for the development of vaccines for bacteria of the type listed in Table 6.

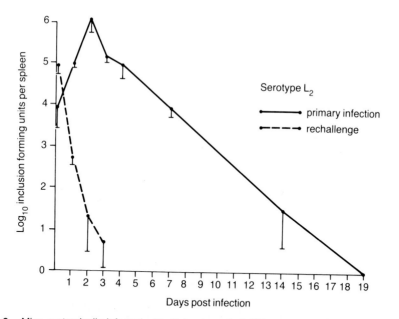

FIG. 6. Mice systemically infected with *C. trachomatis* (LGV-serotype L2) develop acquired resistance. Balb/c mice were challenged intravenously with 1×10^8 IFU *C. trachomatis*. Animals 19 days convalescent from the primary infection were rechallenged intravenously with the same inoculum.

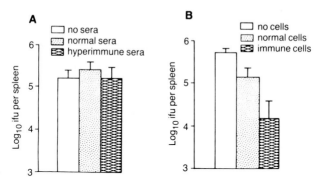

FIG. 7. Passive transfer of immune spleen cells but not of hyperimmune serum protects mice against systemic infection with LGV. Balb/c mice were challenged intravenously with 1×10^8 IFU *C. trachomatis* 2 hr after receiving either 0.5 ml hyperimmune serum (micro IF antibody titer 1:512) or normal serum (titer $< 1:16$) or with 2×10^8 immune spleen cells (6 day post-infection) or normal spleen cells. $p < 0.01$ for immune spleen cells versus normal spleen cells or versus no spleen cells.

T-Cell Responses at Mucosal Sites

Cell-mediated antibacterial activity of macrophages is known to be effective in eliminating bacteria from solid tissues. However, we have no clear idea if or how

TABLE 7. Comparison of the ability of immunization with live or dead
F. tularensis in rats to induce antibody, DTH, macrophage MIF production
and the ability to adoptively transfer resistance[a]

Immunization	Antibody titer	DTH	MIF production	Transfer protection
Live[b]	+ +	+ +	+ +	+ +
Dead[c]	+ +	−	−	−
None	−	−	−	ND[d]

[a]From ref. 75.
[b]4.6×10^6 living F. tularensis.
[c]5×10^8 heat killed F. tularensis.
[d]ND, not done.

TABLE 8. Efficacy of live vaccination in the prevention of tularemia in humans[a]

Vaccine	No. who developed symptomatic tularemia after aerosol challenge/No. given aerosol challenge of virulent F. tularensis			
	Experiment no. 1	p	Experiment no. 2	p
Live, attenuated F. tularensis	ND[b]		3/18	
Killed F. tularensis	8/14	0.65	ND	0.002
None	6/8		8/10	

[a]From refs. 29 and 106.
[b]ND, not done.

well T-cells function on mucosal surfaces, such as the respiratory, genital, or gut epithelia. The histopathology of the jejunum in typhoid fever or of the rectum in lymphogranuloma venereum proctitis suggests that mononuclear phagocytic cell recruitment and activation may occur efficiently in the submucosa of the gut for infections which can and do spread systemically (99,109). For intracellular bacterial pathogens, such as those strains of C. trachomatis which remain localized to the mucosa itself, however, the nature and role of the effector T-cell response is unknown. The host response in this infection includes a prominent submucosal lymphocytic infiltration and lymphoid follicle formation. We have observed that genital infection with C. trachomatis in humans or experimental infection of the salpinx or epididymis in primates results in the induction of a prominent cellular response in peripheral blood mononuclear cells, as detected by antigen-induced lymphocyte blastogenesis during the acute phase of infection (18). In primates with salpingitis, this response appears to be temporally correlated with the intensity of the mononuclear (predominantly lymphocytic) cell infiltrate of the infected fallopian tube (D. Patton and R. Brunham, unpublished). The functional significance of this correlation remains to be determined.

T-cells of the Secretory Immune System

Whether a mucosal or secretory T-cell immune system exists which is distinct from the systemic T-cell system in humans is unknown. Evidence from experiments in animals suggests the existence of such a system. As described previously, unique helper T-cells are found in gut-associated lymphoid tissue (32). Two distinct pools of recirculating T-lymphocytes which preferentially migrate to either lymph node tissue or intestinal epithelium have been seen in sheep (22). Intraepithelial lymphocytes of the mouse intestinal mucosa are predominantly T-lymphocytes with distinctive granular characteristics; under certain antigenic stimuli, these may mature into mucosal mast cells (49). Waldman and Henney (123) have observed that following intrapulmonary immunization, MIF-producing cells are found only in the lung and not in the spleen. Pulmonary infection of rabbits with *L. monocytogenes* or *Str. pneumoniae* results in the local induction of cells which produce MIF when exposed to these organisms *in vitro* and which are detectable in bronchial washings (24). T-cell responses localized to mucosal surfaces do occur. Whether different or similar antibacterial effectors operate at systemic or secretory sites remains to be defined.

K-Lymphocyte Antibacterial Activity

The antibacterial activity of other cells in the lymphoid series is currently the subject of investigation. Antibody-dependent cell-mediated cytotoxicity (ADCC) appears to be an important host immune defense mechanism against some infectious agents, especially viruses. Small lymphocytes lacking specific surface markers for T- or B-cells and possessing high-affinity Fc receptors (K cells) are the mediators for this effect. Lowell et al. (75) have found that K-lymphocytes are bactericidal for *N. meningiditis in vitro* in the presence of specific immune sera but in the absence of complement (see Fig. 8). This activity approximated that of monocytes. The physiologic significance of ADCC is presently unclear; since this activity occurs

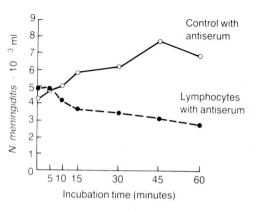

FIG. 8. Antibacterial activity of human lymphocytes. Immune serum lacking complement exerts an antibacterial effect on *N. meningiditis* when in the presence of lymphocytes. (From ref. 75, with permission of the publisher.)

in the absence of complement and is more efficient at lower concentrations of antibody than is granulocyte-mediated cytotoxicity, it may be relatively important in sites deficient in complement components, such as cerebrospinal fluid and secretory surfaces, or in the presence of low concentrations of antibody.

Immunopathology of the Cellular Immune Response

Although important in the antibacterial process, TDTH also may contribute to tissue destruction. At the onset of the antibacterial process in animals experimentally infected with *M. tuberculosis*, granuloma formation and tissue necrosis occur concomitantly (102). Tuberculous cavities, lepra reactions, and syphilitic gummas are examples of clinical events in which such DTH reactions may be harmful. Lymphokine-secreting lymphocytes may mediate the process directly by lymphotoxin production, or the tissue destruction may be consequent to the heightened activity of mononuclear phagocytes. The association of DTH with tuberculous cavity formation has been studied by Yamamura et al. (131). The authors found that 70% of rabbits infected locally in the lung with *M. tuberculosis* developed cavitary lesions. If, however, the development of DTH and MIF-producing cells was prevented by desensitization with tuberculin-active peptide, none developed cavitary disease. A clear correlation between DTH and immunopathology was shown in this model system. Similarly, Godal (42,43) has reported that when patients with borderline leprosy undergo reversal reactions, the *in vitro* correlates of CMI are heightened, and erythematous, edematous cutaneous lesions, and nerve destruction occur with extensive lymphocytic infiltration and granuloma formation. The pathogenesis of reversal reactions is unknown, but such reactions may follow anti-*M. leprae* chemotherapy or may appear spontaneously in the postpartum state. This may relate to a general recovery of CMI competence in these two situations.

IMMUNOPROPHYLAXIS OF BACTERIAL INFECTIONS

Following the introduction of highly efficacious antibiotic therapy for bacterial infections, research into vaccine development had virtually halted. However, the realizations that bacterial infections continue to be important, especially in areas of the world with poor access to medical care, and that bacterial resistance to antibiotics readily occurs prompted further scientific study of immunoprophylaxis.

Four types of bacterial vaccines are either currently in use or are under investigation. These are: (a) whole dead bacteria, (b) live attenuated bacteria, (c) toxoid, and (d) component vaccines. From the foregoing review, certain principles are apparent in designing the appropriate vaccine for a given bacterial disease. A clear understanding of the host-bacterial relationship in humans is needed for vaccine development. For those bacterial infections in which serum antibody appears most important for protection, parenteral vaccination with whole dead bacteria or preferably with a nontoxic but immunogenic component is rational. Presently, infant and childhood infection with *B. pertussis* is effectively prevented by vaccination with whole dead bacteria (2). Polysaccharide vaccines against serogroups A and C of *N. meningiditis* and against 14 serotypes of *Str. pneumoniae* are presently available. Polysaccharide vaccine for *H. influenzae* type b has been developed but currently is not licensed. These vaccines are all highly immunogenic, inducing protective immunity to systemic disease with these agents in children and adults, but are poorly immunogenic in infants. This is a major defect, since infants would benefit most from immunoprophylaxis against certain of these infections.

Similarly, a type III polysaccharide vaccine against group B streptococcus has been produced which is immunogenic in most nonpregnant adults, but its immunogenicity in pregnant women is not yet known. The striking immunogenicity of polysaccharide vaccines in human adults was unexpected, since polysaccharide antigens are notoriously poor immunogens in animals. It may be that immunologic responses of children and adults to bacterial polysaccharide vaccines are secondary in nature, and that priming requires stimulation with a polysaccharide immunogen carrier. This has led to the development of polysaccharide-outer membrane protein complex as a candidate immunogen for *H. influenzae* type b. Further study is needed of the ontogeny of immune responsiveness in early life. Other surface components of bacterial pathogens are currently under study as potential immunogens.

For diseases caused by systemic action of absorbed bacterial toxin, parenteral immunization with inactive toxoid has proved highly efficacious. Tetanus and diphtheria represent two diseases controlled by this means. Other toxin-induced illnesses (such as that caused by exotoxin A-producing *P. aeruginosa*) might be significantly modified by immunization with appropriate toxoids.

For diseases which are localized on or which originate from mucosal surfaces, effective stimulation of the secretory immune response may be critical. Studies in humans are necessary to clearly define optimal ways of inducing a secretory immune response. Live attenuated oral vaccines to enteric pathogens, such as *S. typhi*, *Shigella flexneri*, and *V. cholerae*, show early promise in preventing disease. For many bacterial diseases, the initial step in pathogenesis involves adherence to epithelial cells via surface attachment structures, such as "M" protein with *Str. pyogenes* and pili protein of *N. gonorrheae*. Such structures are being isolated, purified, and evaluated as immunogens for potential vaccines. The appropriate route for immunization with these antigens is not yet defined.

For bacteria which survive within host mononuclear phagocytes, parenteral vaccination with live attenuated bacteria appears to be required for the effective induction of protective immunity. Bacillus Calmette-Guérin (BCG) has long been available as a vaccine to prevent tuberculosis, but its value is controversial. Studies from India currently suggest that immunization of adults with BCG does not prevent the developement of "reactivated" pulmonary tuberculosis (4). Further study of its role in preventing miliary or reactivation tuberculosis following immunization in childhood is awaited. Live attenuated *F. tularensis* vaccine effectively prevents human tularemia (20). Live attenuated rickettsial vaccines are under study. Vaccine development for this group of diseases has proceeded slowly since the development of appropriate attenuated strains is difficult.

MAJOR PROBLEMS IN NEED OF STUDY

The basis for the restriction of cellular immune responses by the major histocompatibility complex remains to be well defined (83). The discovery of major histocompatibility complex restriction has raised fundamental questions about the nature of both T-cell recognition in general and about the relevant antigenic determinants on parasitized or antigen-presenting macrophages. Discoveries made from model systems in animals may help to define the situation in man, especially as relates to the antigenic determinants which induce a CMI reaction.

More accurate and relevant diagnostic tests are needed to measure specific CMI responses to appropriate bacteria and which can practically be performed in a clinical setting (i.e., a CMI test analagous to serologic tests for diagnosis of or susceptibility to disease). Molecular characterization of products of TDTH which activate macrophages may be useful in this regard (16).

Definition of the molecular basis of antibacterial activity of activated macrophages would allow more direct assessment of the efficacy of vaccination for agents such as those listed in Table 6.

The normal physiology of the cellular and humoral aspects of the secretory-mucosal immune system must be further defined in man. More precise study of the secretory immune response in a variety of infections is needed to comprehensively assess the relationship of this response to the natural history and manifestations of bacterial infection.

The regulation of the immune response during the evolution of immune reactions to bacterial infection has not been studied extensively (101). The major histocompatibility complex is involved, but it is not known how. Questions regarding the basis for susceptibility to lepromatous leprosy, for late manifestations of syphilis, or for reactive arthritis following enteric or genital bacterial infection may be answered by this approach.

CONCLUSIONS

The immune responses to bacterial infections are almost as varied as are the bacterial pathogens themselves. It must be remembered that immune reactions serve only to amplify and focus those nonspecific host reactions which usually maintain a stable host-bacteria interaction. Studies of immune reactions have helped in the understanding of the pathogenesis of bacterial infections and have provided methods for effectively preventing many such infections. Many bacterial diseases remain largely unstudied, and many that have been studied could be reexamined in light of the new knowledge and techniques in basic immunology. Effective containment of disease caused by bacteria which involve man alone (e.g., *T. pallidum*, *N. gonorrheae*, *C. trachomatis*, *S. typhi*) should be possible with effective immunoprophylaxis. For bacteria not so limited in host range (e.g., rickettsia, *F. tularensis*), immunotherapy and immunoprophylaxis can still play an important role in effective containment.

ACKNOWLEDGMENTS

Dr. Brunham is a recipient of a fellowship from the Medical Research Council of Canada. Work reported herein has been supported by National Institutes of Health grants AI-14180 and AI-16222.

REFERENCES

1. Andersen, V., Hansen, N. E., Karle, H., Lind, I., Hoiby, N., and Weeke, B. (1976): Sequential studies of lymphocyte responsiveness and antibody formation in acute bacterial meningitis. *Clin. Exp. Immunol.*, 26:469–477.
2. Anonymous (1981): Pertussis vaccine. *Br. Med. J.*, 282:1563–1564.
3. Anonymous (1979): Gut reaction to antigen. *The Lancet*, I:763.
4. Anonymous (1981): BCG vaccination after the Madras study. *The Lancet*, I:309–310.
5. Askernase, P. W., and Atwood, J. E. (1976): Basophils in tuberculin and "Jones-Mote" delayed reactions of humans. *J. Clin. Invest.*, 58:1145–1154.
6. Atkinson, J. P., and Frank, M. M. (1974): The effect of bacillus calmette-guerin-induced macrophage activation on the in vivo clearance of sensitized erythrocytes. *J. Clin. Invest.*, 53:1742–1749.
7. Armstrong, J. A., and Hart, D. P. (1971): Response of cultured macrophages to *Mycobacterium tuberculosis* with observations on fusion of lysosomes with phagosomes. *J. Exp. Med.*, 134:713–740.
8. Balakrishna Sarma, V. N., Malaviya, A. N., Kumar, R., Ghia, O. P., and Bakhtary, M. M. (1976): Development of immune response during typhoid fever in man. *Clin. Exp. Immunol.*, 28:35–39.
9. Banck, G., and Forsgren, A. (1978): Many bacterial species are mitogenic for human blood B lymphocytes. *Scand. J. Immunol.*, 8:347–354.
10. Bayer, A. S., Theofilopoulos, A. N., Eisenberg, R., Dixon, F. J., and Guze, L. B. (1976): Circulating immune complexes in infective endocarditis. *N. Engl. J. Med.*, 295:1500–1505.
11. Bennett, M., and Becker, E. E. (1977): Marrow dependent cell function in early stages of infection with *Listeria* monocytogenes. *Cell. Immunol.*, 33:203–210.
12. Besredka, A. (1927): *Local Immunization*. Williams & Wilkins, Baltimore.
13. Bianco, C., Griffin, F. M., and Silverstein, S. C. (1975): Studies of the macrophage complement receptor. *J. Exp. Med.*, 141:1278–1290.
14. Bienenstock, J., and Befus, A. D. (1980): Mucosal immunology. *Immunology*, 41:249–270.
15. Bjorvatn, B., Barnetson, R. S., and Kronvall, G. (1976): Immune complexes and complement hypercatabolism in patients with leprosy. *Clin. Exp. Immunol.*, 26:388–396.
16. Bloom, B. R. (1980): The unspecificity of cellular reactions. *J. Immunol.*, 124:2527–2529.
17. Brown, E. J., Hosea, S. W., and Frank, M. M. (1981): The role of the spleen in experimental pneumococcal bacteremia. *J. Clin. Invest.*, 67:975–982.
18. Brunham, R. C., Martin, D. H., Kuo, C. C., Wang, S. P., Stevens, C. E., Hubbard, T., and Holmes, K. K. (1981): Cellular immune response during uncomplicated genital infection with *Chlamydia trachomatis* in humans. *Infect. Immunol.*, 34:98–104.
19. Brunham, R. C., Kuo, C. C., Chen, W. J., and Holmes, K. K. (1981): Immunity to *C. trachomatis*. Twenty-third Interscience Conference on Antimicrobial Agents and Chemotherapy, Chicago, Abstr. 520.
20. Burke, D. S. (1977): Immunization against tularemia: Analysis of the effectiveness of live *Francisella tularensis* vaccine in prevention of laboratory-acquired tularemia. *J. Infect. Dis.*, 135:55–60.
21. Burrows, W., and Ward, L. L. (1953): Studies on immunity to Asitica cholera. VII. Prophylactic immunity to experimental enteric cholera. *J. Infect. Dis.*, 92:164–174.
22. Cahill, R. N. P., Poskitt, D. C., Frost, H., and Trnka, Z. (1977): Two distinct pools of recirculating T lymphocytes: Migratory characteristics of nodal and intestinal T lymphocytes. *J. Exp. Med.*, 145:420–428.
23. Campbell, P. A. (1976): Immunocompetent cells in resistance to bacterial infections. *Bacteriol. Rev.*, 40:284–313.
24. Cantley, J. R., and Hand, W. L. (1974): Cell-mediated immunity after bacterial infection of the lower respiratory tract. *J. Clin. Invest.*, 54:1125–1134.

25. Cash, R. A., Music, S. I., Libonati, J. P., Craig, J. P., Pierce, N. F., and Hornick, R. B. (1974): Response of man to infection with *Yibrio cholerae*. II. Protection from illness afforded by previous disease and vaccine. *J. Infect. Dis.*, 130:235–333.

26. Craig, S. W., and Cebra, J. J. (1971): Peyer's patches: An enriched source of precursors for IgA-producing immunocytes in the rabbit. *J. Exp. Med.*, 134:188–200.

27. Crowther, D., Fairley, G. H., and Sewell, R. L. (1969): Lymphoid cellular responses in the blood after immunization in man. *J. Exp. Med.*, 129:849–867.

28. Edelson, P. J., and Erbs, C. (1978): Biochemical and functional characteristics of the plasma membrane of macrophages from BCG-infected mice. *J. Immunol.*, 120:1532–1536.

29. Eigelsbach, H. T., Hornick, R. B., and Tulis, J. J. (1967): Recent studies on live tularemia vaccine. *Med. Ann. Distr. Columbia*, 36:282–286.

30. Eisen, H. (1980): Antibody formation. In: *Microbiology*, third edition, edited by B. A. Davis, R. Dulbecco, H. N. Eisen, and H. S. Ginsberg, pp. 420–450. Harper and Row, New York.

31. Elberg, S. S., Schneider, P. and Fong, J. (1957): Cross-immunity between *Brucella melitensis* and *Mycobacterium tuberculosis*. Intracellular behavior of *Brucella melitensis* in monocytes from vaccinated animals. *J. Exp. Med.*, 106:545–554.

32. Elson, C. O., Heck, J. A., and Strober, W. (1979): T-cell regulation of murine IgA synthesis. *J. Exp. Med.*, 149:632–643.

33. Fauci, A. S., and Pratt, K. R. (1976): Activation of human B lymphocytes. *J. Exp. Med.*, 144:674–684.

34. Fearson, D. T., and Austen, K. F. (1980): Medical intelligence: The alternative pathway of complement—A system for host resistance to microbial infection. *N. Engl. J. Med.*, 303:259–263.

35. Finland, M. (1979): Pneumonia and pneumococcal infections, with special reference to pneumococcal pneumonia. *Am. Rev. Respir. Dis.*, 120:481–502.

36. Flexner, S. (1913): The results of the serum treatment in thirteen hundred cases of epidemic meningitis. *J. Exp. Med.*, 17:553–576.

37. Forsgren, A., and Grubb, A. O. (1979): Many bacterial species bind human IgD. *J. Immunol.*, 122:1468–1472.

38. Freter, R. (1969): Studies of the mechanism of action of intestinal antibody in experimental cholera. *Texas Rep. Biol. Med. [Suppl. 1]*, 27:299–316.

39. Freter, R., De, S. P., Mondal, A., Shrivastava, D. L., and Sunderman, F. W., Jr. (1969): Co-proantibody and serum antibody in cholera patients. *Texas Rep. Biol. Med. [Suppl. 1]*, 27:83–87.

40. Friis, R. (1972): Interaction of L cells and *Chlamydia psittaci*: Entry of the parasite and host response to its development. *J. Bacteriol.*, 110:706–721.

41. Fubara, E. S., and Freter, R. (1973): Protection against eneteric bacterial infection by secretory IgA antibodies. *J. Immunol.*, 111:395–403.

42. Godal, T. (1974): The role of immune responses to *Mycobacterium leprae*. In: *Host Defense and Tissue Damage in Leprosy*, edited by L. Brent and J. Holborow, pp. 161–169. North-Holland, Amsterdam.

43. Godal, T. (1978): Immunological aspects of leprosy—present status. *Prog. Allergy*, 26:211–242.

44. Goldschneider, I. (1976): Bacterial allergy and immunity. In: *Textbook of Immunopathology*, second edition, edited by P. A. Miescher and H. J. Muller-Eberhard, pp. 505–520. Grune & Stratton, New York.

45. Goldschneider, I., Gotschlich, E. C., and Artenstein, M. S. (1969): Human immunity to the meningococcus. I. The role of humoral antibodies. *J. Exp. Med.*, 129:1307–1326.

46. Goldschneider, I., Gotschlich, E. C., and Artenstein, M. S. (1969): Human immunity to the meningococcus. II. Development of natural immunity. *J. Exp. Med.*, 129:1327–1348.

47. Good, R. A., Finstad, J., and Gatti, R. A. (1970): Bulwarks of bodily defense. In: *Infectious Agents and Host Reactions*, edited by S. Mudd, pp. 76–114. Saunders, Philadelphia.

48. Greenwood, A. J., Oduloju, A. J., and Ade-Serrano, M. A. (1979): Cellular immunity in patients with meningococcal disease and in vaccinated subjects. *Clin. Exp. Immunol.*, 38:9–15.

49. Guy-Grand, D., Griscelli, C., and Vassalli, P. (1978): The mouse gut T lymphocyte, a novel type of T cell. Nature, origin, and traffic in mice in normal and graft-versus-host conditions. *J. Exp. Med.*, 148:1661–1677.

49a. Hahn, H., and Kaufman, S. H. E. (1981): The role of cell-mediated immunity in bacterial infection. *Rev. Infect. Dis.*, 3:1221–1250.

50. Hall, J. G., Bede Morris, M. B., Moreno, G. D., and Bessis, M. C. (1965): The ultrastructure and function of the cells in lymph following antigenic stimulation. *J. Exp. Med.*, 121:91–109.

51. Harkiss, G. D., Brown, D. L., and Evans, D. B. (1979): Longitudinal study of circulating immune complexes in a patient with *Staphylococcus albus*-induced shunt nephritis. *Clin. Exp. Immunol.*, 37:228–238.

52. Hopkins, J., McConnell, I., and Lachmann, P. J. (1981): Specific selection of antigen-reactive lymphocytes into antigenically stimulated lymph nodes in sheep. *J. Exp. Med.*, 153:706–719.

53. Hornick, R. B., Greisman, S. E., Woodward, T. E., DuPont, H. L., Dawkins, A. T., and Snyder, M. J. (1970): Typhoid fever: Pathogenesis and immunologic control. *N. Engl. J. Med.*, 283:686–746.

54. Hosea, S. W., Brown, E. J., Hamburger, M. I., and Frank, M. M. (1981): Opsonic requirements for intravascular clearance after splenectomy. *N. Engl. J. Med.*, 304:245–250.

55. Husband, A. J., and Gowans, J. L. (1978): The origin and antigen-dependent distribution of IgA-containing cells in the intestine. *J. Exp. Med.*, 148:1146–1160.

56. Husby, G., van de Rijn, I., Zabriskie, J. B., Abdin, Z. H., and Williams, R. C. (1976): Antibodies reacting with cytoplasm of subthalamic and caudate nuclei neurons in chorea and acute rheumatic fever. *J. Exp. Med.*, 144:1094–1110.

57. Jungi, T. W., and McGregor, D. D. (1978): Allogeneic restriction of acquired antimicrobial resistance in the rat. *J. Immunol.*, 121:449–455.

58. Jungi, T. W., and McGregor, D. D. (1978): Allogeneic restriction of the delayed inflammatory reaction in the rat. *J. Immunol.*, 121:456–463.

59. Kantor, F. S. (1975): Infection, anergy and cell-mediated immunity. *N. Engl. J. Med.*, 292:629–634.

60. Kauffman, C. A., Linnemann, C. C., Jr., Schiff, G. M., and Phair, J. P. (1975): Effect of viral and bacterial pneumonias on cell-mediated immunity in humans. *Infect. Immunol.*, 13:78–83.

61. Kaufmann, S. H. E., Simon, M. M., and Hahn, H. (1979): Specific Lyt 123 T cells are involved in protection against *Listeria monocytogenes* and in delayed-type hypersensitivity to listerial antigens. *J. Exp. Med.*, 150:1033–1038.

62. Koster, F. T., and McGregor, D. D. (1971): The mediator of cellular immunity. III. Lymphocyte traffic from the blood into the inflamed peritoneal cavity. *J. Exp. Med.*, 133:864–876.

63. Koster, F. T., McGregor, D. D., and Mackaness, G. B. (1971): The mediator of cellular immunity. II. Migration of immunologically committed lymphocytes into inflammatory exudates. *J. Exp. Med.*, 133:400–409.

64. Kostiala, A. A. I., and McGregor, D. D. (1975): The mediator of cellular immunity. IX. The relationship between cellular hypersensitivity and acquired cellular resistance in rats infected with *Listeria monocytogenes. J. Exp. Med.*, 141:1249–1260.

65. Kostiala, A. A. I., McGregor, D. D., and Logie, P. S. (1975): Tularaemia in the Rat. I. The cellular basis of host resistance to infection. *Immunology*, 28:855–869.

66. Kutteh, W. H., Koopman, W. J., Conley, M. E., Egan, M. L., and Mestecky, J. (1980): Production of predominantly polymeric IgA by human peripheral blood lymphocytes stimulated in vitro with mitogens. *J. Exp. Med.*, 152:1424–1429.

67. Lagrange, P. H., and Closs, O. (1979): Protective immunity to chronic bacterial infection. *Scand. J. Immunol.*, 10:285–290.

68. Lancefield, R. C. (1933): A serological differentiation of human and other groups of hemolytic streptococci. *J. Exp. Med.*, 57:571–595.

69. Lancefield, R. C., McCarty, M., and Everly, W. N. (1975): Multiple mouse protective antibodies directed against group B streptococci. *J. Exp. Med.*, 142:165–179.

70. Lawy, A. M., Blyth, W. A., and Taverne, J. (1973): Interactions of TRIC agents with macrophages and BHK-21 cells observed by electron microscopy. *J. Hyg. (Lond.)*, 71:515–528.

71. Lee, T. J., Schmoyer, A., Snyderman, R., Yount, W. J., and Sparling, P. F. (1978): Familial deficiencies of the sixth and seventh components of complement associated with bacteremic *Neisseria* infections. In: *Immunobiology of Neisseria gonorrhoeae*, edited by G. F. Brooks, E. C. Gotschlich, K. K. Holmes, W. D. Sawyer, and F. E. Young, pp. 204–206. ASM Publications, Washington, D.C.

72. Leijh, P. C. J., van den Barselaar, M. T., van Zwet, T. L., Daha, M. R., and van Furth, R. (1979): Requirement of extracellular complement and immunoglobulin for intracellular killing of micro-organisms by human monocytes. *J. Clin. Invest.*, 63:772–784.

73. Levy, R. L., and Hong, R. (1973): The immune nature of subacute bacterial endocarditis (SBE) nephritis. *Am. J. Med.*, 54:645–652.
74. Lowell, G. H., Smith, L. F., Griffiss, J. M., and Brandt, B. L. (1980): IgA-dependent, monocyte-mediated, antibacterial activity. *J. Exp. Med.*, 152:452–457.
75. Lowell, G. H., Smith, L. F., Artenstein, M. S., Nash, G. S., and MacDermott, R. P., Jr. (1979): Antibody-dependent cell-mediated antibacterial activity of human mononuclear cells. I. K lymphocytes and monocytes are effective against meningococci in cooperation with human immune sera. *J. Exp. Med.*, 150:127–137.
76. Lumb, J. R. (1979): Perspectives on the in vivo location of cellular interactions in the humoral immune response. *Ann. Rev. Microbiol.*, 33:439–457.
77. Mackaness, G. B. (1964): The behaviour of microbial parasites in relation to phagocytic cells in vitro and in vivo. *Soc. Gen. Microbiol.*, 14:213–240.
78. Mackaness, G. B. (1962): Cellular resistance to infection. *J. Exp. Med.*, 116:381–406.
79. Mackaness, G. B. (1964): The immunological basis of acquired cellular resistance. *J. Exp. Med.*, 120:105–120.
80. Mackaness, G. B. (1967): The relationship of delayed hypersensitivity to acquired cellular resistance. *Br. Med. Bull.*, 23:52–54.
81. Mackaness, G. B. (1969): The influence of immunologically committed lymphoid cells on macrophage activity in vivo. *J. Exp. Med.*, 129:973–992.
82. McDermott, M. R., and Bienenstock, J. (1979): Evidence for a common mucosal immunologic system. I. Migration of B immunoblasts into intestinal, respiratory, and genital tissues. *J. Immunol.*, 122:1892–1898.
83. McDevitt, H. O. (1980): Regulation of the immune response by the major histocompatibility system. *N. Engl. J. Med.*, 303:1514–1517.
84. McGregor, D. M., and Logie, P. S. (1974): Macrophage-lymphocyte interactions in infection immunity. In: *Mononuclear Phagocytes in Immunity, Infection, and Pathology*, edited by E. E. van Firth, pp. 631–651. Blackwell, London.
85. McGregor, D. D., and Kostiala, A. A. I. (1976): Role of lymphocytes in cellular resistance to infection. In: *Contemporary Topics in Immunobiology, Vol. 5*, edited by W. O. Weigle, pp. 237–266.
86. McGregor, D. D., Koster, F. T., and Mackaness, G. B. (1970): The mediator of cellular immunity. I. The life-span and circulation dynamics of the immunologically committed lymphocyte. *J. Exp. Med.*, 133:389–399.
87. Mestecky, J., McGhee, J. R., Arnold, R. R., Michalek, S. M., Prince, S. J., and Babb, J. L. (1978): Selective induction of an immune response in human external secretions by ingestion of bacterial antigen. *J. Clin. Invest.*, 61:731–737.
88. Mosley, W. H. (1969): Vaccines and somatic antigens. The role of immunity in cholera. A review of epidemiological and serological studies. *Texas Rep. Biol. Med. [Suppl. 1]*, 27:227–241.
89. Moxon, E. R., Smith, A. L., Averill, D. R., and Smith, D. H. (1974): *Haemophilus influenzae* meningitis in infant rats after intranasal inoculation. *J. Infect. Dis.*, 129:154–162.
90. Nathan, C. F., Murray, H. W., and Cohn, Z. A. (1980): The macrophage as an effector cell. *N. Engl. J. Med.*, 303:622–626.
91. Niklasson, P. M., and Williams, R. C., Jr. (1974): Studies of peripheral blood T- and B-lymphocytes in acute infections. *Infect. Immunol.*, 9:1–7.
92. North, R. J. (1970): The relative importance of blood monocytes and fixed macrophages to the expression of cell-mediated immunity to infection. *J. Exp. Med.*, 132:521–534.
93. North, R. J. (1973): Cellular mediators of anti-*Listeria* immunity as an enlarged population of short-lived, replicating T cells. Kinetics of their production. *J. Exp. Med.*, 138:342–355.
94. Orlans, E., Peppard, J., Reynolds, J., and Hall, J. (1978): Rapid active transport of immunoglobulin A from blood to bile. *J. Exp. Med.*, 147:588–592.
95. Pichichero, M. E., Hall, C. B., and Insel, R. A. (1981): A mucosal antibody response following systemic *Haemophilus influenzae* type B infection in children. *J. Clin. Invest.*, 67:1482–1489.
96. Pierce, N. F., and Gowans, J. L. (1975): Cellular kinetics of the intestinal immune response to cholera toxoid in rats. *J. Exp. Med.*, 142:1550–1563.
97. Pollack, M. (1980): *Pseudomonas aeruginosa* exotoxin A. *N. Engl. J. Med.*, 302:1360–1362.
98. Pollack, M., and Young, L. S. (1979): Protective activity of antibodies to exotoxin A and lipopolysaccharide at the onset of *Pseudomonas aeruginosa* septicemia in man. *J. Clin. Invest.*, 63:276–286.

99. Quinn, T. C., Goodell, S. E., Mkrtichian, E., Schuffler, M. D., Wang, S. P., Stamm, W. E., and Holmes, K. K. (1981): *Chlamydia trachomatis* proctitis. *N. Engl. J. Med.*, 305:195–200.

100. Read, S. E., Fischetti, V. A., Utermohlen, V., Falk, R. E., and Zabriskie, J. B. (1974): Cellular reactivity studies to streptococcal antigens. Migration inhibition studies in patients with streptococcal infections and rheumatic fever. *J. Clin. Invest.*, 54:439–450.

101. Reinherz, E. L., and Schlossman, S. F. (1980): Regulation of the immune response—Inducer and suppressor T-lymphocyte subsets in human beings. *N. Engl. J. Med.*, 303:370–373.

102. Remold, H., and David, J. R. (1976): Cellular or delayed hypersensitivity. In: *Textbook of Immunopathology*, second edition, edited by P. A. Mieschler and H. J. Mueller-Eberhard, pp. 157–176. Grune & Stratton, New York.

103. Rosen, F. S., and Janeway, C. A. (1966): The gamma globulins. III. The antibody deficiency syndromes. *N. Engl. J. Med.*, 275:709–715.

104. Rosenthal, A. S. (1980): Regulation of the immune response—Role of the macrophage. *N. Engl. J. Med.*, 303:1153–1156.

105. Russell, M. W., Brown, T. A., and Mestecky, J. (1981): Role of serum IgA. Hepatobiliary transport of circulating antigen. *J. Exp. Med.*, 153:968–976.

106. Saslaw, S., Eigelbach, H. T., Prior, J. A., Wilson, H. E., and Carhart, S. (1961): Tularemic vaccine study. II. Respiratory challenge. *Arch. Intern. Med.*, 107:134–146.

107. Schoolnik, G. K., Buchanan, T. M., and Holmes, K. K. (1976): Gonococci causing disseminated gonococcal infection are resistant to the bactericidal action of normal human sera. *J. Clin. Invest.*, 58:1163–1173.

108. Schwab, J. H. (1975): Suppression of the immune response by microorganisms. *Bacteriol. Rev.*, 39:121–143.

109. Sprinz, H., Gangarosa, E. J., Williams, M., Hornick, R. B., and Woodward, T. E. (1966): Histopathology of the upper small intestines in typhoid fever. Biopsy study of experimental disease in man. *Am. J. Dig. Dis.*, II:615–624.

110. Steele, E. J., Chaicumpa, W., and Rowley, D. (1974): Isolation and biological properties of three classes of rabbit antibody to *Vibrio cholerae*. *J. Infect. Dis.*, 130:93–103.

111. Sutter, E. (1956): Interaction between phagocytes and pathogenic microorganisms. *Bacteriol. Rev.*, 20:94–132.

112. Theofilopoulos, A. N., and Dixon, F. J. (1979): The biology and detection of immune complexes. In: *Advances in Immunology, Vol. 28*, edited by F. J. Dixon and H. G. Kunkel, pp. 160–220. Academic Press, New York.

113. Thorley, J. D., Smith, J. W., Luby, J. P., and Sanford, J. P. (1977): Peripheral blood lymphocyte response to acute infections in humans. *Infect. Immunol.*, 16:110–114.

114. Tillett, W. S., and Frances, T. (1929): Cutaneous reactions to polysaccharides and proteins of pneumococcus in lobar pneumonia. *J. Exp. Med.*, 50:687–701.

115. Tomasi, T. B., Larson, L., Challacombe, S., and McNabb, P. (1980): Mucosal immunity: The origin and migration patterns of cells in the secretory system. *J. Allergy Clin. Immunol.*, 65:12–19.

116. Tomasi, T. B., Tan, E. M., Solomon, A., and Prendergast, R. A. (1965): Characteristics of an immune system common to certain external secretions. *J. Exp. Med.*, 121:101–124.

117. Tramont, E. E. (1977): Inhibition of adherence of *Neisseria gonorrhoeae* by human genital secretions. *J. Clin. Invest.*, 59:117–124.

118. Unanue, E. R. (1978): The immune granulomas. In: *Immunological Diseases*, third edition, edited by M. Samter, pp. 297–305. Little, Brown, Boston.

119. Unanue, E. R. (1980): Cooperation between mononuclear phagocytes and lymphocytes in immunity. *N. Engl. J. Med.*, 303:977–985.

120. Van de Rijn, I., Fillit, H., Brandeis, W. E., Reid, H., Poon-King, T., McCarthy, M., Day, N. K., and Zabriskie, J. B. (1978): Serial studies on circulating immune complexes in poststreptococcal sequelae. *Clin. Exp. Immunol.*, 34:318–325.

121. Villarreal, H., Jr., Fischetti, V. A., van de Rijn, I., and Zabriskie, J. B. (1979): The occurrence of a protein in the extracellular products of streptococci isolated from patients with acute glomerulonephritis. *J. Exp. Med.*, 149:459–472.

122. Wagner, H. N., Jr., Iio, M., and Hornick, R. B. (1963): Studies of the reticuloendothelial system (res). II. Changes in the phagocytic capacity of the res in patients with certain infections. *J. Clin. Invest.*, 42:427–434.

123. Waldman, R. H., and Henney, C. S. (1971): Cell-mediated immunity and antibody responses in the respiratory tract after local and systemic immunization. *J. Exp. Med.*, 134:482–494.

124. Weisz-Carrington, P., Roux, M. E., McWilliams, M., Phillips-Quagliata, J. M., and Lamm, M. E. (1979): Organ and isotype distribution of plasma cells producing specific antibody after oral immunization: Evidence for a generalized secretory immune system. *J. Immunol.*, 123:1705–1708.

125. Wemambu, S. N. C., Turk, J. L., Waters, M. F. R., and Rees, R. J. W. (1969): Erythema nodosum leprosum: A clinical manifestation of the arthus phenomenon. *The Lancet*, II:933–935.

126. WHO Scientific Group (1973): Cell-mediated immunity and resistance to infection. *WHO Tech. Rep. Ser.*, no. 519.

127. Wiggins, R. C., and Cochrane, C. G. (1981): Immune-complex-mediated biologic effects. *N. Engl. J. Med.*, 304:518–520.

128. Williams, R. C., and Gibbons, R. J. (1972): Inhibition of bacterial adherence by secretory immunoglobulin A: A mechanism of antigen disposal. *Science*, 177:697–699.

129. Wood, B. W. (1960): Phagocytosis with particular reference to encapsulated bacteria. *Bacteriol. Rev.*, 24:41–49.

130. Wyrick, P. B. Brownridge, E. A., and Ivins, B. E. (1978): Interaction of *Chlamydia psittaci* with mouse peritoneal macrophages. *Infect. Immunol.*, 19:1061–1067.

131. Yamamura, Y., Ogawa, Y., Maeda, H., and Yamamura, Y. (1974): Prevention of tuberculous cavity formation by desensitization with tuberculin-active peptide. *Am. Rev. Respir. Dis.*, 109:594–601.

132. Zabriskie, J. B., Utermohlen, V., Read, S. E., and Fischetti, V. A. (1973): Streptococcus-related glomerulonephritis. *Kidney Int.*, 3:100–104.

133. Ziegler, K., and Unanue, E. R. (1979): The specific binding of *Listeria monocytogenes*-immune T lymphocytes to macrophages. I. Quantitation and role of H-2 gene products. *J. Exp. Med.*, 150:1143–1160.

134. Zinkernagel, R. M., Blanden, R. V., and Langman, R. E. (1974): Early appearance of sensitized lymphocytes in mice infected with *Listeria* monocytogenes. *J. Immunol.*, 112:496–501.

135. Zinkernagel, R. M., Althage, A., Adler, B., Blanden, R. V., Davidson, W. F., Kees, U., Dunlop, M. B. C., and Shreffler, D. C. (1977): H-2 restriction of cell-mediated immunity to an intracellular bacterium. Effector T cells are specific for *Listeria* antigen in association with H-21 region-coded self-markers. *J. Exp. Med.*, 145:1353–1367.

Advances in Host Defense Mechanisms, Vol. 2,
edited by John I. Gallin and Anthony S. Fauci.
Raven Press, New York © 1983.

Role of Lymphoid Cells in Immune Surveillance Against Viral Infection

N. S. Greenspan, D. H. Schwartz, and P. C. Doherty

The Wistar Institute of Anatomy and Biology, Philadelphia, Pennsylvania 19104

The discovery in 1974 that the cytotoxic activity of virus-specific murine thymus-derived (T) cells was restricted by antigens encoded in the major histocompatibility complex (MHC) of the mouse (H-2) (52–54,268–270) initiated a wave of intense research activity in viral immunology, with emphasis on the cell-mediated immune response to viral infection and on the role of MHC gene products in regulating these responses (reviewed in ref. 271). Investigation of humoral immunity to viruses, the classic preoccupation of viral immunologists, continued unabated throughout the 1970s to the present (33,223,224). In addition to cytotoxic T lymphocytes mediating MHC-restricted cytotoxicity (Tc or CTL) and B cell-derived antibody-producing cells, other functionally distinct subsets of lymphoid cells of potential relevance to antiviral immune responses have been described. These subsets include helper T cells (Th), suppressor T cells (Ts), natural killer (NK) cells, and the cells mediating antibody-dependent cellular cytotoxicity (ADCC), referred to as killer (K) cells.

Thus the contemporary viral immunologist is faced with a considerable diversity of types of lymphoid cells and associated immunologic mechanisms that may be involved in the host response to a given virus infection. Nevertheless, particular functional subclasses and/or mechanisms often have been studied in isolation because of the difficulties inherent in performing and interpreting studies of multiple cell types and effector mechanisms. This state of affairs has been reflected in the preponderance of review articles which address themselves to a particular form of antiviral immunity, such as antibody-mediated immune mechanisms (38,223,224) or virus-specific CTL (32,271). Therefore, this review explores in depth a few model virus-host systems in the hope of fostering an integrated view of immune responsiveness to viral infection. The virus-host systems chosen for discussion reflect the authors' areas of greatest expertise but were chosen also with the aim of illustrating for the reader the range of phenomena encountered in viral immunology. In addition, we have tried to maintain a balance between data from experimental animals and human subjects, since one of the avowed aims of this series is to facilitate the transfer of basic knowledge of infectious disease processes to the clinical sphere. Although a paucity of relevant experimental information will, in general, preclude any definite conclusions as to the relative *in vivo* importance of any given subclass of lymphocyte or immunologic mechanism, it is hoped that by surveying the potentially relevant cell types and effector mechanisms, the acquisition of such information will be encouraged.

Before proceeding to the discussions of the individual virus-host systems, it will be useful to briefly review some general aspects of virus-host interactions, the MHC and its role in immune responsiveness, and current understanding of the diversity of functional lymphoid cell subsets.

General Aspects of Virus-Host Interaction

The inherent complexity of the immune response to viral (as well as nonviral) antigens is matched by the complexity of the interaction of virus with host cells. Depending on the virus and the host cell, viral penetration of the target cell may result in productive replication with or without cell death, abortive replication with synthesis of viral antigens but without release of infectious progeny virus, persistent and/or latent infection, or neoplastic transformation (89). Related to the site of infection, viruses employ different modes of spread within the host: (a) in the extracellular fluid (type I), (b) from cell to adjacent cell (type II), and (c) from parent cell to daughter cell (type III) (168). Infected leukocytes, especially macrophages, are responsible for early dissemination of certain viruses (156). Some viruses may employ more than a single type of spread in a given host, and which host immune mechanisms are effective in controlling a given virus infection will depend, in part, on the primary mode(s) of spread utilized by the virus (168). The types of host cells infected by a particular virus may also influence the nature or efficacy of the elicited immune response. Furthermore, that viral infection can alter the functional properties of the immune system in significant ways has been documented with a variety of viruses; in some cases, direct infection of lymphoid cells by the virus may be involved (169,170,251).

Other factors also contribute to the complexity of the interaction between virus and host. Generally, a virus infection will expose the host to a multiplicity of foreign molecules, each of which may possess several antigenic determinants (also referred to as epitopes) (33,43). Furthermore, virus-determined antigens will exist not only on the surface (or inside) of the virion but also on the surface (or inside) of the infected cell (43); the sets of molecules and epitopes expressed on the virion surface and the infected cell surface may not be identical (239,264). Thus antigen-specific effector elements of the immune system may be directed at virions or infected cells, or both, and elements directed at one may not affect the other. Genetic differences in immune responsiveness to viral antigens have been observed among inbred strains of mice (reviewed in ref. 271) and among human individuals (16,151,217), so that the pattern of virus-host interaction may vary with host genotype in a given species. Conversely, genetic variants of a given species of virus may behave in substantially different ways in genetically identical hosts (89). Many or all of the above factors may need to be considered in the course of designing immunologically based preventive or therapeutic protocols if they are to be both safe and effective.

The MHC and Immune Responsiveness

The MHC (H-2 in the mouse and HLA in the human) is a complex genetic region encoding a variety of gene products involved in the expression and regulation of immune responsiveness (130). The loci of the MHC encode three major classes of molecules with differing structural and functional properties (131,244). Class I molecules (H-2K, D, and L or HLA-A, B, and C), which include the classic transplantation antigens, are composed of a 45,000 dalton MHC-encoded polypeptide and a noncovalently linked non-MHC-encoded polypeptide of 11,500 daltons, β_2-microglobulin. The 45,000 dalton chain is polymorphic, glycosylated, and inserts into the cell membrane (190,244). The class I molecules serve as restriction elements (see below) for virus-specific Tc cells (271). Class II molecules (H-2I or HLA-DR) consist of two noncovalently associated glycosylated polypeptide chains of molecular weights 33,000 (α-chain) and 28,000 (β-chain) daltons (234). Both the α- and β-chains insert into the cell membrane (244). Class II molecules serve as restriction elements for Th cells (reviewed in ref. 226). Class III molecules are involved in the complement pathways (219).

The MHC was initially discovered in the mouse (the H-2 region) in the 1930s. It could be detected serologically but was studied more for its influence on graft rejection (130), from which the name derives. It was only in the 1970s, however, that immunologists learned enough about MHC antigens to begin to ascribe to them biologic functions (54). The key observations that led to the development of the current concepts of MHC function were: (a) the genetic control of immune responsiveness by genes located in the MHC (10), (b) the dual specificity of Th cells for antigen and class II molecules (H-2I or HLA-D) (226), and (c) the dual specificity of Tc cells for antigen and class I molecules (50). The necessity for T cells to recognize antigen in conjunction with self MHC-encoded molecules is referred to as MHC restriction (or, for example, H-2 restriction in the mouse). MHC restriction was initially described and analyzed in mice, although it appears to occur in mammals generally (271). The importance of MHC restriction for antiviral immunity is discussed further in the context of particular viruses.

Lymphoid Subpopulations

At present, a variety of classes of lymphocytes can be distinguished, in man or mouse, on the basis of cell surface phenotypes and/or functional characteristics: B cells potentially capable of antibody production and secretion, T cells, NK cells, and K cells capable of mediating ADCC. It is likely that each of these is involved in some antiviral immune responses, although their relative contributions in any given antivirus response may be expected to vary considerably, depending on many variables, such as mode of virus spread, host genotype, and age. A few brief comments on each of the major lymphoid cell classes follow.

In humans and mice, B cells are most easily distinguished from non-B cells by virtue of the cell surface expression of serologically detectable immunoglobulin (Ig) molecules which serve as antigen receptors (252). One obvious approach to subclassifying B lymphocytes would rely on the class (e.g., IgM or IgG) or subclass (e.g., IgGl or IgG2) of the Ig produced by B cells or their clonal progeny. However, attempts to classify B cells on the basis of other cell surface molecules and on functional criteria are underway (reviewed in ref. 96).

Mature peripheral T cells can be routinely identified in mouse and human on the basis of their expression of the Thy (196) and T3 (138) markers, respectively. In addition, human T cells often have been operationally identified by their capacity to form rosettes with sheep red blood cells (SRBC) (78,119). T cells have been subclassified, in both mice and humans, on the basis of serologically detected cell surface markers; in both systems, cell surface phenotype has been correlated with cell function. In the mouse, the most widely used set of T cell markers belongs to the Lyt series (34); in man, the various T antigens (which are defined by monoclonal antibodies) are the most important (199). The chief T cell subsets and their primary markers are as follows: inducer or Th; $Lyt-1^+$ (mouse) and $T4^+$ (human); Ts cells, $Lyt-2,3^+$ (mouse) and $T5^+$ and $T8^+$ (human); and Tc cells (CTL), $Ly-2,3^+$ (mouse) and $T5^+$ and $T8^+$ (human) (34,199). In the mouse, an additional $Lyt-1^+,2^+,3^+$ subset of T cells is of recognized importance (34). These cells are thought to function both as amplifier cells and in feedback suppression, and they may also serve as precursors for the Th, Ts, and Tc cells (87).

In any case, the present classification scheme is certain to be refined as more is learned about the functional implications of the expression of particular cell surface molecules and as new marker antigens are discovered. Some proposed refinements already available cannot be discussed due to space limitations. For further information on T cell subsets in mice or humans, the reader is referred to recent reviews (9,35,199). NK cells are lymphocytes which can lyse certain types of tumor cells and normal cells by a contact-dependent mechanism without manifesting classic immunologic specificity or antigenic memory (249). In both mice and humans, NK cells possess receptors for the Fc region of IgG (FcR) but do not express endogenously produced surface Ig (108). Despite the possession of FcR by NK cells, natural cell-mediated cytotoxicity (CMC) does not appear to depend on IgG (107). Some evidence indicates that NK cells may express certain T cell antigens (Thy 1 in the mouse and the receptor for SRBC in humans) at low levels; it has been suggested therefore, that the NK cell lineage is closely related to the T cell lineage (108). NK cell activity is generally augmented by interferon or interferon inducers in both murine and human systems (108). The factors determining susceptibility or resistance of target cells to lysis by NK cells are still unclear.

It is generally believed that K cells are closely related or identical to NK cells, although ADCC and natural cytotoxicity do appear to represent distinct lytic mechanisms (108), whether mediated by the same or distinct cell types. Like NK cells, K cells also express the FcR, which is directly involved in ADCC, but do not express endogenously synthesized Ig (108). Interferon may enhance K CMC (108,223,249) as well as NK CMC. The immunologic specificity in ADCC is provided by the antibody bound to the target cell and is not an intrinsic property of the K cell (223). Thus K cells would not be expected to possess any antigenic memory. Neither ADCC nor natural CMC is MHC restricted (223). In general, ADCC appears to be much more efficient when mediated by human rather than murine K cells (223).

INFLUENZA VIRUS AND LYMPHOID CELLS

Basic Characterizations of Influenza A Viruses

The influenza A viruses are enveloped viruses with a segmented single-stranded RNA genome of nonmessage polarity (125). They have been thoroughly characterized biochemically, genetically, and serologically (124) and are responsible for significant annual morbidity and mortality (126). Attempts to control the spread of influenza A viruses and the incidence of influenza (the disease) with vaccines have been less than completely successful, at least in part because of the well-known propensity of influenza A viruses to undergo antigenic variation. Two types of variation have been shown to affect the (virion) surface glycoproteins of influenza A viruses: antigenic drift and antigenic shift (248). The first probably represents serial point mutations occurring progressively in the virion surface glycoproteins of related virus strains, all of the same subtype (defined below) (141). Antigenic drift occurs in type B as well as in type A influenza viruses. In contrast, antigenic shift has been observed only for type A influenza viruses; it refers to a major alteration in the antigenic characteristics of the surface glycoproteins resulting in a virus of a subtype distinct from that of the prior virus (248). It has been postulated that antigenic shift occurs as a result of recombination or gene reassortment between human and animal influenza A viruses. Evidence for this mechanism is strongest in the case of the origin of the A/Hong Kong/68 (H3N2) influenza virus (247).

Type A influenza viruses are distinguished from types B and C on the basis of the serologic properties of their respective nucleoproteins (NP); all type A NPs are cross-reactive with one another but not with those of type B or type C viruses (36). The NP and the matrix (M) protein are the major internal protein antigens of the influenza A virion. The M protein is also antigenically similar for all type A influenza viruses. In contrast, subtypes of type A influenza viruses are distinguished from one another on the basis of antigenic differences in the two virion surface glycoproteins, the hemagglutinin (HA) and the neuraminidase (NA) (36). The spikes seen projecting from influenza virions on electron microscopic examination are composed of HA trimers and NA tetramers, with the HA spikes predominating numerically (36). Influenza A epidemics and pandemics are associated with antigenic variation (drift and shift) in the HA and NA (248).

While the antigenic properties of virions are of obvious importance in understanding host immune responsiveness to viral infection, the nature and quantity of virus-determined antigens expressed by infected host cells also have a considerable impact on the host-virus interaction (43). In the case of influenza A virus-infected cells, it is well established that the HA and NA are expressed on the host cell surface in immunologically significant amounts (265). Whether or not infected cells express the internal virion proteins is controversial. Evidence has been reported to indicate that NP (159,239) and M (1,2,13,28,201) can be detected on cell surfaces subsequent to infection by live virus. Other investigators have questioned the expression of M (in significant quantities) on the cell surface (95,264). The relevance of this issue will become clear in the context of the specificity of Tc for influenza-infected cells. At present, the other five virus-encoded molecules found in infected cells (three polymerases also found in the virion and two nonstructural proteins not associated with virions) have not been implicated in any major role in antiviral immunity.

B Cell-Dependent Immunity to Influenza A Viruses

The importance of B cell-derived antibody in host resistance to influenza A infection is well documented (192,212). Natural influenza A virus infection or immunization with influenza A virus vaccines generally induces the production of antibody specific for the virus HA, NA, and NP molecules (207). Antibody specific for the HA can be detected by its ability to inhibit virus-mediated hemagglutination, a property referred to as hemagglutination inhibition (HI) (56). This HI antibody can neutralize virus *in vitro* and inhibit the release of virus from infected cells (57). It has been demonstrated in both humans and mice that anti-HA antibody (either actively acquired or passively administered) can protect individuals from infection upon respiratory tract exposure to virus (154,159,191,237), lessen the severity of infection once the disease process is underway (44,72,159), and decrease the amount of virus shedding (39). It is generally acknowledged that antibody specific for the HA is the most important humoral component preventing influenza A virus reinfection (212).

The specificity characteristics of the anti-HA antibody are of interest. Primary infection or immunization has been shown to elicit HI antibody reactive with the immunizing virus and cross-reactive with related viruses of the same subtype (208). Patients challenged a second time with virus of the same subtype produce cross-reactive antibody (CRA) that reacts with all viruses of the same subtype (but not viruses of unrelated subtypes); they may also produce strain-specific antibody (SSA) reactive with the virus causing the initial infection (142,233). Similar results have been obtained with vaccines in humans (209) and with purified HA in mice (243). In the mouse model, sequential immunization with the related HO and H1 HAs led to the production of CRA reactive with both virus strains and also to the production of SSA, which was specific for the initial immunogen, HO, and unreactive with the H1 in a single radial diffusion test. The SSA response developed with the kinetics of a secondary response. In addition, SSA specific for the secondary immunogen, H1, developed with kinetics intermediate between those typical of primary and secondary humoral responses (240). In all these situations, exposure to the second virus (or HA) elicits some antibody reactive only to the original immunogen, a phenomenon termed "original antigenic sin" (OAS) by Davenport and colleagues (44).

Of potential biologic importance is the finding that homologous antibody is probably more effective in virus neutralization than is CRA (142). In mice, passive transfer of homologous antibody to the HA of the infecting virus proved much more effective in protection against infection than did transfer of heterologous antibody elicited by a related HA (237). This result indicates the greater efficacy of SSA in protection against infection as compared to CRA. If these observations are relevant for human humoral immunity to influenza A viruses, then it becomes easier to understand the relative ineffectiveness of vaccinating with a previous cross-reacting strain instead of with the currently prevalent strain (191).

Although antibody is produced by B cells, other sorts of lymphoid cells may play important roles in generating and effecting humoral immunity. In the case of purified influenza A virus HA antigens, it has been demonstrated that both the CRA and SSA responses in mice are T cell dependent, with the strain-specific (SS) response manifesting a stronger requirement for T cell help (243). In contrast to results in other antigen systems (122), however, Virelizier et al. (243) found that B cell memory for the HA developed in the presumed absence of functional T cells. In fact, these investigators explained OAS on the basis of the ability of a heterologous HA to stimulate SS memory B cells specific for the initial immunizing HA, even though their secreted antibody did not react with the heterologous molecule (240). An intrinsic affinity requirement, more stringent for *in vitro* reactivity than for B cell triggering, has been hypothesized to explain this discrepancy in antigen recognition between soluble and cell-bound antibody (241).

In addition to anti-HA antibody, antibody directed against antigenic determinants on the NA is thought to play a role in immunity to influenza A virus. Experiments performed *in vitro* demonstrated that anti-NA antibody interferes with virus release from infected cells (57). That this effect might have relevance *in vivo* is suggested by observations correlating lower rates of infection (158,225) or illness (164) with titers of antibody specific for the NA of the infecting strain of virus in human volunteers. The ability of anti-NA antibody to lessen the severity of infection has been documented in mice (213) as well. Antibody to NA has also been shown to reduce the transmission of influenza A virus infection in experimental animals (211) and to reduce virus titers in nasal secretions in humans (41). Antibody to internal virion antigens (NP or M) does not appear to have any protective effect in mice (172,242).

Local production of antibody in the respiratory tract, predominantly IgA, has been demonstrated in humans following natural infection (4) or intranasal immunization with live attenuated virus vaccine (40,80,121). It probably contributes to immunity but to a lesser degree than does serum antibody (192).

There are several mechanisms by which antibody might contribute to host defense against influenza A virus infection. Direct neutralization of virus by anti-HA antibody seems likely to play a significant role, given that influenza A virus probably utilizes, at least partially, type I spread [according to the scheme of Notkins et al. (169) outlined earlier]. However, antibody may interact with a number of other factors to facilitate viral inactivation. Complement may enhance the efficiency of virus neutralization (171), and it has been reported in one instance that decomplementation of mice increased the severity of influenzal pneumonia (109). In some instances, binding of antibody to virus may not result in inactivation directly but, by serving as an opsonin, may favor viral destruction by a cooperating phagocytic cell (38). This latter process probably is enhanced if complement has been fixed and C3b deposited on the virus-antibody complex (38). Finally, antibody may serve the host in controlling viral infection by participating in ADCC, leading to the destruction of host cells involved in the production of new virus particles. The nature of the K cells that utilize target cell-bound antibody to mediate cytotoxicity by virtue of Fc receptors (FcR) is not fully known, but a subset of such cells probably consists of lymphoid cells (108,249), at least by current cell surface marker criteria. Greenberg et al. (92) have reported that following immunization of volunteers with influenza A virus, there is a sharp rise in cytotoxicity (to influenza A virus-infected target cells) mediated by FcR$^+$ peripheral blood lymphocytes (PBLs). They presented evidence to support the view that this cytotoxicity was ADCC, the antibody being provided during the course of the assay by plasma cells in the PBL population.

NK Cell Immunity to Influenza A Viruses

The ability of NK cells to lyse virus-infected cells varies considerably with the virus and the type of host cell used for infection. For instance, Sendai virus infection of Vero cells increased their susceptibility to NK cell-mediated lysis, while similarly infected L-929 cells were resistant to lysis by NK cells (250). There is a paucity of information on the activity of NK cells in influenza A virus infection.

The contribution of interferons in the development of host resistance to infection by influenza A virus also remains to be studied in depth. In a study of type I (α) interferon in a variety of viral infections in mice, Gresser et al. (94) found that *in vivo* administration of potent antiserum to type I interferon increased the severity of infections with herpes simplex, Moloney sarcoma, vesicular stomatitis, New castle disease, and encephalomyocarditis viruses while leaving influenza A virus infection unaffected. This result must be interpreted cautiously, however, given the possibility that the antiinterferon antibody may not have reached the tracheobronchial epithelium in adequate concentrations to affect local interferon activity. That local production of interferon in the respiratory tract can occur in conjunction with influenza A virus infection has been demonstrated with human nasal washings (163), and type II (γ) interferon can protect murine macrophages against the cytopathic effects of an influenza A virus (238).

T Cell-Dependent Immunity to Influenza A Viruses

CTL specific for influenza A viruses have been extensively and intensively studied in recent years in both murine and human systems. Before discussing the evidence for the role of cell-mediated immunity (CMI) to influenza A virus infections, it will be useful to review the biologic characteristics and specificity of these cells.

The primary *in vivo* murine CTL response to influenza A viruses conforms to the general pattern found for CTL responses to acute animal virus infections. Maximal spleen cell cytotoxic activity reached by day 5 or 6 after influenza A virus immunization is demonstrated only for target cells that express both influenza A viral antigens and the H-2K or H-2D gene products of the effector cells (27,51,64). Cytotoxic effector spleen cells from mice immunized with influenza A and similar effector spleen cells from mice immunized with influenza B or vaccinia viruses show reciprocal exclusion of cytotoxic activity on appropriately infected histocompatible target cells (60). Thus CTL specific for influenza A virus manifest a degree of specificity comparable to that exhibited by CTL elicited with other viruses (55). Investigation of the requirements for target cell formation disclosed that an essential step in the creation of target cells susceptible to influenza A virus-immune CTL is the integration of the influenza A viral antigens into the target cell plasma membranes; adsorption of virions to the cell surface, without dissemination of viral antigens in the cell membranes, was found to be insufficient for creation of susceptible target cells (139). A similar requirement has been demonstrated for Sendai virus antigens and target cells susceptible to Sendai virus-immune CTL (88,136,210,227). Compatible data also have been produced by a number of laboratories working with poxviruses (3,97,114,134).

The fine specificity characteristics of influenza A virus-immune CTL are of interest because of the divergence between cellular and serologic patterns. Antisera elicited by immunization with one subtype of influenza A virus will generally possess hemagglutination inhibiting or neutralizing capacity for viruses of the same subtype but not for heterologous viruses of other subtypes (212). In contrast, several laboratories observed that primary CTL elicited *in vivo* with virus of one subtype would lyse H-2-compatible target cells infected with virus of any type A influenza subtype (27,60,258,277). One group that failed to observe this cross-reactivity and found a largely subtype-specific CTL response utilized substantially different experimental protocols from those reporting the cross-reactivity (62–64). However, when the primary *in vivo* antiinfluenza A virus CTL response was analyzed further by means of "cold-target" competitive inhibition protocols, evidence for two subpopulations of CTL was obtained (27,60,276). One subpopulation was cross-reactive for histocompatible target cells infected with influenza A virus of any subtype, while the second was relatively specific for virus of the subtype used for immunization (homologous virus). The existence of these subpopulations has been substantiated by analysis of the fine specificity of cloned influenza A virus-specific CTL (30,147). In addition, the data obtained with cloned CTL suggest that subtype-specific CTL can be further classified into cells with specificity for determinants unique to the immunizing virus (virus specific) and cells with specificity for determinants shared by all the viruses of a given subtype (truly subtype-specific) (30).

The characteristics of secondary CTL responses to influenza A viruses differ in some respects from primary CTL responses. If immune mice are rechallenged with the same virus used for initial priming, the secondary CTL response elicited is usually of low magnitude; whereas if the virus used for secondary challenge is of a distinct subtype (compared to that of the priming virus), a vigorous response generally ensues. This potent heterologous secondary CTL population is composed primarily of cross-reactive cells (59). The difficulty encountered in eliciting homologous secondary CTL responses to influenza A virus *in vivo* has been attributed to neutralizing antibody remaining in the circulation following the initial priming, although other factors could be involved as well (suppressor cells?) (145). Nevertheless, if spleen cells from a primed animal are adoptively transferred into an 850 rad-irradiated syngeneic recipient and challenged with the homologous virus, a strong response is observed (59). Such is also the case if the immune spleen cells are restimulated with homologous, virus-infected cells *in vitro* (27,276). In both cases, cross-reactive and subtype-specific CTL are generated. If immune spleen cells are restimulated *in vitro* with isolated HA, however, the resultant response is predominantly subtype specific in nature (29,276).

In view of the different specificity patterns manifested by serum antibody and populations of splenic CTL, it was of interest to determine which molecule(s) carried the epitopes (antigenic determinants) recognized by CTL. A variety of observations have confirmed that the subtype-specific CTL recognize epitopes on the HA. First, isolated HA (from the same virus used for priming) can elicit a highly subtype-specific secondary *in vitro* response. Second, monoclonal hybridoma antibodies with specificity for the HA can partially inhibit subtype-specific CTL-mediated lysis *in vitro* (61); such antibodies can also depress the generation of subtype-specific CTL (to a greater extent than cross-reactive CTL) when administered *in vivo* 3 or more hours after primary challenge with virus (93). Third, subtype-specific or virus-specific clones lyse histocompatible target cells infected with viruses encoding NAs other than the NA of the virus used to generate those clones, but they do not lyse target cells expressing HAs of subtypes other than the immunizing subtype (30).

The identity of the viral molecule(s) that carries the epitope(s) recognized by the cross-reactive or type-specific CTL is controversial. Several investigators reported that M protein could be detected on the surfaces of infected cells (1,2,13,28,201). Since the M protein is antigenically similar (by serologic criteria) for all type A influenza viruses (36), these observations of cell surface expression of the M protein suggested that the M protein might carry the epitope(s) recognized by the cross-reactive CTL. However, all the studies that claimed to demonstrate M protein on the surfaces of infected cells utilized antisera which could have contained minor contaminating populations of antibodies specific for antigenic determinants normally expressed on the surfaces of infected cells. These postulated contaminant antibodies of non-M specificity could have reacted with their respective epitopes on the surfaces of infected cells, leading the investigators to interpret the observed reactions as evidence for the expression of M protein in the infected cell membrane.

More recent reports by Hackett et al. (95) and Yewdell et al. (264) make use of monoclonal hybridoma antibodies specific for the M protein of type A influenza viruses. Their results suggest that M protein may be expressed on the plasma membranes of influenza A virus-infected cells but in signficantly smaller amounts than estimated by Ada and Yap (1). Furthermore, Hackett et al. (95) were unable to block *in vitro* CTL-mediated killing of infected cells with monoclonal or heterogenous antibodies specific for M protein, even in the presence of anti-H-2 antibodies. Monoclonal anti-H-2 antibodies have been demonstrated to markedly enhance *in vitro* inhibition of cross-reactive influenza A-specific CTL by anti-HA monoclonal antibodies (8). It is relevant that the CTL being inhibited in the latter study were cross-reactive. Thus it has been demonstrated that cross-reactive CTL specific for influenza A virus-infected cells have specificity for an epitope(s) on the HA molecule. Koszinowski et al. (132) have also provided evidence that cross-reactive influenza A-specific CTL recognize an antigenic determinant(s) on the HA (or NA) surface glycoprotein. They demonstrated that target cells unable to express M protein by virtue of mutation or methods of preparation were susceptible to lysis by cross-reactive CTL.

Although the available evidence strongly indicates that cross-reactive CTL can recognize an epitope(s) on the HA, the NP has not yet been rigorously excluded as an additional cross-reactive antigen. The NP protein is a noteworthy possibility because, as for the M protein, all type A influenza viruses share serologically similar NP molecules (36). In this context, the detection of the cell surface expression of NP protein by Virelizier et al. (239) and Yewdell et al. (264) is noteworthy. There is no current evidence to suggest a role for the NA as an immunogen or antigen in the CTL response elicited by influenza A virus.

The role of CMI in the pathogenesis of influenza A virus infection has been systematically addressed only in the past few years. Conflicting results were obtained in early experiments, with some investigators inferring a protective role for CMI (212), while others favored no role (110) or even pathologic activity of CMI (222,229). In none of these experiments were the effects of different subsets of T cells assessed separately, and in some, antibody-mediated effects also may have confounded interpretation.

Recently, Yap et al. (259–262) have studied this issue in depth. They found a negative correlation between lung virus titer (following intravenous inoculation of live influenza A virus) and cytotoxic activity in the lungs. Significant numbers of cytotoxic cells sensitive to anti-Thy 1.2 serum plus complement were also recoverable from lungs and bronchoalveolar washings 5 to 7 days following intranasal challenge with live virus. In adoptive transfer experiments, these investigators established that primary or secondary influenza A virus-immune spleen cells could confer significant protection against intranasal challenge with a lethal dose of live virus and substantially reduce lung virus titers as well. They further demonstrated that the cells responsible for the protective effect (and the reduction of virus titers) were T cells restricted by H-2K and/or H-2D antigens and sensitive to anti-Ly 2.1 serum plus complement, and that protective activity correlated with cytotoxic activity. The protective effects of adoptively transferred spleen cells were highest for challenge virus of the same subtype as the virus used to prime the transferred cells, but significant protection could be obtained for heterologous type A challenge viruses. As seen for cytotoxicity assays, no cross-reactivity (cross-protection) was seen between type A and type B influenza viruses. More recently, Lin and Askonas (148) have reported that adoptive transfer of cloned cytotoxic T cells protects syngeneic sublethally irradiated mice against a lethal challenge dose of a homologous type A influenza virus. Additionally, these cloned T cells were demonstrated to reduce lung virus titers in mice infected with a homologous or heterologous type A influenza virus. Based on these observations, CTL may play a role in recovery from influenza A virus infection in the mouse lung.

These studies do not provide any definitive evidence on the role, if any, of CTL in the development of the pulmonary pathology associated with influenza A virus infection in the mouse. Yap et al. (263) obtained evidence suggesting that CTL do not contribute to lung pathology, which follows intranasal infection with A/WSN influenza virus. In their studies, athymic (nude) mice generally had greater degrees of pulmonary consolidation and epithelial proliferation (in areas of consolidation) than normal littermates. Furthermore, adoptive transfer of A/WSN-immune splenic T cells, restimulated *in vitro* to nude mice, improved their survival and did not appear to increase the extent of consolidation. Other investigators, using either A/PR8 (257) or A/HK (228) influenza viruses, found that nude mice had less average lung consolidation and longer average survival than normal littermates. Whether the differences in these results with nude mice can be attributed to the different virus strains used or other factors remains to be determined. In any case, the evidence implicating CTL in recovery from influenza A virus infection appears to be stronger at present than the evidence suggesting their role in causing pathology.

Evidence suggests that another type of T cell, termed Td, responsible for mediating delayed-type hypersensitivity (DTH), may contribute to the development of immunopathology in the lungs of mice infected with influenza A virus. Leung and Ada (144) found that following intranasal inoculation of mice with varying doses of influenza A virus, DTH activity (on adoptive transfer) was proportional to the virus dose and degree of pulmonary consolidation. Furthermore, adoptive transfer of cell populations with high Td and low Tc activities not only failed to protect mice from challenge with a lethal intranasal dose of virus but actually increased mortality. The cells with DTH activity recovered from the lungs of infected mice were type specific and classifiable as Td by virtue of possessing the Ly 1 phenotype and requiring I-region homology between donor and recipient for adoptive transfer of DTH activity.

A number of other functional types of T cells have been described in immune responses to influenza A virus: suppressor cells for Td (146), suppressor cells for Tc (145), and helper cells for Tc (7,200). Their respective roles in determining the outcome of pulmonary infections with influenza A virus in mice remain to be defined.

While evidence now exists to support the notion that virus-specific CTL play a role in recovery from pulmonary infection with influenza A virus in mice, one may wonder whether the murine model has any relevance for the human disease. A definitive answer is not yet available, but evidence suggests that humans are capable of mounting cellular immune responses to influenza A virus comparable to the well-characterized CTL responses of mice.

It has been demonstrated that *in vitro* exposure of human PBL to influenza A virus-infected autologous cells results in the generation of virus-specific CTL (17,152,153). In addition, these CTL have been shown to be restricted by HLA-A- and HLA-B-associated determinants (16,153), in analogy to the H-2K- and H-2D-associated restriction elements recognized in conjunction with exogenous antigen by murine CTL. Human CTL exhibited type specificity. They would lyse autologous target cells infected with the type A virus used for stimulation or another type A virus of a different subtype but not autologous target cells infected with a type B influenza virus (152). Thus human influenza A virus-specific CTL share a number of characteristics with murine CTL specific for the same virus. Nevertheless, further research is required before it will be possible to assess the role of CTL in human influenza, even to the extent achieved for mouse influenza.

One more aspect of the research on influenza A virus-specific CTLs merits discussion. Doherty et al. (49) demonstrated that the ability of mice of different inbred strains to mount CTL responses to an influenza A virus varied with the H-2 genotypes of the mice. This observation has been confirmed and extended for the human CTL response (16,151). Evidence has been accumulating to suggest that control over the magnitude of human CTL responsiveness to influenza A virus-infected cells is determined not only by the genes (HLA-A and HLA-B) encoding the relevant restriction elements but also by other genes in the HLA complex (15,16,151). Thus the role of CTL in the human disease caused by influenza A viruses may depend to some extent on the genotype of the particular host infected. Concepts of the genetic control of immune responsiveness and, potentially, disease susceptibility gained from the study of the antiinfluenza A virus CTL response may apply to other clinically important situations and may become among the most significant results of this line of investigation.

ORTHOPOXVIRUSES

Introduction

Although smallpox (variola) appears to have been eradicated from the human population, investigation of the orthopoxviruses will continue to provide insights of major significance to the understanding of viral-host interactions. Jenner (116), whose pioneering use of cowpox lymph vaccine predated the discovery of viruses by more than a century, predicted the eventual elimination of smallpox. While the urgency of studying the orthopoxviruses has diminished, the ability of these viruses to infect the mouse, rat, rabbit, monkey, and other laboratory animals, as well as cultured cell lines, has made their pathogenesis the subject of intensive study for more than 50 years. Virologists have exploited the unique complexity and cytoplasmic DNA replication of the orthopoxviruses to gain information about genetic regulation (37,111,160). Cellular immunologists, on the other hand, have used ectromelia (mousepox) and vaccinia as tools in dissecting the genetics of the immune system. Much of our recent information about virus-cell interactons is a "by-product" of the recent discoveries (e.g., MHC restriction and Ir genes) (reviewed in ref. 271).

The devastating impact of smallpox and mousepox on nonimmune populations makes it reasonable to assume that orthopoxviruses have had a major evolutionary influence on the vertebrate immune system.

Biochemistry and Morphogenesis

The orthopoxviruses, which include vaccinia, rabbitpox, cowpox, monkeypox, mousepox (ectromelia), and smallpox (variola), are the largest animal viruses and the most complex in terms of nucleic acid content, particle size, and morphology (12,111). All poxviruses are antigenically related by common internal NP, but the orthopoxviruses are further related by shared antigenic determinants on outer coat proteins. This most likely reflects a conserved central region comprising roughly 25% of the total 120 to 145 $\times$ 10^6 dalton double-stranded DNA genome. The DNA is complexed with NP to form a nucleoid surrounded by elliptical (lateral) bodies (which may contain specific DNAse inhibitors) and the lipoprotein membrane of the outer coat. In contrast to the viral envelopes of influenza and other budding viruses, this outer membrane of the classically studied virus form grown *in vitro* appears to be a unique structure, not incorporating any preexisting host membrane. However, the concept of the poxvirus membrane has become more complex with the demonstration of two forms of complete infective particles (5,26,182). Intracellular naked virus (INV) particles comprise >90% of virus recovered *in vitro* from commonly used host cells (180,181). These particles remain within the cytoplasm long after the demise of the cell (180). A more recently discovered minority population of extracellular enveloped virus (EEV) buds from the cell surface or is packaged in the Golgi apparatus (5,26,179,182), thereby acquiring a second membrane and at least eight additional protein components (179), including an 89k HA (180) presumably incorporated from the infected cell membrane where it is expressed as a "late" antigen (90; see below). Payne and Norrby (183) found EEV to be twice as infectious *in vitro* as INV, showing faster penetration and greater resistance to environmental inhibitors. The antigenic distinctiveness of INV and EEV is relevant to studies described below but has been largely overlooked.

No specific viral receptor has been identified on host cells, although adsorption appears to occur prior to phagocytosis and pinocytosis, the main routes of entry (160). There is some uncertainty over the role of membrane-membrane fusion in core injection, since the INV envelope apparently is not absolutely required for infectivity (112). Upon penetration, the viral membrane phospholipid and protein coats are degraded by host enzymes releasing the NP core, which is broken down step-wise in a second stage. Complete uncoating of the viral DNA requires the participation of immediate early messenger RNA (mRNA) transcripts of the viral genome coding for proteolytic enzymes. The delayed early RNAs are transcribed as the full DNA core is uncovered, and only after DNA replication has begun do the late mRNAs appear. Thus complete virus particles are not present until at least

4 hr postinfection, although viral proteins are present in the cell membrane within the first hour. The significance of this "eclipse" phase will be discussed. About 7 hr after infection, a wave of new virus is released and spreads to new sites via blood, lymph, and macrophages, or cell to cell (156).

Pathogenesis

The classic studies of Fenner (73–76) with ectromelia and vaccinia remain the paradigm for poxvirus pathogenesis. Entrance through a break in the skin or footpad inoculation leads to local replication and spread to local draining lymph nodes in the first 24 hr. Dissemination to and replication within deeper regional nodes also may occur during this period. Further replication and lysis results in a primary viremia and dissemination throughout the body, in particular to liver and spleen, by day 3. A secondary viremia follows extensive multiplication in parenchymal cells of these organs and leads to local infection of skin and mucous membranes (the characteristic "pocks") by day 6 or 7. Death or recovery hinges on events in the liver (18–21). The spread of virus via lymph or blood occurs as free particles in the plasma and intracellularly, principally within macrophages. Free virus is cleared from the blood of normal mice within minutes (18,156) by littoral macrophages. This intracellular transport of virus is of fundamental importance, allowing both intracellular replication and access by diapedesis to extravascular host organs (156).

Primary Response

Because of the protective advantage thought to be conferred by high postvaccination Ab titers against reinfection (5,26,156), the protection afforded by some passive immunization protocols (5,26,73,75,76), and the nonvirulence of premixed antiserum plus virus inocula (156), it was traditionally thought that neutralizing antibody was responsible for recovery from primary pox infection. Long before the discovery of T cells, however, it was clear that the kinetics of pathogenesis did not correspond to the primary Ab response which, by most techniques used, does not appear until at least day 6 postinfection and does not peak until approximately day 14 (31,73–76), that is, long after virus has been cleared from the tissues of recovering animals. Downie (58) detected specific Ab in human smallpox only after day 5 of the clinical illness or, since symptoms are preceded by a 12-day incubation period, 17 days after infection. Of course, antibody might be functionally present without appearing in the serum, but Fenner (73,76) found that passive immunization with antivaccinia or antiectromelia sera were, respectively, not protective or only partially protective against ectromelia. Unfortunately, Ab response was monitored in many of these early studies by anti-HA titers, even though INV lacking HA was used as the primary infecting agent. Conversely, incomplete protection against live virus challenge following passive or active immunization against INV cannot be interpreted as evidence against the ability of antibody to provide complete protection.

Thus Appleyard, Boulter, and Andrews (5,26) showed that anti-EEV but not anti-INV antisera protected rabbits from lethal doses of poxvirus.

More recently, Payne (181) tested 13 vaccinia strains in different cell lines for *in vitro* EEV production. With one exception (WR), inability to form EEV *in vitro* correlated with low *in vivo* pathogenicity. In all cases, antisera against the dissociated external envelope protected mice from lethal infection, whereas antisera to inactivated INV did not. Payne (181) sounds exactly the right note of caution:

> Interpretation of the *in vivo* data must be more restrained than for the *in vitro* results since the two systems are not strictly analogous. It must be remembered, for example, that the viraemia of other poxviruses . . . is largely cell associated. It should also be realized that the passively transferred antibody does not act in an immunological vacuum as it does *in vitro*. Antibodies directed at the envelope may not alone be sufficient to cause the regression of the infection. These antibodies may simply slow down virus dissemination long enough to permit the immunologically intact recipient to mobilize its cell-mediated immune defenses. Further work is needed to obtain clarification on this point.

The relative importance of cellular versus humoral immunity in the human primary response to poxviruses (and viruses in general) was suggested by observations of patients with immune deficiency diseases (79). Patients with congenital or acquired agammaglobulinemia can be successfully vaccinated against smallpox and recover from measles and other childhood viral diseases. By contrast, thymus-deficient children have developed severe generalized vaccinia infections following vaccination. These observations could not be fully interpreted prior to the discovery of lymphocyte subsets.

In a series of experiments, Blanden (18–20) established a crucial role for T cells in the primary response to ectromelia. Antithymocyte serum (ATS) injected just prior to inoculation resulted in 100% mortality by day 12, as compared to 20% in control groups receiving normal rabbit serum. Virus titer profiles during the first 2 days of infection were similar for both groups, indicating normal macrophage uptake and migration; but by day 6 to 7, the ATS-treated mice had about three orders of magnitude more virus in spleen and liver. Neutralizing antibody was not detectable in treated or untreated mice until 8 to 10 days and reached the same levels for both groups. Splenic interferon was much higher in ATS-treated mice on days 4 to 6 but afforded inadequate, if any, protection during this critical recovery period.

When Thy-positive, macrophage-depleted spleen cells from hyperimmune mice were adoptively transferred to mice that had received ectromelia 24 hr previously, virus replication was effectively reduced over the following 24 hr. The infected recipients did not have elevated antibody or interferon levels, and the passive transfer of hyperimmune serum to give high titers was much less effective than T cell transfer. A radiation-sensitive recipient cell (presumed to be a monocyte) was implicated, since 800 rad irradiated-infected hosts showed a decreased response to transferred antiviral immune cells or serum. To test this point, neutralizing antibody or immune cells were injected 24 hr after ectromelia into mice that were immunodepressed but had their macrophage function intact. Within 10 hr, mononuclear cells had invaded necrotic foci in the liver and within 24 hr had markedly reduced the amount of virus detectable by immunofluorescence. Similarly infiltrated lesions were observed in normally recovering mice by the sixth day of infection. Immunodepressed infected mice not receiving immune cells or sera did not develop mononuclear invasion of hepatic lesions, and these animals died.

These experiments established a vital if somewhat indirect role for virus-specific T cells as attractors and/or activators of monocyte-mediated virus destruction. Subsequently, a more direct role was posited for T cells as the actual killers of infected cells (21,22,81–84, 133,137). Recent work has focused almost exclusively on this aspect and has been exhaustively reviewed (271). The basic assay to detect virus-specific CTL uses transformed fibroblast lines, macrophages, or lymphocyte blasts of known H-2 haplotypes which are preincubated with radioactive chromium and infected *in vitro*. These cells then are exposed to immune lymphocytes from virus-infected mice at 37° C for 6 to 8 hr at which time the amount of chromium released into medium is measured.

Gardner and colleagues (82–84) first showed that the kinetics of splenic antipox CTL were similar to those described by Blanden (19,20) for transferred protection: first detectable by day 2, peaking at day 6, and disappearing by day 10. Identical kinetics were demonstrated for the appearance of specific CTL in the cerebrospinal fluid after intracerebral injection of virus (98).

The poxvirus-specific T cell-mediated cytotoxic response was shown to follow the rules of MHC restriction (50,70,81–83, 133,273); i.e., poxvirus is recognized by CTL precursors and effectors in the context of private (but not public) determinants on H-2K or H-2D cell-surface glycoproteins. Homology at either K or D is necessary and sufficient for either primary stimulation or effector function. On the other hand, I-region homology is neither necessary nor sufficient, although it may serve some role in amplification of the responses. To demonstrate the restriction to K or D of effector function required merely the appropriate infected and unlabeled competing targets, but to show that the same criteria applied for *in vivo* stimulation required the acute removal of alloreactivity to non-K or -D alloantigens prior to stimulation in the relevant adoptive K- or D-homologous host. This was accomplished by "negative selection" filtration through irradiated intermediary animals (11). For example, B10.D2 (K^dI-A^dD^d) cells filtered through irradiated B10.A(5R) (K^bI-A^bD^d) mice to remove alloresponsiveness to K^b-I-A^b make a strong virus-specific response at H-2D^d, but not H-2K^b, when stimulated in adoptive B10.A(5R) hosts.

Fine analysis with H-2 mutants has revealed certain details of this restriction (23,123,150,266,271,272,275). Thus poxvirus-immune T cells from H-2^{bm1}, H-2^{bh}, and H-2^{bg1} mutants, respectively, lyse the wild-type-infected K^b target poorly, substantially, and completely, as compared with wild-type effectors. These mutants are all killed by third-party anti-H-2K^b alloreactive cells but differ in their interrelatedness, as judged by reciprocal skin-grafting. In general, mutations causing rapid graft rejection abolish antiviral cross-reactivity, even in the presence of third-party allorecognition. This suggests an intimate association between viral antigens and limited areas of the H-2 molecules. Where tested, identical restriction patterns between host and donor with respect to K/D, I, and mutant H-2 molecules have been found for *in vivo* antiviral protection in adoptive transfer systems (123,150).

Differences in the requirements for primary *in vivo* CTL induction versus CTL effector function *in vitro* have also been demonstrated with mutants. Mice carrying the H-2^{db} mutation have a deletion in the L molecule, which is coded in the H-2D^d region and carries public specificities. These mice do not generate a primary *in vivo* response to ectromelia at H-2D, although they respond well at H-2K when tested on appropriate infected targets *in vitro*. Nevertheless, H-2^{db}-infected targets are lysed as well as H-2D^d targets by wild-type effectors (25). This dichotomy between the H-2^{db} stimulator and target is intriguing, especially in light of the subsequent finding of Biddison et al. (14) that H-2^{db} mice make a good *in vivo* response to the closely related vaccinia virus. Unfortunately, the ability of vaccinia- or ectromelia-infected H-2^{db} mice to cross-reactively lyse ectromelia- or vaccinia-infected targets, respectively, was not tested.

The H-2^{db} mutation represents one type of Ir gene leading to low response at H-2D. Other low-responder situations have been found (48,274). There is no stimulation at D^k for any haplotype, regardless of K or I-A alleles; unlike the D^{db} mutation, there is no way to test for suitable target presentation. This could be a case of poor association between virus and H-2D^k. The idea that virus must associate with an MHC molecule in order to be recognized fits with a third type of low-responder situation, in which a K allele determines the level of response at a D allele; i.e., K^k causes low response to D^b plus vaccinia, whereas K^b, K^q, or K^s permit high response. This effect is virus specific and dominant in the F$_1$, but not absolute since low response at D^b can be converted to high response if stimulation is carried out in the absence of K^k (11) or if K^{k}D^b effectors have grown up in a chimeric host not expressing K^k (274). To date, no I-region immune response genes have been found for antiviral CTL, although they are the rule for Th involved in antibody production or responses to Ia-restricted bacterial antigens. Either T help is not crucial in the vaccinia response, or it operates via K/D.

These findings are reasonable if the T cell must "see" a neoantigen-virus in association with K or D, and if K^k has an exceptionally high affinity for vaccinia. This favors a "single" as opposed to a "dual" receptor (one for virus, one for MHC) model of the T cell receptor. It is not within the scope of this review to discuss the merits of each model, but it is important to consider what is being recognized by the "immune surveillance" system.

We have already noted the appearance of early eclipse proteins on the infected cell membrane. That these early proteins can stimulate a primary response and serve as target antigens was demonstrated by Ada and colleagues (3,115) and by Ertl et al. (70,134,135), while Zinkernagel and Althage (267) showed that lysis could occur *in vitro* before infectious progeny were assembled. Obviously, such abortive lysis would be highly beneficial *in vivo*. The cell type requirements for primary stimulation were analyzed *in vitro* by Blanden and colleagues (24). This proved a much more difficult task than 2° *in vitro* restimulation (81); under optimal conditions, however, the primary response paralleled *in vivo* kinetics, and macrophages were crucial in the stimulator population either as stimulators per se or as accessory cells. The difficulty of obtaining good primary responses *in vitro* has limited the use of this system, but it may offer a means of defining the role of Th in the primary response.

Before moving on to the secondary response, some studies by Worthington and colleagues (254–256) must be mentioned. They represent a counterbalance to the idea that T cell-mediated responses are paramount in primary recovery. Their arguments in favor of the role of antibody have been largely ignored but never satisfactorily refuted. Briefly, mice were immunodepressed by either irradiation or cyclophosphamide and infected with vaccinia. Mortality in these mice was 90%, as compared to 20 to 30% in mice also receiving immune antisera on day 3 or 4. Even as late as day 7 postinfection, transferred Ab cut mortality in half. In contrast, immune lymphocytes transferred on day 3 decreased mortality only by half and, if transferred after day 3, had virtually no protective effect. In addition, neonatally thymectomized mice [judged T cell deficient by the absence of T cell-induced mortality after lymphocytic choriomeningitis virus (LCMV) infection] showed no significant mortality after vaccinia injection. It was concluded that antibody was of paramount importance in the primary response. The validity of this conclusion rests on two points: (a) Ab titers comparable to those artificially induced are present by day 3 to 7 in the course of normal infection; and (b) CMI does not play a critical role prior to day 3. The authors demonstrated the first point, but this early appearance of Ab is not in line with other studies (29,56,71–74). The second point is presumably supported by the neonatal thymectomy studies but conflicts with the finding that nu/nu (nude T cell-deficient) mice always succumb to vaccinia (70).

Ontogeny of the Primary Response

Fenner (75) demonstrated that partial protection against primary infection was conferred on mice suckling immune mothers by passively transferred Ab in milk and blood. Recent work in our laboratory (214) suggests that T cell immunity is also important in very young animals. By day 8 of life, baby mice can be primed to give an antivaccinia cytotoxic T cell response which follows the kinetics and H-2 restriction pattern of adults. Mice infected within the first week of life generally die within 2 to 6 days. However, thymocytes from 3-day-old animals adoptively transferred to irradiated, infected adults make a strong primary cytotoxic response, as do transferred spleen cells from donors 8 days old or older. Thus the resistance to virus in the suckling offspring of nonimmune mothers parallels the appearance of competent CTL precursors in the periphery. Of course, Th cells for Ab production may also play a role.

Secondary Response

Although the discriminatory capacity of T cells is generally as fine as that of B cells or antiserum, there are often important differences for *in vivo* responses, reflecting, at the population level, the differences between what the H-2-restricted T cell and the unrestricted B cell clones recognize. Thus, as discussed in preceding sections, T but not B cells make a strong response to cross-reactive determinants of influenza subtypes. In considering the possible role of T cells in protection against secondary poxvirus infection following vaccination, it is important to emphasize that serologically related poxviruses are found to be cross-reactive for T cell recognition as well (82,83).

It has generally been assumed that circulating Ab would frustrate any attempts to generate secondary cytotoxic T cells by neutralizing injected virus. While this has been shown to be the case for homologous influenza strains, it has not been formally demonstrated in the pox literature. This restimulation problem has been circumvented in two ways: (a) restimulation of primed cells in an irradiated adoptive host; and (b) restimulation *in vitro*. Only the latter has been studied for poxviruses (24,81,97,150,173–176,271); the following points emerged. *In vitro*, a secondary rather than a primary response is much easier to elicit. Nevertheless, since the kinetics, pattern of K/D restriction for induction and killing, and H-2K^b mutant reactivity are the same for *in vitro* secondary and *in vivo* primary responses, there would seem to be no change in specificity or affinity. In mice, memory cells capable of being restimulated appeared in the spleen 2 weeks after priming, reached a plateau at 5 to 6 weeks, and persisted for at least 16 months (i.e., the life of the mouse). Ia-positive macrophages were more efficient stimulators than Ia-positive B cells, which in turn were superior to Ia-negative T cells, and infection with ultraviolet or γ-irradiated or gluteraldehyde-fixed nonreplicating virus was sufficient for induction and target presentation. Macrophages were also found to play a nonpresenting accessory role when added as late as day 3 of culture.

Although H-2-I region homology was unnecessary at the stimulatory or effector stage, it did induce a significant virus-specific proliferative response, which could be abrogated by treatment of responders with α-Ly-1 sera. Cytotoxicity of secondary responders was only slightly diminished by this treatment but markedly reduced by α-Ly-2 treatment or by pretreatment of responders with α-Ly-1 prior to secondary stimulation.

These findings (all from one group of investigators) are paradoxical. The need for Ia-positive stimulators and Ly-1$^+$ responders suggests a role for H-2-I-restricted Th cells, but the irrelevance of H-2-I-region homology for induction or killing suggests just the opposite. A similar situation is seen for primary *in vitro* alloreactivity (reviewed in ref. 245) and suggests that H-2-I-restricted cells may be amplifiers rather than absolutely required components of the cytotoxic response.

The *in vitro* demonstration of secondary T cell cytotoxicity is no guarantee of *in vivo* relevance, and a search of the literature reveals a single study in humans addressing this point. Perrin and colleagues (189) inoculated volunteers who had been vaccinated as children with vaccinia virus. The authors were looking for an HLA-restricted cytotoxic T cell response. Instead, they found ADCC, which was virus specific but not HLA restricted. Although high titers of antibody did not develop upon revaccination, a definite enhancement of ADCC was seen when PBLs were incubated with targets and postrevaccination compared to prerevaccination serum. The authors suggested that dose and route of administration could modulate the magnitude of the cytotoxic T cell response.

In the case of orthopoxviruses, there is little solid evidence to support the widely repeated statement that antibody provides the main defense against reinfection. The classic studies of Fenner (73–77) are usually cited as proof, but we have seen that these studies argue just as strongly against the adequacy of antibody. Why, for example, should antivaccinia antibody be considered protective against reinfection when passive immunization with hyperimmune sera is not always protective upon primary exposure? If T cells are responsible for eliminating a primary infection, why should an amnestic cellular defense not suffice for secondary protection? It is well known that IgG titers remain elevated for years after exposure (58), but the same is true of recirculating memory T cells. It is also true that the secondary amnestic Ab response comes up more quickly than the primary, but this still cannot account for protection against the initial viremia. For example, Ab appears 14 days after smallpox exposure in vaccinated individuals, as compared to 17 days in nonvaccinated patients (58). Indeed, even the extrapolation of *in vitro* neutralization to *in vivo* conditions may be an oversimplification. We simply do not know enough about the fate of Ab-virus complexes formed *in vivo*.

An intriguing role for virus-specific antibody in protecting against reinfection is suggested by Veada and Nozima (236) in mice and Shultz et al. (220) in rabbits. The authors found that macrophages from previously immunized animals were highly resistant to viral infection *in vitro*. Furthermore, by either rosetting (236) or elution (220), virus-specific cytophilic macrophage-bound antibody could be demonstrated on resistant but not on normal cells. This resistance was lost after 4 to 7 days in culture, possibly because of Ab elution and degradation. These studies do not address other possible factors, such as increased enzyme activity of activated macrophages; they do suggest, however, in view of the extreme importance of intracellular viral replication and spread (156), a possible critical role for cell-bound Ab which might not even be detectable in serum.

Host-Virus Interaction: A Case Study

At the outset of this discussion, we mentioned the likelihood that poxviruses had exerted significant evolutionary pressure on their hosts. Myxomatosis, while not classified in the genus orthopox, is a closely related poxvirus. First isolated from laboratory rabbits, in which it is almost 100% lethal, it was released as a means of pest control into the wild rabbit populations of Australia (1950) and Europe (1952) (reviewed in ref. 77). The immediate effect was to drastically reduce, without completely eradicating, these populations. With time, the wild populations recovered to some extent, never reaching original levels because of the constant presence of enzootic and occasionally epizootic myxomatosis. Surveys of field strains recovered from wild populations at annual or longer intervals showed the early appearance and persistence of new strains of myxomatosis, all of lesser virulence than the original strain (which in Australia was repeatedly released). The reason for this decrease in virulence is presumably the increased potential transmission; i.e., survival of the fittest virus species does not necessarily mean survival of the most lethal, especially when host vectors are rare. Samples of unexposed wild rabbit populations over the same period revealed increasing resistance to the original virus when tested in laboratory conditions; i.e., with succeeding generations, increasing numbers of nonimmune wild rabbits survived an infection lethal for 100% of laboratory animals. Such genetic resistance may reflect the polymorphism of the MHC if, for example, certain alleles allow good stimulation of the cellular and humoral immune response. Alternatively, it may reflect selection for a particularly efficient set of germ-line variable region combining site genes in linkage disequilibrium. In addition, there are may other aspects of natural immunity (e.g., phagocyte enzyme levels, host membrane virus receptors, host support of viral replication) which undoubtedly are relevant.

Summary

Studies with poxviruses illustrate a wide range of host-virus interactions:

1. Macrophages have a role in the transport, replication, and destruction of viruses as well as the presentation of viral antigen to T cells.

2. Uptake and inactivation of free virus by phagocytes are greatly enhanced by specific antibody which recognizes virus particles in the blood. The role of Ab in recognizing viral proteins on infected cells is unclear but has been demonstrated in humans with ADCC. Complement-mediated lysis is another possibility. In addition to opsonizing virus, Ab seems to interfere with the uncoating of the poxvirus DNA core.

3. In contrast to B cells, T cells recognize poxvirus exposed on cell surfaces in the context of MHC molecules. A role for Th cells restricted to H-2-I-region molecules has not yet been shown for T-T or T-B collaboration, but this may reflect the inadequacy of approaches used so far. The fact that IgG is produced in response to poxviruses suggests the participation of Th in the IgM-IgG switch. The use of Lyt-specific cytotoxic monoclonal Abs in conjunction with adoptive transfer experiments might establish the T cell subtypes involved.

4. Differences in the requirements for primary induction versus target recognition or 2° stimulation have been demonstrated. Whether these are qualitative or quantitative is unclear.

5. The relative importance of humoral versus cellular immunity in the primary and secondary response is unresolved. The ability of T cells to eliminate intracellular virus suggests they may be of greatest importance in the primary response and whenever virus gets past the front-line defense of circulating antibody in the secondary response. Careful examination of vaccinated children's primary T and B cell responses would be extremely useful, but smallpox vaccination may soon be, like the disease itself, a thing of the past.

6. Aspects of natural immunity, such as interferon, NK cells, and levels of hydrolytic activity within macrophages, undoubtedly are important in the overall response but have not been dealt with here.

7. The ability of virus to directly influence the evolution of a wild species over only a few decades has been noted, although the genetic basis for this has not been investigated.

Research on poxviruses has led to the eradication of a major scourge of mankind and raised at least as many important questions about host-virus interactions as it has answered.

ACUTE INFECTION WITH EPSTEIN-BARR VIRUS AND THE IMMUNE RESPONSE

Introduction

The Epstein-Barr virus (EBV), a herpes virus discovered in 1964 (68), is the causative agent of infectious mononucleosis (IM) (47,103,166). It is now clear, however, that infection with EBV can lead to a spectrum of clinical and pathologic states and outcomes ranging from asymptomatic seroconversion to florid, life-threatening immunopathologic processes (66). Furthermore, there is reason to believe that the immune response capabilities of the host are a critical factor in determining the course of the host's encounter with EBV (193–195). The ability of EBV to persist for life in immune hosts in a latent form (91,155), to infect B lymphocytes (42,120,177) and transform them (47) into cells capable of unlimited lifespan *in vitro* [lymphoblastoid cell lines (LCL)], and its strong, possibly causal, associations with African Burkitt lymphoma (BL) (reviewed in ref. 67) and nasopharyngeal carcinoma (NPC) (128) all serve to enhance the relevance and importance of this model for the understanding of virus-immune system interactions. Therefore, emphasis in this section is placed on the immunoregulatory phenomena that determine the nature of the clinical and pathologic manifestations of EBV infection. Because of space limitations, IM will be the main focus, with reference to BL and NPC only when necessary.

Before proceeding with a discussion of the immunopathogenesis of IM, it will be helpful to briefly review the characteristics of EBV-determined antigens. The lymphocyte-defined membrane antigen (LYDMA) was discovered in the course of investigating T CMC against EBV genome-containing B cells *in vitro* (230) and is now thought to be expressed on the surfaces of all EBV genome-carrying cells (127). It is the only EBV-determined antigen not detected serologically (65).

The EB nuclear antigen (EBNA) is present in the nuclei of all EBV genome-positive cells (197). Viral DNA synthesis is not required for its production (65).

Two types of membrane antigens (MA) have been described (69,129,221). An early component (EMA) is found in BL tumor cells *in vivo* and in some cells of virus-producing LCL but not in cells of nonproductive LCL (65). The late MA

(LMA) component is found in cells following EBV DNA synthesis in the late phase of viral replication, and viral capsid antigen (VCA) is expressed concurrently (69,221). MA and VCA are the only EBV-determined antigens known to be present in the mature EB virion; since only MA would be expressed on the surface of the virion subsequent to budding through the host cell plasma membrane (65), it is not surprising that neutralizing activity for EBV is associated with MA-specific antibody (45,46,185,186).

A set of antigens associated with the initiation of EBV replication is collectively referred to as the early antigens (EA) (106). The presence of these antigens implies eventual cell death (65). Two patterns of EA distribution have been noted: (a) diffuse, with antigen in both nucleus and cytoplasm, and (b) restricted, with antigen found only in the cytoplasm (104). The ability of EBV to inhibit the biosynthesis of host cell macromolecules may be effected by the molecule(s) detected as EA (85).

VCA is the building block for the EBV capsid (101). The capsid surrounds the DNA-containing nucleoid and is in turn surrounded by the host cell membrane acquired as a consequence of budding (65). As noted above, VCA is expressed only following viral DNA synthesis in conjunction with LMA (86).

The most common result of natural primary exposure to EBV, generally in childhood in developing countries and in lower socioeconomic groups in developed countries, is inapparent infection (102) followed by lifelong seroconversion and complete immunity to IM (71,103,165,166,188,235,246). If primary infection is delayed until late adolescence or young adulthood, as commonly occurs in the upper socioeconomic groups in developed countries, IM will develop in approximately 50% of such instances (165). The factors that determine this age-dependent difference in the outcome of primary EBV infection remain incompletely understood, although viral dose, mode of entry, and immunologic or other physical parameters are considered to play a role (66). It is clear, however, that while seronegative persons are susceptible to IM, persons possessing circulating antibody specific for EBV (presumably neutralizing anti-MA) are not susceptible (66).

Initiation of EBV Infection in IM

EBV most likely gains entrance into the body in the oropharynx either by infecting oropharyngeal epithelial cells with subsequent infection of B lymphocytes or by directly infecting B cells of Waldeyer's ring (66). To date, the only cell type demonstrated to express receptors for EBV is the B cell (120,177). However, *in situ* cytohybridization studies with EBV nucleic acid have demonstrated EBV genome sequences in normal oropharyngeal squamous cells (143) and in nasopharyngeal carcinoma cells (253), suggesting the possibility that EBV infects and replicates in epithelial cells of the oropharynx in addition to infecting B cells. In any case, productive EBV infection is initiated in the oropharynx, and virus is disseminated throughout the body on the basis of either true viremia with infection of distant B cells or dissemination of B cells infected in or near the initial oropharyngeal focus of viral replication (66). Thus IM is a systemic disease.

Infection of B cells by EBV can result in a productive replication cycle with expression of EA, VCA, or LMA, leading inevitably to cell death, even if the cycle is aborted before viral release. Alternatively, EBV may cause two sorts of nonproductive infections: latent infection and malignant transformation (65). In typical cases of IM, malignant transformation is not considered to have a role. However, latent infection of B lymphocytes occurs during IM, and these cells contain copies of the EBV genome and express LYDMA (105). While relatively large numbers of latently infected B cells are in the circulation during the acute phase of IM (as many as 0.05% of mononuclear leukocytes), the number of such cells falls dramatically by the time of convalescence (205). Nevertheless, a small number of such latently infected cells remains in the host for life, as suggested by the ability to establish continuous EBV-carrying LCL *in vitro* from the blood or lymph node biopsies of seropositive individuals (47,167). Presumably, occasional activation of latent cells results in sufficient production of EBV-determined antigens to account for lifelong antibody titers to VCA, MA, and EBNA (91,155).

T Cell-Mediated Immunity

It is thought that the latently infected B cells expressing LYDMA induce the substantial T cell-proliferative response that is associated with IM (99,178,218) and which is believed to account for the cervical lymphadenomegaly, hepatosplenomegaly, and atypical lymphocytes (in peripheral blood) characteristic of IM (193). A considerable body of evidence now exists which suggests that this increase in T cell number is reflected in a variety of functional activities important in controlling B cell infection and proliferation (66). During the acute phase of IM, PBL-mediated cytotoxic activity specific for EBV-genome-carrying cells (generally LCL) can be demonstrated in the ^{51}Cr release assay (113,149,206,230). This specific cytotoxic activity declines with time as the disease progresses into the stage of convalescence (113). It was later established that the cells mediating the lysis of EBV-transformed LCL were T cells (215). Other investigators (202) demonstrated that T cells from the peripheral blood of acute IM patients could inhibit the outgrowth of fetal mononuclear cell cultures exposed to EBV much more effectively than T cells from seronegative adult donors or cord blood. The authors interpreted this phenomenon in terms of CTL activity directed against EBV-infected fetal cells.

In one of the above studies, the investigators addressed the issue of MHC restriction. Seeley et al. (215) concluded that primary CTL from acute IM patients specific for EBV-transformed LCL target cells were not, in general, restricted by the HLA-A and B antigens, although effectors from eight of 11 donors manifested preferential lytic activity against autologous (versus allogeneic) EBV-positive LCL targets. Seeley et al. (215) postulated, therefore, that in a heterogeneous effector population, some clones may be HLA restricted, while others are not so restricted. Slightly different results were obtained by Lipinski et al. (149). These authors failed to demonstrate HLA restriction (preference for self HLA alleles) of CTL lytic for EBV-transformed LCL, but they did observe a necessity for the expression of HLA-

A, B, and C antigens on the target cell surface for susceptibility to CTL-mediated lysis. This latter requirement was inferred from the low levels of lysis seen with HLA antigen-deficient Daudi cells as targets.

Secondary T cells generated *in vitro* in culture with EBV-infected B cells also have been found to lyse EBV-genome-positive LCL targets in the ^{51}Cr release assay (157) and to inhibit outgrowth of B cells infected with EBV *in vivo* or *in vitro* (161,162,203,204,231). While it has been relatively straightforward to obtain evidence for HLA restriction of these secondary T cells for both the ^{51}Cr release assay (157) and the inhibition of outgrowth assay (204), the relevance of those observations to the clinical situation in IM remains unclear. Since the presumed antigenic target of primary and secondary CTL (LYDMA) cannot yet be detected by a method independent of CTL-mediated lysis, it is not possible to conclude that the EBV-determined epitopes recognized by secondary CTL are the same as those with which primary CTL react. Thus the possibility remains that secondary CTL recognize, in addition to HLA restriction elements, epitopes not relevant *in vivo* during IM.

Although activation of CTL may account in part for the marked lymphocytosis seen in IM, considerable evidence suggests that suppressor T cells are also activated as a consequence of EBV infection of B cells (100,117,198,232). Several groups of investigators (100,198,232) were able to demonstrate suppression of the generation of Ig-secreting cells in response to *in vitro* culture with pokeweed mitogen by T cells from the peripheral blood of acute IM patients. In addition, Reinherz et al. (198) demonstrated deficient *in vitro* T cell-proliferative responses to mitogens, specific antigen, and alloantigen during the acute stage of the disease. It was generally found that suppressor activity was considerably reduced during convalescence (100,117,198), as was observed for CTL activity.

As pointed out above, both cytotoxic and suppressor activities are increased during acute IM and decrease toward normal with convalescence. Of related interest is the correlation of the numbers of circulating atypical lymphocytes in peripheral blood during acute IM with cytotoxic (113,206) and suppressor (100) activity. Therefore, one might wonder if the two activities are the same or at least the manifestations of a single cell type. Reinherz et al. (198) were not able to demonstrate any cytotoxic activity against autologous LCL targets, allogeneic LCL targets, or normal lymphocytes with lymphocytes from an acute IM patient, while this same patient's lymphocytes expressed considerable suppressor activity in *in vitro* cultures. The data presented do not allow the conclusion that cytotoxic T cells were absent from the donor; clearly, no general inference can be drawn regarding the overlap of suppressor and cytotoxic T cell subsets. Johnsen et al. (117) also present evidence suggesting that the suppressive activity of IM T cells is not cytotoxic.

Non-T Cell-Mediated Immunity to IM

What contribution to the control of EBV infection is made by other immune mechanisms? It has been suggested that while T cells, whether cytotoxic or suppressor, are particularly important during the acute stages of IM, antibody and non-T cells may provide the major forces responsible for maintaining the lifelong steady state between host and virus (127). The relatively constant levels of post-IM antibody titers to VCA, EBNA, and MA suggests that in small numbers of EBV-infected host B cells, spontaneously induced lytic cycles lead to production of mature virus particles and free virus antigens upon cell death (66). Intermittent excretion of infectious EBV into the oropharynx of individuals following convalescence, and for the rest of life (91,155), is consistent with this notion. Thus neutralizing (anti-MA) antibody may prevent any significant increase in the population of latently infected cells. Antibody to EBV-determined antigens might also play a role through the mechanism of antibody-dependent cellular cytotoxicity ADCC (184). It has been demonstrated that LCL target cells superinfected with the P_3HR-1 EBV strain are susceptible to lysis by ADCC (118,187), and antibodies reactive in the ADCC assay have been found in sera from patients with IM, BL, and NPC (118,184,187). The importance of ADCC *in vivo* may be difficult to define.

NK cells may also contribute to the host response to acute EBV infection (194). In order for Svedmyr and Jondal (230) to demonstrate EBV-specific cytotoxic T cells, they had to fractionate the effector lymphocyte populations they used (on the basis of complement receptors) to remove a high degree of nonspecific cytotoxicity mediated against LCL target cells, regardless of the expression of EBV-determined antigens. Others have also obtained evidence for nonspecific cytotoxicity, of the NK type, against EBV-infected cells (215). Whether such a mechanism can lyse B cells latently infected with EBV remains to be demonstrated.

Numerous observations linking altered immunologic function with fatal and/or complicated courses of IM emphasize the importance of immune mechanisms in the control of acute EBV infection and IM. Unfortunately, most immunodeficiency states are complex, being associated with deficits of more than one type. Thus in these patients, it is not generally possible to ascribe particular deviations from the normal pattern in host-EBV interactions to a single functional deficit. Nevertheless, studies of numerous patients with various immune deficiencies (194) suggest that defects in immune mechanisms may lead to the development of lymphoma following primary infection with EBV or following reactivation of latent EBV infection. Disordered regulation of various lymphoid subsets may also contribute to a variety of relatively uncommon complications of IM, such as hypogammaglobulinemia, asplastic anemia, and splenic rupture.

CONCLUSIONS AND FUTURE DIRECTIONS

The following are a few of the most significant general principles that might be extracted from a review of three different virus-host systems.

Lymphoid cells generally contribute to the control of virus infections, although the exact role and the net effect of immune responsiveness on the host's survival will vary. In certain cases, lymphoid cell-mediated immunopathology may be more significant than lymphocyte-mediated protective effects or virus-mediated tissue damage, as is the case with LCMV infection of the adult mouse brain (52). The importance of immunologically specific antiviral mechanisms must not be allowed to obscure the importance of the numerous nonspecific defense mechanisms: macrophages, complement, interferon, and the mucociliary blanket may, in given circumstances, participate in essential host resistance mechanisms against viruses.

In different virus-host systems, different subpopulations of lymphocytes may be of primary importance. It is particularly intriguing that in IM, Ts cells may significantly aid in controlling the EBV infection by controlling B cell proliferation, since EBV selectively infects, and is disseminated by, B cells. For a variety of other virus-host systems, it is conceivable that Ts cells serve mostly to prevent excessive B cell or effector T cell responses leading to immunopathologic processes in host tissues. Among other factors, the chief mode of spread of a given virus is likely to influence which types of lymphocytes or immunologic mechanisms are critical for host resistance. Furthermore, the relative importance of lymphocyte subpopulations may differ in primary versus secondary responses to the same virus.

Genetically controlled differences in immune responsiveness may affect, sometimes critically, the nature and outcome of virus-host interactions. A clear instance of this general principle is provided by the X-linked immunodeficiency syndrome which predisposes to fatal IM and malignant lymphoma following infection with EBV (reviewed in ref. 194). The *in vivo* relevance of MHC-determined variation in immune responsiveness to influenza viruses (reviewed in ref. 216) has yet to be determined, but progress in this system could provide valuable clues to understanding the associations of particular MHC alleles with particular diseases.

Viral glycoproteins are generally major determinants of viral pathogenicity and the primary targets, by themselves or in association with products of the MHC, of antiviral immune responses. The central role of these molecules in virus-host relationships is attested to by the highly significant effects of their genetic variation. For example, one may recall the impact of antigenic shift and antigenic drift in influenza viruses on the incidence of the disease (126). Thus greater knowledge of the structure and function of viral glycoproteins may contribute substantially to a fuller understanding of the interactions of lymphocytes and viruses in particular and of viral pathogenesis in general.

In closing, it is appropriate to briefly consider what sort of advances in the understanding of lymphocyte-virus interactions are likely to be witnessed in the near future. Certainly, monoclonal hybridoma antibodies, cloned B and T lymphocytes, and recombinant DNA techniques will play pivotal roles in this field. Experimental strategies employing monoclonal antibodies and cloned genes have already begun to pay dividends in unraveling the structure and function of the influenza A virus HA (140). Results with clones of CTL specific for influenza A viruses (30,148) have placed earlier concepts of CTL specificity on a firmer experimental basis and have opened the way for a rigorous examination of immunoregulation of the CTL response to influenza A viruses. Similar approaches will no doubt prove fruitful in other virus-host systems. Thus modern techniques should allow thorough examination of virus-host interactions at the level of macromolecular structure and function as well as at the level of cell-cell interactions. Ultimately, it should be possible to determine not only which viral glycoproteins are involved in determining a particular characteristic of viral behavior or which molecules are involved as targets of a given class or clone of lymphocytes, but also which amino acids form the active site of a viral receptor for cell surface structures or which amino acids compose the epitope recognized by a particular lymphocyte-borne antigen receptor. Analyses of antiviral immune responses should identify relevant clones of lymphocytes by a variety of criteria: cell surface differentiation antigens, epitope specificity of the antigen receptors, and idiotypes of the antigen receptors. Additionally, it may become possible to rigorously determine, at least for animal models of virus diseases, what roles different kinds of lymphoid cells actually play *in vivo* and how they vary with host or virus genotype. Finally, accumulation of this type of knowledge may bring benefits to the clinical sphere, as suggested by the development of synthetic vaccines (6).

ACKNOWLEDGMENTS

This work was supported by grants AI-15412, AI-14162, and CA-10815 from the National Institutes of Health and the Medical Scientists Training Program at the University of Pennsylvania. We thank the Editorial Department for preparing the manuscript.

REFERENCES

1. Ada, G. L., and Yap, K. L. (1977): Matrix protein expressed at the surface of cells infected with influenza virus. *Immunochemistry*, 14:643–651.
2. Ada, G. L., and Yap, K. L. (1979): The measurement of haemagglutinin and matrix protein present on the surface of influenza virus-infected P815 mastocytoma cells. *J. Gen. Virol.*, 42:541–553.
3. Ada, G. L., Jackson, D. C., Blanden, R. V., Tha Hla, R., and Bowern, N. A. (1976): Changes in the surface of virus-infected cells recognized by cytotoxic T cells. I. Minimal requirements for lysis of ectromelia-infected P-815 cells. *Scand. J. Immunol.*, 5:23–30.
4. Alford, R. H., Rossen, R. D., Butler, W. T., and Kasel, J. A. (1967): Neutralizing and hemagglutination-inhibiting activity of nasal secretions following experimental human infection with A2 influenza virus. *J. Immunol.*, 98:724–731.
5. Appleyard, G., and Andrews, C. (1974): Neutralizing activities of antisera to poxvirus soluble antigens. *J. Gen. Virol.*, 23:197–200.
6. Arnon, R. (1980): Chemically defined antiviral vaccines. *Ann. Rev. Microbiol.*, 34:593–618.
7. Ashman, R. B., and Mullbacher, A. (1979): A T helper cell for antiviral cytotoxic T-cell responses. *J. Exp. Med.*, 150:1277–1282.
8. Askonas, B. A., and Webster, R. G. (1980): Monoclonal antibodies to hemagglutinin and to H-2 inhibit the cross-reactive cytotoxic T cell populations induced by influenza. *Eur. J. Immunol.*, 10:151–156.
9. Bach, M.-A., and Bach, J.-F. (1981): The use of monoclonal anti-T cell antibodies to study T cell imbalances in human diseases. *Clin. Exp. Immunol.*, 45:449–456.
10. Benacerraf, B., and McDevitt, H. O. (1972): Histocompatibility-linked immune response genes. *Science*, 175:273–279.
11. Bennink, J. R., and Doherty, P. C. (1979): Reciprocal stimulation of negatively selected high-responder and low-responder T cells in virus-infected recipients (major histocompatibility complex, Ir genes, H-2 restriction, vaccinia virus). *Proc. Natl. Acad. Sci. USA*, 76:3482–3485.
12. Bergoin, M., and Dales, S. (1971): Comparative observations on poxviruses of invertebrates and vertebrates. In: *Comparative Virology*, edited by K. Maramorosch and E. Korstak, pp. 171–205. Academic Press, New York.

13. Biddison, W. E., Doherty, P. C., and Webster, R. G. (1977): Antibody to influenza virus matrix protein detects a common antigen on the surface of cells infected with type A influenza viruses. *J. Exp. Med.*, 146:690–697.

14. Biddison, W. E., Hansen, T. H., Levy, R. B., and Doherty, P. C. (1978): Involvement of *H-2L* gene products in virus-immune T-cell recognition. Evidence for *H-2L*-restricted T-cell response. *J. Exp. Med.*, 148:1678–1686.

15. Biddison, W. E., Payne, S. M., Shearer, G. M., and Shaw, S. (1980): Human cytotoxic T cell responses in trinitrophenyl hapten and influenza virus. Diversity of restriction antigens and specificity of HLA-linked genetic regulation. *J. Exp. Med.*, 152:2045–2075.

16. Biddison, W. E., and Shaw, S. (1979): Differences in HLA antigen recognition by human influenza virus-immune cytotoxic T cells. *J. Immunol.*, 122:1705–1709.

17. Biddison, W. E., Shaw, S., and Nelson, D. L. (1979): Virus specificity of human influenza virus-immune cytotoxic T cells. *J. Immunol.*, 122:660–664.

18. Blanden, R. V. (1970): Mechanisms of recovery from a generalized viral infection: Mousepox. I. The effects of antithymocyte serum. *J. Exp. Med.*, 132:1035–1054.

19. Blanden, R. V. (1971): Mechanisms of recovery from a generalized viral infection: Mousepox. II. Passive transfer of recovery mechanisms with immune lymphoid cells. *J. Exp. Med.*, 133:1074–1089.

20. Blanden, R. V. (1971): Mechanisms of recovery from a generalized viral infection: Mousepox. III. Regression of infectious foci. *J. Exp. Med.*, 133:1090–1104.

21. Blanden, R. V. (1974): T cell response to viral and bacterial infection. *Transplant. Rev.*, 19:56–88.

22. Blanden, R. V., and Gardner, I. D. (1976): The cell-mediated immune response to ectromelia virus infection. I. Kinetics and characteristics of the primary effector T cell response *in vivo*. *Cell. Immunol.*, 22:271–282.

23. Blanden, R. V., Dunlop, M. B. C., Doherty, P. C., Kohn, H. I., and McKenzie, I. F. C. (1976): Effects of four H-2K mutations on virus-induced antigens recognized by cytotoxic T cells. *Immunogenetics*, 3:541–548.

24. Blanden, R. V., Kees, U., and Dunlop, M. B. C. (1977): *In vitro* primary induction of cytotoxic T cells against virus-infected syngeneic cells. *J. Immunol. Methods*, 16:73–89.

25. Blanden, R. V., McKenzie, I., Kees, U., Melvold, R. W., and Kohn, H. I. (1977): Cytotoxic T cell response to ectromelia virus-infected cells. Different H-2 requirements for triggering precursor T-cell induction or lysis by effector T cells defined by the BALB/c H-2^{db} mutant. *J. Exp. Med.*, 146:869–880.

26. Boulter, E. A., and Appleyard, G. (1973): Differences between extracellular and intracellular forms of poxvirus and their implication. *Prog. Med. Virol.*, 16:86–108.

27. Braciale, T. J. (1977): Immunologic recognition of influenza virus-infected cells. I. Generation of a virus-strain specific and a cross-reactive subpopulation of cytotoxic T cells in the response to type A influenza viruses of different subtypes. *Cell. Immunol.*, 33:423–436.

28. Braciale, T. J. (1977): Immunologic recognition of influenza virus-infected cells. II. Expression of influenza A matrix protein on the infected cell surface and its role in recognition by cross-reactive cytotoxic T cells. *J. Exp. Med.*, 146:673–689.

29. Braciale, T. J. (1979): Specificity of cytotoxicity of T cells directed to influenza hemagglutinin. *J. Exp. Med.*, 149:856–869.

30. Braciale, T. J., Andrew, M. E., and Braciale, V. L. (1981): Heterogeneity and specificity of cloned lines of influenza-virus-specific cytotoxic T lymphocytes. *J. Exp. Med.*, 153:910–923.

31. Briody, B. A. (1959): Response of mice to ectromelia and vaccinia viruses. *Bacteriol. Rev.*, 23:61–95.

32. Burakoff, S. J., Reiss, C. S., Finberg, R., and Mescher, M. F. (1980): Cell-mediated immunity to viral glycoproteins. *Rev. Infect. Dis.*, 2:62–77.

33. Burns, W. H., and Allison, A. C. (1975): Virus infections and the immune responses they elicit. *The Antigens*, 3:479–573.

34. Cantor, H., and Boyse, E. (1977): Regulation of the immune response by T-cell subclasses. *Contemp. Top. Immunobiol.*, 7:47–67.

35. Cantor, H., and Gershon, R. K. (1979): Immunological circuits: Cellular composition. *Fed. Proc.*, 38:2058–2064.

36. Choppin, P. W., and Compans, R. W. (1975): The structure of influenza virus. In: *The Influenza Viruses and Influenza*, edited by E. D. Kilbourne, pp. 15–51. Academic Press, New York.

37. Condit, R. C., and Motyczka, A. (1981): Isolation and preliminary characterization of temperature-sensitive mutants of vaccinia virus. *Virology*, 113:224–241.
38. Cooper, N. R. (1979): Humoral immunity to viruses. In: *Comprehensive Virology, Vol. 15, Virus-Host Interactions: Immunity to Viruses*, edited by H. Fraenkel-Conrat and R. R. Wagner, pp. 123–170. Plenum, New York.
39. Couch, R. B., Douglas, R. G., Jr., Fedson, D. S., and Kasel, J. A. (1971): Correlated studies of a recombinant influenza-virus vaccine. III. Protection against experimental influenza in man. *J. Infect. Dis.*, 124:473–480.
40. Couch, R. B., Douglas, R. G., Jr., Rossen, R., and Kasel, J. A. (1971): Role of secretory antibody in influenza. In: *The Secretory Immunologic System*, edited by D. H. Dayton, Jr., P. A. Small, Jr., R. M. Chanock, H. E. Kaufman, and T. B. Tomasi, pp. 93–112. U.S. Department of Health, Education, and Welfare, Public Health Service, Bethesda, Maryland.
41. Couch, R. B., Kasel, J. A., Gerin, J. L., Schulman, J. L., and Kilbourne, E. D. (1974): Induction of partial immunity to influenza by a neuraminidase-specific vaccine. *J. Infect. Dis.*, 129:411–420.
42. Crawford, D. H., Rickinson, A. B., Finerty, S., and Epstein, M. A. (1978): Epstein-Barr (EB) virus genome-containing, EB nuclear antigen-negative B-lymphocyte populations in blood in acute infectious mononucleosis. *J. Gen Virol.*, 38:449–460.
43. Crumpacker, C. S. (1980): Viral glycoproteins in infectious disease processes. *Rev. Infect. Dis.*, 2:78–103.
44. Davenport, F. M., Hennessy, A. V., and Francis, T., Jr. (1953): Epidemiologic and immunologic significance of age distribution of antibody to antigenic variants of influenza virus. *J. Exp. Med.*, 98:641–656.
45. DeSchryver, A., Klein, G., Hewetson, J., Rocchi, G., Henle, W., Henle, G., and Pope, J. (1974): Comparison of EBV neutralization tests based on abortive infection or transformation of lymphoid cells and their relation to membrane reactive antibodies (anti-MA). *Int. J. Cancer*, 13:353–362.
46. DeSchryver, A., Rosen, A., Gunven, P., and Klein, G. (1976): Comparison between two antibody populations in the EBV systems: Anti-MA versus neutralizing antibody activity. *Int. J. Cancer*, 17:8–13.
47. Diehl, V., Henle, G., Henle, W., and Kohn, G. (1968): Demonstration of herpes group virus in cultures of peripheral leukocytes from patients with infectious mononucleosis. *J. Virol.*, 2:663–669.
48. Doherty, P. C., and Bennink, J. R. (1979): Vaccinia-specific cytotoxicity T-cell responses in the context of H-2 antigens not encountered in thymus may reflect aberrant recognition of a virus-H-2 complex. *J. Exp. Med.*, 149:150–157.
49. Doherty, P. C., Biddison, W. E., Bennink, J. R., and Knowles, B. B. (1978): Cytotoxic T-cell responses in mice infected with influenza and vaccinia viruses vary in magnitude with H-2 genotype. *J. Exp. Med.*, 148:534–543.
50. Doherty, P. C., Blanden, R. V., and Zinkernagel, R. M. (1976): Specificity of virus-immune effector T cells for H-2K or H-2D compatible interactions: Implications for H-antigen diversity. *Transplant. Rev.*, 29:89–124.
51. Doherty, P. C., Effros, R. B., and Bennink, J. (1977): Heterogeneity of the cytotoxic response of thymus-derived lymphocytes after immunization with influenza viruses. *Proc. Natl. Acad. Sci. USA*, 74:1209–1213.
52. Doherty, P. C., and Zinkernagel, R. M. (1974): T cell-mediated immunopathology in viral infection. *Transplant. Rev.*, 19:89–120.
53. Doherty, P. C., and Zinkernagel, R. M. (1975): H-2 compatibility is required for T cell-mediated lysis of target cells infected with lymphocytic choriomeningitis virus. *J. Exp. Med.*, 141:502–507.
54. Doherty, P. C., and Zinkernagel, R. M. (1975): A biological role for the major histocompatibility antigens. *Lancet*, 1:1406–1409.
55. Doherty, P. C., and Zinkernagel, R. M. (1976): Specific immune lysis of paramyxovirus-infected cells by H-2 compatible thymus-derived lymphocytes. *Immunology*, 31:27–32.
56. Douglas, R. G. (1975): Influenza in man. In: *The Influenza Viruses and Influenza*, edited by E. D. Kilbourne, pp. 395–447. Academic Press, New York.
57. Dowdle, W. R., Downie, J. C., and Laver, W. G. (1974): Inhibition of virus release by antibodies to surface antigens of influenza viruses. *J. Virol.*, 13:269–275.
58. Downie, A. W. (1963): Pathogenesis of generalized virus diseases. *Vet. Rec.*, 75:1125–1133.

59. Effros, R. B., Bennink, J., and Doherty, P. C. (1978): Characteristics of secondary cytotoxic T-cell responses in mice infected with influenza A viruses. *Cell. Immunol.*, 36:345–353.
60. Effros, R. B., Doherty, P. C., Gerhard, W., and Bennink, J. (1977): Generation of both cross-reactive and virus-specific T-cell populations after immunization with serologically distinct influenza A viruses. *J. Exp. Med.*, 145:557–568.
61. Effros, R. B., Frankel, M. E., Gerhard, W., and Doherty, P. C. (1979): Inhibition of influenza-immune T cell effector function by virus-specific hybridoma antibody. *J. Immunol.*, 123:1343–1346.
62. Ennis, F. A., Martin, W. J., and Verbonitz, M. W. (1977): Hemagglutinin specific cytotoxic T cell response during influenza infection. *J. Exp. Med.*, 146:893–898.
63. Ennis, F. A., Martin, W. J., and Verbonitz, M. W. (1977): Cytotoxic T lymphocytes induced in mice by inactivated influenza virus vaccine. *Nature*, 269:418–419.
64. Ennis, F. A., Martin, W. J., Verbonitz, M. W., and Butchko, G. M. (1977): Specificity studies on cytotoxic thymus-derived lymphocytes reactive with influenza virus-infected cells; evidence for dual recognition of H-2 and viral hemagglutinin antigens. *Proc. Natl. Acad. Sci. USA*, 74:3006–3010.
65. Epstein, M. A., and Achong, B. G. (1977): Recent progress in Epstein-Barr virus research. *Ann. Rev. Microbiol.*, 31:421–445.
66. Epstein, M. A., and Achong, B. G. (1977): Pathogenesis of infectious mononucleosis. *Lancet*, 2:1270–1273.
67. Epstein, M. A., and Achong, B. G. (1979): The relationship of the virus to Burkitt's lymphoma. In: *The Epstein-Barr Virus*, edited by M. A. Epstein and B. G. Achong, pp. 322–337. Springer-Verlag, Berlin.
68. Epstein, M. A., Achong, B. G., and Barr, Y. M. (1964): Virus particles in cultured lymphoblasts from Burkitt's lymphoma. *Lancet*, 1:702–703.
69. Ernberg, I., Klein, G., Kourilsky, F. M., and Silvestre, D. (1974): Differentiation between early and late membrane antigen on human lymphoblastoid cell lines infected with Epstein-Barr virus. I. Immunofluorescence. *J. Natl. Cancer Inst.*, 53:61–65.
70. Ertl, H. C. J., Gerike, R. H. W., and Koszinowski, U. (1977): Virus-specific T cell sensitization. Requirements for vaccinia virus-specific T cell sensitization *in vivo*. *Immunogenetics*, 4:515–522.
71. Evans, A. S., Niederman, J. C., and McCollum, R. W. (1968): Seroepidemiologic studies of infectious mononucleosis with EB virus. *N. Engl. J. Med.*, 279:1121–1127.
72. Farnik, J., and Bruj, J. (1966): An outbreak of influenza A2 in a population with a known antibody profile. *J. Infect. Dis.*, 116:425–428.
73. Fenner, F. (1949): Studies in mousepox (infectious ectromelia of mice). IV. Quantitative investigations of the spread of virus through the host in actively and passively immunized animals. *Aust. J. Exp. Biol. Med. Sci.*, 27:1–18.
74. Fenner, F. (1949): Studies in mousepox (infectious ectromelia of mice). VI. A comparison of the virulence and infectivity of three strains of ectromelia virus. *Aust. J. Exp. Biol. Med. Sci.*, 27:31–43.
75. Fenner, F. (1949): Studies in mousepox (infectious ectromelia of mice). VII. The effect of the age of the host upon the response to infection. *Aust. J. Exp. Biol. Med. Sci.*, 27:45–53.
76. Fenner, F. (1949): Mousepox (infectious ectromelia of mice): A review. *J. Immunol.*, 63:344–373.
77. Fenner, F. (1979): Portraits of viruses: The poxviruses. *Intervirology*, 11:137–157.
78. Froland, S. S. (1972): Binding of sheep erythrocytes to human lymphocytes. A probable marker of T lymphocytes. *Scand. J. Immunol.*, 1:269–280.
79. Fulginiti, V. A., Kempe, G. H., Hathaway, W. E., Pearlman, D. S., Seiber, O. F., Heller, J. J., Joyner, J. J., and Robinson, A. (1968): Progressive vaccinia in immunologically deficient individuals. In: *Immunologic Deficiency Diseases in Man, National Foundation of Birth Defects, Vol. 4, No. 1*, edited by D. Bergsma and R. Good, pp. 129–151. Williams & Wilkins, Baltimore.
80. Fulk, R. V., Fedson, D. S., Huber, M. A., Fitzpatrick, J. R., and Kasel, J. A. (1970): Antibody responses in serum and nasal secretions according to age of recipient and method of administration of A2/Hong Kong/68 inactivated influenza virus vaccine. *J. Immunol.*, 104:8–13.
81. Gardner, I. D., and Blanden, R. V. (1974): The cell-mediated immune response to ectromelia virus infection. II. Secondary response *in vitro* and kinetics of memory T cell production *in vivo*. *Cell. Immunol.*, 22:283–296.

82. Gardner, I. D., Bowern, N. A., and Blanden, R. V. (1974): Cell-mediated cytotoxicity against ectromelia virus-infected target cells. I. Specificity and kinetics. *Eur. J. Immunol.*, 4:63–67.

83. Gardner, I. D., Bowern, N. A., and Blanden, R. V. (1974): Cell-mediated cytotoxicity against ectromelia virus-infected target cells. II. Identification of effector cells and analysis of mechanism. *Eur. J. Immunol.*, 4:68–72.

84. Gardner, I. D., Bowern, N. A., and Blanden, R. V. (1975): Cell-mediated cytotoxicity against ectromelia virus-infected target cells. III. Role of the H-2 gene complex. *Eur. J. Immunol.*, 5:122.

85. Gergely, L., Klein, G., and Ernberg, I. (1971): Effect of EBV-induced early antigens on host-cell macromolecular synthesis, studied by combined immunofluorescence and radioautography. *Virology*, 45:22–29.

86. Gergely, L., Klein, G., and Ernberg, I. (1971): The action of DNA-antagonists on Epstein-Barr virus (EBV)-associated early antigen (EA) in Burkitt lymphoma lines. *Int. J. Cancer*, 7:293–302.

87. Gershon, R. K., and Cantor, H. (1980): Immunoregulation: A futuristic review. In: *Strategies of Immune Regulation*, edited by E. E. Sercarz and A. J. Cunningham, pp. 43–62. Academic Press, New York.

88. Gething, M. J., Koszinowski, U., and Waterfield, M. (1978): Fusion of Sendai virus with the target cell membrane is required for T cell cytotoxicity. *Nature*, 274:689–691.

89. Ginsberg, H. S. (1980): Pathogenesis of viral infections. In: *Microbiology: Including Immunology and Molecular Genetics*, third edition, edited by B. D. Davis, R. Dulbecco, H. N. Eisen, and H. S. Ginsberg, pp. 1031–1045. Harper and Row, Hagerstown, Maryland.

90. Ginsberg, H. S. (1980): Pox viruses. In: *Microbiology: Including Immunology and Molecular Genetics*, third edition, edited by B. D. Davis, R. Dulbecco, H. N. Eisen, and H. S. Ginsberg, p. 1082. Harper and Row, Hagerstown, Maryland.

91. Golden, H. D., Chang, R. S., Prescott, W., Simpson, E., and Cooper, T. Y. (1973): Leukocyte-transforming agent: Prolonged excretion by patients with mononucleosis and excretion by normal individuals. *J. Infect. Dis.*, 127:471–473.

92. Greenberg, S. B., Six, H. R., Drake, S., and Couch, R. B. (1979): Cell cytotoxicity due to specific influenza antibody production *in vitro* after recent influenza antigen stimulation. *Proc. Natl. Acad. Sci. USA*, 76:4622–4626.

93. Greenspan, N., and Doherty, P. C. (1982): Modification of cytotoxic T cell response patterns by administration of hemagglutinin-specific monoclonal antibodies to mice infected with influenza A viruses. *Hybridoma*, 1:149–159.

94. Gresser, I., Tovey, M. G., Maury, C., and Bandu, M. T. (1976): Role of interferon in the pathogenesis of virus diseases in mice as demonstrated by the use of anti-interferon serum. II. Studies with herpes simplex, Moloney sarcoma, vesicular stomatitis, Newcastle disease and influenza viruses. *J. Exp. Med.*, 144:1316–1323.

95. Hackett, C. J., Askonas, B. A., Webster, R. G., and van Wyke, K. (1980): Quantitation of influenza virus antigens on infected target cells and their recognition by cross-reactive cytotoxic T cells. *J. Exp. Med.*, 151:1014–1025.

96. Hammerling, U. (1981): Differentiation of B lymphocytes in lineage development and in the immune response. *Prog. Allergy*, 28:40–65.

97. Hapel, A. J., Bablanian, R., and Cole, G. A. (1978): Inductive requirements for the generation of virus-specific T lymphocytes. I. The nature of the host cell-virus interaction that triggers secondary poxvirus-specific cytotoxic T lymphocyte induction. *J. Immunol.*, 121:736–743.

98. Hapel, A., and Gardner, I. (1974): Appearance of cytotoxic T cells in cerebro spinal fluid of mice with ectromelia virus-induced meningitis. *Scand. J. Immunol.*, 3:311–319.

99. Haynes, B. F., Schooley, R. T., Payling-Wright, C. R., Grouse, J. E., Dolin, R., and Fauci, A. S. (1979): Characterization of thymus-derived lymphocyte subsets in acute Epstein-Barr virus-induced infectious mononucleosis. *J. Immunol.*, 122:699–702.

100. Haynes, B. F., Schooley, R. T., Grouse, J. E., Payling-Wright, C. R., Dolin, R., and Fauci, A. S. (1979): Emergence of suppressor cells of immunoglobulin synthesis during acute Epstein-Barr virus-induced infectious mononucleosis. *J. Immunol.*, 123:2095–2101.

101. Henle, G., and Henle, W. (1966): Immunofluorescence in cells derived from Burkitt's lymphoma. *J. Bacteriol.*, 91:1248–1256.

102. Henle, G., and Henle, W. (1970): Observations on childhood infections with the Epstein-Barr virus. *J. Infect. Dis.*, 121:303–310.

103. Henle, G., Henle, W., and Diehl, V. (1968): Relation of Burkitt's tumor-associated herpes-type virus to infectious mononucleosis. *Proc. Natl. Acad. Sci. USA*, 59:94–101.

104. Henle, G., Henle, W., and Klein, G. (1971): Demonstration of two distinct components in the early antigen complex of Epstein-Barr virus infected cells. *Int. J. Cancer*, 8:272–282.

105. Henle, W., and Henle, G. (1972): Epstein-Barr virus: The cause of infectious mononucleosis— A Review. In: *Oncogenesis and Herpes viruses*, edited by P. M. Biggs, G. de The, and L. N. Payne, pp. 269–274. IARC, Lyon.

106. Henle, W., Henle, G., Zajac, B., Pearson, G., Waubke, R., and Scriba, M. (1970): Differential reactivity of human sera with early antigens induced by Epstein-Barr virus. *Science*, 169:188– 190.

107. Herberman, R. B., editor (1980): *Natural Cell-Mediated Immunity Against Tumors*. Academic Press, New York.

108. Herberman, R. B. (1981): Natural killer (NK) cell. In: *The Lymphocyte*, edited by K. W. Sell and W. V. Miller, pp. 33–43. Alan R. Liss, New York.

109. Hicks, J. T., Ennis, F. A., Kim, E., and Verbonitz, M. (1978): The importance of an intact complement pathway in recovery from a primary viral infection: Influenza in decomplemented and in C5-deficient mice. *J. Immunol.*, 121:1437–1445.

110. Hirsch, M. S., and Murphy, F. A. (1968): Effects of anti-lymphoid sera on viral infections. *Lancet*, 2:37–40.

111. Holowczak, J. A. (1982): Poxvirus DNA. *Curr. Top. Microbiol. Immunol.*, 97:27–79.

112. Howe, C., Coward, J. E., and Fenger, T. W. (1980): Viral invasion: Morphological, biochemical and biophysical aspects. In: *Comprehensive Virology*, Vol. 16, edited by H. Fraenkel-Conrat and R. R. Wagner, pp. 1–71. Plenum, New York.

113. Hutt, L. M., Huang, Y. T., Dascomb, H. E., and Pagano, J. S. (1975): Enhanced destruction of lymphoid cell lines by peripheral blood leukocytes taken from patients with acute infectious mononucleosis. *J. Immunol.*, 115:243–248.

114. Jackson, D. C., Ada, G. L., Hapel, A. J., and Dunlop, M. B. C. (1976): Changes in the surface of virus-infected cells recognized by cytotoxic T cells. II. A requirement for glycoprotein synthesis in virus-infected target cells. *Scand. J. Immunol.*, 5:1021–1029.

115. Jackson, D. C., Ada, G. L., and Tha Hla, R. (1976): Cytotoxic T cells recognize very early, minor changes in ectromelia virus-infected target cells. *Aust. J. Exp. Biol. Med. Sci.*, 54:349– 363.

116. Jenner, E. (1975): An inquiry into the causes and effects of the variolae vaccinae, a disease discovered in some of the western counties of England, particularly Gloucestershire and known by the name of the Cow Pox. In: *Milestones in Microbiology*, edited by T. H. Brock, p. 121. American Society of Microbiology, Washington, D.C.

117. Johnsen, H. E., Madsen, M., and Kristensen, T. (1979): Lymphocyte subpopulations in man: Suppression of PWM-induced B-cell proliferation by infectious mononucleosis T cells. *Scand. J. Immunol.*, 10:251–255.

118. Jondal, M. (1976): Antibody-dependent cellular cytotoxicity (ADCC) against Epstein-Barr virus-determined membrane antigens. I. Reactivity in sera from normal persons and from patients with acute infectious mononucleosis. *Clin. Exp. Immunol.*, 25:1–5.

119. Jondal, M., Holm, G., and Wigzell, H. (1972): Surface markers on human T and B lymphocytes. I. A large population of lymphocytes forming non-immune rosettes with sheep red blood cells. *J. Exp. Med.*, 136:207–215.

120. Jondal, M., and Klein, G. (1973): Surface markers on human B and T lymphocytes. II. Presence of Epstein-Barr virus receptors on B lymphocytes. *J. Exp. Med.*, 138:1365–1378.

121. Kasel, J. A., Hume, E. B., Fulk, R. V., Togo, Y., Huber, M., and Hornick, R. B. (1969): Antibody responses in nasal secretions and serum of elderly persons following local or parenteral administration of inactivated influenza virus vaccine. *J. Immunol.*, 102:555–562.

122. Katz, D. H., and Benacerraf, B. (1972): The regulatory influence of activated T cells on B cell responses to antigen. *Adv. Immunol.*, 15:1–94.

123. Kees, U., and Blanden, R. V. (1976): A single genetic element in H-2K affects mouse T cell antiviral function in poxvirus infection. *J. Exp. Med.*, 143:450–455.

124. Kilbourne, E. D., editor (1975): In: *The Influenza Viruses and Influenza*. Academic Press, New York.

125. Kilbourne, E. D. (1975): The influenza viruses and influenza—An introduction. In: *The Influenza Viruses and Influenza*, edited by E. D. Kilbourne, pp. 1–14. Academic Press, New York.

126. Kilbourne, E. D. (1975): Epidemiology of influenza. In: *The Influenza Viruses and Influenza*, edited by E. D. Kilbourne, pp. 483–538. Academic Press, New York.

127. Klein, E., Klein, G., and Levine, P. H. (1976): Immunological control of human lymphoma: Discussion. *Cancer Res.*, 36:724–727.

128. Klein, G. (1979): The relationship of the virus to nasopharyngeal carcinoma. In: *The Epstein-Barr Virus*, edited by M. A. Epstein and B. G. Achong, pp. 340–350. Springer-Verlag, Berlin.

129. Klein, G., Clifford, P., Klein, E., and Stjernsward, J. (1966): Search for tumor-specific immune reactions in Burkitt lymphoma patients by the membrane immunofluorescence reaction. *Proc. Natl. Acad. Sci. USA*, 55:1628–1635.

130. Klein, J. (1975): *Biology of the Mouse Histocompatibility-2 Complex. Principles of Immunogenetics Applied to a Single System.* Springer-Verlag, New York.

131. Klein, J. (1978): H-2 mutations: Their genetics and effect on immune functions. *Adv. Immunol.*, 26:55–146.

132. Koszinowski, U. H., Allen, H., Gething, M. J., Waterfield, M. D., and Klenk, H. D. (1980): Recognition of viral glycoproteins in influenza A-specific cross-reactive cytolytic T lymphocytes. *J. Exp. Med.*, 151:945–958.

133. Koszinowski, U., and Ertl, H. (1975): Lysis mediated by T cells and restricted by H-2 antigen of target cells infected with vaccinia. *Nature*, 255:552–554.

134. Koszinowski, U., and Ertl, H. (1976): Role of early viral surface antigens in cellular immune response to vaccinia virus. *Eur. J. Immunol.*, 6:679–683.

135. Koszinowski, U., and Ertl, H. (1977): Cytotoxic interactions of virus specific effector cells with virus-infected targets of different cell type. *J. Immunol.*, 4:107–114.

136. Koszinowski, U., Gething, M. J., and Waterfield, M. (1977): T cell cytotoxicity in the absence of viral protein synthesis in target cells. *Nature*, 267:160–163.

137. Koszinowski, U., and Thomssen, R. (1975): Target cell-dependent T cell-mediated lysis of vaccinia virus-infected cells. *Eur. J. Immunol.*, 5:245–251.

138. Kung, P. C., Goldstein, G., Reinherz, E. L., and Schlossman, S. F. (1979): Monoclonal antibodies defining distinctive human T cell surface antigens. *Science*, 206:347–349.

139. Kurrle, R., Wagner, H., Rollingnoff, M., and Rott, R. (1979): Influenza virus-specific T cell-mediated cytotoxicity: Integration of the virus antigen into the target cell membrane is essential for target cell formation. *Eur. J. Immunol.*, 9:107–111.

140. Laver, G., and Air, G. (1980): *Structure and Variation in Influenza Virus.* Elsevier, New York.

141. Laver, W. G., Air, G. M., Webster, R. G., Gerhard, W., Ward, C. W., and Dopheide, T. A. (1980): The antigenic sites on influenza virus hemagglutinin. Studies on their structure and variation. In: *Structure and Variation in Influenza Virus*, edited by G. Laver and G. Air, pp. 295–306. Elsevier, New York.

142. Laver, W. G., Downie, J. C., and Webster, R. G. (1976): Diversity of the antibody response to the different antigenic determinants on the hemagglutinin subunits of influenza virus. *J. Immunol.*, 116:336–341.

143. Lemon, S., Hutt, L., Shaw, J., Li, J.-L. H., and Pagano, J. S. (1977): Replication of EBV in epithelial cells during infectious mononucleosis. *Nature*, 268:268–270.

144. Leung, K. N., and Ada, G. L. (1980): Cells mediating delayed-type hypersensitivity in the lungs of mice infected with an influenza A virus. *Scand. J. Immunol.*, 12:393–400.

145. Leung, K.-N., Ashman, R. B., Ertl, H. C. J., and Ada, G. L. (1980): Selective suppression of the cytotoxic T cell response to influenza virus in mice. *Eur. J. Immunol.*, 10:803–810.

146. Liew, F. Y., and Russell, S. M. (1980): Delayed-type hypersensitivity to influenza virus. Induction of antigen-specific suppressor T cells for delayed-type hypersensitivity to hemagglutinin during influenza virus infection in mice. *J. Exp. Med.*, 151:799–814.

147. Lin, Y. L., and Askonas, B. A. (1980): Cross-reactivity for different type A influenza viruses of a cloned T-killer cell line. *Nature*, 288:164–165.

148. Lin, Y. L., and Askonas, B. A. (1981): Biological properties of an influenza A virus-specific killer T cell clone. Inhibition of virus replication *in vivo* and induction of delayed-type hypersensitivity reactions. *J. Exp. Med.*, 154:225–234.

149. Lipinski, M., Fridman, W. H., Tursz, T., Vincent, C., Pious, D., and Fellous, M. (1979): Absence of allogeneic restriction in human T-cell-mediated cytotoxicity to Epstein-Barr virus-infected target cells. Demonstration of an HLA-linked control at the effector level. *J. Exp. Med.*, 150:1310–1322.

150. McKenzie, I. F. C., Pang, T., and Blanden, R. V. (1977): The use of H-2 mutants as models for the study of T cell activation. *Immunol. Rev.*, 35:181–230.

151. McMichael, A. (1978): HLA restriction of human cytotoxic T lymphocytes specific for influenza virus. Poor recognition of virus associated with HLA A2. *J. Exp. Med.*, 148:1458–1467.

152. McMichael, A. J., and Askonas, B. A. (1978): Influenza virus-specific cytotoxic T cells in man; induction and properties of the cytotoxic cell. *Eur. J. Immunol.*, 8:705–711.

153. McMichael, A. J., Ting, A., Zweerink, H. J., and Askonas, B. A. (1977): HLA restriction of cell-mediated lysis of influenza virus-infected human cells. *Nature*, 270:524–526.

154. Meiklejohn, G., Kempe, C. H., Thalman, W. G., and Lennette, E. H. (1952): Evaluation of monovalent influenza vaccines. II. Observations during an influenza A-prime epidemic. *Am. J. Hyg.*, 55:12–21.

155. Miller, G., Niederman, J. C., and Andrews, L.-L. (1973): Prolonged oropharyngeal excretion of Epstein-Barr virus after infectious mononucleosis. *N. Engl. J. Med.*, 288:229–232.

156. Mims, C. A. (1964): Aspects of the pathogenesis of virus diseases. *Bacteriol. Rev.*, 28:30–71.

157. Misko, I. H., Moss, D. J., and Pope, J. H. (1980): HLA antigen-related restriction of T lymphocyte cytotoxicity to Epstein-Barr virus. *Proc. Natl. Acad. Sci. USA*, 77:4247–4250.

158. Monto, A. S., and Kendal, A. P. (1973): Effect of neuraminidase antibody on Hong Kong influenza. *Lancet*, 1:623–625.

159. Morris, J. A., Kasel, J. A., Saglam, M., Knight, V., and Loda, F. A. (1966): Immunity to influenza as related to antibody levels. *N. Engl. J. Med.*, 274:527–535.

160. Moss, B. (1974): Reproduction of poxvirus. In: *Comprehensive Virology, Vol. 3*, edited by H. Fraenkel-Conrat and R. R. Wagner, pp. 405–474. Plenum, New York.

161. Moss, D. J., Rickinson, A. B., and Pope, J. H. (1978): Long-term T-cell-mediated immunity to Epstein-Barr virus in man. I. Complete regression of virus-induced transformation in cultures of seropositive donor leukocytes. *Int. J. Cancer*, 22:662–668.

162. Moss, D. J., Rickinson, A. B., and Pope, J. H. (1979): Long-term T-cell-mediated immunity to Epstein-Barr virus in man. III. Activation of cytotoxic T cells in virus-infected leukocyte cultures. *Int. J. Cancer*, 23:618–625.

163. Murphy, B. R., Baron, S., Chalhub, E. G., Uhlendorf, C. P., and Chanock, R. M. (1973): Temperature-sensitive mutants of influenza virus. IV. Induction of interferon in the nasopharynx by wild-type and a temperature-sensitive recombinant virus. *J. Infect. Dis.*, 128:488–493.

164. Murphy, B. R., Kasel, J. A., and Chanock, R. M. (1972): Association of serum anti-neuraminidase antibody with resistance to influenza in man. *N. Engl. J. Med.*, 286:1329–1332.

165. Niederman, J. C., Evans, A. S., Subramanyan, M. S., and McCollum, R. W. (1970): Prevalence, incidence and persistence of EB virus antibody in young adults. *N. Engl. J. Med.*, 282:361–365.

166. Niederman, J. C., McCollum, R. W., Henle, G., and Henle, W. (1968): Infectious mononucleosis. Clinical manifestations in relation to EB virus antibodies. *JAMA*, 203:205–209.

167. Nilsson, K., Klein, G., Henle, W., and Henle, G. (1971): The establishment of lymphoblastoid lines from adult and fetal human lymphoid tissue and its dependence on EBV. *Int. J. Cancer*, 8:443–450.

168. Notkins, A. L. (1974): Immune mechanisms by which the spread of viral infections is stopped. *Cell. Immunol.*, 11:478–483.

169. Notkins, A. L., Mergenhagen, S. E., and Howard, R. J. (1970): Effect of virus infections on the function of the immune system. *Ann. Rev. Microbiol.*, 24:525–538.

170. Oldstone, M. B. A. (1979): Immune responses, immune tolerance and viruses. In: *Comprehensive Virology, Vol. 15*, edited by H. Fraenkel-Conrat and R. R. Wagner, pp. 1–36. Plenum, New York.

171. Oldstone, M. B. A., Sissons, J. G. P., and Fujinami, R. S. (1980): Action of antibody and complement in regulating virus infection. In: *Immunology 80: Progress in Immunology IV*, edited by M. Fougereau and J. Dausset, pp. 599–621. Academic Press, London.

172. Oxford, J. S., and Schild, G. C. (1976): Immunological and physicochemical studies of influenza matrix (M) polypeptides. *Virology*, 74:394–402.

173. Pang, T., and Blanden, R. V. (1976): The cell-mediated immune response to ectromelia virus infection. Secondary response *in vitro*: Specificity, nature of effector and respondent cells and requirements for induction of antigenic changes in stimulator cells. *Aust. J. Exp. Biol. Med. Sci.*, 54:253–264.

174. Pang, T., and Blanden, R. V. (1976): The role of adherent cells in the secondary cell-mediated response *in vitro* to a natural poxvirus pathogen. *Aust. J. Exp. Biol. Med. Sci.*, 54:559–571.

175. Pang, T., McKenzie, F. C., and Blanden, R. V. (1976): Cooperation between mouse T cell subpopulations in the cell-mediated response to a natural poxvirus pathogen. *Cell. Immunol.*, 26:153–159.

176. Pang, T., Andrew, M. E., Melvold, R. W., and Blanden, R. V. (1977): Specificity or affinity of cytotoxic T cells for self H-2K determinants apparently does not change between primary and secondary responses to ectromelia virus infection. *Aust. J. Exp. Biol. Med. Sci.*, 55:39–48.

177. Pattengale, P. K., Smith, R. W., and Gerber, P. (1973): Selective transformation of B lymphocytes by EB virus. *Lancet*, 2:93–94.

178. Pattengale, P. K., Smith, R. W., and Perlin, E. (1974): Atypical lymphocytes in acute infectious mononucleosis. Identification by multiple T and B lymphocyte markers. *N. Engl. J. Med.*, 291:1145–1148.

179. Payne, L. (1978): Polypeptide composition of extracellular enveloped vaccinia virus. *J. Virol.*, 27:28–37.

180. Payne, L. G. (1979): Identification of vaccinia hemagglutinin polypeptide from a cell system yielding large amounts of extracellular enveloped virus. *J. Virol.*, 31:147–155.

181. Payne, L. G. (1980): Significance of extracellular enveloped virus in the in vitro and in vivo dissemination of vaccinia. *J. Gen. Virol.*, 50:89–100.

182. Payne, L. G., and Norrby, E. (1976): Presence of haemagglutinin in the envelope of extracellular vaccinia virus particles. *J. Gen. Virol.*, 32:63–72.

183. Payne, L. G., and Norrby, E. (1978): Adsorption and penetration of enveloped and naked vaccinia virus particles. *J. Virol.*, 27:19–27.

184. Pearson, G. R. (1978): *In vitro* and *in vivo* investigations on antibody-dependent cellular cytotoxicity. *Curr. Top. Microbiol. Immunol.*, 80:65–96.

185. Pearson, G., Dewey, F., Klein, G., Henle, G., and Henle, W. (1970): Relation between neutralization of Epstein-Barr virus and antibodies to cell membrane antigens induced by the virus. *J. Natl. Cancer Inst.*, 45:989–995.

186. Pearson, G., Henle, G., and Henle, W. (1971): Production of antigens associated with Epstein-Barr virus in experimentally infected lymphoblastoid cell lines. *J. Natl. Cancer Inst.*, 46:1243–1250.

187. Pearson, G. R., and Orr, T. W. (1976): Antibody-dependent lymphocyte cytotoxicity against cells expressing Epstein-Barr virus antigens. *J. Natl. Cancer Inst.*, 56:485–488.

188. Pereira, M. S., Blake, J. M., and Macrae, A. D. (1969): EB virus antibody at different ages. *Br. Med. J.*, 4:526–527.

189. Perrin, L. H., Zinkernagel, R. M., and Oldstone, M. B. A. (1977): Immune response in humans after vaccination with vaccinia virus: Generation of a virus-specific cytotoxic activity by human peripheral lymphocytes. *J. Exp. Med.*, 146:949–969.

190. Ploegh, H. L., Orr, H. T., and Strominger, J. L. (1981): Major histocompatibility antigens: The human (HLA-A, -B, -C) and murine (H-2K, H-2D) class I molecules. *Cell*, 24:287–299.

191. Potter, C. W., Jennings, R., Nicholson, K., Tyrrell, D. A. J., and Dickinson, K. G. (1977): Immunity to attenuated influenza virus WRL 105 infection induced by heterologous, inactivated influenza A virus vaccines. *J. Hyg.*, 79:321–332.

192. Potter, C. W., and Oxford, J. S. (1979): Determinants of immunity to influenza infection in man. *Br. Med. Bull.*, 35:69–75.

193. Purtilo, D. T. (1980): Immunopathology of infectious mononucleosis and other complications of Epstein-Barr virus infections. In: *Pathology Annual: 1980*, edited by S. C. Sommers and P. P. Rosen, pp. 253–299. Appleton-Century-Crofts, New York.

194. Purtilo, D. (1981): Immune deficiency predisposing to Epstein-Barr virus-induced lymphoproliferative diseases: The X-linked lymphoproliferative syndrome as a model. *Adv. Cancer Res.*, 34:279–312.

195. Purtilo, D. T., and Sakamoto, K. (1981): Epstein-Barr virus and human disease: Immune responses determine the clinical and pathologic expression. *Hum. Pathol.*, 12:677–679.

196. Raff, M. C. (1970): Two distinct populations of peripheral lymphocytes in mice distinguishable by immunofluorescence. *Immunology*, 19:637–650.

197. Reedman, B. M., and Klein, G. (1973): Cellular localization of an Epstein-Barr virus (EBV)-associated complement-fixing antigen in producer and non-producer lymphoblastoid cell lines. *Int. J. Cancer*, 11:499–520.

198. Reinherz, E. L., O'Brien, C., Rosenthal, P., and Schlossman, S. F. (1980): The cellular basis

for viral-induced immunodeficiency: Analysis by monoclonal antibodies. *J. Immunol.*, 125:1269–1274.

199. Reinherz, E. L., and Schlossman, S. F. (1980): Regulation of the immune response—Inducer and suppressor T-lymphocyte subsets in human beings. *N. Engl. J. Med.*, 303:370–373.

200. Reiss, C. S., and Burakoff, S. J. (1981): Specificity of the helper T cell for the cytolytic T lymphocyte response to influenza viruses. *J. Exp. Med.*, 154:541–546.

201. Reiss, C. S., and Schulman, J. L. (1980): Influenza type A virus M protein expression on infected cells is responsible for cross-reactive recognition by cytotoxic thymus-derived lymphocytes. *Infect. Immun.*, 29:719–723.

202. Rickinson, A. B., Crawford, D., and Epstein, M. A. (1977): Inhibition of the *in vitro* outgrowth of Epstein-Barr virus-transformed lymphocytes by thymus-dependent lymphocytes from infectious mononucleosis patients. *Clin. Exp. Immunol.*, 28:72–79.

203. Rickinson, A. B., Moss, D. J., and Pope, J. H. (1979): Long-term T-cell-mediated immunity to Epstein-Barr virus in man. II. Components necessary for regression in virus-infected leukocyte cultures. *Int. J. Cancer*, 23:610–617.

204. Rickinson, A. B., Wallace, L. E., and Epstein, M. A. (1980): HLA-restricted T-cell recognition of Epstein-Barr virus-infected B cells. *Nature*, 283:865–867.

205. Rocchi, G., de Felici, A., Ragona, G., and Heinz, A. (1977): Quantitative evaluation of Epstein-Barr virus-infected mononuclear peripheral blood leukocytes in infectious mononucleosis. *N. Engl. J. Med.*, 296:132–134.

206. Royston, I., Sullivan, J. L., Periman, P. O., and Perlin, E. (1975): Cell-mediated immunity to Epstein-Barr virus-transformed lymphoblastoid cells in acute infectious mononucleosis. *N. Engl. J. Med.*, 293:1159–1163.

207. Schild, G. C., and Dowdle, W. R. (1975): Influenza virus characterization and diagnostic serology. In: *The Influenza Viruses and Influenza*, edited by E. D. Kilbourne, pp. 315–372. Academic Press, New York.

208. Schild, G. C., Oxford, J. S., Dowdle, W. R., Coleman, M., Pereira, M. S., and Chakraverty, P. (1974): Antigenic variation in current influenza A viruses: Evidence for a high frequency of antigenic "drift" for the Hong Kong virus. *Bull. WHO*, 51:1–11.

209. Schild, G. C., Smith, J. W. G., Cretescu, L., Newman, R. W., and Wood, J. M. (1977): Strain-specificity of antibody to haemagglutinin following inactivated A/Port Chalmers/1/73 vaccine in man: Evidence for a paradoxical strain-specific antibody response. *Dev. Biol. Stand.*, 39:273–281.

210. Schrader, J. W., Henning, R., Milner, R. J., and Edelman, G. M. (1976): The recognition of H-2 and viral antigens by cytotoxic T cells. *Cold Spring Harbor Symp. Quant. Biol.*, 41:547.

211. Schulman, J. L. (1970): Effects of immunity on transmission of influenza: Experimental studies. *Prog. Med. Virol.*, 12:128–160.

212. Schulman, J. L. (1975): Immunology of influenza. In: *The Influenza Viruses and Influenza*, edited by E. D. Kilbourne, pp. 373–393. Academic Press, New York.

213. Schulman, J. L., Khakpour, M., and Kilbourne, E. D. (1968): Protective effects of specific immunity to viral neuraminidase on influenza virus infection of mice. *J. Virol.*, 2:778–786

214. Schwartz, D. H., and Doherty, P. C. (1981): Virus-immune and alloreactive response characteristics of thymocytes and spleen cells from young mice. *J. Immunol.*, 127:1411–1414.

215. Seeley, J., Svedmyr, E., Weiland, O., Klein, G., Moller, E., Eriksson, E., Andersson, K., and Van Der Waal, L. (1981): Epstein-Barr virus selective T cells in infectious mononucleosis are not restricted to HLA-A and B antigens. *J. Immunol.*, 127:293–300.

216. Shaw, S. (1981): Human T-cell-mediated cytotoxicity: The role of HLA. In: *The Lymphocyte*, edited by K. W. Sell and W. V. Miller, pp. 13–30. Alan R. Liss, New York.

217. Shaw, S., Shearer, G. M., and Biddison, W. E. (1980): Human cytotoxic T-cell responses to type A and type B influenza viruses can be restricted by different HLA antigens. Implications for HLA polymorphism and genetic regulation. *J. Exp. Med.*, 151:235–245.

218. Sheldon, P. J., Hemsted, E. H., Papamichail, M., and Holborrow, E. J. (1973): Thymic origin of atypical lymphoid cells in infectious mononucleosis. *Lancet*, 1:1153–1155.

219. Shreffler, D. C. (1976): The S region of the mouse major histocompatibility complex (H-2): Genetic variation and functional role in complement system. *Transplant. Rev.*, 32:140–167.

220. Shultz, R. M., Woan, M. C., and Tompkins, W. A. F. (1974): Macrophage immunity to vaccinia virus: Factors affecting macrophage immunity *in vitro*. *J. Reticuloendothel. Soc.*, 16:37–47.

221. Silvestre, D., Ernberg, I., Neauport-Sautes, C., Kourilsky, F. M., and Klein, G. (1974): Differ-

entiation between early and late membrane antigen on human lymphoblastoid cell lines infected with Epstein-Barr virus. II. Immunoelectron microscopy. *J. Natl. Cancer Inst.*, 53:67–74.

222. Singer, S. H., Noguchi, P., and Kirschstein, R. L. (1972): Respiratory diseases in cyclophosphamide-treated mice. II. Decreased virulence of PR8 influenza virus. *Infect. Immun.*, 5:957–960.

223. Sissions, J. G. P., and Oldstone, M. B. A. (1980): Antibody-mediated destruction of virus-infected cells. *Adv. Immunol.*, 29:209–260.

224. Sissons, J. G. P., and Oldstone, M. B. A. (1980): Killing of virus-infected cells: The role of antiviral antibody and complement in limiting virus infection. *J. Infect. Dis.*, 142:442–448.

225. Slepushkin, A. N., Schild, G. C., Beare, A. S., Chinn, S., and Tyrrell, D. A. J. (1971): Neuraminidase and resistance to vaccination with live influenza A2 Hong Kong vaccines. *J. Hyg.*, 69:571–578.

226. Sprent, J. (1978): Role of H-2 gene products in the function of T helper cells from normal and chimeric mice in vivo. *Immunol. Rev.*, 42:108–137.

227. Sugamura, K., Shimizu, K., and Bach, F. H. (1978): Involvement of fusion activity of ultraviolet light-inactivated Sendai virus in formation of target antigens recognized by cytotoxic T cells. *J. Exp. Med.*, 148:276–287.

228. Sullivan, J. L., Mayner, R. E., Barry, D. W., and Ennis, F. A. (1976): Influenza virus infections in nude mice. *J. Infect. Dis.*, 133:91–94.

229. Suzuki, F., Ohya, J., and Ishida, N. (1974): Effect of antilymphocyte serum on influenza virus infection in mice. *Proc. Soc. Exp. Biol. Med.*, 146:78–84.

230. Svedmyr, E., and Jondal, M. (1975): Cytotoxic effector cells specific for B cell lines transformed by Epstein-Barr virus are present in patients with infectious mononucleosis. *Proc. Natl. Acad. Sci. USA*, 72:1622–1626.

231. Thorley-Lawson, D. A., Chess, L., and Strominger, J. L. (1977): Suppression of in vitro Epstein-Barr virus infection. A new role for adult human T lymphocytes. *J. Exp. Med.*, 146:495–508.

232. Tosato, G., Magrath, I., Koski, I., Dooley, N., and Blaese, M. (1979): Activation of suppressor T cells during Epstein-Barr virus-induced infectious mononucleosis. *N. Engl. J. Med.*, 301:1133–1137.

233. Tyrrell, D. A. J., and Smith, J. W. G. (1979): Vaccination against influenza A. *Br. Med. Bull.*, 35:77–85.

234. Uhr, J. W., Capra, J. D., Vitetta, E. S., and Cook, R. G. (1979): Organization of the immune response genes. *Science*, 206:292–297.

235. University Health Physicians and PHLS Laboratories (1971): Infectious mononucleosis and its relation to EB virus antibody. *Br. Med. J.*, 4:643–646.

236. Veada, S., and Nozima, T. (1973): Delayed hypersensitivity in vaccinia-infected mice. II. Resistance of peritoneal macrophages against vaccinia infection. *Acta Virol.*, 17:41.

237. Virelizier, J. L. (1975): Host defenses against influenza virus: The role of anti-hemagglutinin antibody. *J. Immunol.*, 115:434–439.

238. Virelizier, J. L., Allison, A. C., and De Maeyer, E. (1977): Production by mixed lymphocyte cultures of a type II interferon able to protect macrophages against virus infection. *Infect. Immun.*, 17:282–285.

239. Virelizier, J. L., Allison, A. C., Oxford, J. S., and Schild, G. C. (1977): Early presence of ribonucleoprotein antigen on surface of influenza virus-infected cells. *Nature*, 266:52–53.

240. Virelizier, J. L., Allison, A. C., and Schild, G. C. (1974): Antibody responses to antigenic determinants of influenza virus hemagglutinin. II. Original antigenic sin: A bone marrow-derived lymphocyte memory phenomenon modulated by thymus-derived lymphocytes. *J. Exp. Med.*, 140:1571–1578.

241. Virelizier, J. L., Allison, A. C., and Schild, G. C. (1979): Immune responses to influenza virus in the mouse, and their role in control of the infection. *Br. Med. Bull.*, 35:65–68.

242. Virelizier, J. L., Oxford, J. S., and Schild, G. C. (1976): The role of humoral immunity in host defense against influenza A infection in mice. *Postgrad. Med. J.*, 52:332–337.

243. Virelizier, J. L., Postlethwaite, P., Schild, G. C., and Allison, A. C. (1974): Antibody responses to antigenic determinants of influenza virus hemagglutinin. I. Thymus dependence of antibody formation and thymus independence of immunological memory. *J. Exp. Med.*, 140:1559–1570.

244. Vitetta, E. S., and Capra, J. D. (1978): The protein products of the murine 17th chromosome: Genetics and structure. *Adv. Immunol.*, 26:147–193.

245. Wagner, H., Pfizenmaier, K., and Rollinghoff, M. (1980): The role of the major histocompatibility gene complex in murine cytotoxic T cell responses. *Adv. Cancer Res.*, 31:77–124.

246. Wahren, B., Lantorp, K., Sterner, G., and Espmark, A. (1970): EBV antibodies in family contacts of patients with infectious mononucleosis. *Proc. Soc. Exp. Biol. Med.*, 133:934–939.

247. Webster, R. G., and Bean, W. J., Jr. (1978): Genetics of influenza virus. *Ann. Rev. Genet.*, 12:415–431.

248. Webster, R. G., and Laver, W. G. (1975): Antigenic variation of influenza viruses. In: *The Influenza Viruses and Influenza*, edited by E. D. Kilbourne, pp. 269–314. Academic Press, New York.

249. Welsh, R. M. (1981): Do natural killer cells play a role in virus infections? *Antiviral Res.*, 1:5–12.

250. Welsh, R. M., Jr., and Hallenbeck, L. A. (1980): Effect of virus infections on target cell susceptibility to natural killer cell-mediated lysis. *J. Immunol.*, 124:2491–2497.

251. Wheelock, E. F., and Toy, S. T. (1973): Participation of lymphocytes in viral infections. *Adv. Immunol.*, 16:123–184.

252. Wigzell, H. (1974): On the relationship between cellular and humoral antibodies. *Contemp. Top. Immunobiol.*, 3:77–96.

253. Wolf, H., zur Hausen, H., and Becker, Y. (1973): Epstein-Barr viral genomes in epithelial nasopharyngeal carcinoma cells. *Nature [New Biol.]*, 244:245–247.

254. Worthington, M., Rabson, A. S., and Baron, S. (1972): Mechanism of recovery from systemic vaccinia virus infection I. *J. Exp. Med.*, 136:277–290.

255. Worthington, M. (1973): Mechanism of recovery from systemic infection with vaccinia virus. II. Effects of X-irradiation and neonatal thymectomy. *J. Infect. Dis.*, 127:512–517.

256. Worthington, M. (1973): Mechanism of recovery from systemic infection with vaccinia virus III. Effects of antithymocyte serum. *J. Infect. Dis.*, 127:518–524.

257. Wyde, P. R., Couch, R. B., Mackler, B. F., Cate, T. R., and Levy, B. M. (1977): Effects of low- and high-passage influenza virus infection in normal and nude mice. *Infect. Immun.*, 15:221–229.

258. Yap, K. L., and Ada, G. L. (1977): Cytotoxic T cells specific for influenza virus-infected target cells. *Immunology*, 32:151–160.

259. Yap, K. L., and Ada, G. L. (1978): Cytotoxic T cells in the lungs of mice infected with an influenza A virus. *Scand. J. Immunol.*, 7:73–80.

260. Yap, K. L., and Ada, G. L. (1978): The recovery of mice from influenza virus infection: Adoptive transfer of immunity with immune T lymphocytes. *Scand. J. Immunol.*, 7:389–397.

261. Yap, K. L., and Ada, G. L. (1978): The recovery of mice from influenza A virus infection: Adoptive transfer of immunity with influenza virus-specific cytotoxic T lymphocytes recognizing a common virion antigen. *Scand. J. Immunol.*, 8:413–420.

262. Yap, K. L., Ada, G. L., and McKenzie, I. F. C. (1978): Transfer of specific cytotoxic T lymphocytes protects mice inoculated with influenza virus. *Nature*, 273:238–239.

263. Yap, K. L., Braciale, T. J., and Ada, G. L. (1979): Role of T-cell function in recovery from murine influenza infection. *Cell. Immunol.*, 43:341–351.

264. Yewdell, J. W., Frank, E., and Gerhard, W. (1981): Expression of influenza A virus internal antigens on the surface of infected P815 cells. *J. Immunol.*, 126:1814–1819.

265. Yewdell, J. W., and Gerhard, W. (1981): Antigenic characterization of viruses by monoclonal antibodies. *Ann. Rev. Microbiol.*, 35:185–206.

266. Zinkernagel, R. M. (1976): H-2 compatibility requirement for virus-specific T-cell-mediated cytolysis. The H-2K structure involved is coded by a single cistron defined by H-2K^b mutant mice. *J. Exp. Med.*, 143:437–443.

267. Zinkernagel, R. M., and Althage, A. (1977): Antiviral protection by virus immunocytotoxic T cells: Infected target cells are lysed before infectious virus progeny is assembled. *J. Exp. Med.*, 145:644–651.

268. Zinkernagel, R. M., and Doherty, P. C. (1974): Characteristics of the interaction *in vivo* between cytotoxic thymus-derived lymphocyte and target monolayers infected with lymphocytic choriomeningitis virus. *Scand. J. Immunol.*, 3:287–294.

269. Zinkernagel, R. M., and Doherty, P. C. (1974): Restriction of *in vitro* T-cell-mediated cytotoxicity in lymphocytic choriomeningitis within a syngeneic or semiallogeneic system. *Nature*, 248:701–702.

270. Zinkernagel, R. M., and Doherty, P. C. (1975): H-2 compatibility requirement for T-cell-mediated

lysis of targets infected with lymphocytic choriomeningitis virus. Different cytotoxic T cell specificities are associated with structures coded in H-2K or H-2D. *J. Exp. Med.*, 141:1427–1436.

271. Zinkernagel, R. M., and Doherty, P. C. (1979): MHC-restricted cytotoxic T cells: Studies on the biological role of polymorphic major transplantation antigens determining T-cell restriction-specificity, function and responsiveness. *Adv. Immunol.*, 27:51–177.

272. Zinkernagel, R. M. and Klein, J. (1977): H-2-associated specificity of virus-immune cytotoxic T cells from H-2 mutant and wild-type mice: M523 (H-2K^{ka}) and M505 (H-2K^{bd}) do, M504 (H-2D^{da}) do not crossreact with wild-type H-2K or H-2D. *Immunogenetics*, 4:581–590.

273. Zinkernagel, R. M., and Oldstone, M. B. A. (1976): Cells that express viral antigens but lack H-2 determinants are not lysed by immune T cells but are lysed by other anti-viral immune attack mechanisms. *Proc. Natl. Acad. Sci. USA*, 73:3666–3670.

274. Zinkernagel, R. M., Althage, A., Cooper, S., Kreeb, G., Klein, P. A., Sefton, B., Flaherty, L., Stimpfling, J., Shreffler, D., and Klein, J. (1978): Ir genes in H-2 regulate generation of antiviral cytotoxic T cells: Mapping to K or D and dominance of unresponsiveness. *J. Exp. Med.*, 148:592.

275. Zinkernagel, R. M., Klein, P., and Klein, J. (1978): Host-determined T cell fine-specificity for self H-2 in radiation bone marrow chimeras of standard C57BL/6 (H-2^b), mutant Hzl (H-2^{ba}), and F$_1$ mice. *Immunogenetics*, 7:73.

276. Zweerink, H. J., Askonas, B. A., Millican, D., Courtneidge, S. A., and Skehel, J. J. (1977): Cytotoxic T cells to type A influenza virus; viral hemagglutinin induces A-strain specificity while infected cells confer cross-reactive cytotoxicity. *Eur. J. Immunol.*, 7:630–635.

277. Zweerink, H. J., Courtneidge, S. A., Skehel, J. J., Crumpton, M. J., and Askonas, B. A. (1977): Cytotoxic T cells kill influenza virus infected cells but do not distinguish between serologically distinct type A viruses. *Nature*, 267:354–356.

Advances in Host Defense Mechanisms, Vol. 2,
edited by John I. Gallin and Anthony S. Fauci.
Raven Press, New York © 1983.

The Lymphoid System in Mycotic and Mycobacterial Diseases

Ulysses G. Mason and Charles H. Kirkpatrick

The Conrad D. Stephenson Laboratory for Research in Immunology, Department of Medicine, National Jewish Hospital and Research Center/National Asthma Center, Denver, Colorado 80206

In fungal and mycobacterial infections, the components of the lymphoid system provide both specific immunity mediated by the cellular and humoral immune systems and nonspecific protective or curative processes. The specific immune system is composed of lymphocytes and humoral antibodies. Acting in concert with or triggered by the specific system, the nonspecific system consists of phagocytic cells, the complement system, lymphokines, and plasma factors. Each of these multiple, complex systems is important in host defenses. Their functions often overlap and sometimes are redundant. When a defect occurs in any system, either naturally or induced, susceptibility to infection can occur.

Immunologic reactions to specific antigens in sensitized hosts may be broadly classified as those mediated by antibodies and those mediated by cells (Fig. 1). The latter category is termed cell-mediated immunity. Its functions play the major role in defense and limitation of spread and growth of fungi and mycobacteria. The afferent limb of this process involves macrophages, which facilitate the engagement of antigen-sensitive T-lymphocytes; the mechanisms by which this is accomplished are still being defined. The efferent limb involves release of various soluble factors, which amplify the immune response by promoting phagocytosis of the organisms and enhancing macrophage activity. Despite this important protective and curative role, hypersensitivity responses mediated by cellular immunity can contribute to symptoms and to the pathogenesis of these infections.

In this chapter, we examine host defense mechanisms against fungal infections with particular emphasis on the cellular immune system, explore the role of various fungal infections on functions of the immune system, and discuss treatment and prophylaxis of the diseases.

COMPONENTS OF THE IMMUNE SYSTEM AND THEIR INTERACTIONS WITH FUNGAL AND MYCOBACTERIAL ORGANISMS

T-Lymphocytes

A vast body of evidence indicates that antigen-responsive T-lymphocytes initiate cell-mediated immune responses (8,14,105,109,147,150). The data derive from

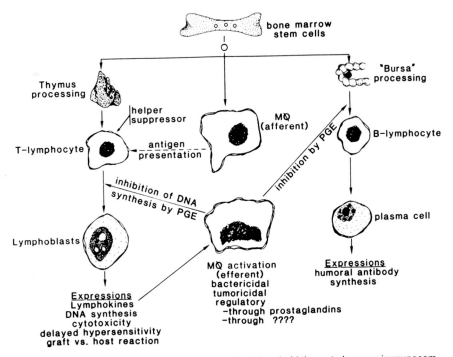

FIG. 1. Processing of stem cells by thymus and gut lymphoid tissue to become immunocompetent T- and B-lymphocytes. Transformation to cells of the lymphoblast and plasma cell series occurs after stimulation. Note the central role of macrophages in processing antigens for presentation and activation of T-lymphocytes and in production of immunoregulatory prostaglandins.

in vivo experiments with passive transfer of immunity with lymphoid cells and *in vitro* activation of macrophages with soluble factors from antigen-activated T-cells. For example, animals that receive immune, but not nonimmune T-cells, are significantly more resistant to challenges with lethal doses of bacteria (53), such as *Listeria* (7), and fungi, such as *Candida albicans* (102) or *Cryptococcus neoformans* (54). Moreover, both the protective effects and the property of transferring delayed hypersensitivity can be abrogated by treating the cell suspensions with anti-Thy 1.2 and complement, a procedure for selectively killing thymus-derived lymphocytes.

The critical role of antigen-sensitive lymphoid cells has also been demonstrated *in vitro*. Patterson and Youmans (114) showed that when lymphocytes from normal or immune mice were added to macrophage cultures that had been infected with tubercle bacilli, multiplication of the organisms was inhibited only in those cultures that received lymphocytes from the immunized animals. Cells from nonimmune donors had no effect. In similar studies of the role of lymphocytes in immunity to *Histoplasma capsulatum*, Howard and Otto (70) found that inhibition of growth of the organism within macrophages was achieved only after immune lymphocytes were added to the cultures.

Recently, Beaman et al. (6) described interactions between murine lymphocytes, macrophages, and *Coccidioides immitis in vitro*. Although peritoneal macrophages from nonimmune mice are able to phagocytose *C. immitis*, the viability of the organisms was unchanged after 4 hr. In contrast, when macrophages were infected in the presence of lymphocytes from immune mice, marked reductions in the viability of the organisms was observed. This effect could also be deleted by treatment of the lymphocytes with anti-Thy 1.2 and complement. Thus experiments with both fungi and tubercle bacilli (26,48) affirm the importance of immune T-lymphocytes in microbicidal cellular responses to certain infections. The T-cells appear to affect the organisms indirectly through activation of macrophages rather than through direct cytotoxic activities.

In contrast to these observations, some investigators were unable to demonstrate an obligate role for thymus-dependent T-cells in protection against candidiasis. Marra and Balish (97) found that progression of disseminated candidiasis in mice could not be correlated with the development of, or increase in, cutaneous hypersensitivity responses.

Cutler (31) showed that congenitally athymic nude mice were more resistant to parenteral infections with *C. albicans* than were their phenotypically normal littermates. In addition, Rogers et al. (123) demonstrated that reconstitution of nude mice with a thymus made them just as susceptible as normal mice to systemic infection by *C. albicans*. These findings are significant because they illustrate the delicate balance of thymus-dependent immune responses in control of resistance to this organism. Presumably, the athymic mouse is less susceptible to lethal challenges with *C. albicans* because other elements of the immune system, such as complement and antibodies, provide adequate protection. Following thymic transplantation, the mice have suppressor cells (as well as other T-lymphocytes); these exert a negative regulatory effect that is involved in increased susceptibility to fatal infections.

Finally, by use of a mouse model in which abscesses were produced in the thighs, Pearsall et al. (115,116) found that passive transfer of lymphoid cells from mice that were sensitized by infection with *C. albicans* afforded no appreciable protection to challenges with lethal doses of organisms, although the lymphoid cells from these mice could transfer delayed hypersensitivity. However, a single dose of 0.5 ml immune serum given intraperitoneally to normal mice a few hours before the initiation of infection resulted in significant ($p < 0.01$) protection at day 22. Normal serum was not protective.

From the results of experiments that demonstrated an important role for T-cells and, in some cases, for serum in immune responses to the microorganisms emerges the issue of the interrelationships between hypersensitivity and immunity. The question is whether the same immune mechanisms that produce the inflammatory reaction of hypersensitivity to a specific antigen (65) are also responsible for the host's resistance to infection with organisms bearing that antigen. Although it is often accepted that delayed hypersensitivity reflects immunocompetence, there are numerous exceptions. The observations by Pearsall et al. (116) and Marra and

Balish (97) described above are examples. Others deal with guinea pigs that were sensitized to extracts of *M. tuberculosis* and which were shown to have delayed hypersensitivity to tuberculin, but were unable to resist infectious challenges with viable organisms (24,120). In human beings, there is evidence of disparate relationships between delayed hypersensitivity and protective immunity. Approximately one-third of patients with chronic mucocutaneous candidiasis have positive delayed skin tests to candida, but the clinical features of their disease are identical to those of immunodeficient patients (79). Youmans (158) has suggested that hypersensitivity and immunity may be separate processes involving separate T-cells and lymphokines and effector mechanisms; a substantial body of evidence supports this position.

Lymphokines

After antigen presentation by macrophages (124), T-lymphocytes become sensitized in peripheral tissues and thymus-dependent areas of lymph nodes that drain the site of antigen. Upon reexposure to the same antigen, the sensitized T-cells produce soluble mediators (lymphokines), such as macrophage migration inhibiton factor (MIF), macrophage activation factor (MAF), chemotactic factors, blastogenic factors, lymphotoxins, interleukin 2, and immune interferon (Table 1). After release at the site of antigen deposition, these mediators act to amplify cell-mediated immune responses. For example, blastogenic factors induce other lymphocytes to undergo DNA synthesis; chemotactic factors attract phagocytic cells into antigen-containing sites; and MAF and MIF activate macrophages. The progress with isolation and purification of individual lymphokines has been limited, and it is still unclear which lymphokine or combination of lymphokines is most effective in mediating resistance and hypersensitivity.

Since the initial observations of inhibition of macrophage migration by Rich and Lewis (122), several investigators have demonstrated the role of lymphocyte-macrophage interactions in this phenomenon. Using spleen fragments from guinea pigs

TABLE 1. *Products of activated lymphocytes*

Product	Function
MIF	Inhibits migration of macrophages *in vitro*
MAF	Induces morphologic, metabolic, and functional changes in macrophages
Chemotactic factor	Recruits a variety of cell types to migrate into sites of inflammatory reactions
Blastogenic factors	Induces lymphocytes to undergo DNA synthesis
Lymphotoxin	Induces cytolysis of a target cell by direct contact or through release of a factor
Interleukin 2	Induces *in vitro* clonal expansion and prolongs growth of cytotoxic T-lymphocytes or helper cells
Immune interferon	Confers on cells resistance to virus infection

that were sensitized to avirulent human tubercle bacilli and later activated by exposure to old tuberculin, Rich and Lewis (122) noted inhibition of migration of macrophages from the explants. Tuberculin had no effect on explants from nonimmune animals. In 1962, George and Vaughan (57) demonstrated a similar inhibition of migration of peritoneal cells from capillary tubes. The work of David et al. (32,33) demonstrated that the migration of peritoneal exudate cells from guinea pigs with delayed hypersensitivity to purified protein derivative (PPD), ovalbumin, or diphtheria toxoid was specifically inhibited by addition of the appropriate antigen. In addition, the authors showed that antigen-dependent inhibition of macrophage migration was demonstrable when only 2.5% of the cells came from a sensitized animal. Bloom and Bennett (9) confirmed these findings with experiments using separated populations of lymphocytes and macrophages. They also found that in the presence of PPD, only a few lymphocytes from PPD-sensitive donors were required to cause inhibition of normal peritoneal exudate cells. In the absence of lymphocytes, antigen did not inhibit migration of macrophages.

In 1970, Heise and Weiser (68), using antilymphocyte and antimacrophage sera, showed that lymphocytes were essential for the migration inhibition response and that decreasing the number of macrophages had no effect on the overall reaction.

Thus the lymphokines provide an important amplification system in which the products of a relatively small number of antigen-responsive lymphocytes may activate other lymphocytes and macrophages and initiate intense but localized inflammatory responses.

Macrophages

The theory of phagocytosis was first proposed by Metchnikoff in 1844 after he observed mobile cells of the starfish larva engulfing solid particles. In mammals, the mononuclear phagocyte system is composed of monocytes and tissue macrophages. As effector cells in the immune response, monocytes and macrophages are generally regarded as the first line of defense against facultative and obligate intracellular organisms, such as *L. monocytogenes*, *M. tuberculosis*, and *C. albicans* (25,143,144). To carry out this function, activation of macrophages by sensitized lymphocytes appears to be a crucial mechanism (82,94–96). Monocytes are aided in phagocytosis by surface receptors for subclasses of IgG and C3, which form attachments to organisms that are opsonized with immunoglobulin or complement.

In 1942, Lurie (93) demonstrated that macrophages were involved in immunity to tuberculosis. Using irritating substances, he induced inflammatory peritoneal exudates in normal and immunized rabbits. After he removed the cells, he mixed them with tubercle bacilli, and phagocytosis was allowed to take place for 1 hr. The infected cell mixtures then were injected into the eyes of rabbits. After 10 to 14 days, the author noted that the number of mycobacteria in the eyes of animals implanted with immune cells was usually lower than the number found in recipients of nonimmune cells. It was concluded that the ability to inhibit proliferation of the bacilli was a unique property of the phagocytic cells.

Studies supporting Lurie's observations were carried out by Suter in 1952 and 1953 (139,140). These showed that intracellular multiplication of tubercle bacilli was retarded or completely inhibited within macrophages from animals primed with Bacillus Calmette-Guérin (BCG), as compared with proliferation of tubercle bacilli within normal macrophages. The presence of immune or normal serum had no effect on the multiplication of tubercle bacilli within normal or immune macrophages.

Evidence for the role of macrophages in immunity to *Candida* comes from several experiments. Baine et al. (3) showed that after injection of *Candida* into rabbits, the organisms were quickly removed from the bloodstream by the lung when the yeasts were injected into a peripheral vein or by the liver when the injection was into the mesenteric vein. When organisms were injected into the perfused liver, they were found in neutrophils and Kupffer cells, indicating that both cell types were responsible for clearance. To investigate the fate of phagocytosed organisms, Peterson and Calderone (117) measured incorporation of tritiated leucine by *C. albicans* and observed a 71 to 93% reduction of protein synthesis by the organisms after ingestion by rabbit alveolar macrophages. Although organisms are readily ingested by macrophages, their relatively poor fungicidal activity has been well documented. Stanley and Hurley (138) showed that mouse peritoneal macrophages readily phagocytosed *C. albicans*. Within several hours, however, more than 90% of the ingested yeast had formed pseudohyphae, which subsequently destroyed the macrophages. Ozato and Uesaka (112) confirmed the ability of *C. albicans* to multiply within mouse peritoneal macrophages.

In cryptococcal infections, Cline and Lehrer (25) showed that only monocytes were able to phagocytose the organisms. Diamond et al. (37) showed that although ingestion of the organisms was not affected by size of the capsule, monocytes were 15% less efficient than neutrophils in killing cryptococci. In a later study, Diamond and Bennett (38) found that human macrophages derived from peripheral blood monocytes and activated *in vitro* by cryptococcal antigens could not kill ingested cryptococci, even though the blood monocytes from which they had been derived could kill the yeast. These studies emphasize the limited capacity of monocytes and activated macrophages to ingest and kill cryptococci.

From the evidence outlined here, it must be concluded that macrophages partially limit but do not eradicate the spread of fungi. In contrast, with tubercle bacilli, macrophages activated through lymphokines elaborated by T-cells bring about marked intracellular inhibition of mycobacterial multiplication.

Unlike their role in deep fungal infections, macrophages do not appear to be important in either limiting or eradicating superficial fungal infections. The organisms multiply and the infection spreads, an interplay which leads to cell-mediated immune damage to the skin, arrest of the spreading infection, and, eventually, sloughing of the skin with the organisms. It appears that monocytes probably cannot completely ingest the long fungal filaments that spread through the upper dermal layers (72).

Antibodies and Immune Complexes

The majority of evidence indicates that circulating antibodies play a minor role in defense against fungal and mycobacterial infections. Exceptions include the experiments by Pearsall et al. (116) and the clinical evidence that suggests that antibodies may be important in limiting cutaneous infections with organisms such as *Candida*. This evidence is indirect and is based on the observation that patients with extensive candidiasis of the skin and mucous membranes essentially never have blood-borne infections of parenchymal organs. It is assumed that antibodies, possibly in conjunction with the complement system, prevent dissemination of the organisms. Conversely, antibodies develop during widespread fungal infections, often at times when delayed hypersensitivity is depressed or absent, and then become undetectable during recovery. Complement-fixing (CF) antibodies are important in diagnosis and prognosis of mycotic infections, such as coccidioidomycosis. The CF antibody titer provides a rough measure of the severity of the disease; the more extensive tissue involvement, the higher the titer. Thus antibodies detected with agglutination tests become an index of the presence and severity of systemic disease.

In studies attempting to elucidate the mechanism of the immunosuppressive activity of plasma, antibodies have also been implicated in histoplasmosis. Newberry et al. (108) and Kirkpatrick et al. (74) suggested that circulating antibody might be involved because sera containing CF antibodies suppressed lymphocyte transformation by normal subjects, and the patients with the highest CF titers demonstrated the most depressed lymphocyte transformation responses. In another study of immunologic responses in histoplasmosis, Cox (27) reported similar correlation between serum-mediated suppression of lymphocyte transformation responses to *Histoplasma* antigens and serum CF antibody titers. Suppression was specific for the *Histoplasma* antigen because responses to mitogens and *Candida* antigen were not affected by the serum. Although the specificity of suppression in Cox's study is most consistent with an effect of antibody, either alone or complexed with antigen, a direct suppressive effect of antibody has not been proved. It is possible that the CF antibody titers may reflect antigen-antibody complexes, despite the absence of demonstrable circulating antigen.

In this regard, immune complexes are known to suppress T-cell-mediated delayed-type hypersensitivity responses (125), inhibit antibody-dependent cell-mediated cytotoxicity (113), and suppress the chemotactic responses of neutrophils (90). Carr et al. (21) found a significantly increased concentration of circulating immune complexes in 68% of patients with active *M. tuberculosis* infections and 58% with active *M. avium-intracellulare* infections by a Clq binding assay. The assay gave positive results in only 15% of cured *M. tuberculosis* patients, 22% of patients with chronic obstructive pulmonary disease, and 3% of healthy controls. Although the clinical significance of the marked prevalence of immune complexes in these patients was unclear, the authors speculated that the complexes might play a pathogenic role by causing granuloma formation by impairing T-cell function.

In coccidioidomycosis, Yoshinoya et al. (156) found circulating immune complexes in 73% of 22 patients with active infections but in only 13% of 13 patients with inactive infections. The temporal relationship between depressed T-cell function and chronic coccidioidomycosis (23,28), coupled with the relationship between CF antibody titers, immune complexes, and disease severity, suggested to the investigators that antigen-antibody complexes provided a negative feedback on T-cell function and adversely affected the course of the disease. Thus one must question the protective role of immunoglobulins and consider whether they might be contributing to the pathogenesis of some systemic fungal and mycobacterial infections.

Nonantibody Plasma Factors

Antigens are only one example of nonantibody plasma factors that can influence cellular immune responses. Fischer et al. (51) described the physiochemical properties of the inhibitory material in the serum of some patients with chronic mucocutaneous candidiasis. The inhibitor was shown to be nondialyzable, thermostable, nonprecipitable with ammonium sulfate, and absorbable on anti-*Candida* antibodies or concanavalin A-coupled agarose columns. These results suggested that the factor was not an immunoglobulin but rather a polysacchride antigen of *C. albicans*. When the polysaccharide antigens were added to cultures of lymphocytes from normal candida-sensitive donors, inhibition of *Candida*-induced lymphocyte transformation was observed. This is not the mechanism of impaired lymphocyte responses in all patients with chronic mucocutaneous candidiasis. The inhibitory plasma factor was found in only six of 23 of the patients of Fischer et al. (51); and many reports (1,69,75) have shown that these patients may have impaired lymphocyte responses, even in the absence of inhibitory plasma factors.

Similar effects have been noted with mycobacterial products. Kleinhenz et al. (80) examined the effects of plasma from anergic tuberculosis patients on PPD-induced DNA synthesis in mononuclear cells from healthy, tuberculin-sensitive subjects. The tuberculous plasma markedly suppressed DNA synthesis by normal cells. This effect was attributed to C-arabino-D-galactan, a polysaccharide component of mycobacterial cell walls. The effect was nonspecific because responses to phytohemagglutinin (PHA) were also suppressed. Of particular interest was the finding that the immunosuppressive effects of the plasma could be blocked by indomethacin, an inhibitor of cyclooxygenase which is essential for conversion of arachidonic acid into prostaglandins. Further experiments showed that the arabinogalactan stimulated macrophages to elaborate a prostaglandin, and it was this product that resulted in the immunosuppressive activity. The authors' work also showed that the suppression was monocyte dependent. In addition, the tuberculous plasma had a direct inhibitory effect on T-lymphocyte responses to PHA; this was also indomethacin reversible. The effects of plasma and polysaccharide were not due to cytotoxicity or altered kinetics of DNA synthesis, and these agents did not generate autonomously functioning suppressor cells. The activities were reversed by washing the cells. The sequence of events appears to begin with stimulation of macrophages by the polysaccharide, followed by elaboration of prostaglandins by the macrophages, and, in turn, suppression of antigen- and mitogen-induced thymidine incorporation by lymphocytes. The advantages of these events to host defense mechanisms or hypersensitivity are unknown.

Other studies have also implicated arachidonic acid derivatives in the immuno-deficiency that often accompanies chronic infectious diseases. The studies of patients with chronic coccidioidomycosis by Catanzaro (22) illustrate the nonspecific im-munosuppressive role of prostaglandins. Mononuclear cells from his patients dem-onstrated subnormal *in vitro* responses to PHA, but addition of indomethacin to the cultures resulted in significant augmentation of the responses. Furthermore, when adherent cells were removed by passage of the mixed mononuclear cells over nylon wool columns, the nonadherent cells responded more vigorously to PHA than did the unseparated cells. The observations probably mean that suppression of the response to PHA is mediated by an activity that is restricted to the adherent cell population, and that indomethacin acts on those cells.

We (98) have examined the influence of the products of arachidonic acid on lymphocyte responses in patients with nontuberculous mycobacterial infections. In nearly every case, the mononuclear cells demonstrated subnormal responses to PPD, candida, other "atypical" mycobacterial antigens, and the mitogen PHA. Addition of indomethacin, an inhibitor of the cyclooxygenase pathway, resulted in signifi-cantly enhanced responses to stimulation with antigens and the mitogen. In contrast, inhibition of the lipoxygenase pathway with nordihydroguiaretic acid (NDGA) pro-duced further impairment of lymphocyte responses (Fig. 2). The results with in-domethacin suggest that enhancement of antigen- and mitogen-dependent T-cell proliferation occurs by preventing formation of cyclooxygenase products and pos-

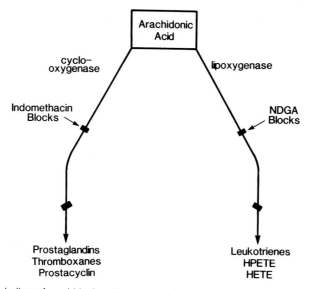

FIG. 2. Metabolism of arachidonic acid occurs via the cyclooxygenase and lipoxygenase path-ways. Indomethacin is a preferential inhibitor of the former, and NDGA is an inhibitor of the latter.

sibly by making more substrate available for production of lipoxygenase products. Since the former pathway leads to production of prostaglandins, prostacyclins, and thromboxanes, and because prostaglandins are known to have immunosuppressive effects, it is likely that the suppressive activity is mediated by prostaglandins or other cyclooxygenase products. Compatible with this model is the effect of the lipoxygenase inhibitor NDGA, which may make more substrate available for production of the inhibitors via the cyclooxygenase pathway. An alternative model proposes that a lipoxygenase derivative provides a stimulatory or supportive effect on lymphocyte DNA synthesis. Inhibition of the cyclooxygenase pathway would avail more substrate to the lipoxygenase system, while NDGA would remove this effect and reduce DNA synthesis. There is currently no direct support for this model.

We have also found immunosuppressive activity in the plasma of some patients with atypical mycobacterial infections. This was demonstrated in experiments in which cells and plasmas from healthy PPD-sensitive donors and patients with atypical mycobacterial infections were studied in all combinations. Plasma from about 80% of the patients would suppress responses by lymphocytes from PPD-sensitive donors by 25 to 70%. When the patients' cells were cultured in normal plasma, however, the responses still were subnormal. Thus in addition to an immunosuppressive activity in the plasma, there is also a hyporesponsiveness that is intrinsic to the lymphocytes. The nature of the plasma factor is unknown.

In summary, a number of plasma-associated factors can suppress lymphocyte transformation responses to antigens and mitogens (67). Some investigations have implicated antibodies, alone or as immune complexes. Other studies have highlighted the suppressive role of the components of antigens which can affect a population of cells that release prostaglandins, which, in turn, cause suppression of thymidine incorporation in lymphocytes. However, the clinical significance of plasma factors is not clear.

Complement

Gelfand et al. (55) defined an antifungal mechanism in which the alternate pathway and late components of the complement system are involved in survival of guinea pigs from sepsis due to *C. albicans*. The kidneys, liver, and spleen from normal guinea pigs, animals with a genetically determined total deficiency of the fourth component of complement (C4D), and animals depleted of late complement components by cobra venom factor were compared after they had been challenged with lethal doses of *C. albicans*. Cobra venom factor-treated animals had a mortality rate of 70% 72 hr after infection. None of the normal or C4-deficient guinea pigs died from the challenge. Colony counts of organs demonstrated that total deficiency of C4 was not associated with increased numbers of organisms in the liver, spleen, or kidney 24 hr after infection. In marked contrast, the animals that were depleted of the alternative pathway and terminal complement components by cobra venom factor had significantly more *Candida* in these tissues. These studies showed that in nonimmune guinea pigs, the classic complement pathway did not play a critical role in defense against intravenous challenges with *Candida*, but defects in the alternative pathway and the late components are accompanied by increased sensitivity to this organism.

In evaluating guinea pigs with cryptococcosis, Diamond et al. (39) found that shortened survival times and increased infection in peripheral blood, lung, and liver were associated with cobra venom treatment, but there were no differences between normal control animals and C4-deficient animals in survival or degree of infection. When taken together, these studies strongly suggest that alternate pathway activation or late complement components make an important contribution to protection from some fungal infections.

Polymorphonuclear Leukocytes

The polymorphonuclear leukocyte is the other principal phagocytic cell of man. It plays a major role in the body's defense against acute infectious processes and is concerned with the elimination of organisms that rely on evasion of phagocytosis for survival. Although leukocytes are similar to macrophages in many aspects of their phagocytic behavior (37,86,87,126), they are not subject to lymphocyte-mediated activation.

Louria and Brayton (92) demonstrated the limited ability of polymorphonuclear leukocytes to control candida infections. After 4 hr of incubation, the fungi formed pseudohyphae, which appeared to penetrate the membrane of viable leukocytes. Although it was possible that killing could have occurred after a longer incubation, the ability of the organism to avoid this outcome was interpreted as a mechanism for proliferation that was unhampered by ordinarily effective cellular defenses.

In vivo observations pertinent to understanding the importance of leukocytes as an integral part of antifungal mechanisms are the common occurrence of deep-seated candidiasis in patients with severe neutropenia and the occasional occurrence in patients whose polymorphonuclear leukocytes have shown impaired candidacidal activity. Oh et al. (110) demonstrated that neutrophils from normal adults and infants killed approximately 30% of the *C. albicans* after 60 min, and that there was virtually no killing of *Candida* by the cells from two patients with chronic granulomatous disease. Lehrer (85) found that leukocyte candicidal deficiency was manifested by eosinophils as well as neutrophils and macrophages. Defective leukocyte candidacidal activity has also been demonstrated in patients with Hodgkin's disease, acute leukemia, and metastatic cancer, suggesting that defects in cellular function, as well as neutropenia, may be important in the acquisition of candidal infection in compromised hosts (89). Thus, even though leukocytes demonstrate poor *in vitro* fungicidal activity, the cells appear to be important *in vivo*.

Evidence for the role of neutrophils is also provided by Diamond and co-workers (41–43), who studied the interaction between neutrophils and pseudohyphal forms of candida. In the absence of serum, neutrophils attached to and spread over the surfaces of partially ingested hyphae, which then appeared to be damaged. Using an assay that measured neutrophil-induced inhibition of uptake of radiolabeled cytosine by *Candida*, damage to the fungus by neutrophils from normal subjects was less in the absence than in the presence of serum, most likely because of the effect of opsonization by low levels of anti-*Candida* IgG in normal sera. Further investigations showed that *Candida* activated neutrophil oxidative microbial mechanisms, as shown by iodination of *Candida* by neutrophils, and chemiluminescence from neutrophils interacting with *Candida*. Contact between neutrophils and hyphal forms of *Aspergillus* and *Rhizopus* also occurred in the absence of serum but not with the *C. neoformans*, an encapsulated yeast, and only minimally with yeast-phase *Candida*. In summary, although *in vitro* studies support a role for leukocytes in host defense against some fungal hyphae, these cells do not appear to be as effective as macrophages.

Summary

Our understanding of the physiology of the lymphoid system and the cellular basis of immune responses has increased greatly in the past 20 years. These responses comprise a complex series of events which occur as a result of the interaction of an immunocompetent cell with antigen. In a general way, one can distinguish between specific mechanisms, such as the reactions of antigen-responsive lymphocytes with antigen, and nonspecific mechanisms, which do not depend on the entry of a foreign substance into the body for activation. Examples of the latter mechanism are the function of cells, monocytes, macrophages, and polymorphonuclear leukocytes, which perform phagocytosis.

The T-cell appears to be the crucial link in the cell-mediated response to fungal and mycobacterial antigens, because ensuing interactions between antigen-activated T-lymphocytes and effector cells result in amplification of the immune response. This is manifested by recruitment of macrophages and neutrophils in cell-mediated reactions, such as delayed-type hypersensitivity and other host defense systems, including phagocytosis, microbicidal activity, and complement cascade.

A major unknown in cellular immune responses is the relationship between delayed hypersensitivity and immunity in mycotic and mycobacterial infections. In candidiasis and tuberculosis, some evidence casts doubt on the role of delayed hypersensitivity in acquired immunity to the disease. Further studies are required in both fungal and mycobacterial infections to unravel the precise relationship between hypersensitivity and immunity.

ROLE OF LYMPHOID SYSTEM IN DEEP MYCOSES

Candidiasis, Coccidioidomycosis, Cryptococcosis, Histoplasmosis

From the immunologic viewpoint, histoplasmosis, coccidioidomycosis, and probably disseminated candidiasis (47) can be discussed as a single group. Furthermore, cryptococcal infections may be handled similarly by the cellular immune system. Assessment of the immunologic responses to *C. neoformans* has been difficult, however, owing in part to the poor antigenicity of the organisms (100). In each of these fungal infections, cellular immune mechanisms play a major role in defense and limitation of spread and growth of the organisms.

Many primary infections with *Histoplasma* and *Coccidioides* (111) organisms are asymptomatic; hypersensitivity and immunity develop, and the growth and spread of the organisms is contained without clinically apparent disease. Despite this protective and curative role, cell-mediated immunity probably plays a pathogenic role in these infections. In the immunologically normal host, symptoms develop about the same time that the cellular immune response appears. Fever, myalgias, cough, chest pain, and, especially in coccidioidomycosis, erythema nodosum, signify localization of the fungus and immunologic response. In immunosuppressed patients, the infection may disseminate rapidly and produce fulminating diseases. If cellular immunity deteriorates or is suppressed, dissemination may occur years after the initial infection (10,34) (Fig. 3).

Because of the clinical association between Hodgkin's disease and cryptococcosis (50,66) and because of the known defects in specific cellular immunity in patients with this lymphoma, it has been proposed that cell-mediated immunity is important in resistance to this infection. It is noteworthy that cryptococcosis patients who do not have underlying diseases may have reduced lymphocyte transformation responses to specific antigens (36). Graybill and Alford (61) described reduced lymphocyte counts and reduced skin test responsiveness to *Candida* and *Histoplasma* antigens in patients who had recovered from disseminated cryptococcosis, suggesting a generalized subnormal responsiveness of the cellular immune system. It is not known if this impairment is related to the predisposition of the patients to cryptococcosis or is a consequence of the infection. The recent studies by Catanzaro (22) in coccidioidomycosis and Kleinhenz et al. (80) in tuberculosis make the latter mechanism quite likely.

Several investigators have tried to define the role of the various blood leukocytes in resistance to cryptococcal infections. In a murine model, Gentry and Remington (56) demonstrated that immunization by infection with the obligate intracellular protozoa *Toxoplasma gondii* and *Besnoitia jellisoni* resulted in activated macrophages and conferred resistance against challenge with *C. neoformans*. Diamond and associates (37) found that macrophages that were derived from human peripheral blood monocytes could not kill ingested cryptococci when activated *in vitro* by cryptococcal antigen, even though the blood monocytes from which they had been derived could kill the organisms. Also, Kalina et al. (73) demonstrated that rabbit peritoneal macrophages formed tight rings around large-capsule cryptococci. The macrophages penetrated the capsules and yeast cytoplasm without phagocytosis of the whole yeast.

Bulmer and co-workers (15–17) have proposed a major role for circulating phagocytes in the pathogenesis of cryptococcal infections. Unencapsulated organisms are inhaled into the lungs where encapsulation occurs. Alveolar macrophages are unable to kill the unencapsulated organisms and wall off the infection. Circulating macrophages are able to destroy unencapsulated cryptococci, but capsular materials

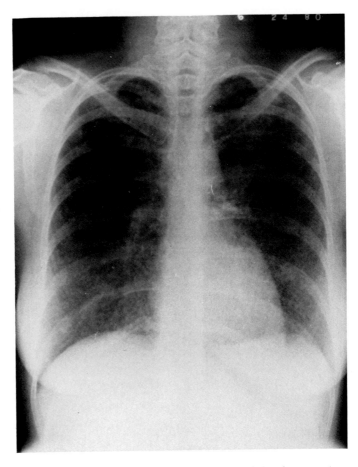

FIG. 3. Patient with cellular immunodeficiency and history of chronic mucocutaneous candidiasis who developed this diffuse nodular pulmonary infiltrate caused by coccidioidomycosis.

inhibit phagocytosis. Thus an early immune response in the lungs may be protective against inhaled organisms; but, since the organisms are walled off and presumably inactive, they may become active and invasive if there are changes in the hosts' defense mechanisms.

Recent studies by Diamond and Allison (40) identified the types of human peripheral blood leukocytes that are capable of killing *C. neoformans* and provided an animal model which shares characteristics with cryptococcosis in humans (36). In the presence of rabbit anticryptococcal antibody, 25% of an inoculum of *C. neoformans* survived incubation for 4 hr in mixed mononuclear cell preparations, 36% in a cell preparation without macrophages, 53% in pure granulocytes, and 97% in the presence of purified T-cells. This study indicated that several types of human leukocytes were capable of antibody-associated fungicidal activity. In an animal model, using guinea pigs that were inoculated intraperitoneally, the authors found that survivors apparently cleared the fungi that had disseminated from extraperitoneal sites, including the brain, rather than prevent dissemination from the peritoneal cavitiy. Moreover, histologic observations suggested that the magnitude of the cellular responses and not fungicidal efficiency of cells determined the outcome of the infections. Although using the intraperitoneal site might not be considered relevant, it did provide a route for delivery of reproducible inoculum and simulated the feature in man of an initially local infection that later disseminates.

Aspergillosis, Mucormycosis

Aspergillosis occurs in three clinical forms: invasive, saprophytic, and allergic bronchopulmonary. The invasive form characteristically occurs as an opportunistic infection in patients whose immune responses are compromised either through underlying diseases, such as leukemia or Hodgkin's disease, or by immunosuppressive agents, such as corticosteroids, irradiation, or azathioprine (18,157). The more common forms of aspergillosis, the saprophytic fungus ball and allergic bronchopulmonary aspergillosis, usually occur in pulmonary tissues that have been damaged by other diseases (Fig. 4). There is no evidence that they occur as a consequence of impaired host defenses.

Immunologic defense mechanisms against *Aspergillus* have not been clearly defined. Some authors have examined pulmonary macrophages of mice that were exposed to inhaled challenges of *Aspergillus* and found that the spores were phagocytosed (49). The spores were also readily phagocytosed *in vitro*, but after 75 min of incubation, no apparent killing was observed. Thus the alveolar macrophages could ingest the organisms and possibly inhibit germination but were not fungicidal (49).

Ford and co-workers (52) injected aspergillus spores intravenously into mice and found that the number of organisms decreased in the liver and spleen. In addition, 4 hr after inoculation and before fungal hyphae appeared, neutrophils also were observed in the liver. In contrast, no neutrophils were seen in the brain or kidneys before the appearance of hyphae. The authors interpreted their results as indicative of a need for a prompt polymorphonuclear leukocyte response to prevent hyphal growth; a delay might permit hyphae to grow beyond the control of the leukocytes.

Data from *in vitro* experiments have not resolved the role of the neutrophil in normal host defense against aspergillosis. Lehrer and Jan (88) were unable to detect killing of spores of *A. fumigatus* by human blood phagocytes (both polymorphonuclear leukocytes and monocytes). Hydrogen peroxide, potassium iodide, and human myeloperoxidase were rapidly fungicidal in a cell-free system, but chloride, which may be the naturally occurring intracellular halide, was unable to substitute for iodide (87).

Mucormycosis, like aspergillosis, is frequently found in patients with underlying diseases, such as diabetes mellitus. Bartrum et al. (5) found 69 cases with pulmonary mucormycosis in the literature. An underlying disease was present in 62 cases, and only one case occurred in a patient who was known to be healthy. It appears that dissemination of this fungus occurs only in seriously compromised hosts.

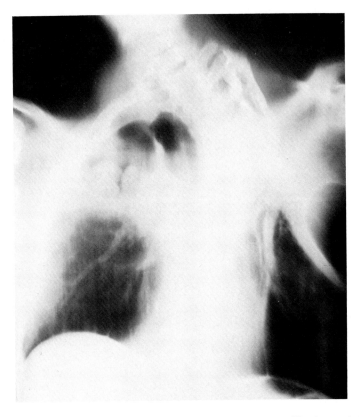

FIG. 4. Anatomic abnormality in the apex of the lung. Note the aspergillus fungus balls in the tuberculous cavity.

Diamond and co-workers (42) examined the interactions of human polymorphonuclear leukocytes with invasive *A. fumigatus* and *R. oryzae* (one of the fungi which commonly cause mucormycosis). Having observed that neutrophils attached to hyphae of *Aspergillus* and *Rhizopus*, they attempted to determine whether neutrophils kill the fungi and to define the cellular mechanisms involved in the interaction. Light and electron microscopic studies, conducted between 1 and 2 hr of incubation, revealed that the hyphae that were in close contact with neutrophils showed dramatic morphologic changes. An assay of neutrophil-induced reduction of uptake of radioisotopes by the hyphae was used to quantitate damage to fungi. Damage to hyphae of *Aspergillus* and *Rhizopus* by neutrophils was inhibited by substances, such as colchicine, cytochalasin B, and 2-deoxygenase, which inhibit neutrophil surface function and motility. Similarly, damage to hyphae was inhibited by compounds, such as theophylline and isoproterenol, which raise levels of 3′,5′-cAMP in neutrophils, although the effect was more pronounced with *Rhizopus* than *Aspergillus*. Hydrocortisone, included in cultures at levels equivalent to pharmacologic doses in humans, also inhibited damage by neutrophils to *Rhizopus* hyphae, but not *Aspergillus*.

In order to define further the cellular mechanisms involved in damage to the organisms, known inhibitors of neutrophil microbicidal functions, such as cyanide, azide, and catalase, were also used; these, too, led to reduction of the damage to hyphae. Because cationic proteins in neutrophils are fungicidal, inhibition of these substances was accomplished by adding anionic amino acid polymers. These agents inhibited damage to *Rhizopus* but not *Aspergillus* hyphae. Lactoferrin was not implicated in damage to the organisms, since damage to hyphae by neutrophils was not inhibited by iron in a concentration 10 times that required to saturate all neutrophil lactoferrin. Lysozyme, which is also present in granules of neutrophils, damaged hyphae but only when they were incubated in distilled water rather than isotonic medium. The effect was more pronounced with *Aspergillus* and *Rhizopus* hyphae. This suggested that lysozyme plays a minor role in damage to the organisms.

The findings of Diamond et al. (42) with *Aspergillus* and *Rhizopus* are similar to their earlier experiments of interactions between neutrophils and *C. albicans* pseudohyphae (41). There was a comparable range of damage to the pseudohyphal and hyphal forms of all the fungi by neutrophils from normal subjects. The significance of their experiments is that neutrophils cause metabolic impairments in hyphae, and this function represents a nonphagocytic mechanism for damage to hyphal forms of fungi. The importance in the intact host remains to be established.

Blastomycosis

As in the deep mycoses, it is generally accepted that cell-mediated immunity plays a part in the mechanism of resistance against blastomycosis. Live cells of *Blastomyces dermatitidis* can effectively induce immunity, as shown by an increase in 50% lethal dose in experimental animals (137). The efficacy of live vaccines has not been a consistent finding. Some have reported no effect of intravenous administration of killed *B. dermatitidis*, whereas others have described protection of mice given an intraperitoneal injection of the fungal suspension against lethal challenges with spore-mycelium suspensions but no protection against challenges with yeast cells (84).

Studies by Cozad and Chang (29) addressed the relationship between host resistance and delayed hypersensitivity in blastomycosis. No protective effect could be detected in mice challenged intraperitoneally 3 days after inoculation with *B. dermatitidis* yeast cells in Freunds incomplete adjuvant. When challenged after 9 days, significant protection was afforded. The protective effect peaked at day 18 and then decreased but was still present 35 days after immunization. The prevailing level of delayed hypersensitivity, as determined by footpad responses, also peaked at day 18 and then waned slightly. The authors concluded that a close parallel relationship existed between host resistance and the level of delayed hypersensitivity.

Paracoccidioidomycosis

This deep-seated mycosis, also known as South American blastomycosis, is caused by *Paracoccidioides brasiliensis* and can lead to a severe, chronic granulomatous condition of skin, mucous membranes, lymph nodes, and internal organs. Paracoccidioidomycosis is endemic to the humid tropical and subtropical areas of continental Latin America and is most frequent in Brazil. Humoral immune responses in infected patients have been investigated and seem to be intact; however, other studies suggest that impaired cell-mediated immunity may occur as part of the illness. For example, Musatti et al. (107) studied the *in vivo* and *in vitro* cellular responses to specific and nonspecific agents in 19 patients with paracoccidioidomycosis. Nearly half of the patients exhibited depressed cell-mediated immune responses, as evaluated by intradermal tests with an antigenic preparation from *P. brasiliensis* and other ubiquitous antigens, including PPD, *Candida*, and *Trichophytin*, and by the reduced ability to develop sensitivity to 2,4-dinitrochlorobenzene (CDNB). When the capacity to react to *P. brasilienis* antigen was compared to the reactions to the other skin test antigens, it was found that those patients who developed delayed hypersensitivity reactions to *P. brasiliensis* had significantly greater responses to the other tests than did patients who were unresponsive to *P. brasiliensis*.

The plasma from the patients was shown to have inhibitory activity on normal lymphocyte responses to PHA. The inhibitory plasmas all came from patients who had negative skin tests with *P. brasiliensis*. In most of these patients, the *in vitro* T-cell proliferation responses to *P. brasiliensis* were improved when normal plasma was substituted for autologous plasma.

Production of macrophage MIF but not lymphocyte transformation in response to *P. brasiliensis* antigen correlated with delayed cutaneous hypersensitivity responses. Finally, there was a reduction in the percentage, but not in the absolute number, of T-cells in the patients compared to normal controls.

To test the hypothesis that symptomatic infection with *P. brasiliensis* caused impaired host cellular immune defenses, Mok and Greer (104) studied responses in 36 patients and 60 controls. After evaluation of skin tests with PPD, *P. brasiliensis*, and histoplasmin and leukocyte migration responses to PHA and PPD, the authors concluded that the prevalence of *P. brasiliensis* skin test positivity was lowest in patients with the longest duration of the disease. This implied a decrease in specific cell-mediated immunity with prolonged active infection. The authors also found that in clinically cured patients, the prevalence of skin sensitivity and lymphocyte transformation to *P. brasiliensis* and PPD increased, suggesting a restoration of cellular immunity upon clinical recovery.

A role of complement in resistance to paracoccidioidomycosis has not been established. Complement activation did not produce fungicidal activity to *P. brasiliensis* in the studies by Calich et al. (19). Despite the ability of the fungus to activate complement and therefore provide a possible explanation for the morphologic skin changes, cobra venom factor-treated mice were able to develop lesions that showed no differences in leukocytes and quantity of cell migration. Furthermore, an intense neutrophil infiltrate was observed in C5-deficient mice that had been treated with cobra factor *in vivo*. Thus there is no direct evidence for complement-dependent mechanisms in the presence of leukocytes in lesions induced by this fungus.

In vitro evidence that suggested a role for polymorphonuclear leukocytes in defense against *P. brasiliensis* was provided by the studies of Goihman-Yahr et al. (58). Cells from patients with the infection were equally capable of phagocytosing *Candida*, being activated by endotoxin, and had the same peroxidase activity as neutrophils from patients with unrelated diseases and healthy controls. Phagocytosis of *P. brasiliensis* was essentially similar in all groups. However, the phagocytic ability of the leukocytes from the patients with paracoccidioidomycosis was significantly lower than the cells from either of the control groups at all times and all intervals tested. These results suggest the role of a phagocytic cell defect in the pathogenesis of paracoccidioidomycosis.

Sporotrichosis

Although this uncommon disease is usually manifested by cutaneous ulceration and regional lymphangitis, more cases of systemic sporotrichosis involving bones, joints, and lungs have been reported recently, especially in the immune-compromised host. Cell-mediated immunity is the component of the lymphoid system that provides immune defenses against sporotrichosis.

Plouffe and co-workers (118) evaluated cellular immunity in six patients with systemic sporotrichosis, with involvement of lungs only in one, joints only in two, both lungs and joints in one, meninges in one, and multiple organs and skin in one. Although disseminated disease developed in one of the patients during drug-induced bone marrow aplasia, no underlying disorders were present in the other five patients. Lymphocyte cultures showed subnormal responses to PHA during the active stage of the infection. Five patients with active sporotrichosis were studied with sporothrix antigen; cells from three patients responded, and cells from two patients did not. Of particular interest was the finding that preincubation of the patients' mononuclear cells, a procedure that removes certain cells with suppressive functions, was accompanied by marked increases in thymidine incorporation in three patients, no change in one patient, and a decrease in thymidine incorporation in one patient. No increases in stimulation indices were noted with PHA or sporothrix antigen when cells were cultured in normal human plasma rather than autologous plasma. All patients had normal peripheral lymphocyte counts with normal percentages of T-cells. Three of six patients were anergic to skin testing with *Candida*, streptokinase-streptodornase, and PPD. The other three patients had positive skin reactions only to PPD. Thus most of these patients had defects in cellular immunity as measured by delayed hypersensitivity skin tests or lymphocyte transformation studies.

Acquired Cellular Immunodeficiency

Recently, there have been several reports (59,99,130) of unusual infections, such as mucocutaneous candidiasis, *Pneumocystis carinii* pneumonia, and nontuberculous mycobacterial infections in previously healthy men. Most of the patients were homosexual and many had histories of drug abuse. Their immunologic evaluations usually disclosed cutaneous anergy. In one report (59), there was virtual elimination of helper/inducer T-cells and an abnormally increased percentage of suppressor/cytotoxic cells. Thus the normal ratio of T-helper cells to T-suppressor cells was inverted. As a number of patients had concurrent infections with herpes virus or cytomegalovirus, and in view of the prevalence of these viruses among male homosexuals and the potential for immunosuppression by these viruses (63), it is possible that the viral infections led to suppression of cellular immunity and predisposition to opportunistic infections, such as oral candidiasis, pneumocystis pneumonia, and "atypical" mycobacterioses. The pathogenesis of this newly recognized disease is still being defined.

ROLE OF LYMPHOID SYSTEM IN SUPERFICIAL MYCOSES

Mucocutaneous Candidiasis

It is generally believed that classic cell-mediated immunity plays a major role in resistance against superficial infections caused by *C. albicans*. The evidence derives from the frequent association of mucocutaneous candidiasis with diseases such as the Di George syndrome, thymus dysplasias, and other disorders in which T-cell functions are subnormal (20,44,79,83,106,119). Detailed studies have shown considerable heterogeneity in the expressions of cellular immunity in these patients, but certain features are common.

Most patients have normal levels of thymopoietin-like activity in their serum (78) and normal numbers of rosette-forming T-cells; however, the ratio of helper to suppressor T-cells may be low (62). At present, studies of T-cell subclasses with specific anti-T-cell antisera have not been reported.

Most patients with chronic mucocutaneous candidiasis have essentially normal lymphocyte responses to nonspecific mitogens, such as concanavalin-A, PHA, and pokeweed mitogen. The most common defect (and this too is somewhat variable) is the impairment of lymphocyte responses to specific antigens, especially antigens of *C. albicans*. The defect is expressed as diminished responses to antigens as assayed by activation of T-cells to cytotoxic activity, antigen-induced DNA synthesis, and lymphokine production.

Antibody-mediated immunity in mucocutaneous candidiasis usually is intact. Although the production of antibody suggests that the afferent components and cell cooperations in the B-cell system are normal, it is not known if the antibodies provide any protective immunity. Axelsen et al. (2) suggested that they may prevent dissemination of mucocutaneous infections to parenchymal organs.

Plasma of candidiasis patients may inhibit *in vitro* responses of lymphocytes to antigens, including candida, as well as mitogens and allogeneic cells. The studies by Fischer et al. (51) provided evidence that, in some cases, the inhibitory substance was a polysaccharide antigen from *C. albicans*.

Abnormal functions of phagocytic cells in this fungal infection are rare. Impaired chemotaxis has been described (45,149,155), and Twomey et al. (146) studied a patient whose monocytes were apparently unable to process or present antigens to lymphocytes. The majority of patients do not demonstrate defects of either chemotaxis or phagocytic activity.

The role of complement in the pathogenesis of the cutaneous lesions was studied by Sohnle et al. (134). When the authors noted that the intense cutaneous inflammatory infiltrates in patients with normal immunologic functions and patients with impaired delayed hypersensitivity were virtually identical, immunofluorescent studies of immunoreactants in normal and lesional skin were done. Deposits of C3 and properidin were found along the basement membranes in cutaneous lesions of three of six patients with mucocutaneous candidiasis, and *Candida* antigen was found with C3 and properidin in the lesions of one. Immunoglobulin or C4 were not found in any specimens.

These observations then were used to examine models of cutaneous candidiasis in guinea pigs. It was found that the initial lesion was an intense infiltration of the infected site with neutrophils. Later, the lesions spontaneously cleared. This event corresponded with the appearance of delayed hypersensitivity to candida and markedly increased epidermal proliferation. The neutrophilic infiltration probably was related to activation of the complement system by soluble polysaccharide antigens from candida. In fact, *in vitro* studies showed that *Candida* could activate the alternative complement pathway and generate chemotactic factors. It was proposed that patients with mucocutaneous candidiasis are susceptible to candida infections because of the defects in cell-mediated immunity, but the inflammation which occurs in the lesions is due to a separate process, i.e., activation of the complement system.

The role of complement components in cutaneous candidiasis was studied by Ray and Wuepper (121). In normal mice, only *C. albicans* and *C. stellatoidea* invaded both the stratum corneum and stratum malpighii, and *C. tropicalis* invaded the stratum malpighii but failed to penetrate the stratum corneum. C5-deficient mice or cobra venom factor-treated mice developed no inflammatory responses to the infections and permitted all *Candida* species to proliferate into the subcutaneous fat. Thus complement-dependent chemotactic factors and neutrophils played a key role in containment of cutaneous candidiasis in this model.

The role of neutrophils in cutaneous candidiasis has been examined in two animal models in which candida infections were induced in guinea pigs by either placing occlusive dressings over the organisms or by applying the organisms directly to the skin without occlusive dressings (133). The response to the cutaneous infection with occlusive dressings was characterized by accumulation of neutrophils in the upper epidermis of the infected skin. The organisms seemed to become trapped in the thick crust, which then was sloughed, removing them from the animal. The role of the neutrophil in defense against this infection was in the formation of the crust rather than by providing any recognizable candidacidal function. In contrast, infections produced without occlusive dressings produced less epidermal infiltration with neutrophils and were influenced by prior immune status of the animal. Clearing of these infections appeared to be a function of delayed hypersensitivity. The following evidence supported this conclusion: (a) scaling of lesions was more prominent in immune than in nonimmune animals; (b) animals immunized by the cutaneous infections had positive delayed-type hypersensitivity skin tests and lymphocyte transformations but weak humoral immunity as evidenced by low anticandida agglutinin titers; (c) immune animals developed histopathologic changes consistent with delayed hypersensitivity reaction; and (d) the ability to increase gross scaling in response to cutaneous infections was transferable from immune to normal animals with washed peritoneal exudate cells. Clearly, acquired cellular immunity and neutrophils are involved in resistance in this model; but whether both are involved in protection against natural cutaneous candida infection remains unanswered. Antibody-mediated mechanisms of immunity do not appear to be operating in this system.

Dermatophytoses

Like the fungi mentioned above, susceptibility to infection by dermatophytic fungi is more common in individuals who are immunosuppressed with malignant lymphomas, Cushing's disease, diabetes mellitus or recipients of immunosuppressive drugs (141,142). Jones et al. (71) reported that cell-mediated immunity to dermatophytic fungi was associated with resistance to infection, whereas absent cellular responses or the presence of both cell-mediated and humoral immunity was associated with susceptibility to chronic dermatophytoses. One of their studies involved three atopic men with no past or current evidence of dermatophytosis who had no reaction to trichophyton skin tests. The men were experimentally infected with *Trichophyton mentagrophytes var granulare*. All developed cellular immunity, and infections in two healed spontaneously. The third subject developed type I humoral immunity, as demonstrated by an elevated IgE level and a wheal and flare response to trychophytin, but his infection did not heal and spread to his feet. The authors suggested that a local antagonism existed between humoral and cellular immunity in which the local antibody-dependent response reacted with fungal antigens to decrease the local cellular immune response. As a result of this lessened immunologic damage, the epidermis remained intact, and the organism spread across the skin surface.

When volunteers with chronic dermatophyte infections elsewhere on their bodies were experimentally infected, Jones et al. (71) observed that the newly infected areas were less inflammatory than similar experimentally induced infections in normal noninfected volunteers. They concluded that the degree of inflammation produced by the experimental infection was partially determined by the host's capacity to respond immunologically.

Other investigators (64,153) have also found delayed cutaneous hypersensitivity as well as immediate wheal reactions to trichophytin. In the studies by Hanifin et al. (64), reactions to antigenic extracts of *Trichophyton mentagrophytes*, *Trichophyton rubrum*, and *Dermatophytin* were compared in 49 patients with dermatophytoses. Twelve of 14 *T. mentagrophytes* patients had delayed skin test reactivity; in each case tested, 48 hr responses were confirmed by lymphocyte reactivity to trichophytin. The retarded delayed reactors showed low levels of lymphocyte reactivity, suggesting a lesser degree of cell-mediated responsiveness to trichophytin. Retesting with trichophytin produced a weak but definite 48 hr reaction. No patient with this infection had an immediate wheal and flare response. Because of these few patients with strong cell-mediated responses who were unable to resolve their chronically infecting dermatophytes, Hanifin suggested that delayed reactivity was not essential for resistance against dermatophyte infections.

T. rubrum-infected patients contrasted sharply with the above group in terms of cutaneous and lymphocyte responses. Often chronically infected for years, these patients seldom manifested delayed skin test responses to trichophytin, and their *in vitro* lymphocyte responses were nonreactive. When tested with other antigens, such as candida, mumps, and PPD, both *in vivo* and *in vitro*, normal reactivity was found (64). Apparently, these patients had trichophytin-specific absence of cell-mediated immunity.

Another characteristic of *T. rubrum*-infected patients was the frequent manifestation of immediate wheal reactions to intradermal trichophytin. In an effort to determine whether a factor causing the immediate reaction might be inhibiting delayed responses, intradermal chlorpheniramine was used to depress the immediate wheal reactions. This failed to unmask delayed responses (64).

Hanifin et al. (64) mentioned several possible mechanisms for the absence of cell-mediated immune responses in these patients: (a) the presence of antibodies or other humoral factors, (b) an overloading of the immune system with antigenic material, and (c) genetic factors which might predispose to dermatophyte infections. Whatever the mechanism, the patients represented a natural model of tolerance and inadequate host resistance to a specific infecting organism.

Walters et al. (151) described a factor from the serum which specifically blocked cellular immunity *in vitro* to *T. rubrum*. Using a leukocyte adherence inhibition assay, the authors observed that both chronically and acutely ill patients with dermatophytosis had cell-mediated immunity to antigens of their infecting organism. In addition, serum from the chronically infected patients specifically blocked the activity of their own leukocytes or the leukocytes of other patients with the same species of infecting organism. Reactivity to PPD was not blocked by serum. Thus it appeared that the continued production of antigen or some other factor interfered with the manifestation of cellular immunity.

Additional studies examining the cell-mediated immune responses in persons with chronic dermatophyte infections were performed by Sorensen and Jones (136). Delayed-type hypersensitivity to seven common antigens was examined in 38 individuals with chronic dermatophytoses and 20 healthy controls. The only significant historic difference between the two groups was a 2.9-fold greater frequency of atopic respiratory disease in the chronically infected subjects. Besides a lower frequency of delayed hypersensitivity to trichophytin, the infected group also showed significant reduction in reactions to intradermal mumps skin test antigen and to a *Rhus* oleoresin patch test. From these data, the authors concluded that a possible defect in cell-mediated immunity in patients with chronic dermatophytosis is relatively selective for trichophytin. The defect was not absolutely antigen specific, however (two subjects were anergic); and there was no evidence of increased susceptibility to or morbidity from other infectious diseases.

In summary, cell-mediated immunity to a dermatophyte group antigen produces the inflammation at an infected site. Deficiency of cell-mediated immunity can be associated with chronic dermatophyte infections.

Genetic factors may be responsible for susceptibility to *T. concentricum*, which causes a superficial skin infection in Papua New Guinea. Serjeantson and Lawrence (129) studied families in the Gogol Valley of that country and presented several lines of evidence for autosomal recessive control of susceptibility to this infection: (a) there was no evidence of concordance in married couples, although the condition can be acquired by bodily contact and close association; (b) formal segregation analysis revealed expected family distributions based on recessive hypotheses; and (c) the frequency of the infection in one of three language groups sharing an apparently common environment was significantly different from the other two. In addition, similar findings were reported by Schofield et al. (127); and in the Fiji Islands, the skin infections were found in Melanesians but rarely in Indians (129). These ethnic and racial differences would be expected if predisposition to the disease is genetically determined.

Tinea Versicolor

Sohnle and Collins-Lech (135) investigated the role of cell-mediated immunity as a form of defense in tinea versicolor. Antigenic extracts were prepared from cultured *Pityrosporum orbiculare*, the presumed etiologic agent. Initial evaluations demonstrated that the extracts were capable of sensitizing guinea pigs when injected in complete Freund's adjuvant and of producing positive lymphocyte transformation responses in the immunized animals. Other studies, using human cord blood lymphocytes, demonstrated that the extracts were not mitogenic but functioned as specific antigens.

In a group of 14 normal subjects and 11 tinea versicolor patients, lymphocyte transformation tests revealed a positive response to *P. orbiculare*. However, lymphocytes from tinea versicolor patients produced significantly less leukocyte MIF activity when stimulated by *C. albicans* and *P. orbiculare* than did lymphocytes from normal subjects. Therefore, although tinea versicolor patients, like the normal control subjects, reacted positively to the extracts, the effector functions of lymphocytes from the patients were either absent or malfunctioning, in that they produced subnormal amounts of MIF in response to the relevant antigen.

Mucous Membrane Defense Mechanisms

That cellular immunologic mechanisms may play a part in both the pathogenesis of and host resistance to experimental candidiasis in the palate derives from studies by Budtz-Jorgensen (11–13). When comparing the primary and secondary inflammatory reactions of candida infections produced in the palatal mucosa of monkeys by inoculating *C. albicans* under acrylic plates, there was histologic evidence for a delayed hypersensitivity reaction. One week after inoculation, a diffuse erythema was seen involving the palatal mucosa in contact with the plate. The inflammation subsided during the following 1 to 2 weeks, even though the animals continued wearing the plates. When the monkeys were reinoculated under the acrylic plate, a more intense erythema appeared, which may indicate that the initial experimental infection gave rise to delayed hypersensitivity. Another important observation was that inoculation on the uncovered palatal mucosa did not result in inflammatory changes. Whether disappearance of the infection was caused by an immunologic reaction of the host and/or insufficient environmental conditions for the propagation of the fungi remains to be determined.

To further define the systemic effects of the local infection, Budtz-Jorgensen (12) examined inhibition of leukocyte migration and found that it developed consistently earlier in normal monkeys than in animals treated with azathioprine. In these monkeys, the cellular immune response was delayed by 2 to 3 weeks, and MIF production was less pronounced. In contrast, the humoral immune response demonstrated a completely different course. Antibody was detected in the normal animals only after the cellular immune response had culminated, and the titer rose while the cellular response declined. In the azathioprine-treated animals, the response was early, of shorter duration, and developed before or concurrently with the cellular response. Clearing of infection occurred in the normal monkeys, while antibody was not detectable. In the immunosuppressed animals, although the antibody response was strong and early, healing did not occur until treatment with azathioprine was terminated and the MIF production responses returned.

Budtz-Jorgensen (13) also evaluated *in vitro* cellular hypersensitivity in subjects with *Candida*-induced stomatitis (general and granular) and trauma-induced lesions in the palatal mucosa. More than 75% of the patients with generalized stomatitis demonstrated cellular hypersensitivity, as determined by the leukocyte migration test. Of these patients with granular stomatitis, however, 28% showed significant inhibition of leukocyte migration. Cellular hypersensitivity was restored with antifungal therapy in some patients.

TREATMENT

Traditionally, patients with chronic fungal or mycobacterial infections are treated with antibiotics, either singly or in complex combinations. The infections are cured in many patients. In others, presumably appropriate treatments fail, or the infections tend to recur after termination of treatment. Both these unfavorable outcomes of treatment have prompted investigation of the possible role of manipulation of the immune system in achieving better results.

Levamisole

Levamisole is widely used for treatment of roundworm infections of man and animals. Through serendipity, it was found to act as an immunomodulator, in that it enhanced antibody responses and expression of delayed-type allergic reactions. Mussati et al. (107) have reported that levamisole was a useful adjunct to amphotericin B in treatment of paracoccidioidomycosis. Following treatment with the drug, a patient who was previously unresponsive to PPD, *P. brasiliensis* antigen, and CDNB subsequently demonstrated positive skin test reactivity.

Singh et al. (131) conducted a placebo-controlled clinical trial of levamisole in patients with tuberculosis. They found that after 3 months of treatment, 48% of the levamisole-treated patients were responsive to levamisole, while similar reactions were seen in only 18% of the placebo-treated patients. Levamisole-treated patients also showed significant improvements in their chest X-rays.

Immunologic Therapy

Transfer factor (TF), injections of thymic extracts, thymus transplantation, and infusions of lymphocytes from immunocompetent donors have been employed in attempts to correct the immunologic defects in patients with fungal and mycobacterial infections (46). Most of the experience has been in patients with chronic mucocutaneous candidiasis or chronic coccidioidomycosis. The long-term effects of treatments such as thymus transplantion, thymic hormones, and leukocyte infusions are uncertain because they have been applied to very few patients, and the long-term data often are not reported. Nonetheless, these studies have shown that it is possible to improve immune functions in the patients. For example, two cases with chronic mucocutaneous candidiasis had subnormal numbers of circulating T-lymphocytes and subnormal *in vitro* lymphocyte responses to T-cell mitogens (4,77). Transplantation of fetal thymus resulted in marked increases in the numbers of T-cells and responses to T-cell mitogens.

After giving injections of thymosin fraction 5 to four patients with chronic candidiasis, Wara and Ammann (152) noted clinical and immunologic responses in a 13-year-old girl with a modest T-cell defect and in a 49-year-old man with subnormal lymphocyte responses to PHA. Two other patients were not evaluated because they had been in the study less than 6 months.

Kirkpatrick et al. (75) and Valdimarsson et al. (148) attempted to reconstitute three candidiasis patients with transfusions of peripheral blood leukocytes from candida-sensitive donors. All recipients improved clinically, and two acquired cell-mediated reactivity to *Candida*.

TF has been used to treat candidiasis patients in at least 50 instances (35,79,128,132). In 15 of the cases, it was the only treatment given; 14 of the patients showed improvements in immunologic functions, but only four patients had clinical benefits (Table 2). Better results were obtained when TF from candida-sensitive donors was used in combination with antifungal antibiotics. Of 19 patients in this group, 16 had improvement in immunologic functions, and 13 of these showed clinical benefits. TF from insensitive donors has been used in seven patients with chronic mucocutaneous candidiasis. No patient had any change in immune functions, but three patients had clinical responses. These data also illustrate the dichotomy between hypersensitivity as expressed by delayed skin test and immunity.

It is our conclusion that the most favorable results occur in patients who receive combination therapy with antifungal antibiotics and TF from candida-sensitive donors. This opinion is supported by the controlled clinical trial of TF in candidiasis patients by Mobacken et al. (103). Only one of their seven patients improved, and this patient received 5-fluorocytosine before entering the trial.

Plouffe et al. (118) gave TF to two patients with disseminated sporotrichosis. Both had subnormal *in vitro* responses to PHA and sporothrix antigen and had negative delayed hypersensitivity skin tests. Treatment with TF resulted in clinical and immunologic improvement.

Graybill (60) reported the results of TF therapy in 55 patients with coccidioidomycosis that were treated by members of the Coccidioidomycosis Cooperative Treatment Group. Twenty-nine patients (52%) were cured or improved after treatment with the combination of TF and amphotericin B. These results were slightly better than those in a historic control group that received only amphotericin B (Table 3). Similar proportions of patients died or failed to improve. Long-term follow-up of 36 patients who received combination therapy showed that 14 patients were cured or still improved; six improved patients had relapsed; seven patients had stable but active coccidioidomycosis; and nine patients were dead. These results are somewhat discouraging, but they may be influenced by the fact that patients with more severe infections tended to receive combination therapy. Indeed, a few patients were probably moribund when they entered the trial; five received no additional amphotericin B, and two received less than 1 g of the drug. Nonetheless, TF in the dosages and schedule used in this trial did not markedly affect the outcome of therapy with amphotericin B.

TABLE 2. *TF therapy of chronic mucocutaneous candidiasis*

Treatment	Immunologic responses	Clinical responses
TF alone (Candida-sensitive donors)	14/15 (93%) (5 not described)	4/20 (20%)
TF (Candida-sensitive donors) with antifungal antibiotics	16/19 (84%)	14/19 (74%)
TF (Candida-insensitive donors) with antifungal antibiotics	0/7	3/7 (43%)

TABLE 3. *TF therapy of coccidioidomycosis*[a]

Outcome	Treatment[b]	
	TF and AB	AB
Probable cure	15 (27%) ⎫	39 (45%)
Improved	14 (25%) ⎭	
Died	14 (25%)	23 (27%)
Unimproved	12 (22%)	24 (28%)
Total	55	86

[a]Data summarized from ref. 60.
[b]TF and AB, combined treatment with TF and amphotericin B; AB, treatment with amphotericin B alone.

IMMUNOLOGIC MANIPULATIONS: PROPHYLAXIS

Preparations of mycobacteria have been used as adjuvants for many years. Muramyl dipeptide, N-acetylmuramyl-L-alanyl-D-isoglutamine (MDP), a synthetic analog of a component of the mycobacterial cell wall, represents the minimal chemical structure required for the adjuvant activity of complete Freund's adjuvant (81). This compound has been found to stimulate primary antibody responses and enhance a variety of macrophage functions. Cummings et al. (30) studied the effect of MDP on macrophages in the intact animal. After subcutaneous administration of MDP to mice, peritoneal macrophages were induced to the activated state, and MDP-treated mice were more resistant to challenges with *C. albicans*. Levy et al. (91) prepared *C. albicans* ribosomes and immunized mice prior to intraperitoneal or intravenous challenges with lethal doses of *C. albicans*. The 30-day survival rate of immunized mice challenged intraperitoneally was 75% and 27% in controls. Intravenously challenged mice had a survival rate of 60% in the immunized animals and no survivors among the controls. Addition of incomplete Freund's adjuvant increased the protection in the intravenous challenge model. Vaccination with ribosomes from the organism has also been shown to protect against experimental infections with *H. capsulatum* (145). Although vaccination with ribosomes has already reached the stage of clinical trials, but only in a bacterial infection, it may prove useful in fungal infections (101).

SUMMARY AND CONCLUSIONS

At present, the balance of the literature indicates that cell-mediated immune mechanisms play the major role in defense and limitation of spread and growth of fungal and mycobacterial organisms. The central feature of cell-mediated immune responses is the interaction of antigen and immunocompetent lymphocytes. In order for the reactions to proceed to completion, however, a number of other cellular interactions are necessary. These include (a) macrophage presentation of antigen to T-lymphocytes and production, by activated macrophages, of factors that influence the T-cell, (b) enhancement of microbicidal activity of macrophages by antigen-activated T-cells, and (c) recruitment of mononuclear and polymorphonuclear leukocytes, again by antigen-activated T-cells. Also, these mechanisms are both local and systemic as well as nonspecific and specific.

In our review of the recent research dealing with the various aspects of host defenses that play a role in resistance against fungal and mycobacterial infections, it should be obvious that disagreement exists with respect to the importance of the various components of the immune system. For example, resistance against mucocutaneous candidiasis rests with the thymus-dependent cellular immune system. Yet little evidence indicates that resistance against the disseminated form of candidiasis is of the same nature. Is it possible that resistance against the mucocutaneous form is mediated by cellular mechanisms, and resistance against systemic candidiasis is dependent on some other mechanism?

Another interesting aspect of host resistance is the apparent effect of the organisms on the ability of the immune system to respond. Evidence indicates that during the course of coccidioidomycosis, tuberculosis, and certain viral infections, immunosuppression occurs. This is probably due to the stimulation of T-suppressor lymphocytes (47) or macrophages with immunosuppressive capabilities. Clarification of this suppressive contribution to the infections may provide clues to the pathogenesis of chronic fungal diseases.

REFERENCES

1. Aronson, K., and Soltani, K. (1976): Chronic mucocutaneous candidiasis. A review. *Mycopathologia*, 60:17–25.
2. Axelsen, N. H., Kirkpatrick, C. H., and Buckley, R. H. (1974): Precipitins to *Candida albicans* in chronic mucocutaneous candidiasis studied by crossed immunoelectrophoresis with intermediate gel. Correlation with clinical and immunological findings. *Clin. Exp. Immunol.*, 17:385–394.
3. Baine, W. B., Koeing, M. G., and Goodman, J. S. (1974): Clearance of *Candida albicans* from bloodstream of rabbits. *Infect. Immunol.*, 10:1420–1425.
4. Ballow, M., and Hyman, L. R. (1977): Combination immunotherapy in chronic mucocutaneous candidiasis. Synergism between transfer factor and fetal thymus tissue. *Clin. Immunol. Immunopathol.*, 8:504–512.
5. Bartrum, R. J., Jr., Watnick, M., and Herman, P. G. (1973): Roentgenographic findings in pulmonary mucormycosis. *Am. J. Roentgenol. Radium Ther. Nucl. Med.*, 117:810–815.
6. Beaman, L., Benjamini, E., and Pappagianis, D. (1981): Role of lymphocytes in macrophage-induced killing of *Coccidioides immitis in vitro*. *Infect. Immunol.*, 34:347–353.
7. Blanden, R. V., and Langman, R. E. (1972): Cell-mediated immunity to bacterial infection in the mouse. Thymus-derived cells as effectors of acquired resistance to *Listeria monocytogenes*. *Scand. J. Immunol.*, 1:379–392.
8. Bloom, B. R. (1971): *In vitro* approaches to the mechanism of cell-mediated reactions. *Adv. Immunol.*, 13:101–208.
9. Bloom, B. R., and Bennett, B. (1966): Mechanism of a reaction *in vitro* associated with delayed-type hypersensitivity. *Science*, 153:80–82.
10. Bodey, G. P. (1966): Fungal infections complicating acute leukemia. *J. Chronic Dis.*, 19:667–687.
11. Budtz-Jorgensen, E. (1971): Denture stomatitis: IV. An experimental model in monkeys. *Acta Odontol. Scand.*, 29:513–526.

12. Budtz-Jorgensen, E. (1973): Immune response to *C. albicans* in monkeys with experimental candidiasis in the palate. *Scand. J. Dent. Res.*, 81:360–371.
13. Budtz-Jorgensen, E. (1973): Cellular immunity in acquired candidiasis of the palate. *Scand. J. Dent. Res.*, 81:372–382.
14. Bullock, W. E., Jr., and Fasal, P. (1971): Studies of immune mechanisms in leprosy. II. The role of cellular and humoral factors in impairment of the *in vitro* immune response. *J. Immunol.*, 106:888–889.
15. Bulmer, G. S., and Sans, M. D. (1967): *Cryptococcus neoformans*. II. Phagocytosis by human leukocytes. *J. Bacteriol.*, 94:1480–1483.
16. Bulmer, G. S., and Sans, M. D. (1968): *Cryptococcus neoformans*. III. Inhibition of phagocytosis. *J. Bacteriol.*, 95:5–8.
17. Bulmer, G. S., and Tacker, J. R. (1975): Phagocytosis of *Cryptococcus neoformans* by alveolar macrophages. *Infect. Immun.*, 11:73–79.
18. Burton, J. R., Zacher, J. B., Bessin, R., Rathbun, H. K., Greenough, W. B., III, Sterioff, S., Wright, J. R., Slavin, R. E., and Williams, G. M. (1972): Aspergillosis in four renal transplant recipients: Diagnosis and effective treatment with Amphotericin B. *Ann. Intern. Med.*, 77:383–388.
19. Calich, V. L. G., Kipnis, T. L., Mariano, M., Neto, C. F., and daSilva, W. D. (1979): The activation of the complement system by *Paracoccidioides brasiliensis in vitro*: Its opsonic effect and possible significance for an *in vivo* model of infection. *Clin. Immunol. Immunopathol.*, 12:20–30.
20. Canales, L., Middlemas, R. O., Louro, J. M., and South, M. A. (1969): Immunological observations in chronic mucocutaneous candidiasis. *Lancet*, 2:567–571.
21. Carr, R. I., Chakraborty, A. K., Brunda, M. J., Davidson, P. T., Damle, P. B., Hardtke, M. A., Gilbride, K. J., and Minden, P. (1980): Immune complexes and antibodies to BCG in sera from patients with mycobacterial infections. *Clin. Exp. Immunol.*, 39:562–569.
22. Catanzaro, A. (1981): Suppressor cells in coccidioidomycosis. *Cell. Immunol.*, 64:235–245.
23. Catanzaro, A., Spitler, L., and Moser, K. M. (1975): Cellular immune responses in coccidioidomycosis. *Cell. Immunol.*, 15:360–371.
24. Choucroun, N. (1947): Tubercle bacillus antigens. Biological properties of two substances isolated from paraffin oil extract of dead tubercle bacilli. *Am. Rev. Tuberc.*, 56:203–226.
25. Cline, M. J., and Lehrer, R. I. (1968): Phagocytosis by human monocytes. *Blood*, 32:423–435.
26. Collins, F. M., Congdon, C. C., and Morrison, N. E. (1975): Growth of *M. bovis* (BCG) in T lymphocyte-depleted mice. *Infect. Immun.*, 11:57–64.
27. Cox, R. A. (1979): Immunologic studies of patients with histoplasmosis. *Am. Rev. Respir. Dis.*, 120:143–149.
28. Cox, R. A., and Vivas, J. R. (1977): Spectrum of *in vivo* and *in vitro* cell-mediated immune responses in coccidioidomycosis. *Cell. Immunol.*, 31:130–141.
29. Cozad, G. C., and Chang, G. T. (1980): Cell-mediated immunoprotection in blastomycosis. *Infect. Immun.*, 28:398–403.
30. Cummings, N. P., Pabpst, M. J., and Johnston, R. B., Jr. (1980): Activation of macrophages for enhanced release of superoxide anion and greater killing of *Candida albicans* by injection of muramyl dipeptide. *J. Exp. Med.*, 152:1659–1669.
31. Cutler, J. E. (1976): Acute systemic candidiasis in normal and congenitally thymic-deficient (nude) mice. *J. Reticuloendothel. Soc.*, 19:121–126.
32. David, J. R., al-Askari, S., Lawrence, H. S., and Thomas, L. (1964): Delayed hypersensitivity *in vitro*. I. The specificity of inhibition of cell migration by antigens. *J. Immunol.*, 93:264–273.
33. David, J. R., and David, R. R. (1972): Cellular hypersensitivity and immunity. Inhibition of macrophage migration and the lymphocyte mediators. *Prog. Allergy*, 16:300–449.
34. Davidson, W., and Sarosi, G. (1981): Disseminated blastomycosis and coccidioidomycosis in the same patient. *Am. Rev. Respir. Dis.*, 124:179.
35. DeSousa, M., Cochran, R., Mackie, R., Parrott, D., and Arala-Chaves, M. (1976): Chronic mucocutaneous candidiasis treated with transfer factor. *Br. J. Dermatol.*, 94:79–83.
36. Diamond, R. D. (1977): Effects of stimulation and suppression of cell-mediated immunity on experimental cryptococcosis. *Infect. Immun.*, 17:187–194.
37. Diamond, R. D., Root, R. K., and Bennett, J. E. (1972): Factors influencing killing of *Cryptococcus neoformans* by human leukocytes *in vitro*. *J. Infect. Dis.*, 125:367–376.
38. Diamond, R. D., and Bennett, J. E. (1973): Disseminated cryptococcosis in man: Decreased

lymphocyte transformation in response to *Cryptococcus neoformans. J. Infect. Dis.*, 127:694–697.

39. Diamond, R. D., May, J. E., Kane, M., Frank, M. M., and Bennett, J. E. (1973): The role of late complement components and the alternate complement pathway in experimental cryptococcosis. *Proc. Soc. Exp. Biol. Med.*, 144:312–315.

40. Diamond, R. D., and Allison, A. C. (1976): Nature of the effector cells responsible for antibody-dependent cell-mediated killing of *Cryptococcus neoformans. Infect. Immun.*, 14:716–720.

41. Diamond, R. D., and Krzesicki, R. (1978): Mechanisms of attachment of neutrophils to *Candida albicans* pseudohyphae in the absence of serum, and of subsequent damage to pseudohyphae by microbicidal processes of neutrophils *in vitro. J. Clin. Invest.*, 61:360–369.

42. Diamond, R. D., Krzesicki, M. S., Epstein, B. A., and Wellington, J. (1978): Damage to hyphal forms of fungi by human leukocytes *in vitro. Am. J. Pathol.*, 91:313–323.

43. Diamond, R. D., Krzesicki, R., and Wellington, J. (1978): Damage to pseudohyphal forms of *Candida albicans* by neutrophils in the absence of serum *in vitro. J. Clin. Invest.*, 61:349–359.

44. DiGeorge, A. M. (1968): Congenital absence of the thymus and its immunologic consequences: Concurrence with congenital hypoparathyroidism. *Birth Defects*, 4:116–121.

45. Djawari, D., Bischoff, T., and Hornstein, O. P. (1978): Impairment of chemotactic activity of macrophages in chronic mucocutaneous candidosis. *Arch. Dermatol. Res.*, 262:247–253.

46. Dwyer, J. M., Gerstenhaber, B. J., and Dobuler, K. J. (1983): Clinical and immunological response to antigen specific transfer factor in a case of drug resistant infection with *Mycobacterium xenopi. Am. J. Med. (in press).*

47. Edwards, J. E., Lehrer, R. I., Stiehm, E. R., Fischer, T. J., and Young, L. S. (1978): Severe candida infections. Clinical perspective, immune defense mechanisms and current concepts of therapy. *Ann. Intern. Med.*, 89:91–106.

48. Ellner, J. J. (1978): Suppressor adherent cells in human tuberculosis. *J. Immunol.*, 121:2573–2579.

49. Epstein, S. M., Verney, E., Miale, T. D., and Sidransky, H. (1967): Studies on the pathogenesis of experimental pulmonary aspergillosis. *Am. J. Pathol.*, 51:769–788.

50. Feld, R., Bodey, G. P., Rodriguez, V., and Luna, M. (1974): Causes of death in patients with malignant lymphoma. *Am. J. Med. Sci.*, 268:97–106.

51. Fischer, A., Ballet, J. J., and Griscelli, C. (1978): Specific inhibition of *in vitro* Candida-induced lymphocyte proliferation by polysaccharide antigens present in serum of patients with chronic mucocutaneous candidiasis. *J. Clin. Invest.*, 62:1005–1013.

52. Ford, S., Baker, R. D., and Friedman, L. (1968): Cellular reactions and pathology in experimental disseminated aspergillosis. *J. Infect. Dis.*, 118:370–376.

53. Frenkel, J. K. (1967): Adoptive immunity to intracellular infection. *J. Immunol.*, 98:1309–1319.

54. Gadebusch, H. H. (1972): Mechanism of native and acquired resistance to infection with *Cryptococcus neoformans. Crit. Rev. Microbiol.*, 1:311–320.

55. Gelfand, J. A., Hurley, D. L., Fauci, A. S., and Frank, M. M. (1978): Role of complement in host defense against experimental disseminated candidiasis. *J. Infect. Dis.*, 138:9–16.

56. Gentry, L. O., and Remington, J. S. (1971): Resistance against cryptococcus conferred by intracellular bacteria and protozoa. *J. Infect. Dis.*, 123:22–31.

57. George, M., and Vaughan, J. H. (1982): *In vitro* cell migration as a model for delayed hypersensitivity. *Proc. Soc. Exp. Biol. Med.*, 111:514–521.

58. Goihman-Yahr, M., Essenfeld-Yahr, E., deAlbornoz, M. C., Yarzabal, L., DeGomez, M. H., Martin, B. S., Ocanto, A., Gil, F., and Convit, J. (1980): Defect of *in vitro* digestive ability of polymorphonuclear leukocytes in paracoccidioidomycosis. *Infect. Immun.*, 28:557–566.

59. Gottlieb, M. S., Schroff, R., Schanker, H. M., Weisman, J. D., Fan, P. T., Wolf, R. A., and Saxon, A. (1981): *Pneumocystis carinii* pneumonia and mucosal candidiasis in previously healthy homosexual men: Evidence of a new acquired cellular immunodeficiency. *N. Engl. J. Med.*, 305:1425–1431.

60. Graybill, J. R. (1977): The clinical course of coccidioidomycosis following transfer factor therapy. In: *Coccidioidomycosis. Current Clinical and Diagnostic Status*, edited by L. Ajello, pp. 335–345. Symposia Specialists, Miami.

61. Graybill, J. R., and Alford, R. H. (1974): Cell-mediated immunity in cryptococcosis. *Cell. Immunol.*, 14:12–21.

62. Gupta, S., Kirkpatrick, C. H., and Good, R. A. (1979): Subpopulations of human T-lymphocytes. XI. T-cells with receptors for IgM and IgG and locomotion of T- and non-T-cells in peripheral

blood from patients with chronic mucocutaneous candidiasis. *Clin. Immunol. Immunopathol.*, 14:86–95.

63. Hamilton, J. R., Overall, J. C., Jr., and Glasgow, L. A. (1976): Synergistic effect on mortality in mice with murine cytomegalovirus and *Pseudomonas aeruginosa, Staphylococcus aureus*, or *Candida albicans* infection. *Infect. Immun.*, 14:982–989.

64. Hanifin, J. M., Ray, L. F., and Lobitz, W. C., Jr. (1974): Immunological reactivity in dermatophytosis. *Br. J. Dermatol.*, 90:1–7.

65. Harboe, M. (1981): Antigens of PPD, old tuberculin, and autoclaved *Mycobacterium bovis* BCG studied by crossed immunoelectrophoresis. *Am. Rev. Respir. Dis.*, 124:80–87.

66. Hart, P. D., Russell, E., Jr., and Remington, J. S. (1969): The compromised host and infection. II. Deep fungal infection. *J. Infect. Dis.*, 120:169–191.

67. Heilman, D. H., and McFarland, W. (1966): Inhibition of tuberculin-induced mitogenesis in cultures of lymphocytes from tuberculous donors. *Int. Arch. Allergy*, 30:58–66.

68. Heise, E. R., and Weiser, R. S. (1970): Tuberculin sensitivity: The effect of antilymphocyte and antimacrophage serum on cutaneous, systemic and *in vitro* reactions. *J. Immunol.*, 104:704–709.

69. Higgs, J. M., and Wells, R. S. (1973): Chronic mucocutaneous candidiasis: New approaches to treatment. *Br. J. Dermatol.*, 89:179–190.

70. Howard, D. H., and Otto, V. (1977): Experiments on lymphocyte-mediated cellular immunity in murine histoplasmosis. *Infect. Immun.*, 16:226–231.

71. Jones, H. E., Reinhardt, J. H., and Rinaldi, M. G. (1974): Immunologic susceptibility to chronic dermatophytosis. *Arch. Dermatol.*, 110:213–220.

72. Jones, H. L., and Harrell, E. R. (1977): Superficial fungus infections of the skin. In: *Infectious Diseases: A Modern Treatise of Infectious Processes*, edited by P. D. Hoeprich, pp. 836–846. Harper and Row, Hagerstown.

73. Kalina, M., Kletter, Y., and Aronson, M. (1974): The interaction of phagocytes and large-sized parasite *Cryptococcus neoformans*: Cytochemical and ultrastructural study. *Cell Tissue Res.*, 152:165–174.

74. Kirkpatrick, C. H., Chandler, J. W., Jr., Smith, T. K., and Newberry, W. M., Jr. (1971): Cellular immunologic studies in histoplasmosis. In: *Histoplasmosis*, edited by A. Balows, pp. 371–379. Charles C Thomas, Springfield.

75. Kirkpatrick, C. H., Rich, R. R., and Bennet, J. E. (1971): Chronic mucocutaneous candidiasis: Model building in cellular immunity. *Ann. Intern. Med.*, 75:955–978.

76. Kirkpatrick, C. H., and Smith, T. K. (1974): Chronic mucocutaneous candidiasis: Immunologic and antibiotic therapy. *Ann. Intern. Med.*, 80:310–320.

77. Kirkpatrick, C. H., Ottesen, E. A., Smith, T. K., Wells, S. A., and Burdick, J. F. (1976): Reconstitution of defective cellular immunity with foetal thymus and dialysable transfer factor. Long term studies in a patient with chronic mucocutaneous candidiasis. *Clin. Exp. Immunol.*, 23:414–428.

78. Kirkpatrick, C. H., Greenberg, L. E., Chapman, S. W., Goldstein, G., Lewis, V. M., and Twomey, J. J. (1978): Plasma thymic hormone activity in patients with chronic mucocutaneous candidiasis. *Clin. Exp. Immunol.*, 34:311–317.

79. Kirkpatrick, C. H., and Sohnle, P. G. (1981): Chronic mucocutaneous candidiasis. In: *Immunodermatology*, edited by B. Safai and R. A. Good, pp. 495–514. Plenum, New York.

80. Kleinhenz, M. E., Ellner, J. J., Spagnuolo, P. J., and Daniel, T. M. (1981): Suppression of lymphocyte responses by tuberculous plasma and mycobacterial arabinogalactan. *J. Clin. Invest.*, 68:153–162.

81. Kotani, S. Y., Watanabe, Y., and Kinoshita, F. (1975): Immunoadjuvant activities of synthetic N-acetyl-muramyl-peptides or -amino acids. *Biken J.*, 18:105–111.

82. Krahenbuhl, J. L., and Remington, J. S. (1974): *In vitro* induction of nonspecific resistance in macrophages by specifically sensitized lymphocytes. *Infect. Immun.*, 4:337.

83. Kretschmer, R., Say, B., Brown, D., and Rosen, F. S. (1968): Congenital aplasia of the thymus gland. *N. Engl. J. Med.*, 279:1295–1301.

84. Landay, M. E., Hotchi, M., and Soares, N. (1972): Effect of prior vaccination on experimental blastomycosis. *Mycopathol. Mycol. Appl.*, 46:61–64.

85. Lehrer, R. I. (1971): Measurement of candidacidal activity of specific leukocyte types in mixed cell populations. II. Normal and chronic granulomatous disease eosinophils. *Infect. Immun.*, 3:800–802.

86. Lehrer, R. I. (1972): Functional aspects of a second mechanism of candidacidal activity by human neutrophils. *J. Clin. Invest.*, 51:2566–2572.

87. Lehrer, R. I. (1975): The fungicidal mechanism of human monocytes. I. Evidence for myeloperoxidase-linked and myeloperoxidase-independent candidacidal mechanisms. *J. Clin. Invest.*, 55:338–346.

88. Lehrer, R. I., and Jan, R. G. (1970): Interaction of *Aspergillus fumigatus* spores with human leukocytes and serum. *Infect. Immun.*, 1:345–350.

89. Lehrer, R. I., and Cline, M. J. (1971): Leukocyte candicidal activity and resistance to systemic candidiasis in patients with cancer. *Cancer*, 27:1211–1217.

90. Leung-Tack, J., Maillard, J., and Voisin, G. A. (1979): Chemotaxis inhibition induced by polymorphonuclear neutrophils by soluble immune complexes. *Int. Arch. Allergy Appl. Immunol.*, 58:365–374.

91. Levy, R., Segal, E., and Eylan, E. (1981): Protective immunity against murine candidiasis elicited by *Candida albicans* ribosomal fractions. *Infect. Immun.*, 31:874–878.

92. Louria, D. B., and Brayton, R. G. (1964): Behavior of candida cells within leukocytes. *Proc. Soc. Exp. Biol. Med.*, 115:93–101.

93. Lurie, M. B. (1942): Studies on the mechanism of immunity in tuberculosis. The fate of tubercle bacilli ingested by mononuclear phagocytes derived from normal and immune animals. *J. Exp. Med.*, 75:247–268.

94. Mackanness, G. B. (1962): Cellular resistance to infection. *J. Exp. Med.*, 116:381–406.

95. Mackanness, G. B. (1964): The immunological basis of acquired cellular resistance. *J. Exp. Med.*, 120:105–120.

96. Mackanness, G. B. (1970): The monocyte in cellular immunity. *Sem. Hematol.*, 7:172–184.

97. Marra, S., and Balish, E. (1974): Immunity to *Candida albicans* induced by *Listeria monocytogenes*. *Infect. Immun.*, 10:72–82.

98. Mason, U. G., III, Greenberg, L. E., Yen, S. S., and Kirkpatrick, C. H. (1982): Indomethacin-responsive mononuclear cell dysfunction in "atypical" mycobacterioses. *Cell. Immunol.* 71:54–65.

99. Masur, H., Michelis, M. A., Greene, J. B., Onorato, I., VandeStouwe, R. A., Holzman, R. S., Wormser, G., Brettman, L., Lange, M., Murray, H. W., and Cunningham-Rundles, S. (1981): An outbreak of community-acquired *Pneumocystis carinii* pneumonia: Initial manifestation of cellular immune dysfunction. *N. Engl. J. Med.*, 305:1431–1438.

100. McIntosh, K. (1978): Immunity to infection. In: *Allergy: Principles and Practices*, edited by E. Middleton, Jr., C. E. Reed, and E. F. Ellis, pp. 177–186. C. V. Mosby, Saint Louis.

101. Michel, F. B., D'Hinterland, L. D., Bousquet, J., Pinel, A. M., and Normier, G. (1978): Immuno-stimulation by a ribosomal vaccine associated with a bacterial cell wall adjuvant in humans. *Infect. Immun.*, 20:760–769.

102. Miyake, T., Takeya, K., Nomoto, K., and Muraoka, S. (1977): Cellular elements in resistance to candida infection in mice. I. Contribution of T lymphocytes and phagocytes at various stages of infection. *Microbiol. Immunol.*, 21:703–725.

103. Mobacken, H., Hanson, L. A., Lindholm, L., and Ljunggren, C. (1980): Transfer factor in the treatment of chronic mucocutaneous candidiasis: A controlled study. *Acta Dermatol. Venereol.*, 60:51–55.

104. Mok, P. W. Y., and Greer, D. L. (1977): Cell-mediated immune responses in patients with paracoccidioidomycosis. *Clin. Exp. Immunol.*, 28:89–98.

105. Morrison, N. E., and Collins, F. M. (1976): Restoration of T-cell responsiveness by thymosin: Development of antituberculous resistance in BCG-infected animals. *Infect. Immun.*, 13:554–563.

106. Moser, S. A., Domer, J. E., and Mather, F. J. (1980): Experimental murine candidiasis: Cell-mediated immunity after cutaneous challenge. *Infect. Immun.*, 27:140–149.

107. Musatti, C. C., Rezkallah, M. T., Mendes, E., and Mendes, N. F. (1976): *In vivo* and *in vitro* evaluation of cell-mediated immunity in patients with paracoccidioidomycosis. *Cell. Immunol.*, 24:365–378.

108. Newberry, W. M., Jr., Chandler, J. W., Jr., Chin, T. D. Y., and Kirkpatrick, C. H. (1968): Immunology of the mycoses. I. Depressed lymphocyte transformation in chronic histoplasmosis. *J. Immunol.*, 100:436–443.

109. North, R. J. (1973): Importance of thymus-derived lymphocytes in cell-mediated immunity to infection. *Cell. Immunol.*, 7:166–176.

110. Oh, M-H. K., Bodey, G. E., Good, R. A., Chilgren, R. A., and Quie, P. G. (1969): Defective

candidacidal capacity of polymorphonuclear leukocytes in chronic granulomatous disease of childhood. *J. Pediatr.*, 75:300–303.

111. Opelz, G., and Scheer, M. I. (1975): Cutaneous sensitivity and *in vitro* responsiveness of lymphocytes in patients with disseminated coccidioidomycosis. *Infect. Dis.*, 132:250–255.

112. Ozato, K., and Uesaka, I. (1974): The role of macrophages in *Candida albicans* infection *in vitro*. *Jpn. J. Microbiol.*, 18:29–35.

113. Pape, G. R., Moretta, L., Troye, M., and Perlmann, P. (1979): Natural cytotoxicity of human Fc-receptor-positive T lymphocytes after surface modulation with immune complexes. *Scand. J. Immunol.*, 9:291–296.

114. Patterson, R. J., and Youmans, G. P. (1970): Demonstration in tissue culture of lymphocyte-mediated immunity to tuberculosis. *Infect. Immun.*, 1:600–603.

115. Pearsall, N. N., and Lagunoff, D. (1974): Immunological responses to *Candida albicans*. I. Mouse-thigh lesion as a model for experimental candidiasis. *Infect. Immun.*, 9:999–1002.

116. Pearsall, N. N., Adams, B. L., and Bunni, R. (1978): Immunologic responses to *Candida albicans*. III. Effects of passive transfer of lymphoid cells or serum on murine candidiasis. *J. Immunol.*, 120:1176–1180.

117. Peterson, E. M., and Calderone, R. A. (1977): Growth inhibition of *Candida albicans* by rabbit alveolar macrophages. *Infect. Immun.*, 15:910–915.

118. Plouffe, J. F., Jr., Silva, J., Jr., Fekety, R., Reinhalter, E., and Browne, R. (1979): Cell-mediated immune responses in sporotrichosis. *J. Infect. Dis.*, 139:152–157.

119. Provost, T., Garretson, T., Zeschke, R., Rose, N., and Tomasi, T. (1973): Combined murine deficiency, autoantibody formation and mucocutaneous candidiasis. *Clin. Immunol. Immunopathol.*, 1:429–445.

120. Raffel, S. (1950): Chemical factors involved in the induction of infectious allergy. *Experientia*, 6:410–419.

121. Ray, T. L., and Wuepper, K. D. (1978): Experimental cutaneous candidiasis in rodents. II. Role of the stratum corneum barrier and serum complement as a mediator of a protective inflammatory response. *Arch. Dermatol.*, 114:539–543.

122. Rich, A. R., and Lewis, M. R. (1932): The nature of allergy in tuberculosis as revealed by tissue culture studies. *Bull. Johns Hopkins Hosp.*, 50:115–131.

123. Rogers, R. J., Balish, E., and Manning, D. D. (1976): The role of thymus-dependent cell-mediated immunity in resistance to experimental disseminated candidiasis. *J. Reticuloendothel. Soc.*, 20:291–298.

124. Rosenthal, A. S., Lipsky, P. E., and Shevach, E. M. (1975): Macrophage-lymphocyte interaction and antigen recognition. *Fed. Proc.*, 34:1743–1748.

125. Rowley, D. A., Fitch, F. W., Stuart, E. P., Kohler, H., and Consenze, H. (1973): Specific suppression of immune responses. *Science*, 181:1133–1141.

126. Sagone, A. L., Jr., King, G. W., and Metz, E. N. (1976): A comparison of the metabolic response to phagocytosis in human granulocytes and monocytes. *J. Clin. Invest.*, 57:1352–1358.

127. Schofield, F. D., Parkinson, A. D., and Jeffrey, D. (1963): Observations on the epidemiology, effects and treatment of tinea imbricata. *Trans. R. Soc. Trop. Med Hyg.*, 57:214–227.

128. Schulkind, M. D., and Ayoub, E. M. (1975): Transfer factor as an approach to the treatment of immune deficiency. *Birth Defects*, 11:436–440.

129. Serjeantson, S., and Lawrence, G. (1977): Autosomal recessive inheritance of susceptibility to tinea imbricata. *Lancet*, 1:13–15.

130. Siegal, F. P., Lopez, C., Hammer, G. S., Brown, A. E., Kornfeld, S. J., Gold, J., Hassett, J., Hirschman, S. Z., Cunningham-Rundles, C., Adelsberg, B. R., Parham, D. M., Siegal, M., Cunningham-Rundles, S., and Armstrong, D. (1981): Severe acquired immunodeficiency in male homosexuals, manifested by chronic perianal ulcerative herpes simplex lesions. *N. Engl. J. Med.*, 305:1439–1444.

131. Singh, M. M., Kumar, P., Malviya, A. N., and Kumar, R. (1981): Levamisole as an adjunct in the treatment of pulmonary tuberculosis. *Am. Rev. Respir. Dis.*, 123:277–279.

132. Snyderman, R., Altman, L. C., Frankel, A., and Blaese, R. M. (1973): Defective mononuclear leukocyte chemotaxis: A previously unrecognized immune dysfunction. *Ann. Intern. Med.*, 78:509–513.

133. Sohnle, P. G., Frank, M. M., and Kirkpatrick, C. H. (1976): Mechanisms involved in elimination of organisms from experimental cutaneous *Candida albicans* infections in guinea pigs. *J. Immunol.*, 117:523–530.

134. Sohnle, P. G., Frank, M. M., and Kirkpatrick, C. H. (1976): Deposition of complement components in the cutaneous lesions of chronic mucocutaneous candidiasis. *Clin. Immunol. Immunopathol.*, 5:340–350.
135. Sohnle, P. G., and Collins-Lech, C. (1978): Cell-mediated immunity to *Pityrosporum orbiculare* in tinea versicolor. *J. Clin. Invest.*, 62:45–53.
136. Sorensen, G. W., and Jones, H. E. (1976): Immediate and delayed hypersensitivity in chronic dermatophytosis. *Arch. Dermatol.*, 112:40–42.
137. Spencer, H. D., and Cozad, G. C. (1973): Role of delayed hypersensitivity in blastomycosis of mice. *Infect. Immun.*, 7:329–334.
138. Stanley, V. C., and Hurley, R. (1969): The growth of candida species in cultures of mouse peritoneal macrophages. *J. Pathol.*, 97:357–366.
139. Suter, E. (1952): The multiplication of tubercle bacilli within normal phagocytes in tissue culture. *J. Exp. Med.*, 96:137–150.
140. Suter, E. (1953): Multiplication of tubercle bacilli within mononuclear phagocytes in tissue cultures derived from normal animals and animals vaccinated with BCG. *J. Exp. Med.*, 97:235–246.
141. Sutton, R. L., Jr., and Waisman, M. (1977): Dermatoses due to fungi. *Cutis*, 19:377–394.
142. Taplin, D. (1976): Superficial mycoses. *J. Invest. Dermatol.*, 67:177–181.
143. Territo, M. C., and Cline, M. J. (1975): Mononuclear phagocyte proliferation, maturation and function. *Clin. Haematol.*, 4:685–703.
144. Territo, M. C., and Cline, M. J. (1976): Macrophages and their disorders in man. In: *Immunobiology of the Macrophage*, edited by D. S. Nelson, pp. 594–616. Academic Press, New York.
145. Tewari, R. P., Sharma, D., Solotorovsky, M., Lafemina, R., and Balint, J. (1977): Adoptive transfer of immunity from mice immunized with ribosomes or live yeast cells of *Histoplasma capsulatum. Infect. Immun.*, 15:789–795.
146. Twomey, J. J., Waddell, C. C., Krantz, S., O'Reilly, R., L'Esperance, P., and Good, R. A. (1975): Chronic mucocutaneous candidiasis with macrophage dysfunction, a plasma inhibitor, and co-existent aplastic anemia. *J. Lab. Clin. Med.*, 85:968–977.
147. Uhr, J. W. (1966): Delayed hypersensitivity. *Physiol. Rev.*, 46:359–419.
148. Valdimarsson, H., Moss, P. D., Holt, P. J. L., and Hobbs, J. R. (1972): Treatment of chronic mucocutaneous candidiasis with leukocytes from HLA compatible sibling. *Lancet*, 1:469–472.
149. VanScoy, R. E., Hill, H. R., Ritts, R. E., and Quie, P. G. (1975): Familial neutrophil chemotaxis defect, recurrent bacterial infections, mucocutaneous candidiasis and hyperimmunoglobulin E. *Ann. Intern. Med.*, 92:766–771.
150. Waldman, R. H., and Henney, C. S. (1971): Cell-mediated immunity and antibody response in the respiratory tract after local and systemic immunization. *J. Exp. Med.*, 134:482–494.
151. Walters, B. A. J., Chick, J. E. D., and Halliday, W. J. (1974): Cell-mediated immunity and serum blocking factors in patients with chronic dermatophytic infections. *Int. Arch. Allergy*, 46:849–857.
152. Wara, D. W., and Ammann, A. J. (1978): Thymosin treatment of children with primary immunodeficiency disease. *Transplant Proc.*, 10:203–209.
153. Whiting, D. A., and Bisset, E. A. (1974): The investigation of superficial fungal infections by skin surface biopsy. *Br. J. Dermatol.*, 91:57–65.
154. Williams, D. M., Krick, J. A., and Remington, J. S. (1977): Pulmonary infection in the compromised host. Part I. In: *Lung Disease: State of the Art*, edited by J. F. Murray, pp. 131–166. American Lung Association, New York.
155. Wright, D. G., Kirkpatrick, C. H., and Gallin, J. I. (1977): Effects of levamisole on normal and abnormal leukocyte motion. *J. Clin. Invest.*, 59:941–950.
156. Yosinoya, S., Cox, R. A., and Pope, R. M. (1980): Circulating immune complexes in coccidioidomycosis: Detection and characterization. *J. Clin. Invest.*, 66:655–663.
157. Young, R. C., Bennett, J. E., Vogel, C. L., Carbone, P. P., and DeVita, V. T. (1970): Aspergillosis: The spectrum of the disease in 98 patients. *Medicine*, 49:147–173.
158. Youmans, G. P., editor (1979): *Tuberculosis.* Saunders, Philadelphia.

Advances in Host Defense Mechanisms, Vol. 2,
edited by John I. Gallin and Anthony S. Fauci.
Raven Press, New York © 1983.

Host-Parasite Relationships: The Role of the Lymphoid System in Protozoan Infections

Anthony C. Allison and Elsie M. Eugui

*Institute of Biological Sciences, Syntex Research,
Palo Alto, California 94304*

Parasites infect hundreds of millions of people and their domestic livestock, contributing to chronic ill health and constraining food production, especially in third world countries. Traditional methods of preventing and treating parasitic diseases, by vector control and chemotherapy, are expensive and often ineffective. Vectors are becoming resistant to insecticides and acaricides, and parasites to widely used drugs. As emphasized by the World Health Organization and the Food and Agriculture Organization, the situation is deteriorating, and alternative ways of controlling parasitic diseases are being considered. One of these is immunoprophylaxis. Sufficient successful examples are available to encourage exploration of others. For many years, cattle have been immunized against the helminth *Dictyocaulus viviparus* (107), the hemoprotozoan *Babesia bovis* (see ref. 99), and the tick-borne protozoan *Theileria annulata* (88).

Vaccines can be developed empirically, as in the case of Jenner's vaccine, which eventually led to the elimination of smallpox. Nevertheless, it is useful to understand the immune responses elicited by different parasites and the mechanisms by which the parasites avoid elimination. Until recently, parasite immunology was concerned largely with a description of parasite antigens and the humoral responses that they elicit. Demonstration of the presence of these antigens and antibodies is useful for diagnosis and immunoepidemiology. Recently, this approach has been refined by the use of monoclonal antibodies not only to recover and characterize individual parasite antigens, as described below, but also to protect animals from infection and inhibit multiplication of parasites in culture. Of special interest is the application of monoclonal antibodies to isolate parasite antigens for immunization (62). This is a valuable way to define protective antigens and opens up a range of possibilities, including the preparation of antigens by recombinant DNA technology or synthesis.

Recombinant DNA technology has already shown its usefulness in the analysis of antigenic variation in African trypanosomes, as discussed briefly below. In this case, there is no doubt that antibodies against the variant-specific glycoprotein of the parasite play an important role in immunity (Table 1). Nevertheless, other mechanisms also are relevant, including nonspecific immunodepression. In several parasitic infections, however, it has been difficult to establish the importance of

TABLE 1. *Principal effector mechanisms in immunity and escape mechanisms of protozoan parasites*

Parasite	Effector mechanism	Escape mechanism
Trypanosoma brucei, vivax, and *congolense*	Antibody against surface glycoprotein	Antigenic variation
Trypanosoma cruzi	Antibody against surface glycoprotein	Intracellular situation
Plasmodium species	Stage-specific antibodies; cell-mediated immunity	Antigenic variation; intracellular location
Leishmania species	T-lymphocyte-dependent macrophage activation	Generation of specific suppressor lymphocytes
Theileria species	Lymphocyte-mediated cytotoxicity of infected cells	Generation of specific suppressor lymphocytes

antibodies in protection, and increasing evidence has accumulated for a role of cell-mediated immunity in host protection, as reviewed in this chapter. Cell-mediated responses depend on T-lymphocytes, which, apart from their helper effects on antibody formation, are thought to bring about recovery from parasitic infections in three ways:

1. Immune T-lymphocytes reacting with antigen release a mediator or mediators able to activate macrophages, so that the latter can limit multiplication of parasites within them. This is believed to be the principal mechanism operating not only against mycobacteria, such as *Mycobacterium leprae*, but also against *Leishmania*, as discussed below (Table 1). This system is applicable when the cells bearing parasites are macrophages, which have a killing mechanism related to the generation of toxic products of oxygen (84). The killing mechanism depends on the presence in cell membranes of cytochrome b5 (98), an enzyme system found in neutrophils and macrophages but not in lymphocytes or cell lines derived from them. Hence it is unlikely that products of activated T-lymphocytes can increase the capacity of lymphoid cells to kill *Theileria* macroschizonts within them.

2. A subpopulation of T-lymphocytes may be able to lyse parasite-infected cells. T-lymphocytes from immune animals are more cytotoxic for virus-infected cells bearing the same major histocompatibility antigens than for allogeneic virus-infected cells (117). Thus the receptors on the cytotoxic lymphocytes appear to recognize complexes of virus antigens and host histocompatibility antigens on the surface of infected cells. As discussed below, this appears to be the major mechanism of protective immunity in theileriosis (Table 1).

3. T-lymphocyte products activate macrophages and/or natural killer (NK) cells, and products of these cell types inhibit the proliferation of intraerythrocytic parasites. This mechanism is discussed in relation to hemoprotozoa (Table 1).

Parasites often establish chronic infections, which are advantageous to the parasite because they prolong the time during which transmission to the vector can occur. Parasites have developed several mechanisms by which they can escape from attack by the immune systems of the host. The principal known escape mechanisms are as follows:

1. *Intracellular location.* Even in macrophages, which have parasiticidal capacity, this is not always effective, as discussed below in the case of *Leishmania*. Parasites in other cell types, such as *Trypanosoma cruzi* in muscle and *Toxoplasma gondii* in several cell types in the body, are sheltered from immune attack. Such cell types usually lack microbicidal capacity and may not have on their surfaces the complexes of parasite antigens and major histocompatibility antigens that are required not only for T-lymphocyte-mediated killing virus-infected cells (117) but also cells bearing protozoan parasites, as in the case of *Theileria*.

2. *Antigenic variation.* The prototype example is African trypanosomes, and recent molecular biologic studies of this remarkable phenomenon are summarized below. Antigenic variation has been demonstrated also in relapsing *Plasmodium knowlesi* infections in *Macaca mulatta* monkeys by variant-specific agglutination of schizont-infected erythrocytes (9). Many antigenic types of *P. falciparum* have been demonstrated by agar gel precipitation (112), and antigenic diversity is thought to be one of the reasons why African children have repeated infections with this parasite.

3. *Nonspecific immunosuppression.* This is a common phenomenon in parasitic, viral, and other infections. It is discussed here briefly for African trypanosome infections, and is observed also in malaria infections.

4. *Specific suppression.* The high susceptibility of the BALB/c strain of mice to *L. tropica* infections has been correlated with the presence of a population of suppressor T-lymphocytes that can abrogate a curative cell-mediated immune response (64). Other mechanisms, including the presence of host antigens on the parasite surface, have been demonstrated for metazoan parasites but not yet for protozoa.

The use of host animals that have inherited or acquired deficiencies in various immune functions, including those of T- or B-lymphocytes, macrophages, and NK cells, has helped to define the role of these functions in recovery from protozoan parasitic infections and resistance to reinfection. Thus parasite immunology is in an exciting phase of development.

AFRICAN SPECIES OF TRYPANOSOMA

The well-known ability of these parasites to undergo antigenic variation appears to be the main explanation for their persistence. In recent years, antigenic variation has been analyzed at the molecular level. In 1969, Vickerman (109) showed that all bloodstream forms of *T. brucei* have a 12 to 15 nm electron-dense surface layer just outside the plasma membrane. This coat covers the entire cell, including the flagellum. It is also found on the infective metacyclic forms from the tsetse salivary gland but is absent from the procyclic forms present in the midgut of the fly. Interestingly, Tetley et al. (103) have recently found that the infective, hypopharyngeal forms of *T. vivax* in the tsetse lack the glycoprotein coat. Biochemical studies reported by Cross (28) showed that the coat is composed of about 10^7 molecules of a unique glycoprotein with a molecular weight of about 65,000. These molecules form a monolayer apparently just outside the plasma membrane. This is probably the only protein exposed on the cell surface and carries all the antigenic determinants of the living trypanosome. Antigenic variation involves replacement of the glycoprotein in the coat with another glycoprotein having different antigenic determinants. The glycoproteins from several variants have been found to exhibit marked differences in amino acid composition (68).

What is the function of the variant-specific glycoprotein? *T. brucei* can be cultured at 37°C, in which case the glycoprotein coat is formed, or at 27°C, when the parasites multiply but do not produce a glycoprotein coat. We found that such uncoated parasites rapidly activate complement by the alternative pathway and are lysed in fresh serum (48). The glycoprotein coat prevents access of serum proteins to the parasite plasma membrane and so protects the parasite. However, the coat glycoproteins themselves are highly immunogenic, and the antibodies formed rapidly lyse the trypanosomes in the presence of complement. Survival of the parasite depends on the antigenic variation. Since antigenic variation occurs *in vivo* during the early stages of infection before antibody is formed (108) and in culture in the absence of antibody (38), the antibody does not appear to induce antigenic variation but to act as a selective agent on preexisting variants.

The variable antigen type (VAT) refers to trypanosomes expressing a particular antigen. The antigen is termed variant-specific glycoprotein (VSG). Many different VATs, all derived from a trypanosome clone, constitute a serodeme. The extent of the VAT repertoire in a serodeme is above 100 but probably finite (16). It was formerly thought that in the metacyclic form, the trypanosome reverts to a single, basic antigenic type. However, several antigenic types of metacyclic can be obtained even from cloned trypanosomes (73). The relative proportions of three major metacyclic types of one clone was the same regardless of what VAT was used to infect the tsetse (57). Thus the repertoire of metacyclic VATs for each serodeme is likely to be small. If this is true for several serodemes, the possibility of vaccination becomes realistic.

During the last few years, progress has been made in elucidating the molecular basis of antigenic variation, which is one of the most interesting problems in contemporary biology. Three different mechanisms have been considered. According to the first, each trypanosome could have a single VSG gene which mutates to give rise to changing gene products. Because of substantial differences in amino acid constitution of VSGs, and for other reasons, this model has been discarded. Second, antigenic variation could involve the rearrangement of chromosomal sequences to create new VSG genes in much the same way as variable and constant regions of immunoglobulins combine to form a wide range of antibodies. There is no evidence for such a mechanism. According to the third mechanism, genes for all the VSGs, in the repertoire are present intact within the chromosome of the parasite. Only one of these genes is expressed at a time, and antigenic variation simply involves the shutting off of one gene and turning on of another.

The use of cloned complementary (cDNAs) prepared from messenger RNAs for VSGs as probes in hybridization studies has provided important information. These DNAs have hybridized with genomic fragments from every VAT tested belonging to the same serodeme (111). These and other experiments have shown that the gene for a VSG is present whether or not that VSG is expressed. The DNA probe hybridizes with a unique messenger RNA only from VATs expressing the VSG corresponding to the probe (61,87); this RNA was absent in other VATs. It can be concluded that although many VSG genes are present in the chromosome of the parasite, only one, which codes for the VSG of the cell, is transcribed. Moreover, the hybridization experiments have shown that when the gene is being transcribed to form messenger RNA, an expression-linked copy is present (61,87). The appearance of an expression-linked copy of a VSG gene seems to involve duplication of the basic copy of the gene and transposition of the duplicate to a new location in the chromosome, where it is transcribed to form messenger RNA. The expression-linked copy of the VSG gene is more susceptible to digestion by DNAase than is the original genomic copy, which is typical of genes being transcribed in other systems. Thus the phenomenon of antigenic variation, which is the major mechanism by which African trypanosomes avoid immune elimination, is at last becoming understood in molecular terms.

Immunosuppression in African Trypanosomiasis

Infections of laboratory rodents by African trypanosomes is accompanied by severe, generalized immunosuppression (25,53,66). Infection by *T. brucei* in mice results in polyclonal proliferation of B-, T-, and null cells in the blood, spleen, peritoneum, and bone marrow (24). An initial phase of increased immune responsiveness is followed by depression of the response to parasite antigens as well as unrelated antigens. Several functions of B- and T- subsets are impaired, although the production of mediators of delayed hypersensitivity continues.

The mechanism underlying the immunosuppression has been investigated. Eardley and Jayawardena (39) attributed the phenomenon to suppressor T-cells, which induce macrophages to become inhibitory. However, because trypanosome infection of nude mice results in marked changes in B-cell function (24), it is unlikely that suppressor T-cells are required.

Grosskinsky and Askonas (55) have presented evidence that peritoneal macrophages following ingestion of opsonized *T. brucei*, when transferred to syngeneic recipients, induce changes in immunologic functions similar to those observed in trypanosome infections. These include (a) an increased number of nonspecific background plaque-forming cells in the spleen, and (b) increase or suppression of the specific immune response to sheep erythrocytes, depending on the timing of antigen challenge. Priming simultaneously with the transfer of trypanosome-containing macrophages increased immune responsiveness, whereas if priming was delayed until 4 days after transfer of parasite-containing macrophages, the immune response to sheep erythrocytes was suppressed. Transfer of macrophages that had ingested opsonized erythrocytes had no such immunomodulatory effects. Treatment of the peritoneal exudate cells with anti-Thy 1.2 and complement before transfer did not affect their capacity to influence immune responses. Thus activation of suppressor T-cells in this population could not account for the observed effects.

These results suggest that macrophages following ingestion of African trypanosomes acquire immunomodulatory capacity and play a major part in the polyclonal activation and immunodepression that are characteristic of African trypanosome infections. This is not a feature of any phagocytic event. Hence the parasite must elaborate some product that influences macrophage activity and suppresses immune responses to parasite antigens as well as unrelated antigens, thereby increasing the changes of parasite survival in the vertebrate host.

LEISHMANIASIS

Leishmaniasis is an infection caused by flagellated protozoa that in the vertebrate host become amastigotes multiplying in cells of the mononuclear phagocyte lineage. The parasites can produce cutaneous, mucocutaneous, or visceral disease, the latter also known as kala azar. Adler (2) suggested that the healing of cutaneous lesions is related to the development of delayed-type hypersensitivity (DTH) reactions to leishmania antigens. Turk and Bryceson (105) postulated that there is a spectrum of host responses in leishmaniasis analogous to that recognized in leprosy. Toward one end of the spectrum, effective cell-mediated immune responses can activate parasiticidal mechanisms which bring about spontaneous recovery and immunity to reinfection (oriental sore); toward the other end of the spectrum, cell-mediated immune responses are ineffective, and persistent diffuse cutaneous or visceral lesions develop. In the latter, high levels of antibodies against parasite antigens are present, suggesting that antibodies detected by conventional methods (immunofluorescence and complement fixation) are not related to protection (60).

The parasites normally survive and replicate within phagolysosomes of macrophages (31). For recovery from infection, the intracellular environment must be changed in such a way as to be unfavorable for parasite growth. This can be achieved by a specific immune response of T-lymphocytes, normally to parasite antigens but experimentally to unrelated antigens. As a result of this specific immune response, products of T-lymphocytes are released, which nonspecifically activate macrophages so that they can limit the replication of parasites within them.

Two models for human cutaneous leishmaniasis are infections with L. tropica in the mouse and L. enrietti (12) in the guinea pig. In both cases, granulomatous lesions that persist in the skin for weeks or months are produced. In most strains of mice, infections with moderate numbers of L. tropica usually produce self-limiting lesions like human oriental sores. The same is true of cutaneous infections in guinea pigs with *L. enrietti*. A role of the T-lymphocytes in recovery is suggested by observations that thymectomy impairs recovery of CBA mice from *L. tropica* infections (90), and that widespread cutaneous infections develop in *L. enrietti*-infected guinea pigs when they are immunosuppressed with antilymphocyte serum (13) or when the primary lesion is in a skin site with interrupted lymphatic drainage (70). Moreover, DTH reactions to unrelated antigens in guinea pigs were found to inhibit the growth of *L. enriettii* (5).

Three phenomena are considered: (a) recognition of leishmania antigens by T-lymphocytes, (b) production by T-lymphocytes of mediators that increase the capacity of macrophages to kill parasites or limit their intracellular growth, and (c) development of specific suppression, as a result of which the protective immune response can be abrogated.

Proliferative responses of human lymphocytes to leishmanial antigens were reported by Wyler et al. (114). When the concentration of leishmanial antigen was 1 μg/ml, only lymphocytes from patients responded. The response was observed in T-cell-enriched populations and should be a useful supplement to DTH tests when studying specific cellular responses in the spectrum of diseases thought to represent varying degrees of efficiency of host defense against the parasite. To analyze T-cell responses of mice to *L. tropica*, Louis et al. (76) adapted a method for the study of T-lymphocyte activation by protein antigens. Parasites were injected into the base of the tail in Freund's complete adjuvant. Lymph node cells, when cultured in the presence of parasites, exhibited strong proliferation. The response was antigen specific and attributable to T-cells, as shown by its elimination with antiserum against mouse T-cells and increase in T-enriched populations. Normal peritoneal cells pulsed with *L. tropica* were able to induce a proliferative response of primed T-cells in the absence of extracellular parasites.

This system was used by Louis et al. (77) to analyze the role of the H-2 gene complex in interactions between antigen-presenting macrophages and *Leishmania*-immune T-lymphocytes. The proliferative response of nylon wool-purified, primed lymph node cells to *L. tropica* parasites *in vitro* could be restored by the addition of either syngeneic or allogeneic adherent spleen cells. These observations suggested the absence of H-2 restriction in eliciting *Leishmania*-specific T-cell responses. When T-blasts generated *in vitro* were separated in a Percoll gradient and maintained for 4 days in T-cell growth factor, however, their response to *L. tropica* was found to be strictly dependent on the presence of syngeneic spleen cells. Further studies using congenic recombinant mice demonstrated that proliferation of parasite-specific blasts required the presence of spleen cells compatible with the corresponding cells in the 1-A region of the major histocompatibility complex (MHC). This requirement for spleen cells compatible with the responding cells in the 1-A region of the MHC was confirmed by treating the cells with monoclonal anti-Ia antibodies and complement. By flow microphotometry, the T-cell phenotype of the *L. tropica*-specific blasts was found to be Thy-1$^+$, Lyt-1$^+$, and Lyt-2$^-$.

Nacy et al. (86) used suspension cultures of resident peritoneal macrophages of C3H/HEN mice, in which infective tissue-derived amastigotes of *L. tropica* can replicate, to study the effects of lymphokines on these cells. Previous studies with *L. tropica* in mouse macrophages and *L. enrietti* in guinea pig macrophages had been with adherent cell cultures, in which the parasites replicate poorly, if at all, and addition of lymphokines had given inconclusive results. Nacy and her colleagues (86) found that treatment of suspended macrophage cultures before exposure to *L. tropica* increased the resistance of the cells to infection; 35% of cells contained intracellular amastigotes compared to medium-treated controls. Macrophage cultures treated with lymphokines after infection developed potent parasiticidal capacity; 75 to 80% of treated macrophages were free of intracellular parasites by 72 hr. Fractionation of lymphokine supernatants showed that the major macrophage-activating component was in a peak of about 65,000 molecular weight, similar to that increasing the capacity of macrophages to kill intracellular *Rickettsia tsutsugamushi* (85) and tumor cells (81). Lower peaks of activity, increasing macrophage microbicidal capacity, were found with molecular weights of about 130,000 and less than 10,000.

Some mice and humans do not recover spontaneously from *Leishmania* infections. Evidence suggests that this is because parasite-specific suppressor T-lymphocytes block the effects of a potentially curative T-cell-mediated immune response. This type of response is under genetic control. The Balb/c strain of mice is exceptional among the strains so far tested in that the infection is dosage independent and progressive, with widespread cutaneous and fatal visceral infection. Howard et al. (63) have shown that this high susceptibility is largely determined by a single autosomal, non-H-2-linked gene, which appears to be distinct from the *Lsh* gene, which determines the susceptibility of mice to *L. donovani* infection (6). Although H-2-linked genetic influences are also detectable in the immune stage of both leishmanial infections, they are relatively minor in the case of *L. tropica*. Thus although progression of disease induced by low infecting doses is slower in congenic Balb/K (H-2^k) than in Balb/c or Balb/B (H-2^b) mice, the eventual outcome is similar in all three (63). Titers of antileishmanial antibodies do not appear to determine either mouse strain susceptibility or inhibition of DTH to parasite antigens during the infection (64); in other words, antibodies do not appear to have either a protective or a blocking role.

Howard et al. (64) presented evidence suggesting that a major component in the susceptibility of the Balb/c strain to *L. tropica* infection is the generation of specific suppressor T-cells that inhibit DTH reactions to parasite antigens and the development of a curative immune response. The main observations included the following: (a) antileishmanial DTH reactions are observed in Balb/c mice only during the early stages of *L. tropica* infections and then become subject to strong suppression; (b) only the T-enriched fraction of cells from the spleens of such suppressed mice, when transferred to normal, syngeneic mice, impairs the induction of leishmania-specific DTH; and (c) adult thymectomized, X-irradiated, bone-marrow-reconstituted Balb/c mice show retardation of lesion growth and even some cures in parallel with the expression of DTH reactivity, in contrast to the converse effects in normally resistant CBA mice. Later, Howard et al. (65) showed that sublethal X-irradiation (550 rads) abrogates suppressor T-cell generation in Balb/c mice and allows the majority of them to recover from *L. tropica* infections.

THEILERIA

In Africa and Asian countries, protozoan parasites of the genus *Theileria* produce diseases of theoretical interest and economic importance. The *T. parva/T. lawrencei* group of parasites produces East Coast fever and corridor disease in East Africa. *T. annulata* has a widespread distribution in North Africa and Asia as far as the Indian subcontinent, and *T. sergenti* is present in Far Eastern countries. In all, many millions of cattle are subject to theileriosis, and the disease frequently has a fatal outcome, especially in the exotic cattle introduced to improve meat and milk production in developing countries.

Theileria infections are academically interesting because the parasites transform lymphoid cells, both *in vivo* and *in vitro*, into cells with uncontrolled proliferation. Parasites multiply with host cells and are distributed to both daughter cells. In this respect, the parasites are like the Epstein-Barr virus, which transforms human B-lymphocytes into cell lines (43). Indeed, theileriosis resembles severe infectious mononucleosis, with transformation of lymphoid cells by the parasite, widespread infiltration of transformed cells into the tissues, and elicitation of a powerful cell-mediated immune response by the host.

Small infective particles (sporozoites) are introduced into the skin with saliva of the tick vector. After 5 or more days (depending on the inoculum), another form of the parasite (macroschizont) appears in the cytoplasm of large lymphoid cells in the lymph nodes of the drainage chain. The parasitized cells increase considerably in number during the next few days.

Lymph nodes studied in light microscopy and ultrastructural analysis (34) showed nonspecific changes and changes characteristic of *T. parva* infection. Nonspecific reactions include germinal center formation, paracortical hyperplasia, and plasmacytosis. The characteristic changes include the presence of large numbers of parasitized large lymphoid cells, mainly in the paracortical areas but also in the sinuses, medullary cords, and stroma. Until about day 12, the predominant picture is of many parasitized, as well as nonparasitized, large lymphoid cells, often in mitosis, so that the node appears lymphomatous. Occasional cytolysis is seen. After day 13, lymphocytolysis becomes much more frequent, so that the lymph node is depleted of cells, and fibrin is deposited. Another characteristic change is panleukopenia, which may cause death. Many degenerating lymphocytes and other leukocytes are seen in peripheral blood smears. From about day 9, there is migration of many infected and uninfected large lymphoid cells into efferent lymphatics to the tracheal lymph duct, where they enter the blood (35).

Other lymph nodes become involved after this time, bronchial and renal nodes severely and mesenteric lymph nodes slightly. Many parasitized cells accumulate in the lungs and bronchial nodes; their presence and the inflammatory response that they elicit may account for the pulmonary edema that is a frequent terminal event. Many parasitized cells accumulate in the lamina propria of the gut (33). The migration pattern of the infected cells thus follows that established for circulating large lymphocytes in the uninfected rat (54). During the third week after infection, microschizonts appear. These infect erythrocytes as the piroplasm form. Ingestion of erythrocytes by the vector tick completes the life cycle.

A major advance was the propagation of *T. annulata* macroschizonts in monolayer culture (106) and in cultures of large lymphoid cells (67). Subsequently, Malmquist et al. (80) succeeded in cultivating macroschizonts of *T. parva* in lines of large lymphoid cells from infected cattle. Brown et al. (8) infected and transformed bovine lymphoid cells with sporozoites from ticks. Lines of infected lymphoid cells containing parasites (7) can be used to establish infections and, in the case of *T. annulata*, for routine immunization against the disease.

The major histocompatibility antigens of cattle appear to constrain cell-mediated immune responses to parasitized cells (see below) and certainly limit analysis of these responses in cattle (which are not highly inbred). It is necessary, therefore, to introduce any desired strain of the parasite into the lymphoid cells of any animal, so that various strains of the parasite can be studied on a syngeneic background. *In vitro* transformation makes that possible.

Immunity in Theileriosis

Cattle immunized against *T. parva* by infection and treatment are solidly immune to challenge with the homologous parasite for at least 3 years (15). They also are fully resistant to some further isolates of the parasite but show varying degrees of susceptibility to others (93). Thus there are strains for which cross protection is complete and others for which it is incomplete.

Attempts to transfer immunity to naive animals by immune serum or gamma-globulin preparations from immune serum (82) or by colostrum feeding (14) have been unsuccessful. In contrast, transfer of large numbers of thoracic duct cells from immune donors to two chimeric twin partners protected them from lethal East Coast fever (40). These results suggest that protective immunity is cell mediated. Evidence has accumulated that protection is correlated with the presence of specific cytotoxic cells that can lyse parasitized cells in a genetically restricted fashion.

Eugui and Emery (46) found the appearance of specific cytotoxic cells in the peripheral blood of immune animals some days after challenge with sporozoites or autologous cells bearing macroschizonts of the same strain of *T. parva*. These lyse autologous but not allogeneic *Theileria*-transformed cells, and they do not lyse YAC-1 cells. Thus they show the genetic restriction and other properties expected of cytotoxic T-lymphocytes. Emery et al. (41) found that the same type of cytotoxic cells appear in peripheral blood 2 weeks after infection and treatment; no nonspecific cytotoxicity was observed in these animals. Emery and co-workers (42) have also found that when cattle are inoculated with allogeneic macroschizont-bearing cells, only the animals developing cytotoxicity against autologous infected cells are immune to challenge with sporozoites. In other words, immunity to challenge with the homologous strain of parasite is well correlated with the presence of specific cytotoxic lymphocytes in all the situations examined.

It is likely that cytotoxic T-lymphocytes recognize *Theileria*-associated surface antigens complexed with SD-antigens on the membrane of infected cells. The former are analogous to the lymphocyte-detected membrane antigens, which are believed to be targets of cytotoxic lymphocytes killing lymphoblastoid cells infected with Epstein-Barr virus (100).

In contrast to this specific cytotoxicity, which is correlated with protection, there is enhanced nonspecific cytotoxicity in primary *Theileria* infections, which may be related to immunopathologic changes. Eugui et al. (47) found that normal bovine peripheral blood lymphocytes (PBL) lyse YAC-1 cells; this is mouse tumor cell line susceptible to lysis by NK cells of other species. In the PBL of animals with primary *T. parva* infections, capacity to lyse YAC-1 cells and allogeneic *Theileria*-infected cell lines increases considerably. By definition, this is enhanced NK-type activity. This is found in animals which are destined to die as well as those which recover from primary infections, so that activation of NK cells is not well correlated with protection.

Ferluga et al. (49) have found that during the course of autologous mixed lymphocyte response (MLRs) stimulated by *Theileria*-transformed cells, nonspecific cytotoxicity is generated. This process is increased by removal of adherent cells or in the presence of indomethacin, suggesting that the production of prostaglandins by adherent cells (presumably monocytes) inhibits the generation of cytotoxicity. It is likely that this reaction is the *in vitro* counterpart of an *in vivo* autologous MLR, with activation of NK cells, occurring during the course of primary *T. parva* infection. Autologous lymphocytes are susceptible to lysis in this system, which is consistent with a role of activated NK cells in the lymphocytolysis and leukopenia which is so prominent in primary *T. parva* infections. NK activation in the bone marrow could result from a reaction to parasitized cells and could inhibit leukopoiesis. Inhibitory effects of NK cells on leukopoiesis are reviewed by Cudkowicz and Hochman (29). Thus the panleukopenia of East Coast fever is due partly to failure of production of leukocytes and partly to their extramedullary destruction. The panleukopenia could predispose animals to superinfection when they are in a state of increased sensitivity to endotoxin (23).

The concept of increased nonspecific cytotoxicity as an immunopathological mechanism leading to lymphocytolysis is novel, but it may be applicable in other infectious diseases, such as lymphocytic choriomeningitis (72) and rinderpest (89). Activation of nonspecific cytotoxicity in virus infections is well known (94).

Reverting to specific immunity, it appears that in animals recovering from primary *T. parva* infections spontaneously or as a result of treatment, a population of memory T-lymphocytes is generated. These remain for the most part in lymphoid organs, such as lymph nodes and the spleen, and are not readily demonstrable in the peripheral blood cells of immune animals until they are challenged with the homologous strain of the parasite. The memory cells then respond to antigenic stimulation; specific cytotoxic cells are generated from precursors and released into efferent lymph and peripheral blood. These cytotoxic cells are able to lyse macroschizont-bearing cells and thereby limit the progress of the infection.

How do *Theileria* parasites escape? Protective immune responses are not readily elicited in untreated infections in exotic *Bos taurus*, although this does happen in many natural infections in East African Zebu cattle *(B. indicus)* (see ref. 115). One explanation is that the generation of protective immunity is inhibited by suppressor mechanisms which are under genetic control. These might be specific suppressor T-lymphocytes, as discussed for *L. tropica* infections. Alternatively, nonspecific suppression could occur in primary *T. parva* infections in susceptible cattle. For example, Ferluga et al. (49) have obtained evidence that release of prostaglandins by monocytes can inhibit cellular responses to *Theileria*-transformed autologous cells. Prostaglandin E2 can activate suppressor T-lymphocytes (50), which nonspecifically inhibit both humoral and cellular immune responses. Third, activation of NK cells occurs in primary *T. parva* infections in susceptible cattle, as described above, and could result in lysis of lymphoblasts specifically responding to stimulation by parasitized cells (47,49). A search should be made for specific suppressor T-lymphocytes that can inhibit the response of lymphocytes to autologous *T. parva*-transformed cells. As Ferluga et al. (49) suggest, the likelihood of eliciting protective immunity based on T-lymphocytes able to lyse autologous parasitized cells may depend on not only inherited factors in the bovine host but also the strain of parasite used. Clearly, a vaccine strain should elicit protective immunity with as little specific or nonspecific suppression as possible.

In wild buffalo infected with *T. lawrencei*, parasites persist and can infect ticks indefinitely. The same happens in some infections by *T. parva* in Zebu cattle (115). Thus the parasites have efficient escape mechanisms, the nature of which has not yet been defined.

HEMOPROTOZOA (PLASMODIUM AND BABESIA)

Hemoprotozoa parasites of the genera *Plasmodium* and *Babesia* multiply in the erythrocytes of many vertebrate species. In the case of *Plasmodium* species, sporozoites introduced by anopheline mosquitoes into mammals initially infect liver cells and later erythrocytes. According to World Health Organization estimates, in Africa alone, at least 100 million persons are infected with malaria parasites every year, and about 1 million die as a result. The resurgence of malaria in several countries where it was formerly controlled is a matter for concern.

Babesia spp. are transmitted by ticks and infect erythrocytes without a preerythrocytic phase. More than 70 species of *Babesia* have been described (74), infecting most domestic animals as well as many wild and laboratory animals. *Babesia* species were formerly thought to be host specific, but several examples of infection of unnatural hosts are now known. Examples are infection of mongolian gerbils with *B. divergens* from blood of cattle (75) and of humans with intact spleens by *B. microti* of wild rodent origin (95).

In many tropical and temperate countries, *B. argentina* (otherwise known as *B. bovis*), *B. bigemina*, and *B. divergens* infect cattle and produce considerable economic loss. *B. canis* is a common cause of tick fever in dogs in some countries. Genetic factors influence susceptibility to *Babesia* infections: for example, *Bos indicus* are more resistant to *Babesia bovis* than are *Bos taurus* (69), and mice of the A strain are more sensitive to *Babesia microti* than are other strains (45).

Because of economic importance of the infection, immunity to *Babesia* in cattle has been repeatedly studied. Recovery of cattle from the acute phase of the infection is accompanied by an immune response that prevents the occurrence of disease after subsequent challenge with the same species. However, relapses of parasitemia can occur and have been associated with changes in antigenic specificity (30). Rodents that have recovered from *B. microti* infections develop lifelong immunity to challenge with parasites of the same species, suggesting that antigenic variation is of minor importance in this case (45).

The role of antibodies in immunity to *Babesia* spp. in cattle is not clear. Some protection against *B. bovis* was transferred from mothers to offspring, presumably by antibodies in colostrum (58). Using serum from donors hyperimmunized by superinfection, Mahoney (78) transferred some protection to splenectomized calves, but not with serum from donors immediately after infection, even though the titer of antibodies was high. The same hyperimmune serum was unable to confer protection to a challenge with the same strain of *B. bovis* stabilized by cryopreservation. Repeated injections of immune serum did not alter the course of *B. microti* infections in mice (17).

B. bovis can be cultured easily in bovine erythrocytes, and supernatants of cultures have been used to elicit protection in cattle against this infection (99). Successful vaccination of cattle against *B. bovis* with a soluble antigen preparation obtained by sonic disintegration of infected erythrocytes has been reported (79).

The role of antibodies in immunity to *Plasmodium* spp. has proved difficult to define and may vary from one host-parasite combination to another. Cohen et al. (26) reported that gammaglobulin fractions from adult Africans could facilitate recovery of West African children from *P. falciparum* infections. In rats, immune IgG protects against *P. berghei* challenge (11,36). The mechanism of such protection has been analyzed by Quin and Wyler (92) and seems to be at least partly due to increased capacity of the spleen to remove parasitized erythrocytes from the circulation.

More recently, a monoclonal antibody against a protein of molecular weight 62,000 in the membrane of *P. berghei* sporozoites has been found to protect mice against mosquito-transmitted infection (116). Other monoclonal antibodies recognizing antigens of the blood forms of *P. yoelii yoelii* can protect mice against blood-transmitted infection (52). Holder and Freeman (62) have used their monoclonal antibodies to identify and purify antigens of *P. y. yoelii* membranes. They found that mice immunized with either a 235,000 molecular weight merozoite-specific protein or a 230,000 molecular weight schizont protein and its derivatives were protected against infection with *P. y. yoelii*. These observations show that antibodies against stage-specific antigens of the parasite can have a protective role, although this does not appear to be exclusive. For example, mice with humoral responses suppressed by neonatal injection of anti-μ serum can be immunized with irradiated sporozoites against mosquito challenge (32).

Our group has long been interested in cellular immune responses in malaria, which was a neglected subject. The saga began with the demonstration that neonatally thymectomized rats are more susceptible to *P. berghei* infections than their intact littermates (10). With the availability of mice congenitally deprived of mature T-lymphocytes (nude or nu/nu mice), and strains of malaria *(P. yoelii)* and babesia *(B. microti)* producing infections from which intact mice recover, the problem was taken up again (18). Escalating parasitemias were observed in nude mice infected with *P. yoelii*. This parasite preferentially invades reticulocytes; in infected mice, there is a progressive increase in susceptible cells, until the animals all succumb with a parasitemia of 70 to 80%.

Weinbaum et al. (110) showed that in mice made B-cell deficient by neonatal injections of anti-μ serum, infections with the normally avirulent *P. yoelii* produce lethal disease. Again, treatment of the B-cell-deficient mice led to a nonsterilizing protective immunity (96). In contrast, with another murine parasite, *P. chabaudi adami*, infection of B-cell-deficient mice was found to activate a T-cell-dependent immune mechanism, which terminated the malaria in a manner similar to that seen in immunologically intact mice (56). The immunized B-cell-deficient mice were resistant to homologous challenge as well as to infections initiated with *P. vinckei* but not to challenge with *P. yoelii* or *P. berghei*.

These observations emphasize the importance of thymus-dependent, antibody-independent mechanisms of immunity to rechallenge with all species of malaria parasites so far tested and the ability of this mechanism to bring about recovery from *P. chabaudi adami* without chemotherapy. It may be relevant that *P. chabaudi* elicits a powerful, thymus-dependent increase in spleen cell cellularity and nonspecific cytotoxic activity (44) and is also more susceptible than *P. berghei* or *P. yoelii* to inhibition by nonspecific stimulators of immunity (Table 2).

TABLE 2. *Susceptibility of asexual erythrocytic forms of murine hemoprotozoa to nonspecific immunity elicited by C. parvum and other agents, and requirement of antibodies for recovery from primary infections*

Parasite	Susceptibility to nonspecific immunity	Requirement for antibodies
B. microti	+ + +	—
B. rodhaini	+ + +	?
P. chabaudi	+ +	—
P. vinckei	+ +	?
P. yoelii	+	+
P. berghei	+	+

Genetic analysis of resistance to infections is an efficient way of revealing underlying mechanisms. Our investigation began with an analysis of the susceptibility of different mouse strains to *P. chabaudi* and *B. microti* (45). It was found that strain A mice are highly susceptible to both infections; in this strain, *P. chabaudi* is nearly always lethal, and the mice do not recover from *B. microti* infections. Investigations of congenic and other strains suggested that susceptibility does not correlate with H-2 haplotype (Table 3). The F_1 offspring of susceptible A and resistant mice are resistant, and some offspring of back-crosses to the susceptible parental strain are susceptible, suggesting that segregation of a major gene has a marked influence on susceptibility. Strain A as well as ICR mice have also been found defective in their response to nonspecific stimulation of immunity against *P. berghei* by *Mycobacterium tuberculosis* BCG or *Corynebacterium parvum* (83).

Strain A mice have two known defects: (a) the capacity of their activated macrophages to kill tumor target cells is decreased (1); and (b) the capacity of their nonadherent spleen cells, so-called NK cells, to kill tumor or other sensitive cells is also less than that of other strains (59,71). In most strains of mice infected with malaria or babesia parasites, there is a rapid increase in the size and number of spleen cells (about fivefold) and in the capacity of their spleen cells to kill tumor cells, expressed in terms of ratio of splenic leukocytes to target cells (45). Thus the total killing capacity of the spleen, a measure of activation of macrophages and NK cells for this property, is considerably augmented. In contrast, strain A mice show little increase in spleen cell number and weight, and capacity to kill tumor cells is slightly, if at all, increased.

Further genetic studies are required to establish whether the macrophage defect of the NK cell defect in the A strain (if these are separate), or some other defect, is responsible for their susceptibility to malaria. The observations of Eugui and Allison (45), which have just been described, show that during the course of hemoprotozoan infections, there is a rapid increase in the number of mononuclear cells, rising to a peak about the time of maximal parasitemia; thereafter, there is a marked increase in the number of erythropoietic precursors (51). In nu/nu mice infected with *P. chabaudi*, the increase in spleen cells and capacity to kill tumor

TABLE 3. *Differences in the susceptibility of various mouse strains to hemoprotozoan infections*

Mouse strain	Haplotype	Persistent B. microti infection	Lethal P. chabaudi infection
A/J Crc	H-2^a	+	+
B10.A/01a	H-2^a	—	—
CBA/CaCrc	H-2^k	—	—
C57B1/10ScSACrc	H-2^b	—	—
Balb/cCrc	H-2^d	—	—
(B10.AxA)F$_1$	H-2^a	—	—

cells does not occur (45). Hence the recruitment and activation of mononuclear cells in malaria infections are thymus dependent. Immune spleen cells placed in diffusion chambers with parasitized erythrocytes elicit a marked macrophage infiltrate around the chamber (3). Presumably, this is due to the liberation of macrophage chemotactic and immobilizing factors. Wyler and Gallin (113) and Coleman et al. (27) have described the presence in the spleens of mice recovering from malaria of a mononuclear chemotactic factor and macrophage migration inhibition factor, which could explain the accumulation of macrophages in the spleens of infected animals. In vaccinated *P. yoelii*-infected mice, mononuclear cells also accumulate in the liver (37).

These observations suggest that sensitized T-cells, reacting with parasite antigens, recruit and activate macrophages and NK cells. Evidence has accumulated that the latter in turn liberate factors that can inhibit the replication of parasites in circulating erythrocytes, leading to degenerate "crisis forms." Such forms were originally described by Taliaferro and Taliaferro (101) in *Cebus capucinus* monkeys recovering from *P. brasilianum*. In mice recovering from *B. microti* infections, such degenerating parasites are observed within circulating erythrocytes (21,22). Similar degenerating intra-erythrocytic parasites are seen in rats recovering from *P. berghei* infections.

Mice inoculated with live *M. tuberculosis* BCG, killed *C. parvum*, and other stimulators of nonspecific immunity are highly resistant to challenge with *B. microti* or *B. rodhaini* (no parasitemia) and resistant also to the normally lethal *P. vinckei* (19,22). Protection by *C. parvum* is thymus independent, since it occurs in nu/nu mice. Evidently, the effector cells can be activated through T-lymphocytes, as in normal infections, or through a mechanism bypassing T-lymphocytes. The presence of degenerate parasites within circulating erythrocytes shows that immunity is not affected by interfering with parasite entry or erythrophagocytosis, as was formerly thought.

Murine hemoprotozoa can be ranked according to the importance of antibodies in recovery from primary infections on the one hand and their susceptibility to nonspecific immunity on the other hand (Table 2). Whether cellular immune mechanisms are important in human malaria and bovine babesiosis is not known.

Recent evidence suggests that the effectomechanism in cell-mediated immunity may be oxidant effects mediated by macrophages or natural killer cells (4,20). When these effectors are appropriately stimulated (e.g. by attachment to malaria parasitized erythrocytes in the absence or presence of antibodies) they show a respiratory burst, as reflected in luminol-enhanced chemiluminiscence. These may produce oxidant stress on parasitized erythrocytes through reactive intermediates such as redox-active metals. The sensitivity of malaria parasites to oxidant stress is illustrated by the effects of agents such as tertiary butylhydroperoxide, which when injected into mice produce the generation of the parasite within erythrocytes analogous to the "crisis forms" observed during recovery. Erythrocytes infected with *P. falcibarum* adhere to endothelial cells of post-capillary venules, where the parasites complete their asexual cycle of replication in a micro environment where the oxygen tension is low. In this way they are protected against oxidant stress. However, if the erythrocytes contain HbS the parasites replicate suboptimally under such conditions, which account for the protected sex of HbS against malaria.

Erythrocytes from persons with thalassemia and glucose-6-phosphate dehydrogenase deficiency are unusually sensitive to oxidant stress. Acquired immunity would be expected to have synergistic effects with such inherited traits. Our recent demonstration (A. C. Allison, C. Laughton and A. Schreiber) that there are two types of vascular endothelial cells is relevant. What we term type 1 endothelial cells are pavement type cells lining most blood vessels and capillaries. Type 2 endothelial cells are found in post-capillary venules of most tissues and in pulmonary and cerebral capillaries. Other cell types such as leukocytes adhere preferentially to type 2 endothelial cells, especially in sites of information. Type 2 endothelial cells respond to mediators of vascular permeability by losing their flat shape, becoming round, and leaving spaces between them through which macromolecules escape into the extravascular compartments. Presumably the same happens in cerebral malaria: excessive numbers of parasitized erythrocytes adhere to type 2 endothelial cells in cerebral capillaries. We have shown (C. Vigo, A. C. Allison, E. M. Eugui, and K. Murphy) that products of activated human lymphocytes as may occur during malaria infections, elicit the release from human peripheral blood mononuclear cells of acetyl glyceryle ether phosphoryl choline (platelet-activating factor), a powerful edemagenic agent. We postulate that platelet-activating factor and other mediators with similar effects, such as the slow-reacting systems of anathylaxis (leukotriene C4, D4, and E4) mediate the increased cerebral vascular permeability in malaria and African trypanosomiasises.

Clark et al. (23) have shown that mice infected with *P. vinckei petteri* and injected with a small dose of endotoxin release interleukin 1, TNF and type 1 interferon into the serum. Thus malaria infections can sensitize mice to endotoxin in the same way as BCG, *C. parvum*, and zymosan. Clark et al. (23) argue that humans with malaria infections might become sensitized in the same way; the presence in the blood of patients of small amounts of material giving endotoxin-like reactivity in the *Limulus* lysate assay has been reported by Tubbs (104). Whether this material comes from the parasite or the gut of the patients is unknown. Clark et al. (23) suggest that material released from parasitized cells at schizogony triggers the release in hosts sensitized by the infection of such mediators as TNF, interferon, interleukin 1, and GAF. These contribute to the pathophysiology of the disease. For example, TNF inhibits the division of stem cells in the bone marrow.

A relationship between macrophage activation and hypercoagulability has been demonstrated. Human monocytes activated by endotoxin, immune complexes, or products of activated lymphocytes release thromboplastin, which initiates blood coagulation (91). This may be happening in patients with malaria, contributing to a consumptive coagulopathy.

Because lipopolysaccharide endotoxins are specialized products of certain gram-negative bacteria, it is unlikely that chemically homologous molecules are present in protozoa. Nevertheless, other structures (e.g., surface-active complex phosphocarbohydrates) in the parasites may be able to trigger the release of mediators from sensitized macrophages and even show activity in the *Limulus* lysate test. Alternatively, small amounts of lipopolysaccharide released from intestinal bacteria could have dramatic effects in individuals whose macrophages are presensitized by malaria or other infections. Another possibility is that parasite antigens released at the time of schizogony form immune complexes which activate mediator release by macrophages. Some of these mediators may also interfere with parasite growth (97,102).

Escape mechanisms vary from one host-parasite combination to another. Mice that have recovered from *P. chabaudi* are immune to challenge with all strains of *P. chabaudi* or *P. vinckei* infections thus far tested; they are also resistant to challenge with virulent *P. yoellii* (45). In this situation, parasite escape mechanisms are inefficient. In *P. knowlesi* infections of *Macaca mulatta*, classic antigenic variation, demonstrable by the sequential appearance of antibodies agglutinating schizont-infected cells, has been demonstrated (9). Children living in endemic areas have repeated *P. falciparum* infections over several years; this is attributed to the presence of many antigenic variants, the existence of which can be shown by precipitation in gels (112).

CONCLUSIONS

The observations reviewed in this chapter illustrate the multiplicity of immune responses elicited by protozoan parasitic infections and of escape mechanisms from the infections. Nevertheless, in each host-parasite combination, it is likely that one type of immune response plays the major role in host protection, and the parasite has one principal mechanism that allows it to escape (Table 1). Understanding both mechanisms is a key to successful vaccination and is of academic interest. Studies such as those being performed on antigenic variation in African trypanosomes, the use of monoclonal antibodies to identify and isolate protective antigens, and the lysis of *Theileria*-parasitized cells by T-lymphocytes are among the most elegant in contemporary immunobiology. The prospects of producing protective antigens by recombinant DNA technology or synthesizing them are already appearing on the horizon. Parasite immunology has emerged from the stage of descriptive phenomenology to become one of the growing points of biologic science. This basic information on the role of the lymphoid system in host-parasite relationships will lead to a better understanding of protozoan infections and, it is hoped, to their control.

REFERENCES

1. Adams, D. O., Marino, P. A., and Meltzer, M. C. (1981): Characterization of genetic defects in macrophage tumoricidal capacity: Identification of murine strains with abnormalities in secretion of cytolytic factors and ability to bind neoplastic targets. *J. Immunol.*, 126:1843–1847.
2. Adler, S. (1958): The relationship between *Leishmania* sp. and their sandfly vectors. *Rev. Bras. Malariol.*, 8:29–32.
3. Allison, A. C., Christensen, J., Clark, I. A., Elford, B. C., and Eugui, E. M. (1979): The role of the spleen in protection against murine babesia infections. In: *The Role of the Spleen in the Immunology of Parasitic Diseases*, edited by G. Torrigiani, pp. 151–182. Schwabe, Basel.

4. Allison, A. C., Eugui, E. M. (1982): A radical interpretation of immunity to malaria parasites. *Lancet*, 2:1431–1433.

5. Behin, R., Mavel, J., and Rowe, D. S. (1977): Mechanisms of protective immunity in experimental cutaneous leishmaniasis of the guinea pig. III. Inhibition of the leishmanial lesions in the guinea pig by delayed hypersensitivity reaction to unrelated antigens. *Clin. Exp. Immunol.*, 29:320–325.

6. Bradley, D. J., Taylor, B. A., Blackwell, J., Evans, E. P., and Freeman, J. (1979): Regulations of *Leishmania* populations within the host. III. Mapping of the locus controlling susceptibility to visceral leishmaniasis in the mouse. *Clin. Exp. Immunol.*, 37:7–14.

7. Brown, C. G. D., Malmquist, W. A., Cunningham, M. P., Radley, D. E., and Burridge, M. J. (1971): Immunization against East Coast fever: Inoculation of cattle with *Theileria parva* schizonts grown in cell culture. *J. Parasitol.*, 57:59–60.

8. Brown, C. G. D., Stagg, D. A., Purnell, R. E., Kanhai, G. K., and Payne, R. C. (1973): Infection and transformation of bovine cells *in vitro* by infective particles of *Theileria parva*. *Nature*, 245:101–103.

9. Brown, K. N. (1977): Antigenic Variation. In: *Immunity in Parasitic Diseases, Vol. 72*, edited by A. Catran and D. Peary, pp. 59–70. Colloque Inserm, Paris.

10. Brown, I. N., Allison, A. C., and Taylor, R. B. (1968): *Plasmodium berghei* infections in thymectomized rats. *Nature*, 219:292–293.

11. Brown, I. N., and Phillips, R. S. (1974): Immunity to *Plasmodium berghei* in rats: Passive serum transfer and role of the spleen. *Infect. Immun.*, 10:1213–1218.

12. Bryceson, A. D. M., Bray, R. S., and Dumonde, D. C. (1974): Experimental cutaneous leishmaniasis. IV. Selective suppression of cell-mediated immunity during the response of guinea pigs to infections with *Leishmania enriettii*. *Clin. Exp. Immunol.*, 16:189–201.

13. Bryceson, A. D., and Turk, J. L. (1971): The effect of prolonged treatment with antilymphocyte serum on the course of infections with BCG and *Leishmania enriettii* in the guinea pig. *J. Pathol.*, 104:153–165.

14. Burridge, M. J., and Kimber, C. D. (1973): Studies on colostral antibodies to *Theileria parva* using the indirect fluorescent antibody test. *Z. Tropenmed. Parasitol.*, 24:305–308.

15. Burridge, M. J., Morzaria, S. P., Cunningham, M. P., and Brown, C. G. D. (1972): Duration of immunity to East Coast fever (*Theileria parva* infection of cattle). *Parasitology*, 64:511–515.

16. Capbern, A., Giroud, C., Baltz, T., and Mattern, D. (1977): *Trypanosoma equiperdum:* Etude des variations antigeniques au cours de la trypanosomose experimentale du lapin. *Exp. Parasitol.*, 42:6–13.

17. Clark, I. A. (1976): *Immunity to Blood Protozoa of Mice with Special Reference to Babesia spp.* Doctoral dissertation, University of London.

18. Clark, I. A., and Allison, A. C. (1974): *Babesia microti* and *Plasmodium berghei yoelii* infections in nude mice. *Nature*, 252:328–329.

19. Clark, I. A., Allison, A. C., and Cox, F. E. G. (1976): Protection of mice against *Babesia* and *Plasmodium* with BCG. *Nature*, 259:309–311.

20. Clark, I. A., Hunt N. H. (1983): Evidence for reactive oxygen intermediates causing hemolysis and parasite death in malaria. *Infect. Immun.*, 39:1–6.

21. Clark, I. A., Richmond, J. E., Wills, E. J., and Allison, A. C. (1977): Intra-erythrocytic death of the parasite in mice recovering from infections with *Babesia microti*. *Parasitology*, 75:189–196.

22. Clark, I. A., Wills, E. J., Richmond, J. E., and Allison, A. C. (1977): Suppression of babesiosis in BCG-infected mice and its correlation with tumour inhibition. *Infect. Immun.*, 17:430–438.

23. Clark, I. A., Virelizer, J. L., Carswell, E. A., and Wood, P. A. (1981): Possible importance of macrophage-derived mediators in acute malaria. *Infect. Immun.*, 32:1058–1066.

24. Clayton, C. E., Sacks, D. L., Olgivie, B. M., and Askonas, B. E. (1979): Membrane fractions of trypanosomes mimic immunosuppressive and mitogenic effects of living parasites on the host. *Parasite Immunol.*, 1:241–249.

25. Clayton, C. E., Selkirk, M. E., Corsini, A. C., Olgivie, B. M., and Askonas, B. A. (1980): Murine trypanosomiasis: Cellular proliferation and functional depletion in the blood, peritoneum and spleen related to changes in bone marrow stem cells. *Infect. Immun.*, 28:824–831.

26. Cohen, S., McGregor, I. A., and Carrington, S. (1961): Gamma-globulin and acquired immunity to human malaria. *Nature*, 192:733–737.

27. Coleman, R. M., Bruce, A., and Rencricca, N. J. (1976): Malaria: Macrophage migration inhibition factor (MIF). *J. Parasitol.* 62:137–138.

28. Cross, G. A. M. (1975): Identification, purification and properties of clone-specific glycoprotein antigens constituting the surface coat of *Trypanosoma brucei*. *Parasitology*, 71:393–417.

29. Cudkowicz, G., and Hochman, P. S. (1979): Do natural killer cells engage in regulated reactions against self to ensure homeostasis? *Immunol. Rev.*, 44:13–41.

30. Curnow, J. A. (1973): Studies on antigenic changes and strain differences in *Babesia argentina* infections. *Aust. Vet. J.*, 49:279–283.

31. Chang, K. P., and Dwyer, D. M. (1976): Multiplication of a human parasite *(Leishmania donovani)* in phagolysosomes of hamster macrophages in vitro. *Science*, 193:678–680.

32. Chen, D. H., Tigelaar, R. E., and Weinbaum, F. I. (1977): Immunity to sporozoite-induced malaria infection in mice. I. The effect of immunization of T and B cell-deficient mice. *J. Immunol.*, 118:1322–1327.

33. De Kock, G. (1957): Studies on the lesions and pathogenesis of East Coast fever (*Theileria parva* infection) in cattle with special reference to the lymphoid tissue. *Onderstepoort J. Vet. Res.*, 27:431–452.

34. De Martini, J. C., and Moulton, J. E. (1973): Responses of the bovine lymphatic system to infection by *Theileria parva*: I. Histology and ultrastructure of lymph nodes in experimentally infected calves. *J. Comp. Pathol.*, 83:281–298.

35. De Martini, J. C., and Moulton, J. E. (1973): Responses of the bovine lymphatic system to injections by *Theileria parva*: II. Changes in the central lymph in experimentally-infected calves. *J. Comp. Pathol.*, 83:299–306.

36. Diggs, C. L., and Osler, A. G. (1969): Humoral immunity in rodent malaria. II. Inhibitions of parasitemia by serum antibody. *J. Immunol.*, 102:298–306.

37. Dockrell, H. M., de Souza, J. B., and Playfair, J. H. L. (1980): The role of the liver in immunity to blood-stage murine malaria. *Immunology*, 41:421–430.

38. Doyle, J. J., Hirumi, H., Hirumi, K., Lupton, G. N., and Cross, G. A. M. (1980): Antigenic variations in clones of animals infective *Trypanosoma brucei* derived and maintained *in vitro*. *Parasitology*, 80:359–369.

39. Eardley, D. D., and Jayawardena, A. N. (1977): Suppressor cells in mice infected with *T. brucei*. *J. Immunol.*, 119:1029–1033.

40. Emery, D. L. (1981): Adoptive transfer between cattle twins of immunity to infections with *Theileria parva* (East Coast fever). *Res. Vet. Sci.*, 30:364–367.

41. Emery, D. L., Eugui, E. M., Nelson, R. T., and Tenywa, T. (1981): Cell-mediated immune responses to *Theileria parva* (East Coast fever) during immunization and lethal infections in cattle. *Immunology*, 43:323–336.

42. Emery, D. L., Morrison, W. I., Nelson, R. T., and Murray, M. (1981): The induction of cell-mediated immunity in cattle inoculated with cell lines parasitized with *Theileria parva*. In: *Advances in the Control of Theileriosis*, edited by A. D. Irvin, M. P. Cunningham, and A. S. Young, pp. 295–310. Martinus Nijhoff, The Hague.

43. Epstein, M. A., and Achong, B., editors (1979): *The Epstein Barr Virus*. Springer, Berlin.

44. Eugui, E. M., and Allison, A. C. (1979): Malaria infections in different strains of mice and their correlation with natural killer activity. *Bull WHO* [Suppl. 1], 57:231–238.

45. Eugui, E. M., and Allison, A. C. (1980): Differences in susceptibility of various mouse strains to haemoprotozoan infections: Possible correlation with natural killer activity. *Parasite Immunol.*, 2:277–292.

46. Eugui, E. M., and Emery, D. L. (1981): Genetically restricted cell-mediated cytotoxicity in cattle immune to *Theileria parva*. *Nature*, 290:251–254.

47. Eugui, E. M., Emery, D. L., Buscher, G., and Khaukha, G. (1981): Specific and non-specific cellular immune responses to *Theileria parva* in cattle. In: *Advances in the Control of Theileriosis*, edited by A. D. Irvin, M. P. Cunningham, and A. S. Young, pp. 289–294. Martinus Nijhoff, The Hague.

48. Ferrante, A., Hirumi, H., Hirumi, K., and Allison, A. C. (1983): Alternative pathway activation of complement by African trypanosomes lacking a glycoprotein coat. *Parasite Immunol. (in press)*.

49. Ferluga, J., Eugui, E. M., and O'Brien, C. (1981): Lymphocyte stimulatory capacities of various *Theileria parva* isolates; potential immunogenic and suppressive determinants associated with parasite antigens and their relevance to vaccines. In: *Advances in the Control of Theileriosis*, edited by A. D. Irvin, M. P. Cunningham, and A. S. Young, pp. 340–347. Martinus Nijhoff, The Hague.

50. Fisher, A., Durandy, A., and Griscelli, C. (1981): Role of prostaglandin E_2 in the induction of nonspecific T lymphocyte suppressor activity. *J. Immunol.*, 126:1452–1455.
51. Freeman, R. R., and Parish, C. R. (1978): Spleen cell changes during fatal and self-limiting malarial infections of mice. *Immunology*, 35:479–484.
52. Freeman, R. R., Trejdosiewicz, A. J., and Cross, G. A. M. (1980): Protective monoclonal antibodies recognizing stage-specific merozoite antigens of a rodent malaria parasite. *Nature*, 284:366–368.
53. Goodwin, L. G., Green, D. G., Guy, N. W., and Voller, A. (1972): Immunosuppression during trypanosomiasis. *Br. J. Exp. Pathol.*, 53:40–43.
54. Gowans, J. L., and Knight, E. J. (1964): The route of recirculation of lymphocyte in the rat. *Proc. R. Soc. Lond. [Biol.]*, 159:257–282.
55. Grosskinsky, C. M., and Askonas, B. A. (1981): Macrophages as primary target cells and mediators of immune dysfunction in African trypanosomiasis. *Infect. Immun.*, 33:149–155.
56. Grun, J. I., and Weidanz, W. P. (1981): Immunity to *Plasmodium chabaudi adami* in the B cell deficient mouse. *Nature*, 290:143–145.
57. Hajduk, S., Cameron, C., Barry, J. D., and Vickerman, K. (1981): Antigenic variation in cyclically transmitted *Trypanosoma brucei*. Variable antigen type composition of metacyclic trypanosome populations from the salivary gland of *Glossina morsitans*. *Parasitology*, 83:595–622.
58. Hall, W. T. K. (1963): The immunity of calves to tick-transmitted *Babesia argentina* infection. *Aust. Vet. J.*, 39:386–389.
59. Herberman, R. B., Nunn, M. E., and Lavrin, D. H. (1975): Natural cytotoxic reactivity of mouse lymphoid cells against syngeneic and allogeneic tumours. I. Distribution of reactivity and specificity. *Int. J. Cancer*, 16:216–229.
60. Heyneman, D. (1971): Immunology of leishmaniasis. *Bull. WHO*, 44:499–514.
61. Hoeijmakers, J. H. J., Fraseh, A. C. C., Bernards, A., Borst, P., and Cross, G. A. M. (1980): Novel expression linked copies of the genes for variant surface antigens in trypanosomes. *Nature*, 284:78–80.
62. Holder, A. A., and Freeman, R. R. (1981): Immunization against blood-stage rodent malaria using purified parasite antigens. *Nature*, 294:361–364.
63. Howard, J. G., Hale, C., and Liew, W. L. C. (1980): Immunological regulation of experimental cutaneous leishmaniasis: I. Immunogenetic aspects of susceptibility to *Leishmania tropica* in mice. *Parasite Immunol.*, 2:303–314.
64. Howard, J. G., Hale, C., and Liew, F. Y. (1980): Immunological regulation of experimental cutaneous leishmaniasis. III. Nature and significance of specific suppression of cell-mediated immunity in mice highly susceptible to *Leishmania tropica*. *J. Exp. Med.*, 152:594–607.
65. Howard, J. G., Hale, C., and Liew, F. Y. (1981): Immunological regulation of experimental cutaneous leishmaniasis. IV. Prophylactic effect of sublethal irradiation as a result of abrogation of suppressor T-cell generations in mice genetically susceptible to *Leishmania tropica*. *J. Exp. Med.*, 153:557–568.
66. Hudson, K. M., and Terry, R. J. (1979): Immunodepression and the course of infection of a chronic *Trypanosoma brucei* infection in mice. *Parasite Immunol.*, 1:317–326.
67. Hulliger, L., Wilde, J. K. H., Brown, C. G. D., and Turner, L. (1964): Mode of multiplication of Theileria in cultures of bovine lymphocytic cells. *Nature*, 203:728–730.
68. Johnson, J. G., and Cross, G. A. M. (1979): Selective cleavage of variant surface glycoproteins from *Trypanosoma brucei*. *Biochem. J.*, 178:689–697.
69. Johnston, L. A. Y. (1967): Epidemiology of bovine babesiosis in northern Queensland. *Aust. Vet. J.*, 43:427–431.
70. Kadivar, D. M., and Soulsby, E. J. (1975): Model for disseminated cutaneous leishmaniasis. *Science*, 190:1198–1200.
71. Kiessling, R., Petranyi, G., Klein, E., and Wigzell, H. (1975): Genetic variations of *in vitro* cytolytic activity and *in vivo* rejection potential of non-immunized semi-syngeneic mice against a mouse lymphoma line. *Int. J. Cancer*, 15:933–940.
72. Lehmann-Grubbe, F. (1971): *Lymphocytic Choriomeningitis*. Springer-Verlag, Wien.
73. Le Ray, D., Barry, J. D., and Vickerman, K. (1978): Antigenic heterogeneity of metacyclic forms of *Trypanosoma brucei*. *Nature*, 273:300–302.
74. Levine, N. E. (1971): Taxonomy of piroplasm. *Trans. Am. Microsc. Soc.*, 90:2–33.
75. Lewis, D., and Williams, H. (1979): Infection of the Mongolian gerbil with cattle piroplasm *Babesia divergens*. *Nature*, 278:170–171.

76. Louis, J., Moedder, E., Behin, R., and Engers, H. (1979): Recognition of protozoan parasite antigens by murine T-lymphocytes. I. Induction of specific T-lymphocyte-dependent proliferative response to *Leishmania tropica*. *Eur. J. Immunol.*, 9:841–847.

77. Louis, J. A., Moedder, E., Mac Donald, H. R., and Engers, H. D. (1981): Recognition of protozoan parasites by immune T-Lymphocytes. II. Role of the H-2 gene complex in interactions between antigen-presenting macrophages and *Leishmania*-immune T-lymphocytes. *J. Immunol.*, 126:1661–1666.

78. Mahoney, D. F. (1964): Bovine babesiosis: The passive immunizations of calves against *Babesia argentina* with special reference to the role of complement fixing antibodies. *Exp. Parasitol.*, 20:119–124.

79. Mahoney, D. F., Wright, I. G., and Goodger, B. V. (1981): Bovine babesiosis: The immunizations of cattle with fractions of erythrocytes infected with *Babesia bovis* (syn. *B. argentina*). *Vet. Immunol. Immunopathol.*, 2:145–156.

80. Malmquist, W. A., Nyindo, M. B. A., and Brown, C. G. D. (1970): East Coast fever: Cultivation *in vitro* of bovine spleen cell lines infected and transformed by *Theileria parva*. *Trop. Anim. Health Prod.*, 2:139–145.

81. Meltzer, M. S., Ruco, L. P., Boraschi, D., and Nacy, C. A. (1979): Macrophage activation for tumour cytotoxicity: Analysis of intermediary reactions. *J. Reticuloendothel. Soc.*, 26:403–415.

82. Muhammed, S. I., Lauerman, J. H., Jr., and Johnson, L. W. (1975): Effect of humoral antibodies on the course of *Theileria parva* infections (East Coast fever) of cattle. *Am. J. Vet. Res.*, 36:399–402.

83. Murphy, J. R. (1981): Host defenses in murine malaria: Non-specific resistance to *Plasmodium berghei* generated in response to *Mycobacterium bovis* infections or *Coerynebacterium parvum* stimulations. *Infect. Immun.*, 33:199–211.

84. Murray, H. W., Juangbhanich, C. W., Nathan, C. F., and Cohn, Z.A. (1979): Macrophage oxygen-dependent antimicrobial activity. II. The role of oxygen intermediates. *J. Exp. Med.*, 150:950–964.

85. Nacy, C. A., Leonard, E. J., and Meltzer, M. S. (1981): Macrophages in resistance to rickettsial infections: Characterization of lymphokines that induce rickettsiacidal activity in macrophages. *J. Immunol.*, 126:204–207.

86. Nacy, C. A., Meltzer, M. S., Leonard, E. J., and Wyler, D. J. (1983): Intracellular replications and lymphokine-induced destruction of *Leishmania tropica* in C3H/HeN mouse macrophages *J. Immunol. (in press)*.

87. Pays, E., Van Meiervenne, N., Le Ray, D., and Steinert, M. (1981): Gene duplication and transposition linked to antigenic variation in *Trypanosoma brucei*. *Proc. Natl. Acad. Sci. USA*, 78:2673–2677.

88. Pipano, E. (1981): Schizonts and tick stages in immunization against *Theileria annulata* infections. In: *Advances in the Control of Theileriosis*, edited by A. D. Irvin, M. P. Cunningham, and A. S. Young, pp. 242–252. Martinus Nijhoff, The Hague.

89. Plawright, W. (1971): *Rinderpest Virus*. Springer-Verlag, Wien.

90. Preston, P. M., Carter, R. L., Leuchars, E., Davies, A. J. S., and Dumonde, D. C. (1972): Experimental cutaneous leishmaniasis. III. Effects of thymectomy on the course of infection of CBA mice with Leishmania tropica. *Clin. Exp. Immunol.*, 10:337–357.

91. Prydz, H., Lyberg, T., Deteix, P., and Allison, A. C. (1979): *In vitro* stimulation of tissue thromboplastin (fact III) activity in human monocytes by immune complexes and lectins. *Thromb. Res.*, 15:465–474.

92. Quin, T. C., and Wyler, P. J. (1979): Intravascular clearance of parasitized erythrocytes in rodent malaria. *J. Clin. Invest.*, 63:1187–1194.

93. Radley, D. E., Brown, C. G. D., Burridge, M. J., Cunningham, M. P., Kirimi, I. M., Purnell, R. E., and Young, A. S. (1975): East Coast fever: 1. Chamoprophylactic immunization of cattle against *Theileria parva* (Muguga) and five theilerial strains. *Vet. Parasitol.*, 1:35–41.

94. Rager-Zisman, B., and Bloom, B. R. (1983): Natural killer (NK) cells in resistance to virus-infected cells. In: *Seminars in Immunopathology*, edited by G. Klein *(in press)*.

95. Ristic, M., and Lewis, G. E. (1974): Babesia in man and wild laboratory-adapted mammals. In: *Parasitic Protozoa, Vol. II*, edited by J. P. Kreier, pp. 53–75. Academic Press, New York.

96. Roberts, D. W., and Weidanz, W. P. (1979): T-cell immunity to malaria in the B-cell deficient mouse. *Am. J. Trop. Med. Hyg.*, 28:1–3.

97. Rzepczyk, C. M., and Clark, I. A. (1981): Demonstration of a lipopolysaccharide-induced cytostatic effect on malarial parasites. *Infect. Immun.*, 33:343–347.

98. Segal, A. W., and Jones, O. T. G. (1980): The cytochrome *b* component of the microbicidal oxidase system of human neutrophils. In: *Biological and Clinical Aspects of Superoxide Dismutase, Developments in Biochemistry*, edited by W. H. Bannister and J. V. Bannister. pp. 231–241. Elsevier, Amsterdam.

99. Smith, R. D., Carpenter, J., Cabrera, A., Gravely, S. M., Erp, E. E., Osorno, M., and Ristic, M. (1979): Bovine babesiosis: Vaccination against tick-borne challenge exposure with culture-derived *Babesia bovis* immunogens. *Am. J. Vet. Res.*, 40:1678–1682.

100. Svedmyr, E., and Jondal, M. (1975): Cytotoxic effector cells specific for B cell lines transformed by Epstein-Barr virus are present in patients with infectious mononucleosis. *Proc. Natl. Acad. Sci. USA*, 72:1622–1626.

101. Taliaferro, W. H., and Taliaferro, L. G. (1944): The effect of immunity on the asexual reproduction of *Plasmodium brasilianum. J. Infect. Dis.*, 75:1–32.

102. Taverne, J., Dockrell, H. M., and Playfair, J. H. (1981): Endotoxin-induced serum factor kills malarial parasites *in vitro. Infect. Immun.*, 33:83–89.

103. Tetley, L., Vickerman, K., and Moloo, S. K. (1981): Absence of a surface coat from a metacyclic *Trypanosoma vivax*: Possible implications for vaccination against vivax trypanosomiasis. *Trans. R. Soc. Trop. Med. Hyg.*, 75:409–414.

104. Tubbs, H. (1980): Endotoxin in human murine malaria. *Trans. R. Soc. Trop. Med. Hyg.*, 74:121–123.

105. Turk, J. L., and Bryceson, A. D. (1971): Immunological phenomena in leprosy and related diseases. *Adv. Immunol.*, 13:209–266.

106. Tsur, I., and Adler, S. (1962): Cultivation of *Theileria annulata* schizonts in monolayer tissue cultures. *Ref. Vet.*, 19:224–225.

107. Urquhart, G. M., Jarrett, W. F. H., and Mulligan, W. (1962): Helminth immunity. *Adv. Vet. Sci.*, 7:87–129.

108. Van Meiervenne, N., Janssens, P. G., and Magnus, E. (1975): Antigenic variations in syringe passaged populations of *Trypanosoma (Trypanozoon) brucei*. Rationalization of the experimental approach. *Ann. Soc. Belg. Med. Trop.*, 55:1–23.

109. Vickerman, K. (1969): On the surface coat and flagellar adhesions in trypanosomes. *J. Cell Sci.*, 5:163–193.

110. Weinbaum, F. I., Evans, C. B., and Tigelaar, R. E. (1976): Immunity to *Plasmodium berghei yoelii* in mice. I. The course of infection in T-cell and B-cell deficient mice. *J. Immunol.*, 117:1999–2005.

111. Williams, R. O., Young, J. R., and Majina, P. A. O. (1979): Genomic rearrangements correlated with antigenic variations in *Trypanosoma brucei. Nature*, 282:847–849.

112. Wilson, R. J. M. (1977): Circulating antigens of parasites. In: *Immunity in Parasitic Diseases, Vol. 72*, edited by A. Cafran and D. Peary, Colloque Inserm, Paris.

113. Wyler, D. J., and Gallin, J. J. (1977): Spleen derived mononuclear cells chemotactic factor in malaria infections: A possible mechanism for splenic macrophage accumulation. *J. Immunol.*, 118:478–484.

114. Wyler, D. J., Weinbaum, F. I., and Herrod, H. R. (1979): Characterization of *in vitro* proliferative responses of human lymphocytes to leishmanial antigens. *J. Infect. Dis.*, 140:215–221.

115. Young, A. S. (1981): The epidemiology of Theileriosis in East Africa. In: *Advances in the Control of Theileriosis*, edited by A. D. Irvin, M. P. Cunningham, and A. S. Young, pp. 38–55. Martinus Nijhoff, The Hague.

116. Yoshida, N., Nussenzweig, R. S., Potocnjak, R., Nussenzweig, V., and Aikawa, M. (1980): Hybridoma produces protective antibodies directed against the sporozoite stage of malaria parasite. *Science*, 207:71–73.

117. Zinkernagel, R. M. (1979): Review: Cellular immune responses to intracellular parasites: Role of the major histocompatibility gene complex and thymus in determining immune responsiveness and susceptibility to disease. *Parasite Immunol.*, 1:91–109

Advances in Host Defense Mechanisms, Vol. 2,
edited by John I. Gallin and Anthony S. Fauci.
Raven Press, New York © 1983.

The Lymphoid System in Infections with Mycobacteria

Ward E. Bullock, Jr.

Division of Infectious Diseases, Department of Internal Medicine, University of Cincinnati College of Medicine, Cincinnati, Ohio 45267

> *Lymphocytes are ordinarily found, often in large numbers, in subacute and chronic inflammatory lesions produced by tubercle bacilli and by other bacteria and irritants, but we have no definite information as to what they are doing there......Congregated often in the more peripheral parts of the lesion, they have the appearance of phlegmatic spectators passively watching the turbulent activities of the phagocytes.*
>
> *Arnold Rich, 1951 (133)*

It can be argued that the science of cellular immunology was ushered in by the classic experiments in which it was shown that delayed-type hypersensitivity (DTH) to simple chemicals and to tuberculin could be transferred to normal animals with cells from the peritoneal exudates of hypersensitive donors (32,86). Historically, the impetus to perform these experiments had been provided, in part, by many previous descriptions of the inflammatory responses evoked in mammalian tissues by tubercle bacilli that could not be transferred to naive recipients by serum. Thus about 17 years prior to discovery of *Mycobacterium tuberculosis*, Virchow (157) commented that nodular tubercles appeared to be made up of a mass of small round cells with their nuclei extending almost to the periphery, as in the case of lymphoid cells of the glands or spleen. In fact, he even regarded the tubercule as a lymphoid follicle, "a lymphoma" that evolved in different forms, sometimes ending in caseation, at other times ending in calcification, fibrosis, or complete resorption. Later, Borrel (16,17) performed careful histopathologic studies on rabbits experimentally infected with tuberculosis and observed that the "tuberculous cell is always a lymphoid cell" and was not derived "in one instance from a lung cell, again from a liver cell or still again from a kidney cell."

In 1891, Koch (83) described the general and focal reactions induced by inoculation of old tuberculin (OT) into the skin of guinea pigs previously infected with *M. tuberculosis*. Although the hope for the clinical use of this material as specific therapy for tuberculosis was never realized, OT and the later semipurified protein derivative (PPD) proved to be valuable reagents for both the diagnosis of tuberculosis and experimental studies of DTH. Using these antigens, Zinsser (168) first clearly differentiated the characteristics of immunologic responses into immediate-type reactions that were antibody or reagin-mediated and those that were of the tuberculin-DTH type.

Zinsser's observation catalyzed many investigations that provided detailed histologic descriptions of the DTH reaction to tuberculin in the skin and lungs of animals experimentally infected with *M-tuberculosis*. Dienes and Mallory (44), in 1932, clearly demonstrated that "a wandering cell infiltration predominately mononuclear in character occurs" in tuberculin reactions of mild to moderate intensity. This observation was confirmed by others, including Martins and Raffel (97), who semiquantitated the relative percentages of various cell populations in the tuberculin reaction sites of guinea pigs at serial intervals after immunization with a heat-killed preparation of Bacillus Calmette-Guérin (BCG) vaccine. Polymorphonuclear leukocytes are the first major elements of the cellular infiltrate to appear during the initial 12-hr of a tuberculin reaction; however, they decline rapidly in number thereafter. After the first 12 hr, large mononuclear cells and lymphocytes become a major component of the DTH lesion, as shown in Fig. 1. Lymphocytes number about 10% of the total mononuclear cell population at 4 hr after OT challenge; at 24 hr, they comprise approximately 30 to 40% of the mononuclear cells present. Even at 6 or 7 days, 10 to 20% of the total cell population are lymphocytes.

A similar shift in cell populations occurs if the lungs of animals sensitized to mycobacterial antigens by a primary immunizing infection are exposed to reinfec-

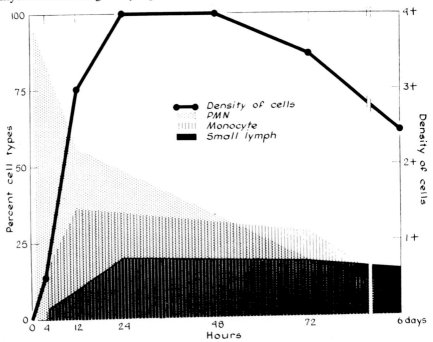

FIG. 1. Relative populations of cells in tuberculin reaction sites at various intervals after tests with tuberculoprotein. (Reprinted from ref. 97 with permission of the publishers.)

tion. Within the lung lesions, there is an initial polymorphonuclear response followed in a few hours by lymphocytic infiltration of the alveolar septa (58,76). Likewise, inhalation of PPD by guinea pigs previously immunized with killed tubercle bacilli induces dominant infiltration of polymorphonuclear cells into the alveolar septa at 3 to 6 hr after exposure. After 24 hr, large numbers of mononuclear cells and lymphocytes appear in the peribronchial and perivascular areas and in alveolar septa (107).

During the early 1960s, the concept began to emerge that DTH may be an immunologic effector mechanism associated closely with acquired resistance to infection that is mediated by lymphoid cells in conjunction with monocytic cells. For example, Lurie (94), after extensive studies on the mechanism of immunity to tuberculosis in rabbits, concluded that "the significant factor in the response to the antigen of the host delayed hypersensitivity is apparently, the marked accentuation of the multiplication and mobilization of the mononuclear phagocytes with enhanced physiological properties." However, it remained for Mackaness (95) and his group to establish the critical link between DTH and cell-mediated immunity (CMI), which, for the purpose of this discussion, may be defined as the acquired enhancement of resistance to infection caused by living microorganisms of the obligate or facultative intracellular type.

In a classic series of experiments, these workers demonstrated conclusively that immunologically committed lymphocytes provide the directive forces which bring mononuclear phagocytic cells to an infected focus and stimulate them to increased microbicidal function. Thus in mice infected with either *Listeria monocytogenes* or BCG, there arises a population of immunologically committed lymphocytes that have the capacity to confer protection as well as a proportionate level of DTH upon normal recipients. The CMI conferred upon recipients results from a specific interaction between the immune lymphoid cells and *L. monocytogenes* or BCG organisms, respectively. This specific interaction in turn leads to a nonspecific activation of host macrophages, as determined by an increased level of microbicidal function (12,95). Since cells from the peritoneal cavity of an animal that received sensitized cells and bacteria by intravenous injection also demonstrated increased microbicidal activity, it was postulated that the peritoneal macrophages must have been activated by soluble products released as a result of the interaction between sensitized lymphocytes and specific antigen.

The assumption by Blanden et al. (12) that molecular mediators of CMI and DTH were operative in their model system was based on an already established body of evidence for the existence of such mediators *in vitro*. Rich and Lewis (134) had observed in 1932 that the migration of cells from splenic explants of tuberculous guinea pigs was inhibited specifically by addition of antigen to the culture medium. More than 30 years later, Bloom and Bennett (13) separated lymphocytes and macrophages from peritoneal exudates induced in tuberculin-sensitized guinea pigs and tested them in a simpler cell migration system developed by George and Vaughan (59). The lymphocytes proved to be the immunologically active cells *in vitro*, whereas the macrophages (through changes in motility) were shown to be the indicator cells. Moreover, Bloom and Bennett (13) and David (41) demonstrated concurrently that if the sensitized peritoneal lymphocytes were interacted *in vitro* with a specific antigen, the cells elaborated a nondialyzable, soluble material that itself was capable of inhibiting the migration of normal exudate cells. This soluble mediator with immunologic activity, so-called migratory inhibitory factor (MIF), was the first of many nonantibody mediators (lymphokines) that have been identified in the culture supernatants of lymphocytes activated by specific antigens, mitogens, or antigen-antibody complexes and presumed to play a role in the *in vivo* phenomena of both DTH and CMI (42).

LYMPHOID CELLS IN DTH LESIONS OF THE SKIN INDUCED BY *MYCOBACTERIA*

The importance of lymphocytes in mediating DTH or cellular resistance to infection with *Mycobacteria* is argued persuasively by *in vitro* studies and by adoptive transfer of protection against a challenge infection. The actual mechanisms by which lymphocytes interact with other cells to resist infection by *Mycobacteria*, however, are understood poorly because the tissue inflammatory response mounted against these organisms is quite complex. Therefore, it is not surprising that more is known concerning the kinetics of cells within the local site of a DTH response to mycobacterial antigens. An important discovery to come from studies of the cellular dynamics within tuberculin-type DTH reactions was that specifically sensitized lymphocytes must interact with cells of the monocyte-macrophage lineage in order for a DTH or CMI response to develop. If the rapidly multiplying precursors of monocytes in the bone marrow are depleted by exposure of experimental animals to sublethal X-irradiation, the irradiated animals can no longer be adoptively sensitized by transfer of lymphocytes from immunized donors (33). On the other hand, if irradiated animals are injected with bone marrow cells from an unimmunized donor and then given specifically sensitized lymphocytes from immunized donors, they regain the ability to express DTH to specific antigenic challenge (93).

Since it was soon recognized that the macrophages are stimulated nonspecifically to antimicrobial activity by specifically sensitized lymphocytes, a considerable effort has been spent in attempting to demonstrate localization of lymphocytes within the site of a tuberculin-type DTH reaction of animals infused intravenously with cells from sensitized donors. Several groups have demonstrated that radioisotopically labeled lymphocytes from tuberculin-sensitized donors do take part in the dermal reaction to tuberculin by recipients of these cells. The donor lymphocytes, however, make relatively little contribution to the cellular infiltrate at the skin test site, since more than 90% of the cells infiltrating the lesion after passive transfer originate in the recipient (99).

Whether the donor cells that accumulate within a tuberculin-skin lesion are those specifically sensitized to the antigen is still a matter of debate. Najarian and Feldman (110) injected guinea pigs with lymphoid cells that had been sensitized to tubercle bacilli and with cells sensitized by skin application of dinitrofluorobenzene (DNFB).

In each transfer experiment, either the tuberculin-sensitized cells or the DNFB-sensitized cells were previously labeled with ³H-thymidine. Immediately after transfusion, the recipients were skin tested with PPD and DNFB. When ³H-thymidine-labeled cells from tuberculin-positive donors were infused along with unlabeled DNFB cells, the total radioactivity recovered per lesion and the concentration of isotope were significantly greater in the PPD lesion than in the DNFB lesion when measured 24 hr after skin testing. The population of labeled cells in the infiltrates ranged from 0.5 to 2.5% of the total cells infiltrating the PPD test site.

In contrast to these findings, other investigators have not been able to demonstrate specific accumulation of radiolabeled cells in DTH lesions with any degree of consistency (79,151). Turk and Oort (153) sought to avoid the nonspecific inflammatory response that occurs during later phases of a tuberculin reaction (i.e., 24 to 48 hr) by careful studies of the early phase of skin test reactivity in guinea pigs sensitized to tuberculin by lymphocyte transfer. Four to 6 hr after skin testing, no significant difference was found in the number of labeled donor cells arriving at the PPD test site and a control site, respectively. It should be pointed out that most studies of this type fail to control for the fact that not all of the isotopically labeled cells infused into recipients are antigen-specific cells.

Notwithstanding the problems associated with attempts to demonstrate selective localization of antigen-specific cells, it is clear that specifically sensitized cells of donor origin do react with antigen at the test site where they serve to trigger the local immune response. That the cells reactive in a tuberculin-DTH lesion are thymus-dependent (T) lymphocytes has been demonstrated in experiments typified by those of Williams and Waksman (162), in which young adult rats were thymectomized, X-irradiated, and injected with bone marrow cells. These animals could not be sensitized to tuberculin by immunization with Freund's adjuvant, and few lymphoid cells could be found at the PPD-skin test site. In contrast, if thymectomized rats were engrafted with hybrid thymuses and then sensitized with Freund's adjuvant, the PPD test was positive, and a substantial proportion (up to 20%) of hybrid thymus-derived cells were found at the test site. Additional evidence that the lymphocytes active in mediating tuberculin type reactions are T cells has been provided by studies in which T lymphocytes within the cell populations of the spleen or lymph nodes from tuberculin-sensitized animals were lysed by treatment with anti-Thy 1.2 and complement. Cells so treated were unable to transfer tuberculin sensitivity to naive recipients (89).

In vitro tests also have been employed to assay the responses to tuberculin by lymphoid cells from humans and animals infected with *Mycobacteria*. Pearmain and co-workers (124) showed that the peripheral blood mononuclear (PBM) cells from Mantoux-positive individuals who had recovered from tuberculosis responded to incubation with PPD *in vitro* by an increase in mitotic activity. Mitoses were absent in the cells from normal subjects who were Mantoux-negative.

Subsequently, Oppenheim (120) employed lymph node cells from guinea pigs sensitized by footpad injection with Freund's adjuvant to demonstrate that the cells responding to tuberculin *in vitro* indeed were lymphocytes. More recently, the association between protective immunity, DTH, and the *in vitro* lymphocyte blastogenic response has been studied during the course of BCG infection after footpad injection of mice (123). Positive responses to the immunizing infection were observed by all three measurements. Blastogenic responses to PPD by lymph node cells draining from the infected footpad peaked from 2 to 4 weeks after infection. Likewise, acquisition of the ability to express DTH to PPD coincided with the emergence of cells capable of responding *in vitro*. On the other hand, lymphocytes capable of conferring antibacterial immunity reached peak activity at a later state (8 weeks) and persisted for at least 3 months. On the basis of these and other studies, it was concluded that a population of large lymphocytes with short lifespan were the predominant cells during the inductive phase of immunity, whereas recirculating, long-lived, small lymphocytes conferred protection during later phases of the immune response.

CELL-MEDIATED IMMUNE REACTIONS TO *MYCOBACTERIA* IN THE LUNG

Since the lung is the major target organ for both primary tuberculous infection and endogenous reactivation of infection, many investigators have studied the pulmonary and local immune responses to infection or immunization by *Mycobacteria*. In 1967, Barclay et al. (9) noted that large numbers of lymphocytes were found in the lungs of mice after immunization by intravenous injection of BCG cell walls in oil. The functional immunologic properties of these cells were further studied by Yamamoto et al. (164), who demonstrated that lymphocytes in the lungs of mice inoculated intravenously with viable BCG 5 weeks previously produced MIF when exposed to PPD *in vitro*. Moreover, the capacity of BCG-immunized mice to resist airborne challenge with viable H37Rv strain of *M. tuberculosis* correlated directly with the degree of MIF activity expressed by the pulmonary lymphocytes. In concurrent studies, Galindo and Myrvik (57) obtained similar results after intravenous injection of rabbits with BCG cell walls in oil. If cell walls or viable BCG were injected locally into the footpad, however, neither preparation was capable of inducing protection against aerosol challenge with H37Rv or of sensitizing pulmonary lymphocytes for MIF production when exposed to PPD *in vitro*.

These results suggested possible compartmentalization of antituberculous immunity, an issue that was explored further by Spencer et al. (145), who immunized guinea pigs via the upper respiratory tract by intranasal installation of viable BCG or H37Rv *M. tuberculosis*. Three weeks later, cells were obtained from the lower respiratory tract by bronchial lavage and tested for the capacity to produce MIF in the presence of specific antigen. MIF production by these cells in response to PPD was significantly higher than that of pulmonary cells from animals which had been immunized by the subcutaneous route only. Conversely, animals immunized by the subcutaneous route developed greater systemic immunity than did those receiving respiratory tract immunization. Thus there appeared to be compartmentalization of the immune response within the lung. The compartmentalization was not absolute, however, and could be overcome partially by delivering higher doses of the immunogen to the lung or to a local subcutaneous site, respectively.

The issue of specificity in the pulmonary granulomatous response to infection with *Mycobacteria* has been addressed by Moore et al. (108). If animals previously injected intravenously with BCG in oil were reinjected with BCG in saline by the same route several weeks later, the pulmonary granulomatous response after the second injection was accelerated greatly. After reinjection, a maximum granulomatous response developed within 4 days, whereas 2 to 4 weeks were required for full development after primary injection. On the other hand, if animals primed by intravenous injection of BCG were then challenged by another granulomogenic organism that did not cross react with BCG (as, for example, *Corynebacterium granulosoum*), an accelerated pulmonary granulomatous response could not be elicited. Pulmonary lavage cells from BCG-sensitized animals failed to produce MIF when exposed to the antigens of *C. granulosoum in vitro* but were triggered to MIF production by PPD stimulation.

Additional evidence that the granulomatous inflammatory responses to mycobacterial antigens within the lung exhibit specificity is derived from experiments in which bentonite particles were coated with soluble antigens and embolized to the lungs of mice previously infected intraperitoneally with *M. tuberculosis* (15). If the bentonite particles were coated with soluble antigens of *M. tuberculosis*, the granulomas that formed around the pulmonary emboli were significantly larger in previously infected mice than those induced by embolization of antigen-coated or uncoated bentonite particles to the lungs of normal control mice. Likewise, particles coated with heterologous antigens prepared from *Histoplasma capsulatum* or *Schistosoma mansoni* failed to induce formation of granulomas larger than controls in tuberculous animals. Enhanced hypersensitivity-type granuloma formation also could be transferred to naive recipients by spleen and lymph node cells from infected donors.

PPD not only triggers MIF production by pulmonary lymphoid cells from animals infected with or sensitized to *M. tuberculosis* but also appears to induce the release of other lymphokines. The best described of these soluble mediators is a factor that is elaborated from cells obtained by bronchial lavage from the lungs of rabbits sensitized by intravenous injection of heat-killed *M. tuberculosis* H37Rv in oil. Supernatants obtained from sensitized alveolar cells incubated with H37Rv or PPD induce fusion of macrophages into giant cells when incubated with nonsensitized alveolar macrophages (55). The macrophage fusion phenomenon appears to be specifically mediated by an immunologic mechanism, since it cannot be elicited with a noncross-reacting antigen. Indirect evidence that the alveolar cells which produce the macrophage-fusion factor are lymphocytes has been provided by experiments in which cell-free supernatant fluids were prepared from BCG-sensitized lymph node cells after incubation with heat-killed BCG. Supernatants from the sensitized lymph node cells, but not control supernatants, induced extensive giant cell formation when incubated with normal alveolar macrophages (56).

In recent studies of the pulmonary immune responses to mycobacterial antigens, Masih et al. (98) have been able to detect MIF-like activity directly within extracts of tissues from guinea pig lungs containing immune granulomas. To produce MIF-containing immune granulomas in the lung, guinea pigs were immunized intravenously with complete Freund's adjuvant and challenged intravenously 5 days later with BCG. MIF activity appeared within the pulmonary granulomas as early as 24 hr after BCG challenge and remained detectable through day 5. As shown in Fig. 2, the lung extracts contained MIF at an early stage of granuloma formation, whereas MIF activity generally could not be measured in extracts from lungs containing mature granulomas that were more than 6 days old. Although these results do not prove that the MIF production actually caused formation of immune granulomas, the fact that MIF was present only during early stages of the granulomatous inflammation suggests that it did enhance the development of granulomas.

At present, little is known concerning the actual identity and functions of the lymphocyte subpopulations that participate in the granulomatous inflammatory response to mycobacterial infection in animals or humans. However, several recent technologic advances will greatly facilitate studies in this area. These advances include (a) the development of fiberoptic bronchoscopy to permit safe collection of alveolar cells from humans by bronchoalveolar lavage, (b) the development of fluorescence microfluorometry and cell-sorting techniques (104), (c) the successful production in mice of alloantibodies to T lymphocyte surface antigens that permit differentiation of cells into various functional subsets (31) and (d) the application of hybridoma technology for the production of monoclonal antibody reagents (84).

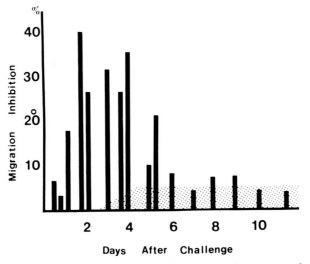

FIG. 2. MIF activity detected in lung extracts obtained at various stages of granulomatous lesions. *Bars,* MIF activity in percent migration inhibition; *dotted area,* approximate histologic development of pulmonary granulomas. (Reprinted from ref. 98 with permission of the publishers.)

By means of the latter technology, exquisitely specific antibodies have been developed that recognize surface antigens on human T cells that correlate with specific functional properties. For example, T cells bearing the so-called T4 or Leu 3a surface antigens, respectively, exert helper activity, whereas cells bearing the T8 or Leu 2a antigen mediate suppressor and cytotoxic activities (88,130).

Application of these technologies has yielded considerable information regarding the lymphoid cell composition of pulmonary granulomas in human sarcoidosis. The percentages of total lymphocytes and T cells in the bronchoalveolar lavage fluid of patients with active sarcoidosis are significantly higher than in the lavage from normal individuals or patients with inactive sarcoidosis (74). More specifically, the T lymphocyte population harvested from the bronchoalveolar lavage fluid of patients with active sarcoidosis contains a higher percentage of the T4$^+$ subset that mediates helper cell activity than do normal lavage fluids. Of considerable interest is the recent observation that the T cells in bronchoalveolar lavage fluids, but not T cells in the peripheral blood of patients with sarcoidosis, secrete a monocyte chemotactic factor that may play a role in the granuloma formation characteristic of this disease (73). As yet, few studies have been published on the cellular composition of lavage fluid from patients with active mycobacterial infections of the lung. Based on extremely limited evidence, it appears that the number of T lymphocytes in lavage fluids from patients with active tuberculosis is increased relative to the number present in lavage from patients with inactive disease (116).

IMMUNE RESPONSES TO MYCOBACTERIA IN T LYMPHOCYTE-DEPLETED ANIMALS

As mentioned previously, it is extraordinarily difficult to investigate the immune functions of lymphoid cells directly within the highly complex microenvironment of granulomas. For these reasons, some investigators have employed T cell-deficient animals to study the course of mycobacterial infections. A prototype of these investigations is the work of Takeya et al. (147), who followed the course of experimental mycobacterial infections in neonatally thymectomized mice. After 4 to 7 weeks of sublethal infection with human tubercle bacilli, the number of culturable *M. tuberculosis* recoverable from the lung, liver, and spleen was much greater in T cell-deficient animals than in thymus-bearing controls. Mice of the thymectomized group also died with tuberculosis much more rapidly than did sham-thymectomized animals. Histologic examination revealed that the granulomatous lesions of T cell-deficient mice were infiltrated primarily by neutrophils and that epithelioid cell formation was minimal, whereas epithelioid cells were well developed in the control group.

The BCG strain of *M. bovis* produces a self-limiting systemic infection in normal mice that is associated with development of tuberculin hypersensitivity and anti-tuberculous immunity. In contrast, BCG infection of congenitally athymic (nude) or neonatally thymectomized mice results in a progressive, systemic infection that is fatal for most animals within 60 days (34,140). Infected thymectomized mice fail to develop detectable tuberculin hypersensitivity, and the pulmonary granulomas do not resolve. On histologic examination, the granulomas contain large numbers of macrophages, many of which are foamy in appearance; few lymphocytes can be seen. Conversely, the granulomas of normal control mice contain large numbers of lymphocytes and far fewer bacilli.

Mycobacteria of low virulence, such as *M. marinum* and *M. leprae*, undergo limited multiplication at the local site of inoculation in experimental animals. Therefore, systemic disease never occurs in rodents after footpad inoculation with *M. leprae* and only to a limited degree after inoculation with *M. marinum*. In congenitally athymic mice, however, multiplication of both *M. leprae* and *M. avium* is approximately 100-fold greater within the footpad than in control animals. Moreover, between 10^5 and 10^6 viable colony-forming units can be recovered from the spleens and livers of the T cell-deficient animals with *M. avium* infection (35,36). The failure of these nonvirulent *Mycobacteria* to achieve more extensive multiplication systemically has been attributed to nonspecific activation of macrophage activity during the course of infection in nude mice and to stimulation of residual T cells in thymectomized animals. If thymectomized mice are given an intraperitoneal injection of 10^8 thymocytes 1 hr before infecting them with *M. tuberculosis*, their capacity to generate antituberculous immunity is largely restored, presumably by provision of T cells capable of activating macrophages in response to the mycobacterial infection (118,119).

LYMPHOCYTE RECIRCULATION: ITS SIGNIFICANCE IN MYCOBACTERIAL INFECTIONS

The Nature of Lymphocyte Recirculation

In an elegant series of experiments, Gowans (65) and co-workers established conclusively that in most mammals, a large pool of cells comprised mostly of T lymphocytes is exchanged constantly between the peripheral blood and lymphoid organs. Recirculation of lymphocytes takes place within both the lymph nodes (including the gut-associated lymphoid tissue) and the spleen. In lymph nodes, lymphocytes traffic from blood to the paracortical regions of the nodes by migration through the specialized cuboidal endothelial cells of the postcapillary venules. Lymphocytes migrate through the nodes to the medullary region and return to blood via the efferent lymphatics and major lymphatic ducts (66). Migration within the spleen is less well defined but appears to take place in the marginal zone of the white pulp areas (i.e., Malphigian corpuscles) via marginal zone-bridging channels (106). The flux of lymphocytes through the lymphoid organs is enormous since it is estimated that, in the rat, about one-half of the small lymphocytes belong to the recirculating pool. These cells migrate through lymph nodes with a modal transit time of 12 to 18 hr and through the spleen with a transit time of 5 to 6 hr (52).

It is now clear that this massive recirculation of cells provides a highly efficient mechanism whereby the small populations of immunocompetent lymphocytes responsive to any given antigen in a nonimmune animal (approximately 1 in 10^5 to 10^6 cells) can be delivered to sites of primary antigenic stimulation within the lymphoid organs in order to initiate and amplify a primary immune response. Likewise, lymphocyte recirculation appears to be responsible for disseminating immunologic memory from the sites of immune responses to other tissues. That cells specifically sensitized to mycobacterial antigens are in fact present within the thoracic duct lymph was first demonstrated by Wesslén (161) who achieved passive transfer of tuberculin DTH to rabbits by local injection of thoracic duct lymphocytes from animals infected 3 to 8 weeks previously with *M. tuberculosis*. Several years later, it was shown that after immunization of rats by BCG infection, populations of lymphocytes specifically sensitized to mycobacterial antigens are delivered to the thoracic duct. Among these cells are long-lived recirculating T lymphocytes that confer a high level of immunity to challenge with virulent *M. tuberculosis* when transferred to a control (90).

Induction of Lymphocyte Trapping in Lymphoid Organs by Mycobacterial Antigens

Not only is it important that immunocompetent cells recirculate extensively through lymphoid organs but, in addition, there must be local retention of these cells if an effective immune response is to be initiated. In fact, injection of a variety of antigenic materials into the drainage area of a lymph node is followed almost immediately by a rapid and substantial fall in the rate at which lymphocytes exit from the node in the efferent lymph (68). The entrapment of recirculating cells lasts for only a few hours. After injection of large doses of antigen into an animal with established delayed hypersensitivity, however, sufficient compartmentalization of the recirculating cells may take place within the lymphoid organs to render the animal unreactive to intradermal antigenic challenge for a period up to 3 days (139). Even longer periods of lymphocyte trapping activity have been observed in some cases. For example, intravenous or subcutaneous injection of mice with viable BCG induces nonspecific trapping of ^{51}Cr-labeled syngeneic lymphocytes in the spleen and draining lymph nodes that persists for 3 weeks or more (165).

The cellular mechanism responsible for the maintenance of the prolonged trapping activity after BCG has not been resolved. Some studies suggest that the trapping phenomenon, especially in lymph nodes, is largely T cell dependent (166); others indicate that activated macrophages may play a central role in prolonged lymphocyte trapping by the spleen and lymph nodes after injection of BCG and certain other adjuvants (53). In the latter studies, selective depletion of B or T lymphocyte populations, as well as nonspecific ablation of lymphocytes by lethal total body X-irradiation, did not reduce trapping. Moreover, nonspecific trapping activity could be induced in lymphoid organs by injection of particulate or high molecular weight substances, regardless of their immunogenicity. This finding also suggests that trapping may be in part a macrophage-dependent phenomenon.

Recent work by Hopkins et al. (72) has demonstrated that in sheep previously sensitized by intramuscular injection of BCG, there is a specific selection of tuberculin-reactive lymphocytes into antigenically stimulated lymph nodes. If the efferent lymphatic from a popliteal lymph node was cannulated, and the cannulated node subsequently challenged repeatedly by injection of PPD into its local drainage site, the response of the drained cells to PPD *in vitro* was eliminated gradually. Skin sensitivity to PPD also was lost in cannulated animals; however, the capacity of the sheep to respond to other antigens to which they had been sensitized remained unimpaired. Control experiments showed that no depletion of the response to PPD occurred in cannulated sheep if the antigen was delivered to a noncannulated node.

The Flux of Recirculating Lymphocytes in Local Granulomas

In contrast to the extensive trafficking of lymphocytes into lymphoid organs, only occasional lymphocytes escape from blood vessels into normal, nonlymphoid tissues. Therefore, major changes must take place within the microenvironment of lesions induced by *Mycobacteria* to permit greater egress of immunocompetent cells from the vasculature if the host is to be successful in limiting the multiplication of organisms by mounting a granulomatous inflammatory response. Support for this assumption has been provided by Smith et al. (143), who established chronic granulomas in the hind limbs of sheep by subcutaneous injection of Freund's adjuvant. As a single lesion developed, the cell output in the afferent lymph draining this lesion increased until a maximum cell output was reached over a period of 2 to 4 weeks that was comparable to the output from a 1 g lymph node. Histologic examination of the lesion revealed numerous small blood capillaries and venules, many of which had high endothelial lining cells similar to those present in the postcapillary venules of lymph nodes. Furthermore, lymphocytes could be identified in all stages of passage across the walls of these small vessels (117,143).

In other experiments of this type, it has been shown that if cells in the afferent lymph from a granuloma that had not passed through a lymph node were radiolabeled with [111]indium and reinjected intravenously, they migrated from blood through the granuloma and back into afferent lymph in large numbers (75). In fact, the modal transit time of labeled cells through a granuloma was about the same as that for a lymph node. If radiolabeled afferent lymph cells from a granuloma were injected intravenously, the specific activity appearing in afferent lymph was five times higher than in the efferent lymph from a normal lymph node not located in the drainage pathway of the granulomatous lesion. Conversely, if efferent cells from the normal node were radiolabeled and injected intravenously, the specific activity appearing in afferent lymph draining the granuloma was one-half that in efferent lymph from the normal node. Since cells from afferent lymphatics also migrated through normal lymph nodes into efferent lymph, at least some labeled afferent cells were considered to be recirculating lymphocytes.

Although there is increasing evidence for selective recruitment of specifically sensitized recirculating lymphocytes into antigen-bearing lymph nodes and subcutaneous granulomas, little is known concerning the recruitment of specifically sensitized cells to sites of actual infection by *Mycobacteria*, as in the lesions of pulmonary tuberculosis (132). Fortunately, the paucity of information in this area is likely to be corrected in the near future, since models are available that can be applied to the study of lymphocyte kinetics in experimental pulmonary infection by *Mycobacteria*. For example, Lipscomb et al. (92) have reported that after intratracheal inoculation of influenza virus into guinea pigs, specific T lymphocytes sensitized to influenza antigens appeared in the lung, coincident with the development of immunity in the hilar lymph nodes and systemic lymphoid tissues. In adoptive transfer experiments, intratracheal inoculation of influenza into nonimmune guinea pigs, followed immediately by intravenous injection of a mixture of ^{3}H-thymidine-labeled syngeneic T-lymphocytes specific for influenza virus and ^{14}C-thymidine-labeled cells specific for an unrelated antigen, resulted in the selective accumulation of virus-specific T cells in the lung. Thus selective recruitment of circulating immune cells by localizing antigen is likely to be one of the mechanisms by which effector cells are provided to mediate immune inflammatory reaction in the lung.

Disturbances of Lymphocyte Traffic in Systemic Mycobacterial Infection

Little is known concerning the kinetics of T cell recirculation in disease states that seriously damage the architecture of the lymphoid organs, despite the fact that the recirculating kinetics of lymphocytes and the routes by which they migrate into lymphoid tissue have been well studied. Since the migration pathways of lymphocytes through the paracortical regions of lymph nodes and the white pulp of spleen are intricate, it is reasonable to assume that pathology involving these areas may exert a profound effect on the trafficking of these cells. A number of microbial pathogens may evoke granulomatous inflammation within lymphoid organs that severely alters their structure. However, it is in patients with lepromatous leprosy that these changes are observed most consistently. The paracortical regions of the lymph nodes are infiltrated by massive numbers of cells belonging to the histiocyte-macrophage series that contain many *M. leprae*. T cells, normally abundant in this area, are largely displaced or depleted (154). Similarly, T cells within the white pulp areas of the spleen may be replaced by masses of histiocytic cells (22,129).

Impaired Lymphocyte Recirculation in M. lepraemurium *Infection*

Granulomatous pathology similar to that observed in lepromatous leprosy also involves the lymphoid organs of rodents experimentally infected with *M. lepraemurium*, the etiologic agent of murine leprosy. Six to 10 weeks after intravenous inoculation of *M. lepraemurium*, both the paracortical regions of lymph nodes and the white pulp areas of the spleen are invaded extensively by macrophages that contain large numbers of acid fast-staining organisms (20). A photomicrograph of the pathology within the white pulp or spleen is illustrated in Fig. 3. Bullock (20,21) utilized this model in a series of experiments designed to study the kinetics of recirculating T cell populations in *M. lepraemurium*-infected Lewis rats. The thoracic ducts of a normal rat and an age-matched animal infected 8 to 10 weeks

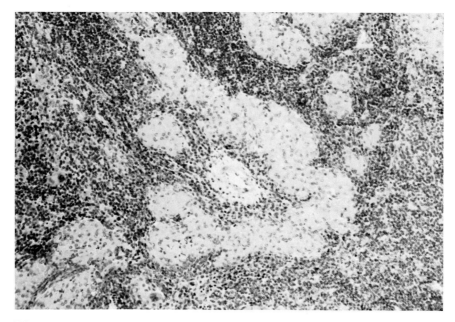

FIG. 3. Infected spleen at 16 weeks after inoculation with *M. lepraemurium*. Area shown depicts invasion of the periarteriolar lymphocyte sheath of white pulp by granulomas containing large histiocytic cells. ×200. (Reprinted from ref. 20 with permission of the publishers.)

previously were cannulated 3 days prior to a recirculation experiment, and a femoral vein cannula was placed for constant perfusion of a nutrient solution. Recirculating lymphocytes were drained from the thoracic duct for 3 days prior to study to reduce the hourly output of cells to a minimum level. On day 0, separate 16 hr collections of thoracic duct lymphocytes (TDL) from normal syngeneic donor rats were pooled, washed, and radiolabeled with either [^{3}H-5] uridine or ^{51}Cr. A mean of 1.6×10^6 labeled TDL/g body weight was given to each member of the experimental pair that had undergone thoracic duct cannulation 3 days previously. After cell infusion, thoracic duct lymph was collected at four intervals in order to quantitate total output of lymphocytes or radioactivity per hour. The results of four experiments are shown in Fig. 4.

During the first 4 hr after infusion of lymphocytes, there was little change in cell output from the thoracic duct. By 8 hr, infused lymphocytes had begun to traffic through the lymphoid organs of normal rats to efferent lymph and thence into the thoracic duct effluent. Lymphocyte output peaked between 12 and 24 hr and then declined to background levels as thoracic duct drainage continued. In contrast, there was little increase in cell output from the thoracic ducts of infected rats throughout the 48 hr period after intravenous injection of lymphocytes. Autoradiographic studies of cells collected from the thoracic ducts of infected rats which had received [^{3}H] uridine-labeled cells also indicated that a large proportion of the labeled lymphocytes given intravenously failed to traverse lymphoid organs into efferent lymph.

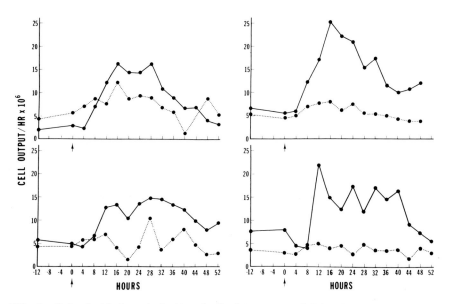

FIG. 4. Cell output in thoracic duct lymph after intravenous administration of syngeneic TDL to four matched pairs of control *(solid lines)* and infected rats *(dashed lines)*. Preparatory reduction in cell output before cell infusion at time-zero *(arrow)* achieved by thoracic duct fistulization on day 3. (Reprinted from ref. 21, part 2, with permission of the publishers.)

Additional studies were performed to exclude the possibility that a factor in the sera of infected rats may have disturbed the traffic of TDL by altering surface properties or other functions. In these experiments, the migration of ^{51}Cr-labeled lymphocytes from infected donor rats was followed through the lymphoid organs of infected rats as well as through two sets of normal recipients, one of which had been injected with pooled serum from infected rats prior to the infusion of labeled cells. TDL from infected donors migrated well through lymphoid organs in normal but not infected rats. Preinjection of normal animals with serum from infected rats did not impair cell migration; instead, it appeared to facilitate migration of lymphocytes from infected donors. In other studies, it was determined that there was no abnormality of cell circulation during the first 2 weeks of infection, but a disturbance was observed after the sixth week. Eight weeks after inoculation with heat-killed *M. lepraemurium*, the disturbance of lymphocyte traffic was minimal. These data suggest that active infection with viable *M. lepraemurium* must be present for more than 2 weeks before a substantial perturbation of lymphocyte traffic can be detected.

The impaired migration of labeled cells to thoracic duct lymph in infected animals might be explained by failure of these cells to gain entry to lymph nodes because of extensive pathology involving the paracortical areas through which lymphocytes traffic. In fact, lymphocytes readily entered the lymphoid organs but then were sequestered for an unknown period (21). If infected rats were splenectomized, the quantity of cells and radioactivity appearing in thoracic duct lymph increased significantly, as compared with the output from infected animals with intact spleens. Nevertheless, the output from splenectomized, infected rats remained well below that of splenectomized control rats. These findings indicated that the spleens of infected rats functioned as a major, but not the only, trap for recirculating lymphocytes. In addition, substantial numbers of cells were trapped by the lymph nodes and a few by the liver as well. Conversely, infused TDL were not trapped by the thymus, lung, gut, bone marrow, muscle, and skin; neither was there any evidence for rapid destruction of labeled cells with excretion of soluble label in the urine or stool.

M. lepraemurium-infected rats develop a blood cytopenia consistent with an increase in cell-sequestering activity by the red pulp of the hypertrophied spleens. To assess the possible role of red pulp hyperfunction in the acute disturbance of lymphocyte circulation, massive splenomegaly and severe hypersplenism were induced in normal rats by repeated intraperitoneal injections of methyl cellulose. Histologic examination revealed extensive involvement of the red pulp by clusters of macrophages in association with a diffuse hyperplasia of the red pulp reticulum; the splenic white pulp was normal, and the lymph nodes also were free of pathology. Remarkably, the T lymphocyte migration through the greatly enlarged spleens of these rats was quite good, being quantitatively only slightly less than in control animals, as determined by cell output and recovery of radioactivity (21). Therefore, entrapment of circulating lymphocytes within the spleens of infected rats probably was not caused by hyperfunction of the red pulp but, rather, was secondary to granulomatous pathology within areas of the white pulp that are utilized for migration by recirculating cells.

Abnormal Lymphocyte Mobilization in M. Lepraemurium Infection

In other experiments, the capacity of *M. lepraemurium*-infected mice to mobilize lymphocytes from lymphoid organs was measured after injection of the synthetic polyanion polymethacrylic acid (PMAA) (28). PMAA produces an absolute lymphocytosis in normal rodents 3 to 4 hr after intravenous injection by rapidly mobilizing lymphocytes to blood from the white pulp of spleen and paracortical areas of lymph nodes; blood lymphocyte levels return to normal within 24 to 48 hr (122). In infected mice, the amount of PMAA-induced lymphocytosis did not differ from control values during the first 10 weeks of infection. Subsequently, there was a progressive decrease in the lymphocytosis stimulated by PMAA that became maximal at approximately 16 weeks. To standardize measurements, a lymphocyte mobilization index was calculated as the ratio of the absolute lymphocyte count in blood at a given time after PMAA injection over the baseline lymphocyte count at zero-time immediately prior to injection. The results of studies on 18 week-infected mice and age-matched controls are summarized in Fig. 5, where it can be seen that the mobilization of lymphocytes to peripheral blood in infected mice was reduced significantly at all time intervals during a 6 hr period after injection of PMAA.

To exclude the possibility that the poor lymphocytic response of infected mice was secondary to depletion of the total endogenous pool from which lymphocytes

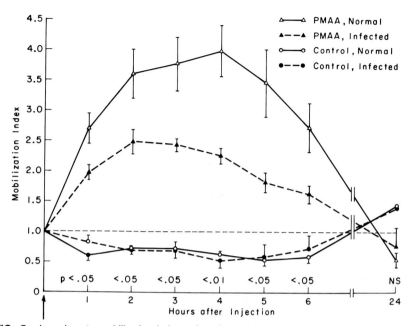

FIG. 5. Lymphocyte mobilization index values in peripheral blood of 18 week-infected C3H mice and age-matched controls after injection of PMAA or buffered saline. Each symbol represents the mean value ± SEM for five mice. *p* values, differences between normal and infected mice after PMAA injection. (Reprinted from ref. 28 with permission of the publishers.)

could be mobilized, normal lymph node cells were harvested from syngeneic donors, labeled with ^{51}Cr, and given intravenously to matched groups of 18 week-infected and control mice. The infused lymphocytes were then allowed to "home" to the lymphoid organs of recipients for 18 to 20 hr, after which PMAA was given intravenously immediately following a control bleeding for the baseline counts of lymphocytes and radioactivity. Subsequent blood samples for counting were obtained at 2, 3, and 6 hr. Similar studies were performed on mice that had been splenectomized or sham-operated 72 hr prior to administration of PMAA. The number of radiolabeled donor lymphocytes mobilized to the blood was expressed as a radioactivity index, defined as the ratio of radioactivity measured per milliliter blood at a given time after injection of PMAA over the baseline level measured at zero-time.

Prior to injection of PMAA, the baseline levels of radioactivity were similar in the blood of normal and infected mice. After PMAA was given, however, the radioactive index in normal controls rose significantly above the index in infected mice at 2, 3, and 6 hr. In splenectomized mice, the index of the normal group again was significantly higher than that of the infected group at each time interval after PMAA. Clearly, a substantial number of donor lymphocytes could not be mobilized to the blood of infected mice even after splenectomy. The only source of mobilizable lymphocytes remaining in splenectomized animals was the lymph node mass from which cells normally are mobilized to blood via the efferent lymphatics. Therefore, many of these cells were retained by the lymph nodes and possibly a few by the liver as indicated previously.

The mechanism for retention of recirculating TDL or lymph node cells in *M. lepraemurium*-infected animals is unknown. Extensive granulomatous pathology might obstruct channels within the fine reticulin network of the spleen and lymph nodes, thereby rendering the egress of lymphocytes more difficult. Alternatively, the large population of macrophages within lymphoid organs of infected animals may play a significant role in the retention of lymphocytes either through a direct cell-to-cell interaction or by local production of factors that could slow the intrinsic ameboid activity of lymphocytes, as has been postulated to occur after injection of certain adjuvants (53).

The biologic significance of the perturbation of T lymphocyte trafficking in *M. lepraemurium*-infected animals remains to be determined. Since recirculation of lymphocytes from blood through lymphoid tissues is essential to facilitate the immune response by interaction with antigen and other immunocompetent cells, however, nonspecific entrapment of these cells may severely restrict their capacity to migrate in response to a variety of antigenic stimuli. Indeed, this phenomenon may account in part for the delayed rejection of skin grafts, the loss of DTH to skin test antigens, and the blockade of experimental allergic encephalitis that has been observed in animals infected with *M. lepraemurium* or other mycobacteria (26,128,136).

Definitive studies to ascertain if similar trapping of immunocompetent lymphocytes occurs within the lymphoid tissues of humans with disseminated mycobacterial infections have not been performed. That such trapping may occur has been suggested by Rook et al. (137), who measured the blastogenic responses to mycobacterial antigens by lymphocytes from the peripheral blood and lymph nodes of patients with severe pulmonary or miliary tuberculosis. Most patients were tuberculin negative; among these, the response to PPD by their peripheral blood lymphocytes was very low. On the other hand, the cells within lymph nodes biopsied from these patients responded well to stimulation with PPD. Putative trapping activity also may partially explain the decrease in numbers of T cells in the peripheral blood that commonly is observed among untreated patients with disseminated mycobacterial infections (40,46,54). Fortunately, the recent introduction of [111]indium has provided a greatly improved radioisotopic label for tracing the circulation of lymphocytes (105,158). It may soon be possible to study the movement from blood to lymphoid organs and/or to granulomatous inflammation of [111]indium-labeled autologous lymphocytes or of homologous cells that have been matched carefully for histocompatibility antigens.

ABERRANT IMMUNOREGULATORY FUNCTION IN MYCOBACTERIAL INFECTIONS

It is now known that an intricate series of cellular interactions are triggered in response to infection with facultative or obligate intracellular microorganisms involving both helper and suppressor immunoregulatory cell populations. In certain aspects, the cellular immune response to these organisms can be viewed as an expression of the net algebraic sum of both helper and suppressor regulatory functions that may be modulated by B cells, T cells, or macrophages (60). In nature, one of the more frequent causes of a severe disturbance in the balance between the helper and suppressor immunoregulatory functions is the prolonged antigenic stimulation provided by slowly progressing infections, of which mycobacterial diseases are a paradigm. Of considerable importance is the fact that in experimental animals or humans with disseminated forms of these infections, the cell-mediated immune response against the infecting organisms frequently is deficient. Moreover, a generalized state of anergy may be present in a substantial proportion of cases (23).

A considerable amount of work performed within the past few years suggests that the ineffective host response associated with disseminated intracellular infection may stem at least as much from intense stimulation of immunosuppressor control mechanisms as it does from a putative deficiency of helper cell-effector functions. A clue that this might be the case in certain mycobacterial infections was provided by studies of antibody responses to sheep erythrocytes (SRBC) in *M. lepraemurium*-infected mice as measured with hemolytic plaque assay techniques (50,135,160). Severe depression of the T lymphocyte-dependent immune response to SRBC was observed consistently as the infection progressed and was attributed to either a lack or dysfunction of cells essential to the immune response.

Characterization of Suppressor Cell Activities in *M. lepraemurium* Infection

In studies by Bullock et al. (25), spleen cells were collected at serial intervals throughout the course of *M. lepraemurium* infection and added to one of two sets of spleen cell cultures from normal littermates; the second set of cultures served as a control. Cultures were immunized *in vitro* with SRBC, and the direct plaque-forming cell (PFC) response to SRBC was measured 4 to 5 days later. In Fig. 6, it may be seen that 5×10^6 spleen cells did not suppress the PFC response of 1×10^7 normal splenocytes during the first 4 weeks of infection, but they did so thereafter. From the fifth through the 10th week, the suppression was mild, with reductions in PFC per culture ranging from 24 to 48%. At 10 to 11 weeks, however, suppressor activity increased greatly; after the 14th week, spleen cells from infected mice consistently reduced the response of normal splenocytes by more than 90%. It is unlikely that immunodepression was caused by the presence of *M. lepraemurium* in cultures, since addition of an equivalent number of bacilli to normal spleen cell cultures induced only a slight reduction in the PFC response. Cells from the peripheral lymph nodes of infected mice did not suppress normal lymph node cells until the infection was terminal, at which time the PFC response was reduced by only 29%. Thus the spleen appeared to be the principal domicile of suppressor cells throughout most of the disease course.

Characterization of the splenic suppressor cells during early infection (5 to 10 weeks) revealed a subpopulation with the properties of macrophages; i.e., they

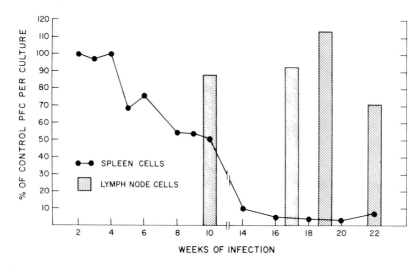

FIG. 6. Effect of 5 × 10⁶ spleen or lymph node cells from infected mice on the primary antibody response to SRBC *in vitro* by 10⁷ lymph node or spleen cells from age-matched, normal control mice. (Reprinted from ref. 25 with permission of the publishers.)

were adherent to nylon wool columns and glass, 95% phagocytized latex particles, and more than 90% stained positively for nonspecific esterase activity. Nylon-passed splenic lymphocytes were not suppressive during this early stage. In addition to these macrophage-like cells, a second population of suppressor cells was identified in the spleen during the 10th to the 11th week of infection and throughout the remaining lifespan. These cells were T lymphocytes, since they readily passed nylon wool columns and treatment with anti-Thy 1.2 serum plus complement abolished most of the suppressor activity, whereas sham anti-Thy 1.2 treatment did not (25).

In the C3H mouse and some other inbred strains, *M. lepraemurium* infection appears to be held in check until about the 10th to 11th week, at which time the spleen begins to enlarge rapidly, and organ counts of *M. lepraemurium* increase steadily. Of interest is the observation that although 4 week-infected mice can express DTH to proteins of *M. lepraemurium* or to SRBC after immunization, they become anergic to these antigens at approximately 10 to 11 weeks of infection (127; W. E. Bullock, *unpublished observations*). Therefore, the antigenic stimulation of early infection appears to activate helper T lymphocytes that in turn stimulate the antimicrobial activity of macrophages. It is tempting to speculate that under the constant stimulus of proliferating helper T cells, activated macrophages may acquire suppressor properties, perhaps secondary to an increase in surface area. Consequently, the macrophage may present more surface receptors capable of adsorbing putative helper factors produced by T lymphocytes. Activated macrophages also might inhibit immunocompetent cells by direct contact or by producing a soluble suppressor substance.

A major subpopulation of lymphocytes with the capacity to function in a bidirectional manner is present in the spleen and thymus but not in lymph nodes of mice (62,163). The immunoregulatory function of these cells depends largely on the activity of the cells being regulated. When the latter are responding at a high level, the activity of regulatory lymphocytes tends to be suppressive; conversely, it enhances when immune activity is low. As a group, the immunoregulatory lymphocytes appear to be less mature, i.e., have not achieved terminal differentiation, are thymus dependent, and are relatively short-lived (61). These cells bear the surface antigen phenotype Ly-1, 2, 3^+ (30,51). Possibly, it is this regulatory subpopulation that is driven to function in a suppressor rather than helper mode by the continuing immunostimulation of chronic *M. lepraemurium* infection. Thus the appearance of suppressor T cells at 10 to 11 weeks (when suppressor activity begins to increase greatly in infected mice) may signal a "switchover" by the Ly-1, 2, 3^+ subpopulation to generation of T suppressor effector cells as a critical level of maximal helper immune function is reached. Although this construction of events is purely hypothetical, advances in the ability to characterize T lymphocyte subpopulations more precisely by monoclonal antibody technology and fluorescence-activated cell sorting clearly will permit this hypothesis to be tested.

Immunoregulatory Disturbances in Other Experimental Mycobacterial Infections

The onset of anergy in association with the evolution of suppressor cell activity in experimental infection by no means is confined to the murine leprosy model (23). Several investigators have demonstrated a persistent suppressor cell effect in mice infected with viable BCG. In general, the immunosuppression is nonspecific, since responses to nonmycobacterial antigens and to substances mitogenic for both T and B cells appear to be reduced (2,37,82,111,121). The identity of cells in the spleens of BCG-infected animals that mediate immunosuppression is a matter of debate. Two groups find that suppression is exerted by T cells only (37,111), whereas other investigators claim that suppressor activity is confined to a macrophage-like cell population (2,82); still others find evidence for both T cell- and macrophage-mediated suppressor function (121,150).

Clearly, these conflicting observations must be resolved by careful attention to experimental variables within the model systems, such as route of infection, source and dosage of BCG, and mouse strain employed. In addition, great care must be taken to minimize cross-contamination of cell populations during separation procedures. The importance of precise control over strain variation within a given species of *Mycobacterium* is underscored by an intriguing report by Cunningham and Collins (39) on the suppressor and helper T cell populations in the spleens of B6D2 F_1 hybrid mice infected intravenously with different strains of *M. kansasii*. Splenic T cells of mice injected 30 days previously with *M. kansasii*, TMC 1203, exhibited substantially reduced responses to phytohemagglutinin (PHA) and concanavalin A (Con A) and in mixed leukocyte culture. In contrast, splenic T cells from animals infected with *M. kansasii*, TMC 1214, exhibited an enhanced level of response to these stimuli *in vitro*. These findings suggest that in the model system employed, strain variation within the same species of organism may be critical in determining whether the cellular immune response of the host will be characterized by a predominance of either helper or suppressor T cell activity.

If one makes the assumption that suppressor cell populations generated within granulomatous infiltrates of the spleen may act to prevent or hinder development of an effective antimycobacterial immune response, it then becomes important to determine if chemotherapy can achieve sufficient reduction in antigen load and healing of the granulomas to permit reversal of suppressor activity. Several species of *Mycobacteria* employed for experimental infections are quite resistant to chemotherapy, as is *M. lepraemurium*. On the other hand, BCG infection can be treated effectively, as reported by Collins and Watson (38), who found that the immunosuppressive effect of spleen cells from BCG-infected mice could be prevented if the animals were placed on isoniazid and rifampin therapy within 24 hr after inoculation. If treatment was delayed for 28 days and then administered for 30 days, however, the depressed splenic T cell responses to PPD *in vitro* could not be reversed, despite a rapid reduction in the number of viable BCG in the spleen. These data suggest that once T suppressor cells are generated in the spleen, the persistence of such cells may be maintained by a much smaller antigenic load that is present within lymphoid tissues in a nonrecognizable form. Of interest will be future investigations to determine if prolonged therapy of experimental mycobacterial infections can restore immune responses to normal levels. Conversely, will interruptions of therapy to produce relapsing infection be associated with cyclic reactivation of suppressor cell activity? In addition, investigation is needed regarding the effect on host survival of immunotherapeutic ablation of T suppressor cell populations by administration of cyclophosphamide (1) or monoclonal antibodies to specific cell subsets.

Immunoregulatory Disturbances in Mycobacterial Diseases of Humans

Leprosy

Of the human mycobacterial diseases, leprosy has been the most studied by far in regard to associated abnormalities of the lymphoid system (24). Nevertheless, despite a massive investigational effort productive of an equally massive literature, we have gained no more than a rudimentary understanding of the basic immunologic defect(s) that permits an individual with lepromatous leprosy to harbor as many as 10^{12} *M. leprae*. Perhaps the only immunologic abnormality in lepromatous leprosy about which there is consensus agreement is the universal anergy displayed by patients to the antigens of *M. leprae* both *in vivo* and *in vitro*. Furthermore, it is unusual for lepromatous patients to develop vigorous DTH-type reactivity to *M. leprae* antigens, even though successful therapy may have eradicated all identifiable bacillary forms from biopsy specimens. In contrast, patients with tuberculoid forms of leprosy are capable of mounting DTH responses to *M. leprae* (109).

Many patients with lepromatous leprosy, in addition to being anergic to *M. leprae*, also experience a generalized, nonspecific impairment of CMI. Manifestations of this nonspecific depression range from significant prolongation of skin homograft survival and diminished lymphocyte transfer reactions (69,70) to depression of DTH responses to skin tests with bacterial antigens (18,19,67) and impaired responses to sensitizing haptenic chemicals (19,159). Likewise, the blastogenic response of lymphocytes from lepromatous patients frequently is abnormally low in response to stimulation by T cell mitogens and nonmycobacterial antigens (27,109,115). The nonspecific depression of CMI generally is less severe than the impairment of reactivity to *M. leprae*; as the tissue load of lepra bacilli is reduced by prolonged antimicrobial therapy, the nonspecific component of anergy tends to be ameliorated or reversed (19,103,112). It has not been determined if these nonspecific abnormalities of the immune response reflect the deficiency of host response that permits unchecked multiplication of *M. leprae* or if they are epiphenomena arising from a specific defect in CMI against *M. leprae*.

To date, all attempts to establish a correlation between susceptibility to lepromatous leprosy and histocompatibility genes have yielded inconsistent results (43,148). Other postulates that lepromatous patients lack *M. leprae*-specific T lymphocytes, i.e., are tolerant (64), or that they have a specific defect of macrophage function (8,71) also lack rigorous experimental verification. The most recent theory to be advanced is that lepromatous patients may respond to infection by preferential induction of *M. leprae*-specific T suppressor cell activity, which may act both specifically and nonspecifically to suppress cell-mediated immune responses. Thus a reduction in the load of mycobacterial antigen by chemotherapy might reduce the intensity of nonspecific suppressor T cell activity. Conversely, the low concentrations of mycobacterial antigens that probably remain in the reticuloendothelial system for life may continue to induce differentiation of specific suppressor T cells that chronically suppress the CMI response to *M. leprae*.

Not unexpectedly, the few studies that have been performed to explore the suppressor cell hypothesis in human leprosy are somewhat conflicting. Mehra et al. (101) have reported that if PBM cells from treated lepromatous patients are exposed to a preparation of Dharmendra-lepromin, T suppressor cell activity is induced that nonspecifically depresses the blastogenic response to Con A by allogeneic PBM cells from normal donors. The particular T cell subset that mediated suppression was identified by reaction with a xenogeneic antihuman T cell serum that defines a surface antigen (TH_2) which is associated with suppressor activity (102,131). TH_2 + T cells obtained from patients with tuberculoid leprosy or normal individuals did not suppress blastogenic responses to Con A. Using different experimental conditions, Nath and Singh (114) studied autologous cell cultures from leprosy patients who were untreated, as contrasted with those studied by Mehra. Addition of *M. leprae* antigens to cultures of PBM cells from patients with tuberculoid leprosy unequivocally induced suppression of the response to stimulation with Con A in 17 of 21 cases. On the other hand, *M. leprae* antigens induced suppression in only six of 15 cell cultures from lepromatous patients; the response to Con A was enhanced in nine.

In another study, Bahr et al. (7) observed that soluble antigens prepared from *M. leprae* and from several other species of *Mycobacteria* all induced suppression of the proliferative response to a variety of antigens by PBM cells cultured from patients with tuberculoid and lepromatous leprosy as well as from healthy donors. Suppression appeared to be mediated by a cell found in the erythrocyte-rosetting fraction of PBM cells, and its ability to suppress was lost after 48 hr in culture. Finally, Stoner et al. (146) preincubated PBM cells from healthy contacts of leprosy patients with *M. leprae* antigens, PPD, BCG, or streptokinase-streptodornase (SKSD) for 7 days. The preincubated cells were added to fresh autologous cells that also were stimulated with the same antigens. Cells primed with *M. leprae* antigens, PPD, or SKSD suppressed the response to the corresponding antigen and also suppressed the responses of secondary cultures to the other antigens. These data suggest that suppressor lymphocytes can be induced by *M. leprae* antigens in PBM cell cultures from healthy individuals as well as from lepromatous patients. This work also lends support to previous studies in which it was found that antigens other than those of *M. leprae* can induce suppression of the lymphoproliferative response *in vitro* (7,144).

Incubation of normal human PBM cells with Con A induces proliferation of a resting T lymphocyte subset that can suppress both antigen-specific and mitogen-stimulated proliferative responses of allogeneic responder cells from healthy donors (141). Therefore, the subset of cells activated to suppressor activity by Con A may play a role in modulating the normal immune response. Two groups have evaluated Con A-induced suppressor activity in human leprosy; both demonstrated that the ability of Con A-pretreated PBM cells from lepromatous patients to suppress the response of normal allogeneic or autologous PBM cells to mitogens and antigens was reduced significantly, as compared with cells from tuberculoid patients or normal individuals (4,113). Con A-inducible suppressor cell function appears to be diminished in some lepromatous patients.

Of interest in regard to the above findings is the fact that lepromatous leprosy is associated with polyclonal hypergammaglobulinemia and an increased incidence of autoantibody formation (152). Patients with lepromatous leprosy also are reported to have significantly higher isohemagglutinin titers and higher serum agglutinin titers against *Candida albicans* than either those with tuberculoid leprosy or normal controls (18). In addition, the antibody response of lepromatous patients to immunization with extrinsic antigens at least equals, and may exceed, the responses of healthy controls (3,77). In aggregate, these findings suggest that T cell-mediated immunoregulatory control over B cell function may be abnormal in patients with lepromatous disease.

To explore this issue further, Bullock et al. (29) employed a reverse hemolytic PFC assay to measure the number of PBM cells from lepromatous patients and controls that respond to pokeweed mitogen (PWM) stimulation *in vitro* by immunoglobulin secretion. As shown in Fig. 7, the PWM-induced PFC responses by PBM cells from patients with lepromatous leprosy (median, 33,000 PFC/10^6 cells in culture) were significantly greater ($p < 0.01$) than those mounted by cells from healthy controls (median, 7,100 PFC/10^6) and by cells from four patients with tuberculoid leprosy (median, 6,625 PFC/10^6 cells).

Further investigations to determine if the blood of lepromatous patients contained large numbers of B lymphocytes spontaneously secreting immunoglobulins on day 0 showed this not to be the case. The numbers of immunoglobulin-secreting PFC on day 0 from lepromatous patients were not significantly higher than the spontaneous PFC in healthy controls. The mean absolute lymphocyte count in the blood of lepromatous patients was lower than that of healthy controls, whereas the count of B lymphocytes was somewhat higher than normal. The differences were not significant. The mean number of T lymphocytes in lepromatous blood samples was significantly lower than normal ($p < 0.01$), as were both the number of cells in the T4$^+$ helper subpopulation and the T8$^+$ suppressor subpopulation.

To differentiate between a possible deficiency of T8$^+$ suppressor cell function on the one hand and hyperfunction of T4$^+$ helper cells on the other in lepromatous patients, T4$^+$ or T8$^+$ cell subpopulations from normals or patients were cocultured with B-enriched cells from normal allogeneic donors. Cultures containing only a B cell-enriched population from either normal or lepromatous donors produced few plaques. However, coculture of 10^4 normal allogeneic T4$^+$ cells with 10^6 normal B-enriched cells resulted in a vigorous PFC response to PWM (Fig. 8). Coculture of 10^4 normal T4$^+$ cells with 10^6 B-enriched lymphocytes from the lepromatous donors also resulted in PFC responses equivalent to the controls. Moreover, coculture of up to 10^6 lepromatous T4$^+$ cells with 10^6 normal B-enriched cells did

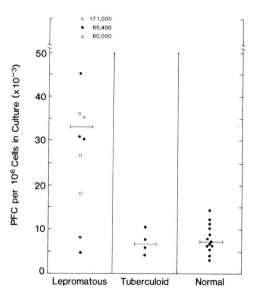

FIG. 7. PWM-stimulated responses of PBM cells from patients with lepromatous ($N = 9$) or tuberculoid ($N = 4$) leprosy and healthy controls ($N = 13$). Two assays, separated by at least 4 weeks, were performed on three lepromatous patients; in each case, results of both assays are indicated by the paired symbols (*circles*, *triangles*, and *squares*, respectively). *Horizontal bars*, median PFC response. (Reprinted from ref. 29 with permission of the publishers.)

not drive the response to supranormal levels under the experimental conditions employed. In Fig. 8 are shown the results obtained in a typical experiment when increasing numbers of T8+ cells from normal donors or from lepromatous patients were cocultured with a mixture of 10^6 B-enriched cells and 10^4 T4+ helper cells from normal allogeneic donors. As the number of normal T8+ cells in coculture was increased from 10^4 to 10^6, the PFC response was suppressed greatly. In marked contrast, all concentrations of T8+ cells from lepromatous patients failed to suppress the response of the normal B cell plus T4+ cell mixture.

The reason for the failure of T8+ cells from lepromatous donors to exert normal suppressor activity *in vitro* is unknown. Additional studies indicate that lepromatous B cells themselves probably are not defective in their responses to T suppressor cell signals. Still to be explored is the possibility that the functional deficit could stem from the loss of an auxiliary cell population *in vivo* that may be necessary to permit expression of efferent-acting T8+ suppressor cells. Alternatively, the sera of lepromatous patients may contain factors that can abrogate or block T suppressor cell function, as has been demonstrated to occur in some patients with active systemic lupus erythematosus (138,155). Whether this *in vitro* phenomenon bears any relationship to immunoregulatory events *in vivo* remains to be determined. Nevertheless, it does suggest a possible mechanism that may explain, in part, the immunopathogenesis of hypergammaglobulinemia in leprosy and perhaps certain other chronic granulomatous infections.

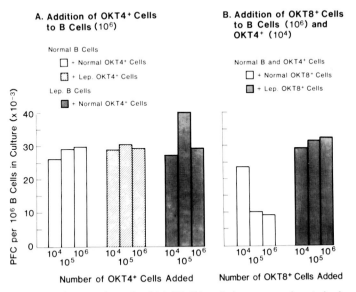

FIG. 8. Representative experiment in which **(A)**, T4+ cells from a normal control or lepromatous patient were cocultured with B-enriched cells from a normal allogeneic donor, and lepromatous T4+ cells were also cultured with normal B cells; **(B)**, T8+ cells from the normal or patient cocultured with a mixture of normal B cells plus T4+ cells.

Tuberculosis

In the past few years, it has become apparent that the well-established concept of an immunopathologic spectrum of leprosy can be applied to the clinical investigation of tuberculosis, although chronologically, the evolution of immunopathology in tuberculosis usually is more rapid. Individuals with miliary disease might be considered as having "lepromatous" forms of tuberculosis; those with micronodular, localized tuberculosis of the lung may be counterparts of patients with tuberculoid leprosy (91,142). The majority of those with miliary tuberculosis are anergic to PPD by both skin testing and *in vitro* studies of lymphocyte transformation, although titers of serum antibodies to mycobacterial antigens frequently are high (11,40,91). Generalized impairment of cell-mediated immune responses can be demonstrated in a substantial percentage of these patients by similar techniques using chemical haptens and a variety of recall antigens (11,40,156). Patients with severe pulmonary tuberculosis also may be anergic to PPD and other antigens (96,100), whereas the majority of patients with well-localized diseases are tuberculin positive. PBM cells from these patients respond well *in vitro* to PPD and to other antigenic stimuli (40,91).

Unlike patients with lepromatous leprosy who remain anergic to *M. leprae* despite prolonged therapy, most people with severe tuberculosis recover cell-mediated immune responses to *M. tuberculosis* within a few months after institution of appropriate chemotherapy (96,100,156,167). The reason for this fundamental difference in the capacity to recover from a state of anergy is speculative. A point worth emphasizing is that most patients with generalized forms of tuberculosis are able to destroy tubercle bacilli and to eliminate antigenic material from the lymphoreticular system once mycobacterial stasis and killing has been achieved by chemotherapy. Patients with lepromatous leprosy, on the other hand, have difficulty in eliminating nonviable *M. leprae*, as evidenced by the persistence of microbial carcasses within tissues for years after initiation of effective antimicrobial therapy. It seems that the more rapid recovery of immune responsiveness in treated patients with miliary tuberculosis parallels directly the accelerated rate at which the granulomatous pathology resolves within the lymphoid organs and other tissues.

As in leprosy, current investigations on the possible mechanism for anergy in tuberculosis have focused on the suppressor immunoregulatory functions of the lymphoid system. Bona and Chedid (14) observed that PBM cells enriched for erythrocyte rosette-forming lymphocytes from BCG-vaccinated healthy adults responded better to PPD stimulation *in vitro* than did unfractionated PBM cells. If lymphocytes depleted of erythrocyte rosette-forming cells were added back to autologous T lymphocytes, responses to PPD were depressed, leading the authors to assume that suppression was mediated by B cells, despite the fact that macrophages were present in the B cell-enriched preparation. Tsuyuguchi et al. (149) observed that when PBM cells from patients with advanced, refractory pulmonary tuberculosis of long standing were stimulated with PPD *in vitro*, the number of cells bearing IgG Fc receptors increased. These cells suppressed the proliferative response of autologous PBM cells to PPD and nonspecifically suppressed PWM-induced IgG synthesis by B cells *in vitro*. PPD stimulation did not expand the IgG Fc receptor-bearing cell subset in PBM cells from patients with newly diagnosed tuberculosis. Since both groups of patients were tuberculin positive by skin test, the authors concluded that the T cells responding in a cutaneous reaction to tuberculin might be different from those responding in antituberculous immunity.

Ellner (48) studied a subpopulation of patients with newly diagnosed pulmonary tuberculosis who had negative tuberculin skin tests. *In vitro*, the PBM cells of these patients responded well to PHA but poorly to PPD and to nonmycobacterial antigens. Depletion of adherent monocytes resulted in marked enhancement of the T-lymphocyte responses to PPD but not to other antigens. Therefore, suppressor activity inducible by specific antigen and mediated by adherent cells appeared to be superimposed on a nonspecific T lymphocyte hyporeactivity to antigens but not to mitogens. Additional studies by Kleinhenz et al. (80) suggested that the specific inhibition of T cell responses to PPD may be caused by mycobacterial polysaccharides (particularly arabinogalactan) in the serum that stimulate adherent mononuclear cells to suppressor activity through increased prostaglandin production. The mechanism for T lymphocyte hyporeactivity to nonmycobacterial antigens in the anergic patients remains to be clarified.

Of interest in regard to the issue of the specificity of suppression mediated by adherent mononuclear cells is a study by Katz et al. (78), who employed a hemolytic PFC assay to measure production of antibody to SRBC by PWM-stimulated PBM cells from tuberculous patients and normal controls. The PFC responses were extremely low in tuberculous patients who were either untreated or treated for 4 to 6 weeks, as compared with the responses of lymphocytes from normal controls. However, removal of adherent cells from PBM cells of tuberculous patients greatly improved the PFC responses of the monocyte-depleted cells, especially in cultures prepared from treated patients.

Disseminated tuberculosis may be associated with severe neutropenia as well as other hematologic disorders (63). Speculation as to the mechanism of neutropenia has included hypersplenism, increased neutrophil demand, and "marrow failure." Another possible mechanism has been suggested recently by Bagby and Gilbert (6), who detected greatly reduced colony growth of marrow cells during neutropenia in two patients with disseminated tuberculosis. Removal of lymphocytes enhanced clonal cell growth in both patients, whereas removal of adherent cells had no effect. T cells from both the peripheral blood and bone marrow of one patient inhibited cell cluster growth when added back to T-depleted cells. In one patient restudied after recovery, inhibitory T cell activity was absent and could not be induced by exposure of T cells to PPD. This study is the first to present evidence that suppressor cells are generated within the lymphoid system during mycobacterial infection that are capable of exerting a potentially lethal effect on the host. If this work is confirmed, it will be of interest from a therapeutic standpoint to determine if the

T cells that inhibit granulopoiesis are of the cytotoxic suppressor subset bearing the $T8^+$ surface antigenic marker, as has been shown in some other cases of bone marrow failure mediated by T lymphocytes (5).

Lymphoid Cells In Tuberculous Effusions

Unlike *M. leprae*, which has a predilection for the dermis and Schwann cells of nerves, *M. tuberculosis* not infrequently infects serosal surfaces, thereby inducing an inflammatory response that evolves within the potential spaces bounded by these membranes. In the pleural space, the result is an exudation of fluid with high protein content in which the white blood count usually ranges between 500 and $8,000/mm^3$. More than 90% of these cells are lymphocytes in the majority of cases of culturally documented tuberculous pleurisy (10). There are no "normal" values for the numbers of T and B lymphocytes in effusions for obvious reasons. Nevertheless, it is known that both the percentage and absolute numbers of T cells in pleural fluid obtained from patients with connective tissue diseases, congestive heart failure, and non-specific pleurisy do not differ significantly from those of peripheral blood (45,125). B cell numbers may be either increased or decreased relative to blood in these effusions.

In tuberculous pleurisy, the absolute number of T cells in the pleural fluid is significantly higher than in peripheral blood, whereas the number of B lymphocytes tends to be lower (49,125). Ellner (47) reported vigorous blastogenic responses to PPD by mononuclear cells cultured from the pleural fluid of three patients with tuberculosis pleurisy. PBM cells from two patients responded poorly to PPD stimulation *in vitro*; however, the same cells depleted of adherent cells responded much better. These findings led the author to postulate that lymphocytes specifically reactive to tuberculin had become compartmentalized within the pleural fluid space and that suppressor mononuclear cells had been excluded. In a larger study, Fujiwara et al. (53a) confirmed and extended Ellner's (47) findings by preparing cells enriched for T lymphocytes from the pleural fluid and blood of patients with tuberculous pleurisy. The T cells were stimulated by PPD in cultures to which various numbers of X-irradiated autologous adherent cells had been added. Pleural fluid T cells showed a greater response than blood T cells from the same patient, irrespective of the numbers of adherent cells added.

It is tempting to conclude from these studies that large numbers of specifically sensitized T cells may be recruited to the pleural fluid in response to the presence of various antigenic materials. At present, however, there is no firm evidence that this is true in tuberculous pleurisy or in other inflammatory conditions of the pleural space that consistently are associated with high percentages of T cells in the effusion (49). Alternatively, T cells specifically reactive to PPD may accumulate nonspecifically within an area of inflammation in a fashion similar to the nonspecific entry of T cells into peritoneal exudates that has been demonstrated to occur in experimental animals immunized against *L. monocytogenes* (85).

The cellular exudate in tuberculosis meningitis contains a high percentage of lymphocytes, as do other forms of chronic meningitis. Unfortunately, virtually nothing is known regarding the immune mechanisms responsible for accumulation of these cells. In the few reported cases in which assays of the blastogenic response to PPD by lymphocytes were performed simultaneously on samples of cerebrospinal fluid (CSF) and blood from patients with tuberculous meningitis, the blastogenic responses of cells in the CSF were higher (81,126). In addition, oligoclonal immunoglobulin has been detected in the CSF but not the serum of patients with tuberculous meningitis (81,87). These fragments of information might be cited as evidence for antigen-specific selection and compartmentalization of T and B lymphocytes within the CSF. As is the case with tuberculous pleural effusions, however, nonspecific mechanisms for lymphocyte accumulation into an inflammatory site cannot be excluded. Since human tuberculous meningitis is extremely difficult to study in a comprehensive manner, animal models may be of help in gaining a better understanding of the immunopathogenesis of this unique form of tuberculous inflammation.

In concluding this chapter on the lymphoid system in mycobacterial infections, one cannot help but view with some astonishment the progress of cellular immunology in the short span since Rich (133) mused with great puzzlement over the role of lymphocytes in granulomatous inflammation. We now know that, far from being "phlegmatic spectators," these cells busily communicate by a remarkably sophisticated system of language with a variety of cell types that participate in the immune response. As our comprehension of this language begins to improve in the years to come, there is every reason to believe that it will become possible to interdict signals which may be inimical to the host defense against mycobacterial diseases by judicious and selective immunotherapy.

ACKNOWLEDGMENTS

This work was supported in part by NIH grants AI 16308 and AI 17339.

The author expresses his appreciation to Mrs. Barbara Huber for editorial assistance, to Dr. Susan Watson for helpful discussions and review of the manuscript, and to Dr. Jan Schwarz for translations from German.

REFERENCES

1. Alexander, J. (1978): Effect of cyclophosphamide treatment on the course of mycobacterium lepraemurium infection and development of delayed-type hypersensitivity reactions in C57BL and BALB/c mice. *Clin. Exp. Immunol.*, 34:52–58.
2. Allen, E. M., and Moore, V. L. (1979): Suppression of phytohemagglutinin and lipopolysaccharide responses in mouse spleen cells by Bacillus Calmette-Guérin. *J. Reticuloendothel. Soc.*, 26:349–356.
3. Almeida De, J. O., Brandao, H., and De Lima, E. G. (1964): Enhanced serologic response of lepromatous patients to antityphoid vaccination. *Int. J. Lepr.*, 32:292–296.
4. Artz, R. P., Jacobson, R. R., and Bullock, W. E. (1980): Decreased suppressor cell activity in disseminated granulomatous infections. *Clin. Exp. Immunol.*, 41:343–352.
5. Bagby, G. C. (1981): T lymphocytes involved in inhibition of granulopoiesis in two neutropenic patients are of the cytotoxic/suppressor (T3+T8+) subset. *J. Clin. Invest.*, 68:1597–1600.
6. Bagby, G. C., and Gilbert, D. N. (1981): Suppression of granulopoiesis by T-lymphocytes in two patients with disseminated mycobacterial infection. *Ann. Intern. Med.*, 94:478–481.
7. Bahr, G. M., Rook, G. A., and Stanford, J. L. (1981): Inhibition of the proliferative response of

peripheral blood lymphocytes to mycobacterial or fungal antigens by co-stimulation with antigens from various mycobacterial species. *Immunology*, 44:593–598.

8. Barbieri, T. A., and Correa, W. M. (1967): Human macrophage culture: The leprosy prognostic test (LPT). *Int. J. Lepr.*, 35:377–381.

9. Barclay, W. R., Anacker, R., Brehmer, W., and Ribi, E. (1967): Effects of oil-treated mycobacterial cell walls on the organs of mice. *J. Bacteriol.*, 94:1736–1745.

10. Berger, H. W., and Mejia, E. (1973): Tuberculous pleurisy. *Chest*, 63:88–92.

11. Bhatnagar, R., Malaviya, A. N., Narayanan, S., Rajgopalan, P., Kumar, R., and Bharandwaj, O. P. (1977): Spectrum of immune response abnormalities in different clinical forms of tuberculosis. *Am. Rev. Respir. Dis.*, 115:207–212.

12. Blanden, R. V., Lefford, M. J., and Mackaness, G. B. (1969): The host response to Calmette-Guérin bacillus infection in mice. *J. Exp. Med.*, 129:1079–1100.

13. Bloom, B. R., and Bennett, B. (1966): Mechanism of a reaction in vitro associated with delayed type hypersensitivity. *Science*, 153:80–82.

14. Bona, C., and Chedid, L. (1976): Stimulation of lymphocytes by purified protein derivative: Suppression by cells from humans vaccinated with Bacille-Calmette-Guérin. *J. Infect. Dis.*, 133:465–468.

15. Boros, D. L., and Warren, K. S. (1973): The bentonite granuloma. Characterization of a model system for infectious and foreign body granulomatous inflammation using soluble mycobacterial, histoplasma and schistosoma antigens. *Immunology*, 24:511–529.

16. Borrel, A. (1893): Tuberculose pulmonaire expérimentale. *Ann. Inst. Pasteur*, 7:593–627.

17. Borrel, A. (1894): Tuberculose expérimentale du rein. *Ann. Inst. Pasteur*, 8:65–82.

18. Buck, A. A., and Hasenclever, H. R. (1963): Influence of leprosy on delayed-type skin reactions and serum agglutination titers to Candida albicans. *Am. J. Hyg.*, 77:305–316.

19. Bullock, W. E. (1968): Studies on immune mechanisms in leprosy. I. Depression of delayed allergic response to skin test antigens. *N. Engl. J. Med.*, 278:298–304.

20. Bullock, W. E., Jr. (1976): Perturbation of lymphocyte circulation in experimental murine leprosy. I. Description of the defect. *J. Immunol.*, 117:1164–1170.

21. Bullock, W. E., Jr. (1976): Perturbation of lymphocyte circulation in experimental murine leprosy. II. Nature of the defect. *J. Immunol.*, 117:1171–1178.

22. Bullock, W. E. (1978): Leprosy: A model of immunological perturbation in chronic infection. *Infect. Dis.*, 137:341–354.

23. Bullock, W. E. (1979): *Mechanisms of Anergy in Infectious Diseases in Immunological Aspects of Infectious Diseases*, edited by G. Dick, pp. 269–294. University Park Press, Baltimore.

24. Bullock, W. E. (1981): Immunobiology of Leprosy. In: *Immunology of Human Infection, Part I*, edited by A. J. Nahmias and J. R. O'Reilly, pp. 369–390. Plenum, New York.

25. Bullock, W. E., Carlson, E. M., and Gershon, R. K. (1978): The evolution of immunosuppressive cell populations in experimental mycobacterial infection. *J. Immunol.*, 120:1709–1716.

26. Bullock, W. E., Evans, P. E., and Filameno, A. R. (1977): Impairment of cell-mediated immune responses by infection with Mycobacterium lepraemurium. *Infect. Immun.*, 18:157–164.

27. Bullock, W. E., and Fasal, P. (1971): Studies of immune mechanisms in leprosy. III. The role of cellular and humoral factors in impairment of the in vitro immune response. *J. Immunol.*, 106:888–889.

28. Bullock, W. E., and Vergamini, M. S. (1977): Impairment of lymphocyte mobilization from lymphoid organs by granulomatous infection. *Cell. Immunol.*, 29:337–346.

29. Bullock, W. E., Watson, S., Nelson, K. E., Schauf, V., Makonkawkeyoon, S., and Jacobson, R. R. (1982): Aberrant Immunoregulatory Control of B Lymphocyte Function in Lepromatous Leprosy. *Clin. Exp. Immunol.*, 49:105–114.

30. Cantor, H., and Boyse, E. A. (1977): Regulation of cellular and humoral immune response by T-cell subclasses. *Cold Spring Harbor Symp. Quant. Biol.*, XLI:23–32.

31. Cantor, H., Sheb, F. W., and Boyse, E. A. (1976): Separation of helper T cells from suppressor T cells expressing different Ly components. II. Activation by antigen: After immunization, specific suppressor and helper activities are mediated by distinct T cell subclasses. *J. Exp. Med.*, 143:1391–1401.

32. Chase, M. W. (1945): The cellular transfer of cutaneous hypersensitivity to tuberculin. *Proc. Soc. Exp. Biol.*, 59:134–135.

33. Coe, J. E., Feldman, J. D., and Lee, S. (1966): Immunologic competence of thoracic duct cells: I. Delayed hypersensitivity. *J. Exp. Med.*, 123:267–281.

34. Collins, F. M., Congdon, C. C., and Morrison, N. E. (1975): Growth of Mycobacterium bovis (BCG) in T-lymphocyte depleted mice. *Infect. Immun.*, 11:57–64.
35. Collins, F. M., Montalbine, F., and Morrison, N. E. (1975): Growth of *Mycobacterium marinum* in the footpads of T-cell-depleted mice. *Infect. Immun.*, 11:1088–1093.
36. Colston, M. J., and Hilson, G. R. F. (1976): Growth of Mycobacterium leprae and M. marinum in congenitally athymic (nude) mice. *Nature*, 262:399–400.
37. Collins, F. M., and Watson, S. R. (1979): Suppressor T-cells in BCG-infected mice. *Infect. Immun.*, 25:491–496.
38. Collins, F. M., and Watson, S. R. (1980): Effect of chemotherapy on suppressor T-cells in BCG-infected mice. *Immunology*, 40:529–537.
39. Cunningham, D. S., and Collins, F. M. (1981): Suppressor and helper T-cells populations in mycobacterium kansasii-infected spleens. *Immunology*, 44:473–480.
40. Daniel, T. M. (1980): The immunology of tuberculosis. *Clin. Chest Med.*, 1:189–201.
41. David, J. R. (1966): Delayed hypersensitivity in vitro: Its mediation by cell-free substances formed by lymphoid cell-antigen interaction. *Proc. Natl. Acad. Sci. USA*, 56:72–77.
42. David, J. R., and Rocklin, R. E. (1978): Lymphocyte mediators: The "lymphokines." In: *Immunological Diseases*, edited by M. Samter, pp. 307–324. Little, Brown, Boston.
43. de Vries, R. R. P., Lai, A., Fat, R. F. M., Nijenhuis, L. E., and van Rood, J. J. (1976): HLA-linked genetic control of host response to *Mycobacterium leprae. Lancet*, 2:1328–1330.
44. Dienes, L., and Mallory, T. B. (1932): Histological studies of hypersensitive reactions. *Am. J. Pathol.*, 8:689–710.
45. Djeu, J. Y., McCoy, J. L., Cannon, G. B., Reeves, W. J., West, W. H., and Herberman, R. B. (1976): Lymphocytes forming rosettes with sheep erythrocytes in metastatic pleural effusions. *J. Natl. Cancer Inst.*, 56:1051–1052.
46. Dwyer, J. M., Bullock, W. E., and Fields, J. P. (1973): Disturbance of the blood T:B lymphocyte ratio in lepromatous leprosy. *N. Engl. J. Med.*, 228:1036–1039.
47. Ellner, J. J. (1978): Pleural fluid and peripheral blood lymphocyte function in tuberculosis. *Ann. Intern. Med.*, 89:932–933.
48. Ellner, J. J. (1978): Suppressor adherent cells in human tuberculosis. *J. Immunol.*, 121:2573–2579.
49. Falcào, R. P., and Bottura, C. (1981): A comparative study of lymphocytes in effusions of patients with tuberculosis or malignant disease. *Clin. Exp. Immunol.*, 45:201–204.
50. Favila, L., and Jiménez (1975): In vitro studies of the humoral immune response of mice infected with mycobacterium lepraemurium. *Rev. Lat. Amer. Microbiol.*, 17:101–103.
51. Feldman, M., Beverly, P. C. L., Woody, J. D., and McKenzie, I. F. C. (1977): T-T interactions in the induction of suppressor and helper T cells: Analysis of membrane phenotype of precursor and amplifier cells. *J. Exp. Med.*, 145:793–801.
52. Ford, W. L., and Gowans, J. L. (1969): The traffic of lymphocytes. *Sem. Haematol.*, 6:67–83.
53. Frost, P., and Lance, E. M. (1974): The cellular origin of the lymphocyte trap. *Immunology*, 26:175–186.
53a. Fujiwara, H., Okunda, Y., Fukukawa, T., and Tsuyuguchi, I. (1982): In vitro tuberculin reactivity of lymphocytes from patients with tuberculous pleurisy. *Infect. Immun.*, 35:402–409.
54. Gajl-Peczalska, K. J., Soo Duk Lim, Jacobson, R. R., and Good, R. A. (1973): B lymphocytes in lepromatous leprosy. *N. Engl. J. Med.*, 288:1033–1035.
55. Galindo, B. (1972): Antigen-mediated fusion of specifically sensitized rabbit alveolar macrophages. *Infect. Immun.*, 5:583–594.
56. Galindo, B., Lazdins, J., and Castillo, R. (1974): Fusion of normal rabbit alveolar macrophages induced by supernatant fluids from BCG sensitized lymph node cells after elicitation by antigen. *Infect. Immun.*, 9:212–216.
57. Galindo, B., and Myrvik, Q. N. (1970): Migration inhibition response of granulomatous alveolar cells from BCG-sensitized rabbits. *J. Immunol.*, 105:227–237.
58. Gardner, L. U. (1926): A comparative study of the blood cells in experimental tuberculous primary and reinfections of the lung. *Trans. Natl. Tuberc. Assoc.*, 22:257.
59. George, M., and Vaughan, J. H. (1962): In vitro cell migration as a model for delayed hypersensitivity. *Proc. Soc. Exp. Biol.*, 111:514–521.
60. Gershon, R. K. (1974): T cell control of antibody production. *Contemp. Top. Immunbiol.*, 3:1–40.

61. Gershon, R. K., Eardley, D. D., Naidorf, K. F., and Ptak, W. (1977): The hermaphrocyte: A suppressor-helper T cell. *Cold Spring Harbor Symp. Quant. Biol.*, XLI:85–91.

62. Gershon, R. K., Lance, E. M., and Kondo, K. (1974): Immunoregulatory role of spleen localizing thymocytes. *J. Immunol.*, 112:546–554.

63. Glasser, R. M., Walker, R. I., and Herion, J. C. (1970): The significance of the blood in patients with tuberculosis. *Arch. Intern. Med.*, 125:691–695.

.64. Godal, T., Myklestad, B., Samuel, D. R., and Myrvang, B. (1971): Characterization of the cellular defect in lepromatous leprosy: A specific lack of circulating Mycobacterium leprae-reactive lymphocytes. *Clin. Exp. Immunol.*, 9:821–831.

65. Gowans, J. L. (1959): The recirculation of lymphocytes from blood to lymph in the rat. *J. Physiol. (Lond.)*, 146:54–69.

66. Gowans, J. L., and Knight, E. J. (1964): The route of recirculation of lymphocytes in the rat. *Proc. R. Soc. [Biol.]*, 159:257–282.

67. Guinto, R. S., and Mabalay, M. A. (1962): Note on tuberculin reaction in leprosy. *Int. J. Lepr.*, 30:278–283.

68. Hall, J. G., and Morris, B. (1965): The immediate effect of antigens on the cell output of a lymph node. *Br. J. Exp. Pathol.*, 46:450–454.

69. Han, S. H., Weiser, R. S., and Kau, S. T. (1971): Prolonged survival of skin allografts in leprosy patients. *Int. J. Lepr.*, 39:1–6.

70. Han, S. H., Weiser, R. S., Tseng, J. J., and Kau, S. T. (1971): Lymphocyte transfer reactions in leprosy patients. *Int. J. Lepr.*, 39:715–718.

71. Hirschberg, H. (1978): The role of macrophages in the lymphoproliferative response to Mycobacterium leprae in vitro. *Clin. Exp. Immunol.*, 34:46–51.

72. Hopkins, J., McConnell, I., and Lachmann, P. J. (1981): Specific selection of antigen-reactive lymphocytes into antigenically stimulated lymph nodes in sheep. *J. Exp. Med.*, 153:706–719.

73. Hunninghake, G. W., and Crystal, R. G. (1981): Pulmonary sarcoidosis: A disorder mediated by excess helper T-Lymphocyte activity at sites of disease activity. *N. Engl. J. Med.*, 305:429–434.

74. Hunninghake, G. W., Gadek, J. E., Young, R. C., Jr., Kawanami, O., Ferrans, V. J., and Crystal, R. G. (1980): Maintenance of granuloma formation in pulmonary sarcoidosis by T lymphocytes within the lung. *N. Engl. J. Med.*, 302:594–598.

75. Issekutz, T. B., Chin, W., and Hay, J. B. (1980): Lymphocyte traffic through granulomas: Differences in the recovery of Indium-111-labeled lymphocytes in afferent and efferent lymph. *Cell. Immunol.*, 54:79–86.

76. Jensen, K. A., and Bindslev, G. (1937): Experimental studies on the development of tuberculous infection in allergic and non-allergic animals. II. Development of tuberculous infection in the lungs after inhalation of low-virulent and high-virulent tubercle bacilli. *Acta Tuberc. Scand.*, 11:101–129.

77. Jha, P., Balakrishnan, K., Talwar, G. P., and Bhutani, L. K. (1971): Status of humoral immune responses in leprosy. *Int. J. Lepr.*, 39:20–24.

78. Katz, P., Goldstein, R. A., and Fauci, A. S. (1979): Immunoregulation in infection caused by Mycobacterium tuberculosis: The presence of suppressor monocytes and the alteration of subpopulations of T-lymphocytes. *J. Infect. Dis.*, 140:12–21.

79. Kay, K., and Rieke, W. O. (1963): Tuberculin hypersensitivity: Studies with radioactive antigen and mononuclear cells. *Science*, 139:487–490.

80. Kleinhenz, M. E., Ellner, J. J., Spagnuolo, P. J., and Daniel, T. M. (1981): Suppression of lymphocyte responses by tuberculous plasma and mycobacterial arabinogalactan. *J. Clin. Invest.*, 68:153–162.

81. Kinnman, J., Frydén, A., Eriksson, S., Möller, E., and Link, H. (1981): Tuberculous meningitis: Immune reactions within the central nervous system. *Scand. J. Immunol.*, 13:289–296.

82. Klimpel, G. R., and Henney, C. S. (1978): BCG-induced suppressor cells. I. Demonstration of a macrophage-like suppressor cell that inhibits cytotoxic T cell generation in vitro. *J. Immunol.*, 120:563–569.

83. Koch, R. (1891): Weitere mittheilung über das tuberkulin. *Dtsch. Med. Wochenschr.*, 17:1189–1192.

84. Kohler, G., and Milstein, C. (1975): Continuous cultures of fused cells secreting antibody of predefined specificity. *Nature*, 256:495–497.

85. Koster, F. T., McGregor, D. D., and Mackaness, G. B. (1971): The mediator of cellular immunity.

II. Migration of immunologically committed lymphocytes into inflammatory exudates. *J. Exp. Med.*, 133:400–409.

86. Landsteiner, K., and Chase, M. W. (1942): Experiments on transfer of cutaneous sensitivity to simple chemical compounds. *Proc. Soc. Exp. Biol.*, 49:688–690.

87. Laterre, E. C. (1965): *Les Protéines du Liquide Céphalorachidien á l'état Normal et Patologique.* Arscia, Brussels.

88. Ledbetter, J. A., Evans, R. L., Lipinski, M., Cunningham-Rundles, C., Good, R. A., and Herzenberg, L. A. (1981): Evolutionary conservation of surface molecules that distinguish T lymphocyte helper/inducer and cytotoxic/suppressor subpopulations in mouse and man. *J. Exp. Med.*, 153:310–323.

89. Lefford, M. J. (1975): Transfer of adoptive immunity to tuberculosis in mice. *Infect. Immun.*, 11:1174–1181.

90. Lefford, M. J., McGregor, D. D., and Mackaness, G. B. (1973): Properties of lymphocytes which confer adoptive immunity to tuberculosis in rats. *Immunology*, 25:703–715.

91. Lenzini, L., Rottoli, P., and Rottoli, L. (1977): The spectrum of human tuberculosis. *Clin. Exp. Immunol.*, 27:230–237.

92. Lipscomb, M. F., Lyons, C. R., O'Hara, R. M., and Stein-Streilein, J. (1982): The antigen induced selective recruitment of specific T lymphocytes to the lung. *J. Immunol.*, 128:111–115.

93. Lubaroff, D. M., and Waksman, B. H. (1968): Bone marrow as a source of cells in reactions of cellular hypersensitivity. I. Passive transfer of tuberculin sensitivity in syngeneic systems. *J. Exp. Med.*, 128:1425–1435.

94. Lurie, M. B. (1964): *Resistance to Tuberculosis: Experimental Studies in Native and Acquired Defensive Mechanisms.* Harvard University Press, Cambridge.

95. Mackaness, G. B. (1969): The influence of immunologically committed lymphoid cells of macrophage activity in vivo. *J. Exp. Med.*, 129:973–992.

96. Malaviya, A. N., Sehgal, K. L., Kumar, R., and Dingley, H. B. (1975): Factors of delayed hypersensitivity in pulmonary tuberculosis. *Am. Rev. Respir. Dis.*, 112:49–52.

97. Martins, A. B., and Raffel, S. (1964): Cellular activities in hypersensitive reactions. I. Comparative cytology of delayed 'Jones-Mote,' and Arthus reactions. *J. Immunol.*, 93:937–947.

98. Masih, N., Majeska, J., and Yoshida, T. (1979): Studies on experimental pulmonary granulomas. I. Detection of lymphokines in granulomatous lesions. *Am. J. Pathol.*, 95:391–406.

99. McCluskey, R. T., Benacerraf, B., and McCluskey, J. W. (1963): Studies on the specificity of cellular infiltrate in delayed hypersensitive reactions. *J. Immunol.*, 90:466–477.

100. McMurray, D. N., and Echeverri, A. (1978): Cell-mediated immunity in anergic patients with pulmonary tuberculosis. *Am. Rev. Respir. Dis.*, 118:827–834.

101. Mehra, V., Mason, L. H., Fields, J. P., and Bloom, B. R. (1979): Lepromin-induced suppressor cells in patients with leprosy. *J. Immunol.*, 123:1813–1817.

102. Mehra, V., Mason, L. H., Rothman, W., Reinherz, E., Schlossman, S. F., and Bloom, B. R. (1980): Delineation of a human T cell subset responsible for lepromin-induced suppression in leprosy patients. *J. Immunol.*, 125:1183–1188.

103. Mehra, V. L., Talwar, G. P., Balakrishnan, K., and Bhutani, L. K. (1972): Influence of chemotherapy and serum factors on the mitogenic response of peripheral leukocytes of leprosy patients to phytohaemagglutinin. *Clin. Exp. Immunol.*, 12:205–213.

104. Melamed, M. R., Mullaney, P. F., and Mendelsohn, M. L., editors (1979): *Flow Cytometry and Sorting.* Wiley, New York.

105. Miller, R. A., Coleman, C. N., Fawcett, H. D., Hoppe, R. T., and McDougall, I. R. (1980): Sézary syndrome: A model for migration of T lymphocytes to skin. *N. Engl. J. Med.*, 303:89–92.

106. Mitchell, J. (1973): Lymphocyte circulation in the spleen. Marginal zone bridging channels and their possible role in cell traffic. *Immunology*, 24:93–107.

107. Miyamoto, T., Kabe, J., Noda, M., Kobayashi, N., and Miura, K. (1971): Physiologic and pathologic respiratory changes in delayed type hypersensitivity reaction in guinea pigs. *Am. Rev. Respir. Dis.*, 103:509–515.

108. Moore, V. L., Myrvik, Q. N., and Leake, E. S. (1973): Specificity of a BCG-induced pulmonary granulomatous response in rabbits. *Infect. Immun.*, 7:743–746.

109. Myrvang, B., Godal, T., Ridley, D. S., Fröland, S. S., and Song, Y. K. (1973): Immune responsiveness to Mycobacterium leprae and other mycobacterial antigens throughout the clinical and histopathological spectrum of leprosy. *Clin. Exp. Immunol.*, 14:541–553.

110. Najarian, J. S., and Feldman, J. D. (1963): Specificity of passively transferred hypersensitivity. *J. Exp. Med.*, 118:341–352.

111. Nakamura, R. M., and Tokunaga, T. (1980): Induction of suppressor T cells in delayed-type hypersensitivity to Mycobacterium bovis BCG in low responder mice. *Infect. Immun.*, 28:331–335.

112. Nath, I., Curtiss, J., Sharma, A. K., and Talwar, G. P. (1977): Circulating T-cell numbers and their mitogenic potential in leprosy—Correlation with mycobacterial load. *Clin. Exp. Immunol.*, 29:393–400.

113. Nath, I., Narayanan, R. B., Mehra, N. K., Sharma, A. K., and Gupta, M. D. (1979): Concanavalin A induced suppressor activity in human leprosy. *J. Clin. Lab. Immunol.*, 2:319–324.

114. Nath, I., and Singh, R. (1980): The suppressive effect of M. leprae on the in vitro proliferative responses of lymphocytes from patients with leprosy. *Clin. Exp. Immunol.*, 41:406–414.

115. Nelson, D. S., Nelson, M., Thurston, J. M., Waters, M. F. R., and Pearson, J. M. H. (1971): Phytohemagglutinin-induced lymphocyte transformation in leprosy. *Clin. Exp. Immunol.*, 9:33–43.

116. Niaudet, P., Venet, A., Even, P., and Bach, J. F. (1979): Study of human lymphocyte populations obtained by bronchoalveolar lavage. *Bull. Eur. Physiopathol. Respir.*, 15:27.

117. Nightingale, G., and Hurley, J. V. (1978): Relationship between lymphocyte emigration and vascular endothelium in chronic inflammation. *Pathology*, 10:27–44.

118. North, R. J. (1973): Importance of thymus-derived lymphocytes in cell-mediated immunity to infection. *Cell. Immunol.*, 7:166–176.

119. North, R. J. (1974): T-cell dependence of macrophage activation and mobilization during infection with Mycobacterium tuberculosis. *Infect. Immun.*, 10:66–71.

120. Oppenheim, J. J. (1968): Relationship of in vitro lymphocyte transformation to delayed hypersensitivity in guinea pigs and man. *Fed. Proc.*, 27:21–28.

121. Orbach-Arbouys, S., and Poupon, M. F. (1978): Actual suppression of *in vitro* reactivity of spleen cells after BCG treatment. *Immunology*, 34:431–437.

122. Ormai, S., Hagenbeek, A., Palkovits, M., and van Bekkum, D. W. (1973): Changes of lymphocyte kinetics in the normal rat, induced by the lymphocyte mobilizing agent polymethacrylic acid. *Cell Tissue Kinet.*, 6:407–423.

123. Patel, P. J., and Lefford, M. J. (1978): Antigen specific lymphocytes transformation, delayed hypersensitivity and protective immunity. I. Kinetics of the response. *Cell. Immunol.*, 37:315–326.

124. Pearmain, G., Lycette, R. R., and Fitzgerald, P. H. (1963): Tuberculin-induced mitosis in peripheral blood leucocytes. *Lancet*, 1:637–638.

125. Petterson, T., Klockars, M., Hellstrom, P. E., Riska, H., and Wangel, A. (1978): T and B lymphocytes in pleural effusions. *Chest*, 73:49–51.

126. Plouffe, J. F., Silva, J., Fekety, R., and Baird, J. (1979): Cerebrospinal fluid lymphocyte transformations in meningitis. *Arch. Intern. Med.*, 139:191–194.

127. Poulter, L. W., and Lefford, M. J. (1978): Relationship between delayed-type hypersensitivity and the progression of mycobacterium lepraemurium infection. *Infect. Immun.*, 20:530–540.

128. Ptak, W., Gaugas, J. M., Rees, R. J. W., and Allison, A. C. (1970): Immune responses in mice with murine leprosy. *Clin. Exp. Immunol.*, 6:117–124.

129. Rea, T. H., Bevans, L., and Taylor, C. R. (1980): The histopathology of the spleen from a patient with lepromatous leprosy. *Int. J. Lepr.*, 48:285–290.

130. Reinherz, E. L., Kung, P. C., Goldstein, G., and Schlossman, S. F. (1979): Separation of functional subsets of human T cells by a monoclonal antibody. *Proc. Natl. Acad. Sci. USA*, 76:4061–4065.

131. Reinherz, E. L., and Schlossman, S. F. (1979): Con A-inducible suppression of MLC: Evidence for mediation by the TH_2^+ T cell subset in man. *J. Immunol.*, 122:1335–1341.

132. Reynolds, H. Y., and Merrill, W. W. (1981): Pulmonary immunology: Humoral and cellular immune responsiveness of the respiratory tract: In: *Current Pulmonology*, edited by P. H. Simmons, vol. 3, pp. 381–422. Wiley, New York.

133. Rich, A. (1951): *The Pathogenesis of Tuberculosis*. Charles C Thomas, Springfield.

134. Rich, A. R., and Lewis, M. R. (1932): The nature of allergy in tuberculosis as revealed by tissue culture studies. *Bull. Johns Hopkins Hosp.*, 50:115–128.

135. Rojas-Espinosa, O., Casoluengo-Méndez, M., and Villanueva-Díaz, G. (1976): Antibody-me-

diated immunity in CFW mice infected with mycobacterium lepraemurium. *Clin. Exp. Immunol.*, 25:381–387.

136. Rook, G. A. W. (1975): The immunological consequences of antigen overload in experimental mycobacterial infections of mice. *Clin. Exp. Immunol.*, 19:167–177.

137. Rook, G. A. W., Carswell, J. W., and Stanford, J. L. (1976): Preliminary evidence for the trapping of antigen-specific lymphocytes in the lymphoid tissue of "anergic" tuberculosis patients. *Clin. Exp. Immunol.*, 26:129–132.

138. Sagawa, A., and Abdou, N. I. (1979): Suppressor-cell antibody in systemic lupus erythematosus: Possible mechanism for suppressor cell dysfunction. *J. Clin. Invest.*, 63:536–539.

139. Schlossman, S. F., Levin, H. A., Rocklin, R. E., and David, J. R. (1971): The compartmentalization of antigen-reactive lymphocytes in desensitized guinea pigs. *J. Exp. Med.*, 134:741–750.

140. Sher, N. A., Chaparas, S. D., Greenberg, L. E., Merchant, E. B., and Vickers, J. H. (1975): Response of congenitally athymic (nude) mice to infection with Mycobacterium bovis (strain BCG). *J. Natl. Cancer Inst.*, 54:1419–1424.

141. Shou, L., Schwartz, S. A., and Good, R. A. (1976): Suppressor cell activity after concanavalin A treatment of lymphocytes from normal donors. *J. Exp. Med.*, 143:1100–1110.

142. Skinsnes, O. K. (1968): Comparative pathogenesis of mycobacterioses. *Ann. NY Acad. Sci.*, 154:19–31.

143. Smith, J. B., McIntosh, G. H., and Morris, B. (1970): The migration of cells through chronically inflamed tissues. *J. Pathol.*, 100:21–29.

144. Sören, L. (1979): Suppressor cells induced by purified protein derivative of tuberculin (PPD): The suppression is mediated by cells that proliferate in response to stimulation with PPD. *Scand. J. Immunol.*, 10:171–178.

145. Spencer, J. C., Waldman, R. H., and Johnson, J. E. (1974): Local and systemic cell-mediated immunity after immunization of guinea pigs with live or killed *M. tuberculosis* by various routes. *J. Immunol.*, 112:1322–1328.

146. Stoner, G. L., Touw, J., Atlaw, T., and Belehu, A. (1981): Antigen-specific suppressor cells in subclinical leprosy infection. *Lancet*, 2:1372–1377.

147. Takeya, K., Mori, R., Nomoto, K., and Nakayama, M. (1967): Experimental mycobacterial infections in neonatally thymectomized mice. *Am. Rev. Respir. Dis.*, 96:469–477.

148. Thorsby, E., Godal, T., and Myrvang, B. (1973): HLA antigens and susceptibility to diseases. II. Leprosy. *Tissue Antigens*, 3:373–377.

149. Tsuyuguchi, I., Shiratsuchi, H., Teraoka, O., and Hirano, T. (1980): Increase of T-cells bearing IgG Fc receptor in peripheral blood of patients with tuberculosis by in vitro stimulation with purified protein derivative. *Am. Rev. Respir. Dis.*, 121:951–957.

150. Turcotte, R. (1981): Evidence for two distinct populations of suppressor cells in the spleens of mycobacterium bovis BCG-sensitized mice. *Infect. Immun.*, 34:315–322.

151. Turk, J. L. (1962): The passive transfer of delayed hypersensitivity in guinea pigs by the transfusion of isotopically labeled lymphoid cells. *Immunology*, 5:478–488.

152. Turk, J. L., and Bryceson, A. D. M. (1971): Immunological phenomena in leprosy and related diseases. *Adv. Immunol.*, 13:209–266.

153. Turk, J. L., and Oort, J. (1963): A histological study of the early stages of the development of the tuberculin reaction after passive transfer of cells labeled with ³H thymidine. *Immunology*, 6:140–147.

154. Turk, J. L., and Waters, M. F. R. (1971): Immunological significance of changes in lymph nodes across the leprosy spectrum. *Clin. Exp. Immunol.*, 8:363–376.

155. Twomey, J. J., Laughter, A. H., and Steinberg, A. D. (1978): A serum inhibitor of immune regulation in patients with systemic lupus erythematous. *J. Clin. Invest.*, 62:713–715.

156. Uberoi, S., Malaviya, A. N., Chattopadhyay, C., Kumar, R., and Shrinivas (1975): Secondary immunodeficiency in miliary tuberculosis. *Clin. Exp. Immunol.*, 22:404–408.

157. Virchow, R. (1865): *Die Krankhaften Geschwülste*. Verlag von August, Hirschwald.

158. Wagstaff, J., Gibson, C., Thatcher, N., Ford, W. L., Sharma, H., Benson, W., and Crowther, D. (1981): A method for following human lymphocyte traffic using indium-111 oxine labeling. *Clin. Exp. Immunol.*, 43:435–442.

159. Waldorf, D. S., Sheagren, J. N., Trautman, J. R., and Block, J. B. (1966): Impaired delayed hypersensitivity in patients with lepromatous leprosy. *Lancet*, 2:773–775.

160. Watson, S. R., Šljivić, V. S., and Brown, I. N. (1975): Defect of macrophage function in the

antibody response to sheep erythrocytes in systemic mycobacterium lepraemurium infection. *Nature*, 26:206–208.

161. Wesslén, T. (1952): Passive transfer of tuberculin hypersensitivity by viable lymphocytes from the thoracic duct. *Acta Tuberc. Scand.*, 26:38–53.

162. Williams, R. M., and Waksman, B. H. (1969): Thymus-derived cells in the early phase of delayed tuberculin reactions. *J. Immunol.*, 103:1435–1437.

163. Wu, C.-Y., and Lance, E. M. (1974): Immunoregulation by spleen-seeking thymocytes. II. Role in the response to sheep erythrocytes. *Cell. Immunol.*, 13:1–11.

164. Yamamoto, K., Anacker, R. L., and Ribi, E. (1970): Macrophage migration inhibition studies with cells from mice vaccinated with cell walls of Mycobacterium bovis: Relationship between inhibitory activity of lung cells and resistance to airborne challenge with Mycobacterium tuberculosis H37Rv. *Infect. Immun.*, 1:595–599.

165. Zatz, M. M. (1976): Effects of BCG on lymphocyte trapping. *J. Immunol.*, 116:1587–1591.

166. Zatz, M. M., and Gershon, R. K. (1974): Thymus dependence of lymphocyte trapping. *J. Immunol.*, 112:101–106.

167. Zeitz, S. J., Ostow, J. H., and van Arsdel, P. P., Jr. (1974): Humoral and cellular immunity in the anergic tuberculosis patient. *J. Allergy Clin. Immunol.*, 53:20–26.

168. Zinsser, H. (1925): Bacterial allergy and tissue reactions. *Proc. Soc. Exp. Biol.*, 22:35–39.

Advances in Host Defense Mechanisms, Vol. 2,
edited by John I. Gallin and Anthony S. Fauci.
Raven Press, New York © 1983.

Lymphoid Cells in Immune Surveillance Against Malignant Transformation

Ronald B. Herberman

Laboratory of Immunodiagnosis, National Cancer Institute, National Institutes of Health, Bethesda, Maryland 20205

The role of the immune system in resistance against tumor growth has been the subject of intense interest during the last 10 to 15 years. To a large extent, attention was focused on this issue by the convincing documentation that some tumors in mice had tumor-associated antigens that could be recognized by the host and could thereby induce specific resistance against progressive tumor growth (63,90,143,203). In addition to such tumor-associated transplantation antigens, early workers in tumor immunology looked for and described tumor-specific antigens, i.e., antigens on tumor cells which appeared to be qualitatively different from those on normal cells. Such antigens were reported to be present on a variety of human tumors (91; for reviews, see refs. 107 and 113) as well as on tumors of experimental animals. A further impetus to the field was provided by the development of *in vitro* assays for detecting humoral and cell-mediated immune responses to tumor-associated cell surface antigens. Considerable reactivity was detected in tumor-bearing or tumor-immune individuals, which was often assumed to be directed against the tumor-associated transplantation antigens (reviewed in refs. 106 and 107). These findings led to extensive efforts at immunotherapy and immunodiagnosis of cancer, based on the expectation that these immunologic approaches would rapidly lead to major advances in the clinical management of patients with cancer.

The actual progress in this direction has been generally disappointing; this has led to considerable skepticism regarding the relevance of the immune system to cancer. To realistically appraise the situation and the problems, however, it is important to realize that several different and separate issues are involved. Among the issues of major clinical relevance are: (a) the possible importance of immune surveillance in prevention of detectable tumor development and growth; (b) the possible efficacy of immunotherapy; (c) the possible value of immunologic tests and tumor markers for the detection, diagnosis, and management of cancer patients; and (d) the possible immunosuppressive effects of tumor growth, which could compromise immunologic reactivity against a wide range of microbial and other antigens. This review focuses primarily on the implications related to immune surveillance.

IS THE IMMUNE SURVEILLANCE HYPOTHESIS VALID?

The general role of the immune system in preventing or limiting tumor growth has been emphasized by many investigators, perhaps beginning with Ehrlich (52). Burnet (28) stated that:

> It is by no means inconceivable that small accumulations of tumor cells may develop and because of the possession of new antigenic potentialities provoke an effective immunological reaction with regression of the tumor and no clinical hint of its existence.

Thomas (254) extended the concept further, postulating that the mechanisms for homograft rejection evolved primarily as a natural defense against neoplasia. This theory of immune surveillance has generated many experimental studies and much discussion and controversy. One of the reasons for the controversy is that the concept is rather complex and leads to a series of predictions. For adequate discussion, it is best to consider the available evidence related to each of the predictions. Some of the major predictions are as follows: (a) Tumor cells have antigens, i.e., structures that could be recognized by the immune system and result in reactivity of the host against the tumor, leading to its eventual elimination. (b) The part of the immune system that is involved in the resistance against tumor growth is the same as that involved in rejection of transplants of normal tissues. (c) Immune depression is a necessary antecedent event to the development of detectable tumors. Along this line, (d) immunosuppression would be expected to cause increased susceptibility to tumor development; and (e) one requisite action of carcinogens and/or tumor promoters might be to suppress host defenses.

The main support for the immune surveillance hypothesis has come from evidence related to prediction (d), since naturally occurring or induced immunodepression has been associated with a higher incidence of some types of tumors. In experimental animals, this has been most clearly demonstrated with tumors induced by oncogenic viruses. Polyoma virus is widespread in nature, yet wild mice do not develop polyoma tumors (126). However, administration of the virus to newborn mice of some inbred strains, when their immune system is not fully developed, results in neoplastic growth. Suppression of immunity, particularly by procedures that affect thymus-dependent immune responses, has been shown to greatly increase the incidence of polyoma tumors (4,6,153–155).

Similarly, neonatal thymectomy of chickens results in an increased frequency of tumors in strains that are genetically resistant to the malignant effects of Marek disease virus (194). Treatment with antilymphocyte serum potentiated murine leukemia virus-induced tumors and shortened the latent period of spontaneous leukemia in AKR mice (6). There is also considerable clinical evidence that immunodepression is associated with an increased incidence of immune deficiency diseases and lymphomas and leukemia (47,65). Gatti and Good (70) estimated that the incidence of tumors in these patients was about 10,000 times that seen in the general age-matched population. Allograft recipients receiving immunosuppressive agents, mainly prednisone and azathioprine, have also been found to have an increased incidence (approximately 100 times that of the general age-matched population) of tumors (87,195). Again lymphomas have been prominent, but the majority of the tumors have been of epithelial origin.

Patients with Hodgkin's disease or other types of cancer or patients with arthritis or other benign diseases who received chemotherapeutic (mainly alkylating) agents have been subsequently found to develop primary malignancies, mainly leukemias and lymphomas, with relatively high frequency (32,129,204,206,217,251).

The effects of immunosuppression on tumor induction in experimental animals by chemical carcinogens have been even less clear-cut (242). In some studies, an increased incidence of tumors was seen (e.g., refs. 12 and 86). Lappé (152), in a study involving isografts of methylcholanthrene-treated skin, found fewer tumors in immunocompetent mice and also found evidence for microscopic regressions of tumors. Haran-Ghera and Lurie (103), however, did not find an increased incidence of tumors due to dimethylbenzanthracene in mice treated with antilymphocyte serum. Similarly, there has been a general failure to observe more rapid tumor growth or even higher incidences of carcinogen-induced tumors in nude mice (243). One possible explanation for such negative findings has been that the carcinogenic agents themselves are immunosuppressive, and additional suppression may not have an incremental effect. The data on this point [prediction (e)], in regard to the possible effects on mature T cells and humoral immunity, have been conflicting (summarized in ref. 242).

A likely explanation for many of the discrepant results regarding the possible association of immune depression and tumor development is that various effector mechanisms might be involved in host resistance. Results might vary with the type of effector mechanism that plays a predominant role with each form of cancer and with the nature and extent of the immune deficiency.

Such a likelihood of diversity of effector mechanisms that might be involved in immune surveillance may be offered as a response to most of the criticisms that have been raised against the hypothesis. When information about thymus-dependent immunity became known, and particularly when T cells were found to play a central role in allograft rejection, the immune surveillance hypothesis was modified to stress the key role of this effector mechanism in antitumor resistance (29). Related to this has been the emphasis placed on expression in tumors of tumor-associated transplantation antigens, since such structures would have to be recognized by T cells in order to get effective T cell-mediated resistance to tumor growth. It has only been possible to obtain strong evidence for a major *in vivo* role of T cells in immunity to virus-induced tumors (21,37,77,81), however, and little comparable evidence exists for spontaneous tumors or even for transplantable chemical carcinogen-induced tumors. Much attention has been given to the decreased incidence of mouse mammary tumors in neonatally thymectomized mice (241,271). There also has been a failure to detect tumor-associated transplantation antigens on many spontaneous tumors (117).

These observations have led to the suggestion (141) that immune surveillance may be operative only against tumors induced by oncogenic viruses, which have strong transplantation antigens and for which immune T cells have been shown to be important in resistance. Other investigators have reacted to such information in a more pessimistic way; e.g., Nossal (180) suggested that immune surveillance and tumor immunology in general were moribund if not terminally ill. The major exceptions to the central role of immune T cells in resistance to tumor growth have even led to a countertheory of immunostimulation (202), suggesting that the immune system may have mainly enhancing effects on tumor induction and growth. When T cell-mediated immunity is viewed as only one of a series of possible host defense mechanisms, however, the evidence summarized above need not be viewed in such a negative light. Target cell structures other than tumor-associated transplantation antigens might be involved in recognition by other types of effector cells; and in T cell-deficient individuals, the other effector mechanisms might still be functional and capable of resisting tumor growth.

What then are the likely alternatives to T cell-mediated immunity in antitumor resistance and immune surveillance? There are a variety of possibilities, including macrophages, natural killer (NK) cells, other related natural effector cells, and antibody-dependent cellular cytotoxicity (ADCC). The evidence in support of a role of each is summarized below.

POSSIBLE ROLE OF MACROPHAGES IN IMMUNE SURVEILLANCE

The observations that activated macrophages could have substantial cytotoxicity against a variety of tumor cell lines and the evidence that transformed cells were selectively susceptible to such attack led rapidly to suggestions by many investigators that macrophages might play an important role in antitumor defenses and might be primarily responsible for immune surveillance against tumors (1,10,41,61,118,121–123). It has been pointed out by several authors that an immune surveillance role of macrophages would overcome most of the arguments that have been raised against the immune surveillance hypothesis (1), and that the characteristics of cytotoxicity by macrophages fit most of the requirements for an ideal model antitumor effector cell (121).

To continue to consider seriously a possible role for macrophages in antitumor defenses, it is important to go beyond the theoretical considerations and generate experimental data in support of various testable predictions regarding an important role for macrophages. Among such predictions are the following: (a) macrophages should be able to enter the site of tumor growth; (b) selective depression of macrophage function should be associated with an increased incidence of tumors; (c) selective augmentation of macrophage function, or selective adoptive transfer of macrophages, should be associated with a decreased incidence of tumors; and (d) one of the requisite effects of carcinogen-inducing tumors controlled by macrophages should be to depress macrophage function. It would be particularly important to obtain experimental data concerning these predictions in regard to the development of spontaneous or carcinogen-induced primary tumors. However, most of the available information has been from studies with transplantable tumor lines and often with a therapy protocol rather than a protocol for prevention of tumor development. Nevertheless, it is worthwhile to consider the available data and their limitations and then discuss the types of further experiments that are needed.

There is abundant evidence that macrophages can accumulate in considerable numbers in a variety of transplantable tumors (51,55) and in many primary tumors (2,71,156). The possibility of a functional antitumor role for such cells was supported by observations that the degree of *in situ* infiltration of primary tumors by macrophages was inversely correlated with a tendency toward metastatic spread of the tumors (2). More extensive examination of this issue has resulted in a considerable amount of contradictory evidence, however, indicating no correlation between the number of macrophages within a tumor and the metastatic potential of the tumor (summarized in ref. 58). This had led to the opposite suggestion, that the presence of macrophages within some tumors may promote their growth and metastasis (56,57).

A frequent experimental approach has been to examine the effects of macrophage-depressive treatments on the growth of tumors. Growth of some transplantable tumors, and particularly their tendency to metastasize, was found to be increased when the recipients were treated with silica, carrageenan, trypan blue, or gold salts (59,75,135,174,237), agents that have been shown to deplete macrophages or interfere with their functions (5,74,119,120). Similarly, Wood and Gillespie (269) showed that *in vitro* damage to macrophages in a tumor inoculum resulted in an increased incidence of metastases. Such treatments also have been shown to augment the development of some primary tumors. Silica treatment of mice during the period of exposure to ultraviolet light was shown to increase the incidence of resultant skin tumors (179); treatment with silica, carrageenan, or antimacrophage serum enhanced Friend virus-induced leukemogenesis (171). Similarly, repeated inoculations of silica into AKR mice resulted in earlier development of spontaneous leukemia (35).

It should be noted that there are some major limitations to such evidence: (a) Silica and carrageenan, and possibly the other depressive treatments as well, may not be entirely selective in their effects. In fact, they may cause increases in some functions, particularly suppressor activity, by macrophages or other cells (40); and these agents can directly or indirectly depress the functions of other cell types, e.g., NK cells (45,183). (b) The effects of such treatments on tumor growth are not always in the same direction, even with the same tumor. For example, Mantovani et al. (170) found that treatment of mice with silica or carrageenan increased the incidence of pulmonary metastases but inhibited the growth of the primary tumors. By using another treatment, sublethal irradiation with 400 rads, which resulted in a decrease for several weeks in the macrophage content in fibrosarcomas, Evans (57) observed a parallel retardation of growth of the tumors.

The converse line of evidence, indicating a decrease in tumor growth after treatment with agents that can stimulate the function of macrophages, has often been taken as a further demonstration of the important role of macrophages in antitumor defenses (156). For example, administration of pyran copolymer (179) has been shown to inhibit the development of ultraviolet light-induced skin tumors. However, a major limitation to such an approach is that almost all the agents used for stimulation of macrophages also can have substantial effects on the activity of other potential effector mechanisms. In particular, such treatments usually cause interferon production and a consequent augmentation of NK activity (109,110).

A more direct approach has involved the adoptive transfer of activated macrophages. Fidler (60) showed that transfer of macrophages that had been activated *in vitro* could interfere with the metastatic spread of tumor cells. Similarly, transfer of *in vivo* activated macrophages had protective effects (158,237). However, even such data do not conclusively demonstrate a direct effector role for macrophages, since activated macrophages are known to produce interferon and other products that might act to stimulate other effector cells, particularly NK cells (45).

Other suggestive pieces of evidence must be considered in regard to the possible role of macrophages in antitumor defenses. Although there are some exceptions, there is generally higher reticuloendothelial activity in strains of mice with low tumor incidence than in high tumor incidence strains (summarized in ref. 238). It is also noteworthy that a variety of agents that are taken up by the reticuloendothelial system and that have been shown to be macrophage toxic can induce tumors. Administration of trypan blue to mice has been shown to cause hepatic sarcomas of the Kupffer cells (192) and reticulum cell sarcomas (76). Carrageenan, polyvinylpyrrolidone, dextran, and CM cellulose have been shown to induce sarcomas, reticulum cell sarcomas, or lymphosarcomas (127,128,267). However, these results may not bear on the issue of the involvement of macrophages in immune surveillance, since at least some of the tumors appear to involve macrophages themselves and therefore seem to be a reflection of transformation following direct damage to this cell population. Of greater interest is whether other types of carcinogens, which cause tumors of other cell types, cause depression of macrophage function during the latent period, prior to the detectable appearance of tumors. Most such studies on this point measured reticuloendothelial clearance or phagocytosis by macrophages *in vitro* rather than macrophage-mediated cytotoxicity or other functions; the results of these studies have been mixed. Some carcinogens (methylcholanthrene and acetylaminofluorene) have been shown to decrease reticuloendothelial functions (8,59,238,253,256), whereas others (dimethylbenzanthracene, urethane, and methylnitrosourea) have had no detectable effects (64,273).

Overall, the available evidence regarding a role of macrophages in immune surveillance is fragmentary and incomplete. Adams and Snyderman (1) have summarized the current status well:

> The extant data support but do not controvert the hypothesis that macrophages exert surveillance. However, the experiments to test this proposition vigorously have not been performed.

What then are the needed experiments? Perhaps the most compelling series of experiments would be to produce a selective depression in macrophage function, or to utilize animals with a selective genetic defect in macrophage function, and to determine whether such animals have an increased incidence of spontaneous tumors or of carcinogen-induced tumors. To overcome the likelihood that in most cases the abnormalities would not be limited to macrophages, it then would be important to show that selective reconstitution of the animals with macrophages could decrease or eliminate any increased incidence of tumors. Another approach would be to obtain extensive evidence as to whether carcinogens cause a decrease in macrophage functions, especially cytotoxic activity, during the latent period and, if so, whether a selective restoration of macrophage function would interfere with carcinogenesis. Yet another direction would be to identify treatments that could selectively increase macrophage functions without altering other effector functions (e.g., noninterferon-inducing agents) and then to determine whether this would be associated with a decrease in the incidence of spontaneous or carcinogen-induced tumors.

Possible Role of NK Cells or Other Related Natural Effector Cells in Immune Surveillance

There is substantial evidence for an important role of NK cells in *in vivo* resistance against established cell lines of tumors, particularly those that show susceptibility to *in vitro* cytolysis by NK cells.

A major approach has been to look for correlations between *in vivo* resistance to the growth of the tumor cell lines and the levels of NK activity in the recipients. In several different situations, a good correlation was observed. Some NK-sensitive tumor lines have produced a lower incidence of tumors and have grown more slowly in nude or thymectomized mice than in euthymic mice with the same genetic background (111,140,214). Fewer transplantable tumors also have been induced in 5- to 10-week-old mice at the peak of NK activity than in older mice with low NK activity (111,229).

Some recent studies have examined the effects of age on growth of several transplantable tumors in nude mice. A much higher incidence of metastases, after either intravenous or subcutaneous transplantation, was seen in 3-week-old nude mice that had low NK activity than in 6-week-old nude mice that had high NK activity. A high rate of pulmonary metastases in young nude recipients was seen with xenogeneic as well as allogeneic tumor cell lines (99,101). Augmentation of NK activity in the 3-week-old nude mice, by treatment with poly I:C or *C. parvum*, inhibited the development of metastases. The apparent major role for NK cells in resistance in nude mice against growth of transplantable tumors and the ability to circumvent this by using nude mice with low NK activity have practical implications for the strong interest in utilizing nude mice for growth of human tumors. Many investigators have noted the difficulty to grow some tumors in nude mice and the rarity of metastases, even when metastatic deposits of human tumors were transplanted (33,167,190,224,227,231). The findings that some human tumor cells are susceptible to mouse NK activity (96,181) are consistent with a role for NK cells in this resistance.

Kiessling and his associates (139,197) performed an extensive series of experiments which demonstrated a correlation between the levels of NK activity in different strains of mice and the resistance of F_1 hybrids between each strain and A mice to the A strain lymphoma, YAC, the cultured line of which is highly sensitive to NK activity. Mice that were thymectomized, irradiated, and reconstituted with fetal liver also showed this resistance (140). Haller et al. (97) extended this approach by transferring bone marrow cells from high or low NK strains to lethally irradiated low NK recipients. Recipients of cells from high NK donors developed high NK activity and had increased resistance to growth of YAC.

The various types of correlation described above have been observed only with tumor lines with some susceptibility to lysis by NK cells. The growth of completely NK-resistant cell lines has not been affected by the levels of NK activity in the recipients (214). It is of interest in this regard that in a study of two sublines of a mouse lung tumor, the metastatic subline was resistant to NK activity, whereas the nonmetastatic subline showed some susceptibility (82).

Beige mice, with low NK activity associated with their recessive point mutation (218), also have provided a convenient model for examining the role of NK cells in resistance to growth of transplantable tumor lines. Talmadge et al. (249) found that an NK-susceptible syngeneic melanoma cell line grew more rapidly and produced more metastases in beige compared to normal mice. This difference was not seen with an NK-resistant subline of the same tumor. Using a similar approach, Kärre et al. (133) found that two NK-susceptible syngeneic lymphomas produced a higher incidence of tumors and grew more rapidly in beige than in normal heterozygous littermates.

Another approach to the *in vivo* role of NK cells in the growth of transplantable tumors has been the attempt to transfer increased resistance by NK cell-enriched populations. Kasai et al. (134) enriched Ly 5^+ spleen cells and depleted Thy 1^+ and B cells and showed that this small subpopulation of cells had high NK activity. Mixture of these Ly 5^+ cells with an NK-sensitive lymphoma cell line resulted in reduced tumor incidence after transplantation. Similarly, local adoptive tranfer of NK-1^+ cells suppressed growth of the YAC lymphoma (250). Systemic adoptive transfer of cells, with the characteristics of NK cells, from normal or nude mice was also found in an immunochemotherapy model system to increase protection against a transplantable leukemia (34).

In an alternative approach that utilized information about selective markers on mouse NK cells, Habu et al. (93) administered antiasialo GM1 to nude mice. The treated mice had almost no detectable NK activity and showed increased susceptibility to transplantation of syngeneic, allogeneic, and human tumors.

Although the above studies point to a significant role of NK cells in resistance against tumor growth, they do not show conclusively that NK cells are the actual *in vivo* effector cells. Since these studies relied on measurement of tumor incidence or growth rate at a considerable time after tumor challenge, one cannot rule out the possibility that NK cells helped to induce or recruit other effector mechanisms, such as T cells or activated macrophages. To obtain more direct information about the role of NK cells in the direct and rapid *in vivo* elimination of tumor cells, ^{125}I-iododeoxyuridine ([125]IUdR)-labeled tumor cells were inoculated intravenously, and clearance from the lungs and other organs was measured (210,212,213). In young mice of strains with high NK activity, there was a greater clearance of radioactivity when measured at 2 to 4 hr after inoculation than was seen in strains with low reactivity. In parallel with the decline of NK activity in mice after 10 to 12 weeks of age, *in vivo* clearance of intravenously inoculated tumor cells was also found to decrease. Furthermore, treatment of mice with a variety of agents that produced augmented or decreased *in vitro* reactivity also resulted in similar shifts in *in vivo* reactivity. Such correlations were observed with several NK-susceptible tumor lines and not with some completely NK-resistant lines (213).

As further confirmation of the role of NK cells in resistance to growth of NK-susceptible transplantable tumors, transfer of NK cell-containing populations into mice with cyclophosphamide-induced depression of NK activity was shown to significantly restore both *in vivo* clearance and NK reactivity (209,211). The effectiveness of the transfer correlated with the levels of NK activity of donor cells in a variety of situations: (a) NK-reactive spleen cells were able to transfer reactivity, whereas NK-unreactive thymus cells were ineffective; (b) spleen cells from young mice of high NK strains were considerably more effective than cells from older mice or from strains with low NK activity; (c) the cells responsible for transfer had the characteristics of NK cells, being nonadherent, nonphagocytic, expressing asailo GM1 and lacking easily detectable Thy 1 antigen; and (d) cells from donors with drug-induced depression of NK activity were unable to transfer reactivity. These results extend the recent findings of Hanna and Fidler (100), who showed that the transfer of NK-reactive spleen cells to cyclophosphamide-treated mice could decrease the number of metastases developing in the lungs after challenge with NK-susceptible solid tumor cells.

A similar pattern of results was obtained when radiolabeled cells were inoculated subcutaneously into the footpads of mice (83). Clearance correlated in several ways with the levels of NK activity in the recipients, and cells with the characteristics of NK cells were effective in local adoptive transfer. In contrast to NK activity and the results with intravenously inoculated tumor cells, however, no decrease in clearance was observed in older or beige mice. Those results suggest that other effector cells also may be involved in reactivity in subcutaneous tissues [e.g., the natural cytotoxic cells described by Stutman et al. (191,245,246)], or that in some situations, local factors may augment the NK cell activity.

Although the results in some studies, particularly those with intravenously inoculated radiolabeled tumor cells, suggested that NK cells may be particularly involved in resistance against hematogenous metastatic spread of tumors (100), the results with the footpad assay (83) and the various demonstrations of NK-related differences in outgrowth of subcutaneous tumors indicate that natural effector cells can enter and be active at sites of local tumor growth. This is supported by the direct demonstration of NK cells in cell suspensions prepared from small tumors growing at subcutaneous or intramuscular locations (72). Thus NK cells have the potential to be involved in the primary line of defense against both the local outgrowth as well as the metastatic spread of transplanted tumors. However, the effectiveness of this natural resistance mechanism is rather limited. Even with tumor cells that are highly susceptible to NK activity, development of progressively growing tumors can occur in animals with high NK activity.

From the evidence summarized above, it is likely that NK cells play an important role in resistance to growth and metastatic spread of some tumor cell lines. Although such results are encouraging, they do not indicate whether NK cells also can have a similar role in defense against growth and metastasis of primary tumors. To obtain evidence in support of such a function, it would be desirable to document the following predictions: (a) Primary tumor cells should have some demonstrable susceptibility to recognition by NK cells. (b) The NK cells of tumor-bearing individuals should be able, under some circumstances, to interact with the autologous tumor. (c) Selective alterations in NK activity in tumor-bearing individuals should affect the growth or degree of metastatic spread of the tumors.

Unfortunately, information relevant to any of these points is scanty, and, to my knowledge, no clear data exist for the last prediction. Before reviewing the available evidence regarding NK reactivity against primary tumor cells, I point out the difficulties that would be anticipated if NK cells were playing a significant role in growth of primary tumors. For such studies, one would have to obtain tumors of sufficient size to prepare adequate numbers of tumor cells. By definition, such tumors had to have been at least relatively successful in evading host defense mechanisms. Therefore, if NK cells play an important role in resistance, tumor outgrowth would only occur in the face of relative resistance to lysis by NK cells and/or depression of NK activity. Thus the observation most consistent with these qualifications of the earlier stated predictions would be detectable but low levels of interaction between NK cells and tumor cells.

Some evidence has accumulated in this direction. The majority of spontaneous mammary tumors of C3H mice (230) and of spontaneous lymphomas in AKR mice (182) have been found to have detectable, albeit low, susceptibility to lysis by NK cells. Similarly, some human leukemias (9,222,272), a myeloma (9), and some carcinomas, sarcomas, and melanomas (169,262) have been significantly lysed by NK cells. Such lysis has been appreciably augmented and thereby evident with a higher proportion of tumors when the effector cells were pretreated with interferon (9,169,262,272). As further support for the ability of NK cells to recognize primary tumor cells, Ortaldo et al. (188) showed that a variety of human tumor cells could cold target inhibit the lysis of radiolabeled K562 cells. Most of these positive results were obtained with NK cells from normal allogeneic donors. In fact, Vánky et al. (262) detected NK reactivity only against allogeneic human tumor cells and concluded that the NK cells of the tumor-bearing individual lacked the ability to recognize the autologous tumor cells. The authors postulated that recognition of foreign histocompatibility antigens was involved in lysis by NK cells, particularly those stimulated by interferon. If correct, their hypothesis would virtually preclude a role for NK cells in resistance against primary tumor growth. However, such restriction of NK reactivity to allogeneic tumors does not fit the many examples of tumor cell lines being susceptible to syngeneic NK cells (114,138).

Likewise, normal C3H mice have been found to be reactive against some syngeneic mammary tumors (230), and some cancer patients also have had detectable, interferon-augmentable NK activity against their autologous tumor cells (169). The reasons for the discrepancies among the human studies are not clear. The positive results were obtained with ovarian carcinoma cells, mainly in 20 hr cytotoxicity assays (169), whereas the allorestricted results involved other types of tumors, tested only in 4 hr assays. The greater sensitivity of the prolonged assay would seem sufficient to account for the differences. In addition, it is possible that the subpopulation of NK cells that are required to interact with certain types of tumors may be selectively inhibited in the autologous tumor-bearing host.

Another line of evidence in support of the possibility of NK cells interacting *in vivo* with autologous primary tumor cells is the demonstration that NK cells can enter and accumulate at the site of tumor growth. They have been detected in small spontaneous mouse mammary carcinomas (72) and in small primary mouse tumors induced by murine sarcoma virus (17,72). In contrast, NK activity usually has been undetectable in large tumors in mice (72) or in clinical tumor specimens. This may be due, at least in part, to the presence of suppressor cells, which have been demonstrated in some cell suspensions from some tumors (3,54,72,73,266).

To further support the possible role of NK cells in resistance against the growth of primary tumors, the effects of selective alterations of NK activity in tumor-bearers should be examined. However, few experiments specifically designed to examine this issue have been reported. Suggestive evidence has come from the administration of indomethacin to mice bearing primary murine sarcoma virus-induced tumors (25). With a treatment schedule that augmented the depressed NK reactivity, tumor incidence and size were reduced, and a higher proportion of tumors completely regressed. Also, one could invoke the therapeutic efficacy of interferon for some primary tumors, a treatment known to augment NK reactivity. The limitations of such data are that such agents have pleiotropic effects, and it is not possible to determine whether the alterations in other functions had the more important influence on tumor growth. Studies with more selective alterations in NK activity will be needed to settle this issue. Such experiments probably should be performed in individuals with only a small amount of tumor present, to allow the detection of effects on tumor growth that might be more likely during a phase when the host is not already overwhelmed by extensive tumor burden.

Of paramount interest is whether NK cells may be involved in immune surveillance against the initial development of spontaneous or carcinogen-induced tumors. Thus far, few well-designed experiments have been performed to directly address this issue. Before turning to those, it is of interest to summarize several pieces of circumstantial evidence that are consistent with, or suggestive of, a role for NK cells: (a) NK activity has been shown to be substantially augmented by retinoic acid (79), which has been reported to retard the development of some primary tumors (160). In support of this possibility, cells with the characteristics of NK cells have been found to inhibit the *in vitro* proliferation of autologous Epstein-Barr virus (EBV)-infected B cells (235). (b) Patients with the genetically determined

Chediak-Higashi syndrome have a high risk of development of lymphoproliferative diseases (44). In recent detailed studies on several patients with this disease (219,220), all were found to have profound deficits in NK and K cell activities, whereas a variety of other immune functions, including cytotoxicity against tumor cells by T cells, monocytes, and granulocytes, were essentially normal. (c) Beige mice, which have an analogous genetic defect, also have a substantial (218,221), but incomplete (25,39), selective deficiency in NK activity. A small colony of aged beige mice have been reported to have a high incidence of lymphomas (163). (d) Another human genetic abnormality, X-linked lymphoproliferative disease (205), has been associated with a defect in the ability to control proliferation of B cells infected with EBV. Recently, low NK activity has been found in such individuals, and this deficit has been suggested to be involved in the pathogenesis of the disease (247). (e) Patients on immunosuppressive therapy after kidney allotransplants have a high risk of developing reticuloendothelial tumors and a variety of carcinomas (195). Patients on such treatment regimens have been found to have low NK activity; this has been suggested as a contributing factor to the subsequent development of tumors (159,261). Each of these lines of evidence fits one of the major predictions of the immune surveillance theory, that tumor development would be associated with, and in fact preceded by, depressed immunity.

In regard to the prediction of the immune surveillance theory that carcinogenic agents would cause depressed immune function, the initial and still fragmentary data in relation to NK cells are promising. (a) Urethane, which produces lung tumors in only some strains of mice, caused transient and marked depression of NK activity in a susceptible strain (84) but not in resistant strains (85). Administration of normal bone marrow cells, which as discussed earlier can reconstitute NK activity, to urethane-treated mice reduced the subsequent development of lung tumors (144; E. Gorelik and R. B. Herberman, *unpublished observations*). Also, infection during the latent period with various viruses, each known to induce interferon and thereby augment NK activity, also reduced the incidence of lung tumors induced by urethane. (b) Carcinogenic doses of dimethylbenzanthracene also were found to produce depression of NK activity during the latent period (53). (c) Sublethal irradiation of mice has been found to cause considerable depression of NK activity (124). Of particular interest, the schedule of multiple low doses of irradiation of C57BL mice, which has been highly effective in inducing leukemia in this strain, was found to produce a substantial deficit in NK activity (193; E. Gorelik and R. B. Herberman, *unpublished observations*). The depressed NK activity could be restored by transfer of normal bone marrow cells (E. Gorelik and R. B. Herberman, *unpublished observations*), a procedure that has been reported to interfere with radiation-induced leukogenesis (132). In contrast, transfer of bone marrow from beige mice did not restore NK activity. (d) NK activity also has been strongly inhibited by two different classes of potent tumor promoters: phorbol esters (79,136) and teleocidin (R. H. Goldfarb, T. Sugimura, and R. B. Herberman, *unpublished observations*). All these observations support the possibility that one of the requisites for tumor induction by carcinogenic agents may be interference with host defenses, including those mediated by NK cells.

Further studies are needed to more directly demonstrate a role for NK cells in immune surveillance. Ideally, one would like to show increased tumorigenesis when NK activity is selectively depressed and reduced tumor formation when such deficiencies are selectively reconstituted or normal levels of reactivity are selectively augmented.

Several practical problems limit vigorous pursuit of such experimental protocols. In addition to the long periods of time needed for such studies and the difficulties in identifying the most relevant experimental carcinogenesis models, completely selective and sustained alterations of NK activity are not easily found or produced. For example, as discussed above, much attention is currently being given to the beige mouse model as a test system for oncogenesis in NK-deficient animals. However, beige mice have some residual NK activity, which can be augmented by interferon (25) and which can approach normal levels upon prolonged incubations with target cells (39). Furthermore, they appear to have normal levels of natural cytotoxic (NC) activity *in vitro* against some monolayer tumor target cells (30) and *in vivo* against subcutaneous inoculations of both lymphoma and carcinoma cell lines (79). In addition, the rate of cytotoxicity by macrophages is somewhat retarded (168), so that an increased tumor incidence in beige mice could not be definitively attributed to the deficit in NK activity. Conversely, induction of interferon or other procedures to augment NK activity generally alter other immune functions as well. Yet another, and perhaps the most central, limitation to the use of beige mice or other NK-deficient mice to evaluate the role of NK cells in prevention of carcinogenesis is that many of the carcinogens themselves can strongly inhibit NK activity. Thus after treatment with a carcinogen, the normal recipients may have as low NK activity as the beige mice; therefore, differences in tumor development might not be seen. The most convincing protocol might be to reconstitute animals with depressed NK activity by adoptive transfer of purified NK cells and determine the effects on carcinogenesis.

In addition to the above evidence for a role of NK cells in antitumor defenses, there are some recent indications for a possible role of the related NC cells of mice that have been found to react primarily with solid tumor cell lines (30,191,244). A good correlation has been seen between *in vitro* susceptibility to lysis by NC cells of recently derived transplantable, chemically induced fibrosarcomas and the cell dose required to produce local tumors *in vivo* (245). These investigators also tested the prediction that if NC cells were involved in immune surveillance, tumors induced *in vivo* by chemical carcinogens would be more resistant to lysis by NC cells than would *in vitro* transformed cells not exposed to such selective pressure by *in vivo* NC cells. Indeed, several *in vitro* transformed lines were quite susceptible to lysis by NC cells. A further tested prediction was that NC cells should be able to enter the site of locally growing tumors; indeed, they were detected within two transplantable sarcomas (246). Such evidence clearly is scanty and does not bear directly on the possible involvement in immune surveillance but does support the possible involvement of NC cells in *in vivo* antitumor resistance.

POSSIBLE ROLE OF ADCC IN IMMUNE SURVEILLANCE

In addition to any direct cytotoxic effects on tumor cells, macrophages (104,137), polymorphonuclear cells (PMNs) (68,94,157), and NK (K) cells (150,186,257) may also act in cooperation with antibodies to produce ADCC. ADCC has been detected against a variety of experimental (22,102,104,148,149,200) and human (95,131) tumors. Also, phagocytosis of tumor cells by macrophages or PMNs may occur and be dependent on the presence of antitumor antibodies (137); but there is very little evidence for a significant role of ADCC or antibody-dependent phagocytosis in *in vivo* antitumor resistance. This is probably due in large part to difficulties in distinguishing between ADCC and the direct antitumor effects of antibodies or various effector cells.

In a variety of experimental tumor systems (reviewed in refs. 116 and 258), *in vivo* administration of antibodies has resulted in some protection against progressive tumor growth, and it has often been suggested that ADCC was a major mechanism for the observed effects. However, in only a few studies has evidence been provided to support this possibility. Furthermore, most of the supportive data are indirect and not conclusive. For example, tumor cells isolated from antibody-producing mice have been shown to be coated with antibodies and thereby susceptible to cytotoxicity by macrophages (104). Also, mice inoculated with tumor-protective hyperimmune serum along with an ascites tumor cell line have been shown to have considerable numbers of rosettes of macrophages with tumor cells (151); this correlated with *in vitro* evidence for macrophage-mediated ADCC. Phagocytosed tumor cells within macrophages also have been noted at the site of tumor growth (137).

Shin and his associates (232–234) used a somewhat more direct approach to support an *in vivo* role for ADCC by alloantibodies. IgG antibodies were shown to have limited effects on mice with larger tumor burdens. This appeared to be related to a shortage of macrophages at the tumor site, since efficacy could be restored by local addition of macrophages. Although it has been difficult to obtain convincing evidence for an *in vivo* antitumor role of ADCC, the following approach might be expected to provide substantially better insight into the possible importance of this mechanism. In a tumor system in which *in vivo* administration of antibodies could be shown to have protective effects, normal recipients of antibodies and tumor cells could be compared with animals selectively depleted of one or another type of potential effector cells. Loss of efficacy of antibodies, for example, in animals with selective deficits in NK cells or macrophages would point toward an important collaboration between these components of the immune system. Further evidence for mediation of antitumor effects by ADCC would be provided by restoration of antibody activity by adoptive transfer of a purified effector cell population into the deficient recipients.

Clearly, since there is such a paucity of evidence for an *in vivo* role of ADCC with tumor cell lines, the question of a possible involvement of this mechanism in immune surveillance becomes highly speculative. This effector mechanism should at least be kept in mind, and appropriate investigative studies should be done. This is particularly relevant for the natural effector cells, since treatments that alter their direct cytotoxic activity have also tended to cause a parallel alteration in their capacity for ADCC. Furthermore, in addition to the possible role for antibodies specifically induced by tumor-associated antigens, natural antitumor antibodies have been demonstrated (35,36,125,172,175), which might interact with effector cells and mediate ADCC. It should be noted that virtually all the evidence discussed above for a possible role of macrophages or NK cells in immune surveillance would also be compatible with the mediation of their effects by collaboration with such natural antibodies.

MECHANISMS BY WHICH TUMORS MAY ESCAPE IMMUNE ATTACK

Despite the multiplicity of potential antitumor effector mechanisms, it is important to note that once tumors become detectable, they usually grow progressively and result in the death of the host. Therefore, attention must be given to the mechanisms for the frequent failure of the immune system to adequately control tumor growth. A variety of mechanisms have been observed or suggested to account for insufficient host defenses, and these are briefly discussed below.

Immunoresistance of Tumor Cells

One major factor may be resistance of tumor cells to attack by immune mech-anisms, rather than an actual lack of the necessary structures and factors for possible recognition and interaction. It has been found in a number of studies that for tumor cells to be able to react with antibodies or immune cells, they must have sufficient quantities or densities of the relevant tumor-associated cell surface antigens (142,259). Tumor cells with subthreshold amounts of these antigens are immunoresistant. The loss or rapid shedding of cell surface antigens from tumor cells has been suggested as a possible explanation for the failure of such antigens to function as tumor-associated transplantation antigens (11). One well-studied mechanism in this area is antigenic modulation (187). This mechanism was originally described with TL antigen. This tumor-associated surface antigen is quite immunogenic in some strains of mice but does not function as a transplantation antigen, since exposure of tumor cells to anti-TL antibody causes a reversible loss of antigen. Some oncofetal antigens have been shown to undergo antigenic modulation (189); this may explain why they usually fail to be involved in resistance against tumor growth. Similarly, surface antigens associated with Gross leukemia virus have been found to be lost, or at least decreased in expression, during *in vivo* growth of tumors but returned upon *in vitro* cultivation (7,130).

This issue of immunoresistance has been shown to be relevant for the interaction of NK cells with tumors. Even highly NK-susceptible tumor lines become relatively NK-resistant after growth *in vivo* (18,49). The nature of this resistance is not well defined, but there have been some indications for reversibility (18), thereby making such examples apparently analogous to antigenic modulation. In other instances, growth *in vivo* may select for a stable resistant tumor cell variant (49). Treatment of some NK-resistant cell lines with inhibitors of RNA or protein synthesis has been found to make them sensitive to lysis by NK cells (38,147). Interferon is one of the mediators of induction of NK resistance of target cells, since pretreatment of some NK-sensitive target cells with interferon can render the cells resistant (260,268).

Resistance of tumor cells to lysis by NC cells (246) or by macrophages (207) has been found to occur. This may also be associated with more efficient tumor growth.

Inhibition of Effector Functions

Another major category of possible mechanisms for lack of effective host resistance is deficiency or inhibition of effector functions. As discussed earlier, the tumor-bearing state, or even the latent period prior to overt tumor growth, is often associated with some immunodepression. Although in some instances there may be a decrease in a particular effector cell population or an intrinsic defect in its function, more often the depressed reactivity has been found to be attributable to inhibition or suppression of function, either by host-derived suppressor cells or factors or by tumor-produced suppressor factors.

Suppressor Cells

Almost all effector mechanisms have been found to be well regulated, with cells or factors inhibiting their activity as well as other cells or factors acting in an accessory or augmenting capacity.

Suppression of T Cell-Mediated Immunity to Tumor Antigens

There is substantial evidence for suppressor cells that can either specifically or nonspecifically inhibit immune responses to tumor-associated antigens (112). The specific suppressor cells have been found mainly to be within a particular subpopulation of T cells, and such suppressor T cells have been found to be involved in several experimental tumor systems (20,42,62,66,67,248). A particularly well-studied tumor system in which suppressor T cells appear to play a central role in tumor development is that of ultraviolet light-induced tumors in mice (42,62). Such tumors are highly antigenic and usually are rejected upon transplantation into normal syngeneic recipients (145). However, these tumors grow progressively in mice treated with ultraviolet light (146). Spleen and lymph node cells from ultraviolet light-treated mice were shown to contain suppressor T cells that could adoptively tranfer inhibition of tumor rejection by normal recipients (42,62). The T suppressor cells in this and some other tumor systems appear to bear antigens of the I-J region of the major histocompatibility complex, with *in vivo* administration of antiI-J sera interfering with the suppressor cell activity and leading to some retardation of tumor growth (88,196).

Macrophages represent the other category of suppressor cells for antitumor immune responses. Macrophage suppressor cells have been shown to nonspecifically inhibit lymphoproliferative responses to tumor-associated antigens (reviewed in refs. 108,115, and 185), the primary or secondary generation of antitumor cytotoxic T cells (184), and the production of lymphokines (263,264). In contrast to the above evidence for an *in vivo* role of T suppressor cells, however, there is little comparable evidence for an important role of suppressor macrophages in interfering *in vivo* with antitumor T cell immunity.

There is considerable evidence for the presence of suppressor macrophages in cancer patients which can inhibit antitumor lymphoproliferative responses as well as responses to mitogens or alloantigens (reviewed in ref. 108). In contrast, there is little documentation of suppressor T cells in cancer patients which can specifically inhibit antitumor responses. Vose (265) recently reported that suppressor lymphocytes, and particularly T cells, were present at the site of growth of some human tumors and in regional lymph nodes which could suppress mixed lymphocyte-tumor cell interactions.

Suppression of NK Activity

Much of the inhibition in NK activity that is seen after *in vivo* treatment with a variety of agents appears to be due to the presence of suppressor cells. Suppressor cells have been detected in mice after treatment with carrageenan, corticosteroids, X-irradiation, adriamycin, *C. parvum*, pyran copolymer, and other immune adjuvants (40,162,225,226). The nature of the suppressor cells in these various situations has not been adequately defined, but adherent cells usually have been found to be responsible. The suppressor cells induced by pyran copolymer appear to be phagocytic as well as adherent and therefore are presumed to be macrophages (225). The mechanism(s) by which these suppressor cells inhibit NK activity has not been defined, but with pyran-induced suppressor cells, soluble factors appear to be involved (225).

In considering the effects of some agents on NK activity, it is important to note that either augmentation or inhibition can be produced, depending on a variety of circumstances (226). Such opposite effects by the same agent have been seen with *C. parvum*, BCG, pyran copolymer, adriamycin, and glucan. The route of inoculation appears to be an important variable with some agents [e.g., *C. parvum*, glucan (161,162)], with depression of NK activity particularly associated with intravenous inoculation and boosting of reactivity mainly seen after intraperitoneal inoculation. It is possible that, depending on the route, different cells come in contact with the agent; consequently, different effects may be seen.

This is not the entire explanation for opposite results, however, since treatment by the same route and with the same dose of an agent can result in both augmentation and depression of NK activity. This may be due in part to differences in the kinetics of augmenting and depressing effects. Augmentation tends to occur early, within

1 to 4 days after treatment, whereas induction of depression tends to occur later. With the macrophage-activating agents, this may be related to the more rapid induction of IFN production than the activation of suppressor activity. Also, as seen with pyran copolymer and adriamycin (226), the status of the recipients may in some way determine the direction of the effect of the same treatment on NK activity. There are some indications that this may be related to the baseline levels of activity of NK and suppressor cells. At various sites and times, NK cells may vary in their responsiveness to augmentation by IFN or to depression. Similarly, macrophages and other suppressor cells may vary in their ability to be activated. More information is required in this area before one can predict with confidence the magnitude, or even the direction, of a response to a particular *in vivo* treatment. Understanding of such variables is likely to provide insight into the basic factors involved in regulation of NK activity.

In addition to induction of suppressor cells by various treatments, suppressor cells for NK activity have been detected in some natural situations. The low NK activity in newborn mice (40; A. Santoni, C. Riccardi, and R. B. Herberman, *unpublished observations*) may be attributable in part to the presence of suppressor cells. Furthermore, some strains of mice with genetically determined low NK activity have suppressors for NK activity. In careful kinetic studies of NK activity in A and SJL mice of various ages, it has been noted that 4- to 6-week-old mice have levels of NK activity comparable to those of other strains, but that by 8 weeks of age, their reactivity is substantially depressed (211). Adherent spleen cells of normal SJL mice inhibit the NK activity of spleen cells of high NK strains (211). In *in vivo* studies of adoptive transfer of NK activity, SJL recipients inhibit full expression of the reactivity of donor NK cells (211; G. Cudkowicz, *personal communication*). It is of interest that other investigators have independently noted that the macrophages of SJL mice are functionally hyperactive (69).

Suppressor cells for NK activity have been found in some tumor-bearing individuals with low NK activity. For example, mice bearing progressively growing primary tumors induced by murine sarcoma virus had low or undetectable NK activity *in situ*, but removal of adherent or phagocytic cells led to a marked increase in activity (73). A role for suppressor macrophages within the tumor was supported by mixing experiments, in which cells from the tumor inhibited the activity of normal spleen cells. Similar evidence for suppressor cells has been obtained with some human tumors (54,72,265).

In studies of the maintenance of mouse NK activity upon overnight incubation at 37° C, a role for suppressor cells from normal mice has been detected (26). Peritoneal macrophages from normal mice, resident cells either obtained without any stimuli or elicited by various materials, markedly suppressed NK activity of effector cells incubated alone or with IFN. This suppressor activity appeared restricted to peritoneal macrophages, since splenic adherent cells were inactive. The peritoneal macrophages of several strains had suppressor activity, including those from high NK strains and from nude mice. This type of suppressor activity was distinct from that seen with activated macrophages. The normal peritoneal cells did not suppress the effector phase of NK activity, and peritoneal macrophages from *C. parvum*-treated mice, which were cytotoxic and able to suppress lymphoproliferative responses, had diminished ability to suppress the *in vitro* maintenance of NK activity (27).

Immunosuppressor Products of Tumor Cells

Another factor to be considered for the depressed immunity and ineffective host defenses to some tumors is immunosuppression by the tumor cells or products of the tumors. In some transplantable tumors in experimental animals, the inhibitory properties of the tumor cells could be attributed to contamination by passenger viruses (23,31). In addition, tumor cells are able to produce a variety of immunosuppressive factors (43,176,198,208) which might play an important role in evading host defenses. Some tumor cells also may make considerable amounts of prostaglandins (19,50,89), which, as discussed below, can be immunosuppressive. Little evidence is available, however, that such tumor-produced factors contribute to progressive tumor growth *in vivo*.

Other Inhibitory Factors

Inhibition by Serum Factors

Serum from tumor-bearing individuals has frequently been found to inhibit various antitumor effector mechanisms. In regard to specific cell-mediated cytotoxicity against tumor-associated antigens, serum factors specifically or nonspecifically interfere with reactivity (10,13,78,105,236). Although most serum-blocking factors, particularly those that appeared to act specifically, were initially thought to be antibodies, increasing evidence for a role of circulating antigens and antigen-antibody complexes has been obtained (178,201,255).

Serum-blocking factors have been described in other assays of specific cell-mediated immunity to tumor antigens, with sera of tumor-bearing individuals able to inhibit lymphoproliferative responses (92,173,239) and production of lymphokines (98).

Serum factors are able to inhibit NK activity. Nair et al. (177) reported that preincubation of normal mouse spleen cells in serum could interfere with their cytotoxic activity, and that sera from tumor-bearing individuals were more inhibitory than those from normal donors. Studies of Sulica et al. (246a) with human NK cells have indicated an inhibitory role of monomeric cytophilic IgG. Incubation of cells with serum or IgG inhibited reactivity, whereas incubation in medium lacking IgG led to an increase in NK activity.

There have been some indications that antibodies or other serum factors could interfere with host resistance *in vivo*. Administration of serum from tumor bearers often has been shown to cause enhancement of growth of syngeneic tumors (reviewed in ref. 258). Although in most instances the mechanisms for enhancement have not been elucidated, there have been a few suggestions of a correlation between enhancing activity and serum factors blocking specific cell-mediated cytotoxicity (14). Furthermore, "unblocking" sera from tumor-free individuals, with the ability to counteract the serum-blocking factors in cytotoxicity assays, were found to have some protective effects upon *in vivo* transfer to tumor bearers (15).

Such observations have led to some clinical approaches to treatment of cancer patients. A trial with patients with malignant melanoma was initiated to examine the effects of repeated infusion of sera found to contain unblocking factors (270), but no clinical benefits have been reported. Another approach has been to pass the plasma of cancer patients over columns containing *Staph. aureus* protein A to remove some circulating IgG. Such a protocol has had some antitumor effects in dogs with spontaneous tumors (252), and clinical trials are now under way in several institutions. It should be noted, however, that the nature of the alteration in the plasma that may lead to reduction in tumor size has not been defined, and the mechanism involved might be quite different from removal of blocking antibodies or immune complexes.

Prostaglandins

Prostaglandins, particularly of the E series (PGE), may be produced by stimulated macrophages or by tumor cells and have various immunosuppressive effects. Indomethacin, an inhibitor of prostaglandin synthesis, has been shown to reverse some of the suppression by monocytes or macrophages of lymphoproliferative responses of tumor-bearing mice or cancer patients (80,115). PGE also may inhibit cytostatic activity of macrophages (228) or interfere with the maintenance of their cytolytic activity (223). Similarly, PGE and some other prostaglandins are inhibitors of both spontaneous and interferon-boosted human and mouse NK activity (24,48).

Production of prostaglandins *in vivo* may have a significant effect on tumor growth. Administration of inhibitors of prostaglandin synthesis (either indomethacin or aspirin) to mice bearing murine sarcoma virus-induced tumors led to partial restoration of their NK activity (24) and also to reduced tumor growth (24,240). Such treatment has been shown to reduce the growth of several other experimental tumors and to augment the antitumor effects of some immunostimulants (165,166,199). Conversely, administration of prostaglandins has been found to facilitate carcinogenesis in mice by methylcholanthrene (164).

Neuroendocrine Factors

Neuroendocrine factors have inhibitory effects on various immune functions. For example, with NK cells, corticosteroids (46,183), transportation stress (113), and left cerebral decortication (16) inhibit cytotoxic reactivity. Similarly, Riley (216) has found that stress-induced elevation in circulating corticosteroids was associated with suppression of T cell numbers and functions. The most impressive indication that this may have important implications for *in vivo* host resistance to tumor growth has come from a study of spontaneous mammary carcinogenesis in mice maintained under low or high stress conditions (215). Mice exposed to chronic stress had an incidence of mammary tumors at 400 days of age of 92%, whereas only 7% of mice housed in a low stress, protective environment developed tumors by that time. However, the latter group later developed tumors with high frequency, with a median latent period of 566 days.

CONCLUDING REMARKS

This chapter points out the heterogeneity of immunologic effector mechanisms that are potentially important for host resistance against tumor growth. It is not realistic to try to decide which among these mechanisms is generally most important, but rather it is best to consider the possibility that several or even all may be involved. One effector mechanism may predominate for some tumors, and a different one may be more important for others. Also, several different effector mechanisms may act in concert in the defense against some type of tumors. This may provide a back-up system in the event of escape from the predominant or first-line effector mechanism. Thus considerations regarding immunologic defenses against tumors may need to be quite complicated and multifocal. This may require more detailed and prolonged investigations to adequately understand the host-tumor interactions. However, this complexity may add considerable flexibility to the system; and, in terms of attempts to augment host resistance against tumors, it may be possible to favorably alter the balance by affecting any one of the several effector mechanisms that are involved.

REFERENCES

1. Adams, D. O., and Snyderman, R. (1979): Do macrophages destroy nascent tumors? *J. Natl. Cancer Inst.*, 62:1341–1345.
2. Alexander, P. (1976): The functions of the macrophage in malignant disease. *Annu. Rev. Med.*, 27:207–224.
3. Allavena, P., Introna, M., Mangioni, C., and Mantovani, A. (1981): Inhibition of natural killer activity by tumor-associated lymphoid cells from ascitic ovarian carcinomas. *J. Natl. Cancer Inst.*, 67:319–325.
4. Allison, A. C. (1970): Potentiation of viral carcinogenesis by immunosuppression. *Br. Med. J.*, 4:419–420.
5. Allison, A. C., Hammington, J. S., and Birbeck, M. (1966): An examination of the cytotoxic effects of silica on macrophages. *J. Exp. Med.*, 124:141–153.
6. Allison, A. C., and Law, L. W. (1968): Effects of antilymphocyte serum on virus oncogenesis. *Proc. Soc. Exp. Biol. Med.*, 127:207–211.
7. Aoki, T., and Johnson, P. A. (1973): Suppression of G (Gross) leukemia cell surface antigens: A kind of antigenic modulation. *J. Natl. Cancer Inst.*, 49:183–189.
8. Argus, M. F., Hudson, M. T., Seepe, T. L., Kane, J. F., and Ray, F. E. (1962): Effect of rapid tissue growth on the uptake of fluorene-2,7-di(sulfonamide-2-napthalene)-S^{35} by the liver and spleen of rats and hamsters. *Br. J. Cancer*, 16:494–499.
9. Axberg, I., Gidlund, M., Orn, A., Pattengale, P., Reisenfeld, I., Stern, P., and Wigzell, H. (1980): In: *Thymus, Thymic Hormones and T Lymphocytes*, edited by F. Aiuti, pp. 154–164. Academic Press, New York.
10. Baldwin, R. W. (1976): Role of immunosurveillance against chemically induced rat tumors. *Trans. Rev.*, 28:62.
11. Baldwin, R. W., and Price, M. R. (1976): Immunobiology of rat neoplasia. *Ann. NY Acad. Sci.*, 276:3–10.
12. Balner, H., and Dersjant, H. (1969): Increased oncogenic effect of methylcholanthrene after treatment with anti-lymphocyte serum. *Nature*, 224:376–378.

13. Bansal, S. C., Bansal, B. R., and Boland, J. P. (1976): Blocking and unblocking factors in neoplasia. *Curr. Top. Microbiol. Immunol.*, 75:45–63.

14. Bansal, S. C., Hargreaves, R., and Sjögren, H. (1972): Facilitation of polyoma tumor growth in rats by blocking sera and tumor eluate. *Int. J. Cancer*, 9:97–106.

15. Bansal, S. C., and Sjogren, H. (1972): Counteraction of the blocking of cell-mediated tumor immunity by inoculation of unblocking sera and splenectomy. Immunotherapeutic effects on primary polyoma tumor in rats. *Int. J. Cancer*, 9:490–499.

16. Bardos, P., Biziere, K., Degenne, D., and Renoux, G. (1982): Regulation of NK activity by the cerebral neocortex. In: *NK Cells: Fundamental Aspects and Role in Cancer. Human Cancer Immunology, Vol. 4*, edited by B. Serrou, C. Rosenfeld, and R. B. Herberman. Elsevier, Amsterdam, pp. 1–6.

17. Becker, S. (1980): Intratumor NK reactivity. In: *Natural Cell-Mediated Immunity Against Tumors*, edited by R. B. Herberman, pp. 985–996. Academic Press, New York.

18. Becker, S., Kiessling, R., Lee, M., and Klein, G. (1978): Modulation of sensitivity to natural killer cell lysis after *in vitro* explantation of a mouse lymphoma. *J. Natl. Cancer Inst.*, 61:1495–1498.

19. Bennett, A., Deltacia, M., Stamford, I. F., and Zebro, T. (1977): Prostaglandins from tumours of human large bowel. *Br. J. Cancer*, 35:881–884.

20. Berendt, M. J., and North, R. J. (1980): T cell-mediated suppression of anti-tumor immunity. An explanation for progressive growth of an immunogenic tumor. *J. Exp. Med.*, 151:69–80.

21. Berenson, J. R., Einstein, A. B., Jr., and Fefer, A. (1975): Syngeneic adoptive immunotherapy and chemotherapy of Friend leukemia: Requirement for T cells. *J. Immunol.*, 115:234–238.

22. Blair, P. B., Lane, M. A., and Mar, P. (1976): Antibody in the sera of tumor-bearing mice that mediates spleen cell cytotoxicity toward the autologous tumor. *J. Immunol.*, 116:606–609.

23. Bonnard, G. D., Manders, E. K., Campbell, D. A., Jr., Herberman, R. B., and Collins, M. J., Jr. (1976): Immunosuppressive activity of a subline of the mouse EL-4 lymphoma. Evidence for minute virus of mice causing the inhibition. *J. Exp. Med.*, 143:187–205.

24. Brunda, M. J., Herberman, R. B., and Holden, H. T. (1980): Inhibition of murine natural killer cell activity by prostaglandins. *J. Immunol.*, 124:2682–2687.

25. Brunda, M. J., Holden, H. T., and Herberman, R. B. (1980): Augmentation of natural killer cell activity of beige mice by interferon and interferon inducers. In: *Natural Cell-Mediated Immunity Against Tumors*, edited by R. B. Herberman, pp. 411–415. Academic Press, New York.

26. Brunda, M. J., Taramelli, D., Holden, H. T., and Varesio, L. (1982): Peritoneal macrophages from normal mice suppress natural killer cell activity. *Fed. Proc.*, 40:1094.

27. Brunda, M. J., Taramelli, D., Holden, H. T., and Varesio, L. (1982): Effects of resting and activated macrophages on natural killer cell activity and lymphoproliferation. *Proc. Am. Assoc. Cancer Res.*, 22:310.

28. Burnet, F. M. (1957): Cancer—a biological approach. *Br. Med. J.*, 1:779–786; 841–847.

29. Burnet, F. M. (1970): The concept of immunological surveillance. *Prog. Exp. Tumor Res.*, 13:1–27.

30. Burton, R. C. (1980): Alloantisera selectivity reactive with NK cells: Characterization and use in defining NK cell classes. In: *Natural Cell-Mediated Immunity Against Tumors*, edited by R. B. Herberman, pp. 19–35. Academic Press, New York.

31. Campbell, D. A., Jr., Manders, E. K., Oehler, J. R., Bonnard, G. D., Oldham, R. K., and Herberman, R. B. (1977): Inhibition of *in vitro* lymphoproliferative responses by *in vivo* passaged rat 13762 mammary adenocarcinoma cells. I. Characteristics of inhibition and evidence for an infectious agent. *Cell. Immunol.*, 33:364–377.

32. Canellos, G. P., DeVita, V. T., and Arsenau, J. C. (1974): Carcinogenesis by cancer chemotherapeutic agents: Second malignancies complicating Hodgkin's disease in remission. *Recent Results Cancer Res.*, 49:108–114.

33. Castro, J. E. (1972): Human tumors grown in mice. *Nature [New Biol.]*, 239:83–84.

34. Cheever, M. A., Greenberg, P. D., and Fefer, A. (1980): Therapy of leukemia by nonimmune syngeneic spleen cells. *J. Immunol.*, 124:2137–2142.

35. Chow, D. A., Greene, M. I., and Greenberg, A. H. (1979): Macrophage-dependent, NK cell-independent natural surveillance of tumors in syngeneic mice. *Int. J. Cancer*, 23:788–797.

36. Chow, D. A., Wolosin, L. B., and Greenberg, A. H. (1981): Immune natural anti-tumor antibodies. II. The contribution of natural antibodies to tumor surveillance. *Int. J. Cancer*, 27:459–469.

37. Collavo, D., Colombatti, A., Chieco-Bianchi, L., and Davis, A. J. S. (1974): T lymphocyte requirement for MSV tumour prevention or regression. *Nature*, 249:169–170.
38. Collins, J. L., Patek, P. Q., and Cohn, M. (1981): Tumorigenicity and lysis by natural killers. *J. Exp. Med.*, 153:89–106.
39. Cudkowicz, G. (1982): Role of natural killer cells in natural resistance against bone marrow transplants. In: *Symposium on Role of Natural Killer Cells, Macrophages and Antibody Dependent Cellular Cytotoxicity in Tumor Rejection and as Mediators of Biological Response Modifiers Activity*, edited by M. A. Chirigos. Raven Press, New York *(in press)*.
40. Cudkowicz, G., and Hochman, P. S. (1979): Do natural killer cells engage in regulated reactions against self to ensure homeostasis? *Immunol. Rev.*, 44:13–52.
41. Currie, G. A. (1976): Immunological aspects of host resistance to the development and growth of cancer. *Biochim. Biophys. Acta*, 458:135–162.
42. Daynes, R. A., and Spellman, C. W. (1977): Evidence for the generation of suppressor cells by ultraviolet radiation. *Cell. Immunol.*, 31:182–187.
43. DeLustro, F., and Argyris, B. F. (1976): Mechanism of mastocytoma-mediated suppression of lymphocyte reactivity. *J. Immunol.*, 117:2073–2080.
44. Dent, P. B., Fish, L. A., White, J. F., and Good, R. A. (1966): Chediak-Higashi syndrome. Observations on the nature of the associated malignancy. *Lab. Invest.*, 15:1634–1641.
45. Djeu, J. Y., Heinbaugh, J. A., Holden, H. T., and Herberman, R. B. (1979): Role of macrophages in the augmentation of mouse natural killer cell activity by poly I:C and interferon. *J. Immunol.*, 122:182–188.
46. Djeu, J. Y., Heinbaugh, J., Vieira, W. D., Holden, H. T., and Herberman, R. B. (1979): The effect of immunopharmacological agents on mouse natural cell-mediated cytotoxicity and on its augmentation by poly I:C. *Immunopharmacology*, 1:231–244.
47. Doll, R., and Kinlen, L. (1970): Immunosurveillance and cancer: Epidemiological evidence. *Br. Med. J.*, 4:420–422.
48. Droller, M. J., Schneider, M. V., and Perlmann, P. (1978): A possible role of prostaglandins in the inhibition of natural and antibody-dependent cell-mediated cytotoxicity against tumor cells. *Cell. Immunol.*, 39:165.
49. Durdik, J. M., Beck, B. N., and Henney, C. S. (1980): The use of lymphoma cell variants differing in their susceptibility to NK cell mediated lysis to analyze NK cell-target cell interactions. In: *Natural Cell-Mediated Immunity Against Tumors*, edited by R. B. Herberman, pp. 805–17. Academic Press, New York.
50. Easty, G. C., and Easty, D. M. (1976): Prostaglandins and cancer. *Cancer Treat. Rev.*, 3:217–225.
51. Eccles, S. A., and Alexander, P. (1974): Macrophage content of tumors in relation to metastatic spread and host immune reaction. *Nature*, 250:667–668.
52. Ehrlich, P. (1957): Über den jetzigen Stand der Karzinomforschung. In: *The Collected Papers of Paul Ehrlich, Vol. II*, edited by F. Himmelweit, pp. 550–562. Pergamon Press, London.
53. Ehrlich, R., Efrati, M., and Witz, I. P. (1980): Cytotoxicity and cytostasis mediated by splenocytes of mice subjected to chemical carcinogens and of mice bearing primary tumors. In: *Natural Cell-Mediated Immunity Against Tumors*, edited by R. B. Herberman, pp. 997–1010. Academic Press, New York.
54. Eremin, O. (1980): NK cell activity in the blood, tumour-draining lymph nodes and primary tumours of women with mammary carcinoma. In: *Natural Cell-Mediated Immunity Against Tumors*, edited by R. B. Herberman, pp. 1011–1029. Academic Press, New York.
55. Evans, R. (1972): Macrophages in syngeneic animal tumors. *Transplantation*, 14:468–472.
56. Evans, R. (1978): Macrophage requirement for growth of murine fibrosarcoma. *Br. J. Cancer*, 37:1080–1088.
57. Evans, R. (1979): Host cells in transplanted murine tumors and their possible relevance to tumor growth. *J. Reticuloendothel. Soc.*, 26:427–432.
58. Evans, R., and Haskill, S. (1983): Activities of macrophages within and peripheral to the tumor mass. In: *The Reticuloendothelial System: A Comprehensive Treatise, Vol. 8: Cancer*, edited by R. B. Herberman and H. Friedman. Plenum Press, New York *(in press)*.
59. Faraci, R. P., Marrone, J. C., Lesser, G. R., and Ketcham, A. S. (1975): The effect of splenectomy on tumor immunity and the metastatic spread of a murine reticulum cell sarcoma. *Panminerva Med.*, 17:59–62.

60. Fidler, I. J. (1974): Inhibition of pulmonary metastases by intravenous injection of specifically activated macrophages. *Cancer Res.*, 34:1074–1079.

61. Fidler, I. J., Gerstein, D. M., and Hart, I. R. (1978): The biology of cancer invasion and metastasis. *Adv. Cancer Res.*, 28:149–175.

62. Fisher, M. S., and Kripke, M. L. (1978): Further studies on the tumor-specific suppressor cells induced by ultraviolet radiation. *J. Immunol.*, 121:1139–1144.

63. Foley, E. J. (1953): Antigenic properties of methylcholanthrene-induced tumors in mice of the same strain. *Cancer Res.*, 13:835–837.

64. Franceschi, C., Perocco, P., DiMarco, A. T., and Prodi, G. (1972): Lack of correlation between immunodepression and reticuloendothelial system activity in urethan or 7,12-dimethylbenz(a)-anthracene-treated rats. *J. Reticuloendothel. Soc.*, 12:592–598.

65. Fraumeni, J. F. (1969): Constitutional disorders of man predisposing to leukemia and lymphoma. *Natl. Cancer Inst. Monogr.*, 32:221–232.

66. Fujimoto, S., Greene, M. I., and Sehon, A. H. (1976): Regulation of the immune response to tumor antigens. I. Immunosuppressor cells in tumor-bearing hosts. *J. Immunol.*, 116:791–799.

67. Fujimoto, S., Greene, M. I., and Sehon, A. H. (1976): Regulation of the immune response to tumor antigens. II. The nature of immunosuppressor cells in tumor-bearing hosts. *J. Immunol.*, 116:800–806.

68. Gale, R. P., Zighelboim, J., Ossorio, C., and Fahey, J. (1974): Western section immunology and connective tissue. *Clin. Res.*, 22:180A.

69. Gallily, R., and Haran-Ghera, N. (1979): Macrophage functions in high and low cancer incidence strains of mice. A comparative study. *Dev. Comp. Immunol.*, 3:523–536.

70. Gatti, R. A., and Good, R. A. (1971): Occurrence of malignancy in immunodeficiency diseases. A literature review. *Cancer*, 28:89–98.

71. Gauci, C. L., and Alexander, P. (1975): The macrophage content of some human tumors. *Cancer Lett.*, 1:20–25.

72. Gerson, J. M. (1980): Systemic and in situ natural killer activity in tumor-bearing mice and patients with cancer. In: *Natural Cell-Mediated Immunity Against Tumors*, edited by R. B. Herberman, pp. 1047–1062. Academic Press, New York.

73. Gerson, J. M., Varesio, L., and Herberman, R. B. (1982): Systemic and in situ natural killer and suppressor cell activities in mice bearing progressively growing murine sarcoma virus-induced tumors. *Int. J. Cancer*, 27:243–248.

74. Ghaffar, A., McBride, W. H., and Cullen, R. T. (1976): Interaction of tumor cells and activated macrophages *in vitro*: Modulation by *Corynebacterium parvum* and gold salts. *J. Reticuloendothel. Soc.*, 20:283–290.

75. Ghose, T. (1957): Effect of the blockade of reticuloendothelial system on tumor growth and metastasis. *Indian J. Med. Sci.*, 11:900–906.

76. Gillman, T., Kinns, A. M., Hallowes, R. C., and Lloyd, J. B. (1973): Malignant lymphoreticular tumors induced by trypan blue and transplanted in inbred rats. *J. Natl. Cancer Inst.*, 50:1179.

77. Glaser, M., Lavrin, D. H., and Herberman, R. B. (1976): *In vivo* protection against syngeneic Gross virus-induced lymphoma in rats: Comparison with *in vitro* studies of cell-mediated immunity. *J. Immunol.*, 116:1507–1511.

78. Glaser, M., Ting, C. C., and Herberman, R. B. (1976): *In vitro* inhibition of cell-mediated cytotoxicity against syngeneic Friend virus-induced leukemia by immunoregulatory alpha globulin. *J. Natl. Cancer Inst.*, 55:1477–1479.

79. Goldfarb, R. H., and Herberman, R. B. (1981): Natural killer cell reactivity: Regulatory interactions among phorbol ester, interferon, cholera toxin, and retinoic acid. *J. Immunol.*, 126:2129–2135.

80. Goodwin, J. S., Messner, R. P., Bankhurst, A. D., Peake, G. T., Saiki, J. H., and Williams, R. C., Jr. (1977): Prostaglandin-producing suppressor cells in Hodgkin's disease. *N. Engl. J. Med.*, 297:963–968.

81. Gorczynski, R. M., and Norbury, C. (1974): Immunity to murine sarcoma virus induced tumours. III. Analysis of the cell populations involved in protection from lethal tumour progression of sublethally irradiated, MSV inoculated, mice. *Br. J. Cancer*, 30:118–128.

82. Gorelik, E., Fogel, M., Feldman, M., and Segal, S. (1979): Differences in resistance of metastatic tumor cells and cells from local tumor growth to cytotoxicity of natural killer cells. *J. Natl. Cancer Inst.*, 63:1397–1404.

83. Gorelik, E., and Herberman, R. B. (1981): Radioisotope assay for evaluation of *in vivo* natural

cell-mediated resistance of mice to local transplantation of tumor cells. *Int. J. Cancer*, 27:709–720.

84. Gorelik, E., and Herberman, R. B. (1981): Inhibition of the activity of mouse NK cells by urethane. *J. Natl. Cancer Inst.*, 66:543–548.

85. Gorelik, E., and Herberman, R. B. (1981): Carcinogen-induced inhibition of NK activity in mice. *Fed. Proc.*, 40:1093.

86. Grant, G., Roe, F. J. C., and Pike, M. C. (1966): Effect of neonatal thymectomy on the induction of papillomata and carcinomata by 3,4-benzopyrene in mice. *Nature*, 210:603–604.

87. Greene, M. H., Young, T. I., and Clark, W. H., Jr. (1981): Malignant melanoma in renal transplant recipients. *Lancet*, 1:1196–1198.

88. Greene, M. I., Dorf, M. E., Pierres, M., and Benacerraf, B. (1977): Reduction of syngeneic tumor growth by an anti-I-J alloantiserum. *Proc. Natl. Acad. Sci. USA*, 74:5118–5121.

89. Grinwich, K. D., and Plescia, O. H. (1977): Tumor-mediated immunosuppression: Prevention by inhibitors of prostaglandin synthesis. *Prostaglandins*, 14:1175–1182.

90. Gross, L. (1943): Intradermal immunization of C3H mice against a sarcoma that originated in an animal of the same line. *Cancer Res.*, 3:326–333.

91. Gutterman, J. U., Hersh, E. M., Freireich, E. J., Rossen, R. D., Butler, W. T., McCredie, K. B., Bodey, G. P., Sr., Rodriguez, V., and Mavligit, G. M. (1973): Cell-mediated and humoral response to acute leukemia cells and soluble leukemia antigen—relationship to immunocompetence and prognosis. *Natl. Cancer Inst. Monogr.*, 37:153–156.

92. Gutterman, J. U., Rossen, R. D., Butler, W. T., McCredie, K. B., Bodey, G. P., Freireich, E. J., and Hersh, E. M. (1973): Immunoglobulin on tumor cells and tumor-induced lymphocyte blastogenesis in human acute leukemia. *N. Engl. J. Med.*, 288:169–173.

93. Habu, S., Fukui, H., Shimamura, K., Kasai, M., Nagai, Y., Okumura, K., and Tamaoki, N. (1981): *In vivo* effects of anti-asialo GM1. I. Reduction of NK activity and enhancement of transplanted tumor growth in nude mice. *J. Immunol.*, 127:34–38.

94. Hafeman, D. G., and Lucas, Z. J. (1979): Polymorphonuclear leukocyte-mediated, antibody-dependent, cellular cytotoxicity against tumor cells: Dependence on oxygen and the respiratory burst. *J. Immunol.*, 123:55–62.

95. Hakala, T. R., Lange, P. H., Castro, A. E., Elliott, A. Y., and Fraley, E. E. (1974): Antibody induction of lymphocyte-mediated cytotoxicity against human transitional-cell carcinomas of the urinary tract. *N. Engl. J. Med.*, 291:637–641.

96. Haller, O., Kiessling, R., Örn, A., Kärre, K., Nilsson, K., and Wigzell, H. (1977): Natural cytotoxicity to human leukemia mediated by mouse non-T cells. *Int. J. Cancer*, 20:93–103.

97. Haller, O., Kiessling, R., Örn, A., and Wigzell, H. (1977): Generation of natural killer cells: An autonomous function of the bone marrow. *J. Exp. Med.*, 145:1411–1416.

98. Halliday, W. J. (1972): Macrophage migration inhibition with mouse tumor antigens: Properties of serum and peritoneal cells during tumor growth and after tumor loss. *Cell. Immunol.*, 3:113–121.

99. Hanna, N. (1980): Expression of metastatic potential of tumor cells in young nude mice is correlated with low levels of natural killer cell-mediated cytotoxicity. *Int. J. Cancer*, 26:675–680.

100. Hanna, N., and Fidler, I. J. (1980): The role of natural killer cells in the destruction of circulating tumor emboli. *J. Natl. Cancer Inst.*, 65:801–809.

101. Hanna, N., and Fidler, I. J. (1981): Expression of metastatic potential of allogeneic and xenogeneic neoplasms in young nude mice. *Cancer Res.*, 41:438–444.

102. Harada, M., Pearson, G., Redmon, L., Winters, E., and Kasuga, S. (1975): Antibody production and interaction with lymphoid cells in relation to tumor immunity in the Moloney sarcoma virus system. *J. Immunol.*, 114:1318–1322.

103. Haran-Ghera, N., and Lurie, M. (1971): Effect of heterologous antithymocyte serum on mouse skin tumorigenesis. *J. Natl. Cancer Inst.*, 46:103–112.

104. Haskill, J. S., and Fett, J. W. (1976): Possible evidence for antibody-dependent macrophage-mediated cytotoxicity directed against murine adenocarcinoma cells *in vivo*. *J. Immunol.*, 117:1992–1998.

105. Hellström, K. E., and Hellström, I. (1976): Immunological enforcement of tumor growth. *In: Mechanisms of Tumor Immunity*, edited by I. Green, S. Cohen, and R. T. McCluskey, pp. 276–89. Wiley, New York.

106. Herberman, R. B. (1974): Cell-mediated immunity to tumor cells. In: *Advances in Cancer Research, Vol. 19*, edited by G. Klein and S. Weinhouse, pp. 207–63. Academic Press, New York.

107. Herberman, R. B. (1979): Tests for tumor associated antigens and their clinical value. In: *Clinical Immunology Update*, edited by E. C. Franklin, pp. 23–55. Elsevier, New York.

108. Herberman, R. B. (1982): Cells suppressing cell-mediated immune responses of cancer patients. In: *Human Suppressor Cell*, edited by B. Serrou, pp. 179–211. North Holland, Amsterdam.

109. Herberman, R. B., Brunda, M. J., Cannon, G. B., Djeu, J. Y., Nunn-Hargrove, M. E., Jett, J. R., Ortaldo, J. R., Reynolds, C., Riccardi, C., and Santoni, A. (1981): Augmentation of natural killer (NK) cell activity by interferon and interferon-inducers. In: *Progress in Cancer Research and Therapy, Vol. 16. Augmenting Agents in Cancer Therapy*, edited by E. Hersh, M. A. Chirigos, and M. J. Mastrangelo, pp. 253–265. Raven Press, New York.

110. Herberman, R. B., Djeu, J. Y., Kay, H. D., Ortaldo, J. R., Riccardi, C., Bonnard, G. D., Holden, H. T., Fagnani, R., Santoni, A., and Puccetti, P. (1979): Natural killer cells: Characteristics and regulation of activity. *Immunol. Rev.*, 44:43–70.

111. Herberman, R. B., and Holden, H. T. (1978): Natural cell-mediated immunity. *Adv. Cancer Res.*, 27:305–377.

112. Herberman, R. B., Holden, H. T., Djeu, J. Y., Jerrells, T. R., Varesio, L., Tagliabue, A., White, S. L., Oehler, J. R., and Dean, J. H. (1980): Macrophages as regulators of immune responses against tumors. In: *Macrophages and Lymphocytes, Part B*, edited by M. R. Escobar and H. Friedman, pp. 361–369. Plenum, New York.

113. Herberman, R. B., and McIntire, K. R., editors (1979): *Immunodiagnosis of Cancer (Part 1 and Part 2)*. Marcel Dekker, New York.

114. Herberman, R. B., Nunn, M. E., and Lavrin, D. H. (1975): Natural cytotoxic reactivity of mouse lymphoid cells against syngeneic and allogeneic tumors. I. Distribution of reactivity and specificity. *Int. J. Cancer*, 16:216–229.

115. Herberman, R. B., Ortaldo, J. R., Djeu, J. Y., Holden, H. T., Jett, J., Lang, N. P., and Pestka, S. (1980): Role of interferon in regulation of cytotoxicity by natural killer cells and macrophages. *Ann. NY Acad. Sci.*, 350:63–71.

116. Herlyn, D. M., Steplewski, Z., Herlyn, M. F., and Koprowski, H. (1980): Inhibition of growth of colorectal carcinoma in nude mice by monoclonal antibody. *Cancer Res.*, 40:717–721.

117. Hewitt, H. B., Blake, E. R., and Walder, A. S. (1976): A critique of the evidence for active host defense against cancer, based on personal studies of 27 murine tumours of spontaneous origin. *Br. J. Cancer*, 33:241–259.

118. Hibbs, J. B., Jr. (1974): Discrimination between neoplastic and non-neoplastic cells *in vitro* by activated macrophages. *J. Natl. Cancer Inst.*, 53:1487–1493.

119. Hibbs, J. B., Jr. (1974): Heterocytolysis by macrophages activated by bacillus Calmette-Guérin: Lysosome exocytosis into tumor cells. *Science*, 184:468–471.

120. Hibbs, J. B. (1975): Activated macrophages as cytotoxic effector cells. I. Inhibition of specific and nonspecific tumor resistance by trypan blue. *Transplantation*, 19:77–81.

121. Hibbs, J. B., Jr., Chapman, H. A., Jr., and Weinberg, J. B. (1978): The macrophage as an antineoplastic surveillance cell; biological perspectives. *J. Reticuloendothel. Soc.*, 24:549–570.

122. Hibbs, J. B., Jr., Lambert, C. H., Jr., and Remington, J. S. (1972): Control of carcinogenesis: A possible role for the activated macrophage. *Science*, 177:998–1000.

123. Hibbs, J. B., Jr., Lambert, L. H., Jr., and Remington, J. S. (1972): Possible role of macrophage mediated nonspecific cytotoxicity in tumor resistance. *Nature [New Biol.]*, 235:48–49.

124. Hochman, P. S., Cudkowicz, G., and Dausset, J. (1978): Decline of natural killer cell activity in sublethally irradiated mice. *J. Natl. Cancer Inst.*, 61:265–268.

125. Houghton, A. N., Taormina, M. C., Ikeda, H., Watanabe, T., Oettgen, H. F., and Old, L. J. (1980): Serological survey of normal humans for natural antibody to cell surface antigens of melanoma. *Proc. Natl. Acad. Sci. USA*, 77:4260–4264.

126. Huebner, R. J. (1963): Tumor virus study systems. *Ann. NY Acad. Sci.*, 108:1129–1148.

127. Hueper, W. C. (1959): Carcinogenic studies on water-soluble and water-insoluble macromolecules. *Arch. Pathol.*, 67:589–595.

128. Hueper, W. C. (1961): Bioassay of polyvinyl pyrrolidones with limited molecular weight range. *J. Natl. Cancer Inst.*, 6:229–237.

129. Hyman, G. A. (1969): Increased incidence of neoplasm in association with chronic lymphocytic leukemia. *Scand. J. Haematol.*, 6:99–104.

130. Ioachim, H., Keller, S., Dorsett, B., and Pearse, A. (1974): Induction of partial immunologic tolerance in rats and progressive loss of cellular antigenicity in Gross virus lymphoma. *J. Exp. Med.*, 139:1382–1394.

131. Jondal, M., and Gunven, P. (1977): Antibody-dependent cellular cytotoxicity (ADCC) against Epstein-Barr virus-determined antigens. III. Reactivity in sera from patients with Burkitt's lymphoma in relation to tumour development. *Clin. Exp. Immunol.*, 29:11–15.

132. Kaplan, H. S., Brown, M. B., and Paull, J. (1953): Influence of bone marrow injections on involution and neoplasia of mouse thymus after systemic irradiation. *J. Natl. Cancer Inst.*, 14:303–316.

133. Kärre, K., Klein, G. O., Kiessling, R., Klein, G., and Roder, J. C. (1980): Low natural *in vivo* resistance to syngeneic leukaemias in natural killer-deficient mice. *Nature*, 284:624–626.

234. Kasai, M., Leclerc, J. C, McVay-Boudreau, L., Shen, F. W., and Cantor, H. (1979): Direct evidence that natural killer cells in nonimmune spleen cell populations prevent tumor growth *in vivo. J. Exp. Med.*, 149:1260–1264.

135. Keller, R. (1976): Promotion of tumor growth *in vivo* by anti-macrophage agents. *J. Natl. Cancer Inst.*, 57:1355–1367.

136. Keller, R. (1979): Suppression of natural antitumor defence mechanisms by phorbol esters. *Nature*, 282:729–731.

137. Key, M., and Haskill, J. S. (1982): Macrophage-mediated, antibody-dependent destruction of tumor cells: *In vitro* identification of an in situ mechanism. *J. Natl. Cancer Inst.*, 66:103–110.

138. Kiessling, R., Klein, E., and Wigzell, H. (1975): "Natural" killer cells in the mouse. I. Cytotoxic cells with specificity for mouse Moloney leukemia cells. Specificity and distribution according to genotype. *Eur. J. Immunol.*, 5:112–117.

139. Kiessling, R., Petranyi, G., Klein, G., and Wigzell, H. (1975): Genetic variation of *in vitro* cytolytic activity and *in vivo* rejection potential of nonimmunized semisyngeneic mice against a mouse lymphoma line. *Int. J. Cancer*, 15:933–940.

140. Kiessling, R., Petrányi, G., Klein, G., and Wigzell, H. (1976): Non-T-cell resistance against a mouse Moloney lymphoma. *Int. J. Cancer*, 17:275–281.

141. Klein, G., and Klein, E. (1977): Rejectability of virus induced tumors and non-rejectability of spontaneous tumors—a lesson in contrasts. *Transplant. Proc.*, 9:1095–1104.

142. Klein, G., Klein, E., and Haughton, G. (1966): Variation of antigenic characteristics between different mouse lymphomas induced by the Moloney virus. *J. Natl. Cancer Inst.*, 36:607–621.

143. Klein, G., Sjögren, H. O., Klein, E., and Hellström, K. E. (1960): Demonstration of resistance against methylcholanthrene-induced sarcomas in the primary autochthonous host. *Cancer Res.*, 20:1561–1572.

144. Kraskovsky, G., Gorelik, L., and Kagan, L. (1973): Abrogation of the immunosuppressive and carcinogenic action of urethan by transplantation of syngeneic bone marrow cells from normal mice. *Proc. Acad. Sci. BSSR*, 11:1052–1053.

145. Kripke, M. L. (1974): Antigenicity of murine skin tumors induced by ultraviolet light. *J. Natl. Cancer Inst.*, 53:1333–1336.

146. Kripke, M. L., and Fisher, M. S. (1976): Immunologic parameter of ultraviolet carcinogenesis. *J. Natl. Cancer Inst.*, 57:211–215.

147. Kunkel, L. A., and Welsh, R. M. (1981): Metabolic inhibitors render "resistant" target cells sensitive to natural killer cell-mediated lysis. *Int. J. Cancer*, 27:73–79.

148. Lamon, E. W., Skurzak, H. M., Andersson, B., Whitten, H. D., and Klein, E. (1975): Antibody-dependent lymphocyte cytotoxicity in the murine sarcoma virus system: Activity of IgM and IgG with specificity for MLV determined antigen(s). *J. Immunol.*, 114:1171–1176.

149. Landazuri, M. O., Kedar, E., and Fahey, J. L. (1974): Antibody-dependent cellular cytotoxicity to a syngeneic Gross virus-induced lymphoma. *J. Natl. Cancer Inst.*, 52:147–152.

150. Landazuri, M. O., Silva, A., Alvarez, J., and Herberman, R. B. (1979): Evidence that natural cytotoxicity and antibody dependent cellular cytotoxicity are mediated in humans by the same effector cell populations. *J. Immunol.*, 123:252–258.

151. Langlois, A. J., Matthews, T., Roloson, G. J., Thiel, H.-J., Collins, J. J., and Bolognesi, D. P. (1981): Immunologic control of the ascites form of murine adenocarcinoma 755. V. Antibody-directed macrophages mediate tumor cell destruction. *J. Immunol.*, 126:2337–2341.

152. Lappé, M. A. (1971): Evidence for immunological surveillance during skin carcinogenesis. Inflammatory foci in immunologically competent mice. *Isr. J. Med. Sci.*, 7:52–65.

153. Law, L. W. (1965): Neoplasms in thymectomized mice following room infection with polyoma virus. *Nature*, 205:672–673.

154. Law, L. W. (1966): Studies of thymic functions with emphasis on the role of the thymus in oncogenesis. *Cancer Res.*, 26:551–574.

155. Law, L. W., and Ting, R. C. (1965): Immunologic competence and induction of neoplasms by polyoma virus. *Proc. Soc. Exp. Biol. Med.*, 119:823–830.
156. Levy, M. H., and Wheelock, E. F. (1974): The role of macrophages in defense against neoplastic disease. *Adv. Cancer Res.*, 20:131–163.
157. Levy, P. C., Yhaw, G. M., and LoBuglio, A. (1979): Human monocyte, lymphocyte, and granulocyte antibody-dependent cell-mediated cytotoxicity toward tumor cells. *J. Immunol.*, 123:594–599.
158. Liotta, L. A., Gattozzi, C., Kleinerman, J., and Saidel, G. (1977): Reduction of tumour cell entry into vessels by BCG-activated macrophages. *Br. J. Cancer*, 36:639–641.
159. Lipinski, M., Tursz, T., Kreis, H., Finale, Y., and Amiel, J. L. (1980): Dissociation of natural killer cell activity and antibody-dependent cell-mediated cytotoxicity in kidney allograft recipients receiving high-dose immunosuppressive therapy. *Transplantation*, 29:214–218.
160. Lotan, R. (1980): Effects of vitamin A and its analogs (retinoids) on normal and neoplastic cells. *Biochim. Biophys. Acta*, 605:33–37.
161. Lotzová, E. (1980): C. parvum-mediated suppression of the phenomenon of natural killer and its analysis. In: *Natural Cell-Mediated Immunity Against Tumors*, edited by R. B. Herberman, pp. 735–752. Academic Press, New York.
162. Lotzová, E., and Gutterman, J. U. (1979): Effect of glucan on natural killer (NK) cells: Further comparison between NK cell and bone marrow effector cell activities. *J. Immunol.*, 123:607–612.
163. Loutit, J. F., Townsend, K. M. S., and Knowles, J. F. (1980): Tumour surveillance in beige mice. *Nature*, 285:66.
164. Lupulescu, A. (1978): Enhancement of carcinogenesis by prostaglandins. *Nature*, 272:634–636.
165. Lynch, N. R., Castes, M., Astoin, M., and Salomon, J. C. (1978): Mechanism of inhibition of tumour growth by aspirin and indomethacin. *Br. J. Cancer*, 38:503–512.
166. Lynch, N. R., and Salomon, J. C. (1979): Tumor growth inhibition and potentiation of immunotherapy by indomethacin in mice. *J. Natl. Cancer Inst.*, 62:117–125.
167. Maguire, H., Jr., Outzen, H. C., Custer, R. P., and Prehn, R. T. (1976): Invasion and metastasis of a xenogeneic tumor in nude mice. *J. Natl. Cancer Inst.*, 57:439–442.
168. Mahoney, K. H., Morse, S. S., and Morahan, P. S. (1980): Macrophage functions in beige (Chediak-Higashi syndrome) mice. *Cancer Res.*, 40:3934–3939.
169. Mantovani, A., Allavena, P., Biondi, A., Sessa, C., and Introna, M. (1982): Natural killer activity in human ovarian carcinoma. In: *NK Cells: Fundamental Aspects and Role in Cancer. Human Cancer Immunology, Vol. 4*, edited by B. Serrou, C. Rosenfeld, and R. B. Herberman. North-Holland, Amsterdam, pp. 123–138.
170. Mantovani, A., Giavazzi, R., Polentarutti, N., Spreafico, F., and Garattini, S. (1980): Divergent effects of macrophage toxins on growth of primary tumors and lung metastasis. *Int. J. Cancer*, 25:617–622.
171. Marcelletti, J., and Furmanski, P. (1978): Spontaneous regression of Friend virus induced erythroleukemia. III. The role of macrophages in regression. *J. Immunol.*, 120:1–9.
172. Martin, S. E., and Martin, W. J. (1975): Anti-tumor antibodies in normal mouse sera. *Int. J. Cancer*, 15:658–664.
173. Mavligit, G. M., Gutterman, J. U., McBride, C. M., and Hersh, E. M. (1973): Cell-mediated immunity to human solid tumors: *In vitro* detection by lymphocyte blastogenic responses to cell-associated and solubilized tumor antigens. *Natl. Cancer Inst. Monogr.*, 37:167–176.
174. McBride, W. H., Tuach, W., and Marmion, B. P. (1975): The effects of gold salts on tumor immunity and its stimulation by *Corynebacterium parvum*. *Br. J. Cancer*, 32:558–565.
175. Menard, S., Colnaghi, M. I., and Della Porta, G. (1977): Natural anti-tumor serum reactivity in BALB/c mice. I. Characterization and interference with tumor growth. *Int. J. Cancer*, 19:267–274.
176. Mizel, S. B., Delarco, J. E., Todaro, G. J., Farrar, W. L., and Hilfiker, M. L. (1980): *In vitro* production of immunosuppressive factors by murine sarcoma virus-transformed mouse fibroblasts. *Proc. Natl. Acad. Sci. USA*, 77:2205–2208.
177. Nair, P. N. M., Fernandes, G., Onoe, K., Day, N. K., and Good, R. A. (1980): Inhibition of effector cell functions in natural killer cell activity (NK) and antibody-dependent cellular cytotoxicity (ADCC) in mice by normal and cancer sera. *Int. J. Cancer*, 25:667–677.
178. Nepom, J. T., Hellström, I., and Hellström, K. E. (1976): Purification and partial characterization of a tumor specific blocking factor from sera of mice with growing chemically induced sarcoma. *J. Immunol.*, 117:1846–1854.

179. Norbury, K. C., and Kripke, M. L. (1979): Ultraviolet-induced carcinogenesis in mice treated with silica, trypan blue, or pyran copolymer. *J. Reticuloendothel. Soc.*, 26:827–832.

180. Nossal, G. J. V. (1980): The case history of Mr. T. I. Terminal patient or still curable? *Immunol. Today*, 1:5–9.

181. Nunn, M. E., and Herberman, R. B. (1979): Natural cytotoxicity of mouse, rat and human lymphocytes against heterologous target cells. *J. Natl. Cancer Inst.*, 62:765–771.

182. Nunn, M. E., Herberman, R. B., and Holden, H. T. (1977): Natural cell-mediated cytotoxicity in mice against nonlymphoid tumor cells and some normal cells. *Int. J. Cancer*, 20:381–387.

183. Oehler, J. R., and Herberman, R. B. (1978): Natural cell-mediated cytotoxicity in rats. III. Effects of immunopharmacologic treatments on natural reactivity and on reactivity augmented by polyinosinic-polycytidylic acid. *Int. J. Cancer*, 21:221–229.

184. Oehler, J. R., and Herberman, R. B. (1979): Evidence for long-lasting tumor immunity in a syngeneic rat lymphoma model: Correlation of *in vitro* findings with *in vivo* observations. *J. Natl. Cancer Inst.*, 62:525–529.

185. Oehler, J. R., Herberman, R. B., and Holden, H. T. (1978): Modulation of immunity by macrophages. *Pharmacol. Ther.*, 2:551–593.

186. Ojo, E., and Wigzell, H. (1978): Natural killer cells may be the only cells in normal mouse lymphoid populations endowed with cytolytic ability for antibody-coated tumor target cells. *Scand. J. Immunol.*, 7:297–306.

187. Old, L. J., Stockert, E., Boyse, E. A., and Kim, J. H. (1968): Antigenic modulation. Loss of TL antigen from cells exposed to TL antibody. Study of the phenomenon *in vitro*. *J. Exp. Med.*, 127:523–539.

188. Ortaldo, J. R., Oldham, R. K., Cannon, G. C., and Herberman, R. B. (1977): Specificity of natural cytotoxic reactivity of normal human lymphocytes against a myeloid leukemia cell line. *J. Natl. Cancer Inst.*, 59:77–82.

189. Ortaldo, J. R., Ting, C. C., and Herberman, R. B. (1974): Modulation of fetal antigen(s) in mouse leukemia cells. *Cancer Res.*, 34:1366–1371.

190. Ozzello, L., Sordat, B., Merenda, C., Carrel, S., Hurlimann, J., and Mach, J. P. (1974): Transplantation of a human mammary carcinoma cell line (BT 20) into nude mice. *J. Natl. Cancer Inst.*, 52:1669–1672.

191. Paige, C. J., Figarella, E. F., Cuttito, M. J., Cahan, A., and Stutman, O. (1978): Natural cytotoxic cells against solid tumors in mice. II. Some characteristics of the effector cells. *J. Immunol.*, 121:1827–1835.

192. Papacharalampous, N. X. (1960): Zur frage der experimentellen induktion von tumoren am retothelialen system der ratte nach langfristigen versuchen mit intraperitonealen injektionen von trypanblau. *Frankf. Z. Pathol.*, 70:598–604.

193. Parkinson, D. R., Brightman, R. P., and Waksal, S. D. (1981): Altered natural killer cell biology in C57BL/6 mice after leukemogenic split-dose irradiation. *J. Immunol.*, 126:1460–1464.

194. Payne, L. N. (1972): Pathogenesis of Marek's disease—a review. In: *Oncogenesis and Herpesviruses*, edited by P. M. Briggs, G. Dethé, and L. N. Payne, pp. 21–37. International Agency for Research on Cancer, Lyon.

195. Penn, I., and Starzl, T. E. (1972): A summary of the status of de novo cancer in transplant recipients. *Transplant. Proc.*, 4:719–732.

196. Perry, L. L., Kripke, M. L., Benecerraf, B., Dorf, M. E., and Greene, M. I. (1980): Regulation of the immune response to tumor antigen. VIII. The effects of host specific anti-I-J antibodies on the immune response to tumors of different origin. *Cell. Immunol.*, 51:349–359.

197. Petrányi, G., Kiessling, R., Povey, S., Klein, G., Herzenberg, E., and Wigzell, H. (1976): The genetic control of natural killer cell activity and its association with *in vivo* resistance against a Moloney lymphoma isograft. *Immunogenetics*, 3:15–28.

198. Pike, M. C., and Snyderman, R. (1977): Macrophage migratory dysfunction in cancer. A mechanism for subversion of surveillance. *Am. J. Pathol.*, 88:727–739.

199. Plescia, O. J., Smith, A. H., and Grinwich, K. (1975): Subversion of immune system by tumor cells and role of prostaglandins. *Proc. Natl. Acad. Sci. USA*, 72:1848–1851.

200. Pollack, S., Heppner, G., Brawn, R. J., and Nelson, K. (1972): Specific killing of tumor cells *in vitro* in the presence of normal lymphoid cells and sera from hosts immune to the tumor antigens. *Int. J. Cancer*, 9:316–324.

201. Prather, S. O., and Lausch, R. N. (1976): Membrane-associated antigen from the SV40-induced

hamster fibrosarcoma, PARA-7. I. Role in immune complex formation and effector cell blockade. *Int. J. Cancer*, 18:820–828.

202. Prehn, R. T., and Lappé, M. A. (1971): An immunostimulation theory of tumor development. *Transplant. Rev.*, 7:26–54.

203. Prehn, R. T., and Main, J. M. (1957): Immunity to methylcholanthrene-induced sarcomas. *J. Natl. Cancer Inst.*, 18:769–775.

204. Puri, H. C., and Campbell, R. (1977): Cyclophosphamide and malignancy. *Lancet*, 1:1306.

205. Purtilo, D. T., De Florio, D., Hutt, L. M., Bhawan, J., Yang, J. P. S., Otto, R., and Edwards, W. (1977): Variable phenotypic expression of an X-linked recessive lymphoproliferative syndrome. *N. Engl. J. Med.*, 297:1077–1081.

206. Reimer, R. R., Hoover, R., Fraumeni, J. F., Jr., and Young, R. C. (1977): Acute leukemia after alkylating-agent therapy of ovarian cancer. *N. Engl. J. Med.*, 297:177–181.

207. Rhodes, J. (1980): Resistance of tumor cells to macrophages. *Cancer Immunol. Immunother.*, 7:211–217.

208. Rhodes, J., Bishop, M., and Benfield, J. (1978): Tumor surveillance: How tumors may resist macrophage-mediated host defense. *Science*, 203:179–181.

209. Riccardi, C., Barlozzari, T., Santoni, A., Herberman, R. B., and Cesarini, C. (1981): Transfer to cyclophosphamide-treated mice of natural killer (NK) cells and *in vivo* natural reactivity against tumors. *J. Immunol.*, 126:1284–1289.

210. Riccardi, C., Puccetti, P., Santoni, A., and Herberman, R. B. (1979): Rapid *in vivo* assay of mouse NK cell activity. *J. Natl. Cancer Inst.*, 63:1041–1045.

211. Riccardi, C., Santoni, A., Barlozzari, T., Cesarini, C., and Herberman, R. B. (1982): *In vivo* role of NK cells against neoplastic or non-neoplastic cells. In: *NK Cells: Fundamental Aspects and Role in Cancer. Human Cancer Immunology, Vol. 4*, edited by B. Serrou, C. Rosenfeld, and R. B. Herberman. North-Holland, Amsterdam, pp. 57–68.

212. Riccardi, C., Santoni, A., Barlozzari, T., and Herberman, R. B. (1980): Role of NK cells in rapid *in vivo* clearance of radiolabeled tumor cells. In: *Natural Cell-Mediated Immunity Against Tumors*, edited by R. B. Herberman, pp. 1121–1139. Academic Press, New York.

213. Riccardi, C., Santoni, A., Barlozzari, T., Puccetti, P., and Herberman, R. B. (1980): *In vivo* natural reactivity of mice against tumor cells. *Int. J. Cancer*, 25:475–486.

214. Riesenfeld, I., Orn, A., Gidlund, M., Axberg, I., Alm, G. V., and Wigzell, H. (1980): Positive correlation between *in vivo* NK activity and *in vivo* resistance towards AKR lymphoma cells. *Int. J. Cancer*, 25:399–403.

215. Riley, V. (1975): Mouse mammary tumors: Alteration of incidence as apparent function of stress. *Science*, 189:465–467.

216. Riley, V. (1981): Psychoneuroendocrine influence on immunocompetence and neoplasia. *Science*, 212:1100–1109.

217. Roberts, M. M., and Bell, R. (1976): Acute leukemia after immunosuppressive therapy. *Lancet*, 2:768–770.

218. Roder, J., and Duwe, A. (1979): The beige mutation in the mouse selectively impairs natural killer cell function. *Nature*, 278:451–453.

219. Roder, J. C., Haliotis, T., Klein, M., Korec, S., Jett, J. R., Ortaldo, J., Herberman, R. B., Katz, P., and Fauci, A. S. (1980): A new immunodeficiency disorder in humans involving NK cells. *Nature*, 284:553–555.

220. Roder, J. C., Laing, L., Haliotis, T., and Kozbor, D. (1982): Genetic control of human NK function. In: *NK Cells: Fundamental Aspects and Role in Cancer. Human Cancer Immunology, Vol. 4*, edited by B. Serrou, C. Rosenfeld, and R. B. Herberman. North-Holland, Amsterdam, pp. 169–186.

221. Roder, J. C., Lohmann-Matthes, M.-L., Domzig, W., and Wigzell, H. (1979): The beige mutation in the mouse. II. Selectivity of the natural killer (NK) cell defect. *J. Immunol.*, 123:2174–2181.

222. Rosenberg, E. B., Herberman, R. B., Levine, P. H., Halterman, R. H., McCoy, J. L., and Wunderlich, J. R. (1972): Lymphocyte cytotoxicity reactions to leukemia-associated antigens in identical twins. *Int. J. Cancer*, 9:648–658.

223. Russell, S. (1982): In: *Symposium on Role of Natural Killer Cells, Macrophages and Antibody Dependent Cellular Cytotoxicity in Tumor Rejection and as Mediators of Biological Response Modifiers Activity*, edited by M. A. Chirigos. Raven Press, New York, pp. 49–56.

224. Rygaard, J., and Poulsen, C. O. (1969): Heterotransplantation of a human malignant tumor to nude mice. *Acta Pathol. Microbiol. Scand.*, 77:758–760.

225. Santoni, A., Riccardi, C., Barlozzari, T., and Herberman, R. B. (1980): Suppression of activity of mouse natural killer (NK) cells by activated macrophages from mice treated with pyran copolymer. *Int. J. Cancer*, 26:837–843.

226. Santoni, A., Riccardi, C., Barlozzari, T., and Herberman, R. B. (1980): Inhibition as well as augmentation of mouse NK activity by pyran copolymer and adriamycin. In: *Natural Cell-Mediated Immunity Against Tumors*, edited by R. B. Herberman, pp. 753–763. Academic Press, New York.

227. Schmidt, M., and Good, R. A. (1976): Cancer xenografts in nude mice. *Lancet*, 1:39.

228. Schultz, R. M., Stoychkov, J. N., Pavlidis, N., Chirigos, M. A., and Olkowski, Z. L. (1979): *J. Reticuloendothel. Soc.*, 26:93–102.

229. Sendo, F., Aoki, T., Boyse, E. A., and Buafo, C. K. (1975): Natural occurrence of lymphocytes showing cytotoxic activity to BALB/c radiation-induced leukemia RL♂1 cells. *J. Natl. Cancer Inst.*, 55:603–609.

230. Serrate, S., and Herberman, R. B. (1981): Natural cell-mediated cytotoxicity against primary mammary tumors. *Fed. Proc.*, 40:1007.

231. Sharkey, F. E., and Fogh, J. (1979): Metastasis of human tumors in athymic nude mice. *Int. J. Cancer*, 24:733–738.

232. Shin, H. S., Economou, J. S., Pasternack, G. R., Johnson, R. J., and Hayden, M. (1976): Antibody mediated suppression of grafted lymphoma. IV. Influence of time of tumor residency *in vivo* and tumor size upon the effectiveness of suppression by syngeneic antibody. *J. Exp. Med.*, 144:1274–1283.

233. Shin, H. S., Hayden, M. L., Langley, S., Kaliss, N., and Smith, M. R. (1975): Antibody-mediated suppression of grafted lymphoma. III. Evaluation of the role of thymic function, non-thumus-derived lymphocytes, macrophages, platelets and polymorphonuclear leukocytes in syngeneic and allogeneic hosts. *J. Immunol.*, 114:1255.

234. Shin, H. S., Johnson, R. J., Pasternack, G. R., and Economou, J. S. (1978): Mechanisms of tumor immunity: The role of antibody and nonimmune effectors. *Prog. Allergy*, 25:163–210.

235. Shope, T. C., and Kaplan, J. (1979): Inhibition of the *in vitro* out growth of Epstein-Barr virus-infected lymphocytes by T$_G$ lymphocytes. *J. Immunol.*, 123:2150–2155.

236. Sjögren, H. O. (1974): Blocking and unblocking of cell-mediated tumor immunity. *Methods Cancer Res.*, 10:19–32.

237. Sones, P. D. E., and Castro, J. E. (1977): Immunological mechanisms in metastatic spread and the antimetastatic effect of *C. parvum*. *Br. J. Cancer*, 35:519–526.

238. Stern, K. (1983): Control of tumors by the RES. In: *The Reticuloendothelial System. A Comprehensive Treatise, Vol. VIII, Cancer*, edited by R. B. Herberman and H. Friedman. Plenum, New York *(in press)*.

239. Stjernswärd, J., and Vánky, F. (1972): Stimulation of lymphocytes by autochthonous cancer. *Natl. Cancer Inst. Monogr.*, 35:237–242.

240. Strausser, H. R., and Humes, J. L. (1975): Prostaglandin synthesis inhibition: Effect on bone changes and sarcoma tumor induction in BALB/c mice. *Int. J. Cancer*, 15:724–730.

241. Stutman, O. (1975): Tumor development after polyoma infection in athymic nude mice. *J. Immunol.*, 114:1213–1217.

242. Stutman, O. (1975): Immunodepression and malignancy. In: *Advances in Cancer Research, Vol. 22*, edited by G. Klein, S. Weinhouse, and A. Haddow, pp. 261–422. Academic Press, New York.

243. Stutman, O. (1979): Chemical carcinogenesis in nude mice: Comparison between nude mice from homozygous matings and heterozygous matings and effect of age and carcinogen dose. *J. Natl. Cancer Inst.*, 62:353–358.

244. Stutman, O., Dien, P., Wisun, R., Pecoraro, G., and Lattime, E. C. (1980): Natural cytotoxic (NC) cells against solid tumors in mice: Some target cell characteristics and blocking of cytotoxicity by D-mannose. In: *Natural Cell-Mediated Immunity Against Tumors*, edited by R. B. Herberman, pp. 949–961. Academic Press, New York.

245. Stutman, O., Figarella, E. F., Paige, C. J., and Lattime, E. C. (1980): Natural cytotoxic (NC) cells against solid tumors in mice: General characteristics and comparison to natural killer (NK) cells. In: *Natural Cell-Mediated Immunity Against Tumors*, edited by R. B. Herberman, pp. 187–229. Academic Press, New York.

246. Stutman, O., Figarella, E. F., and Wisun, R. (1980): Natural cytotoxic (NC) cells in tumor-bearing mice. In: *Natural Cell-Mediated Immunity Against Tumors*, edited by R. B. Herberman, pp. 1073–1079. Academic Press, New York.

246a.Sulica, A., Gherman, M., Galatiuc, C., Manciulea, M., and Herberman, R. B. (1982): Inhibition of human natural killer cell activity by cytophilic immunoglobulin G[1]. *J. Immunol.*, 128:1031–1036.

247. Sullivan, J. L., Byron, K. S., Brewster, F. E., and Purtilo, D. T. (1980): Deficient natural killer cell activity in X-linked lymphoproliferative syndrome. *Science*, 210:543–545.

248. Takei, F., Levy, J. G., and Kilburn, D. G. (1976): *In vitro* induction of cytotoxicity against syngeneic mastocytoma and its suppression by spleen and thymus cells from tumor-bearing mice. *J. Immunol.*, 116:288–293.

249. Talmadge, J. E., Meyers, K. M., Prieur, D. J., and Starkey, J. R. (1980): Role of NK cells in tumour growth and metastasis in beige mice. *Nature*, 284:622–624.

250. Tam, M. R., Emmons, S. L., and Pollack, S. B. (1980): FACS analysis and enrichment of NK effector cells. In: *Natural Cell-Mediated Immunity Against Tumors*, edited by R. B. Herberman, pp. 265–276. Academic Press, New York.

251. Tchernia, G., Mielot, F., and Subtil, E. (1976): Acute myeloblastic leukemia after immunodepressive therapy for primary nonmalignant diseases. *Blood Cells*, 2:67–80.

252. Terman, D. S. (1981): Tumoricidal responses in spontaneous canine neoplasms after extracorporeal perfusion over immobilized protein A. *Fed. Proc.*, 40:45–49.

253. Tewari, R. P., Balint, J. P., and Brown, K. A. (1979): Suppressive effect of 3-methylcholanthrene on phagocytic activity of mouse peritoneal macrophages for Torulopsis glabrata. *J. Natl. Cancer Inst.*, 62:983–990.

254. Thomas, L. (1959): Discussion. In: *Cellular and Humoral Aspects of the Hypersensitive State*, edited by H. S. Lawrence, pp. 529–530. Harper, New York.

255. Thomson, D. M. P. (1975): Soluble tumour-specific antigen and its relationship to tumour growth. *Int. J. Cancer*, 15:1016–1029.

256. Thor, D. E., Reichert, D. F., and Flippen, J. H. (1977): The interaction of chemical carcinogens and the immune responses. *J. Reticuloendothel. Soc.*, 22:243–252.

257. Timonen, T., Ortaldo, J. R., Bonnard, G. D., and Herberman, R. B. (1982): Cultures of human natural killer cells in the presence of T cell growth factor (TCGF) containing medium (CM). In: *Proceedings of the 14th International Leukocyte Culture Conference (in press)*.

258. Ting, C. C., and Herberman, R. B. (1976): Humoral host defense mechanisms against tumors. In: *International Review of Experimental Pathology, Vol. 15*, edited by G. W. Richter and M. A. Epstein, pp. 93–152. Academic Press, New York.

259. Ting, C. C., Lavrin, D. H., Takemoto, K. K., Ting, R. C., and Herberman, R. B. (1972): Expression of various tumor-specific antigens in polyoma virus-induced tumors. *Cancer Res.*, 32:1–6.

260. Trinchieri, G., and Santoli, D. (1978): Anti-viral activity induced by culturing lymphocytes with tumor-derived or virus-transformed cells. Enhancement of human natural killer cell activity by interferon and antagonistic inhibition of susceptibility of target cells to lysis. *J. Exp. Med.*, 147:1314–1333.

261. Tursz, T., Dokhelar, M.-C., Lipinski, M., and Amiel, J.-L. (1982): Low natural killer (NK) cell activity in patients with malignant lymphoma or with a high risk of lymphoid tumors. In: *NK Cells: Fundamental Aspects and Role in Cancer. Human Cancer Immunology, Vol. 4*, edited by B. Serrou, C. Rosenfeld, and R. B. Herberman. North-Holland, Amsterdam, pp. 241–248.

262. Vánky, F. T., Argov, S. A., Einhorn, S. A., and Klein, E. (1980): Role of alloantigens in natural killing. Allogeneic but not autologous tumor biopsy cells are sensitive for interferon-induced cytotoxicity of human blood lymphocytes. *J. Exp. Med.*, 151:1151–1165.

263. Varesio, L., Herberman, R. B., Gerson, J. M., and Holden, H. T. (1979): Suppression of lymphokine production by macrophages infiltrating murine virus-induced tumors. *Int. J. Cancer*, 24:97–102.

264. Varesio, L., Holden, H. T., and Taramelli, D. (1980): Mechanism of lymphocyte activation. II. Requirements for macromolecular synthesis in the production of lymphokines. *J. Immunol.*, 125:2810–2817.

265. Vose, B. M. (1980): Natural killers in human cancer: Activity of tumor-infiltrating and draining node lymphocytes. In: *Natural Cell-Mediated Immunity Against Tumors*, edited by R. B. Herberman, pp. 1081–1097. Academic Press, New York.

266. Vose, B. M., and Moore, M. (1979): Suppressor cell activity of lymphocytes infiltrating human lung and breast tumors. *Int. J. Cancer*, 24:579–585.

267. Walpole, A. L. (1962): Observations upon the induction of subcutaneous sarcomas in rats. In:

The Morphological Precursors of Cancer, edited by L. Severi, pp. 83–88. University of Perugia Division of Cancer Research.

268. Welsh, R. M., Jr., and Kiessling, R. W. (1980): Natural killer cell response to lymphocytic choriomeningitis virus in beige mice. *Scand. J. Immunol.*, 11:363–367.

269. Wood, G. W., and Gillespie, G. Y. (1973): Studies on the role of macrophages in regulation of growth and metastases of murine chemically induced fibrosarcomas. *Int. J. Cancer*, 16:1022–1029.

270. Wright, P. W., Hellstrom, K. E., and Hellstrom, I. (1976): Serotherapy of malignant disease. *Med. Clin. North Am.*, 60:607–630.

271. Yunis, E. J., Martinez, C., Smith, J., Stutman, O., and Good, R. A. (1969): Spontaneous mammary adenocarcinoma in mice: Influence of thymectomy and reconstitution with thymus grafts or spleen cells. *Cancer Res.*, 29:174–178.

272. Zarling, J. M., Eskra, L., Borden, E. C., Horoszewicz, J., and Carter, W. A. (1979): Activation of human natural killer cells cytotoxic for human leukemia cells by purified interferon. *J. Immunol.*, 123:63–70.

273. Zwilling, B. S., Filippi, J. A., and Chorpenning, F. W. (1978): Chemical carcinogenesis and immunity: Immunologic studies of rats treated with methylnitrosourea. *J. Natl. Cancer Inst.*, 61:731–738.

Advances in Host Defense Mechanisms, Vol. 2,
edited by John I. Gallin and Anthony S. Fauci.
Raven Press, New York © 1983.

Nutrition, Host Defenses, and the Lymphoid System

Gerald T. Keusch, *Carla S. Wilson, and **Samuel D. Waksal

*Division of Geographic Medicine, Department of Medicine, Tufts-New England
Medical Center, Boston, Massachusetts 02111*

The functional integrity of the immune system is significantly altered by dietary factors. The advances in immunology over the past two decades have broadened its importance for other scientific disciplines. At the same time, the influence of such factors as nutrition is becoming increasingly important for the understanding of immunologic events. There is ample clinical evidence of concomitant depression of host defense mechanisms and increased infectious disease problems in mal-nourished individuals (63,83,107,108,127,140,143,175,176,182,191,192,204,208, 212,232,238,248,258). These observations support the *in vitro* and experimental data on the interaction of nutritional deficiencies and immune function. The specific biochemical mechanisms involved are not known, but recent experimental studies in animals have begun to elucidate the alterations associated with mononutrient deficiency states. Such experiments can be expected to reveal a great deal of information about the biochemical pathways involved in differentiation, maturation, and regulation of specific subsets of lymphoid and phagocytic cells or the production of individual proteins or regulator molecules which function in various immunologic phenomena. It is not unreasonable to expect that dietary manipulations ultimately may be used to selectively affect individual components of the immune system for therapeutic benefit. One example of this approach is the recent evidence that restricted protein intake can depress and delay the development of autoimmune disease manifestations in the NZB/W f_1 hybrid mouse and prolong its survival (90,91).

This chapter focuses on the effects of nutritional alterations on lymphocyte biology. The earlier works are not reviewed extensively because this has been adequately done by others in the past few years (55,83,110,140,269). Instead, we focus on the research over the last decade, largely because of the tremendous progress in immunology over this time. Indeed, methodology and the ability to dissect out the components of lymphocyte function have advanced so far that early studies may no longer be interpretable in the light of current notions of the organization of the immune system; at worst, they may be misleading.

Current address: Department of Nutrition and Food Science, Massachusetts Institute of Technology, Cambridge, Massachusetts 02111; **Department of Pathology, Mt. Sinai Medical Center, 1 Gustave Levy Place, New York, New York 10029

We also attempt to be critical rather than encyclopedic, in the hope that we thus may point out needs for future investigation and the potential pitfalls likely to be encountered in either human or experimental research. In this context, we begin with an overview of both immunologic and nutritional considerations.

IMMUNOLOGIC CONSIDERATIONS

Long before the thymus gland was discovered to be a critical factor in the differentiation of the T lymphocyte system, it was known that malnutrition resulted in a rapid loss of thymic mass, depletion of thymic lymphocytes, and dramatic alteration of thymic architecture. Historic highlights include the publications by Simon in 1845 (244), Jackson in 1925 (130), and Vint in 1937 (264) and the subsequent use of the term "nutritional thymectomy" (249).

The link between nutrition, the thymus, and disease has been investigated since the beginning of this century. For example, in 1914, Rous (230) studied the effect of limited feeding (dietary restriction) on the susceptibility to the growth of transplantable tumors in mice. The results were variable; but in many instances, tumors failed to progress. In considering the possible mechanisms, the author noted that the resistance elicited in the host by the tumor was probably involved: "Through the instability that it (resistance) introduces, it may have been responsible for the sensitiveness to alterations in the host diet by the transplanted mouse tumors." However, he then went on to deny the possibility that diet could stimulate and/or alter immune processes in the host. Thirty years later, Saxton and colleagues (233) showed that underfeeding inbred AKR mice, which develop a high incidence of spontaneous lymphoid leukemia, resulted in a sharply diminished incidence of disease (from 65 to 10%). Because of the thymic involution associated with the dietary regimen, they considered that the critical events might be mediated through the thymus gland. McEndy et al. (180) then examined the effect of thymectomy in young adult mice and again found a dramatic decrease in leukemia incidence. In retrospect, it was these studies that pioneered the work on the central role of the thymus in the development of the immune response. The complexity of the interactions between nutrition, the thymus, and disease is further demonstrated by more recent experiments, which show that, in some cases, underfeeding can augment many T lymphocyte-mediated immune responses in mice (61,62). These responses are involved in the host response to tumors, to autoimmune diseases, and to infection.

The studies of the past two decades in animals, particularly inbred strains of mice, but also in humans with genetic and acquired immunodeficiencies, have literally revolutionized our understanding of lymphocyte development and function. The chapters in this volume represent a contemporary and detailed view of lymphocyte biology in health and disease. In order to discuss the impact of nutrition on the lymphocyte, it will be helpful to briefly outline our own concepts and thus the perspective we have used in organizing the following material. Thus our bias in areas of controversy will be made clear, and the reader can better assess the validity of the conclusions we have drawn. This is particularly important because of the divergent results that have been obtained in human versus animal experiments. Some authors have spoken of this as a paradox, but perhaps this paradox has a basis in fact.

The effects of nutritional deprivation on the immune system must be understood in terms of the interactions of the subpopulations of cells involved in the immunologic network (Fig. 1). This network consists of interacting thymus-derived lymphocytes (T cells), antibody-forming cell precursors (B cells), and macrophage-like antigen-presenting cells (APCs). The interactions between these cell types and their ability to respond to various antigens is controlled by genes of the major histocompatibility complex (MHC) of humans and animals (30). These genes encode for cell surface determinants (HLA-D in humans and Ia in the murine model). Antigens are presented by APCs in conjunction with Ia molecules (229). At the same time, these macrophage-like cells produce interleukin-1 (IL-1), which triggers the response of helper T cell populations (228). This subpopulation of T cells, which expresses the differentiation antigen Leu 3 in humans and Lyt 1 in the murine system, responds to antigen presented by Ia-positive APCs. T cells of this subclass then respond to this signal by proliferating and subsequently producing interleukin-2 (IL-2). IL-2 nonspecifically stimulates both the generation of cytotoxic T cells, which effect cell-mediated lympholysis, and B cells, which differentiate into antibody-secreting plasma cells (265).

Cytotoxic T cells, induced by IL-2, express the Lyt 2,3 phenotype in the murine system and Leu 2 in humans (45,132) (Table 1). They are able to lyse allogeneic or virus-infected cells in association with the antigens encoded by the K or D end of the murine MHC or the equivalent HLA-A, B, or C in humans. IL-2 also acts on B cells to signal the proliferation and differentiation of antigen-specific precursor cells into secretory plasma cells. These signals are nonspecific and can induce both T and B cell responses to any antigen. There is also a specific component of the response which is linked to the Ig-variable region and encodes for the antigen-specific receptor on both T and B cells. The expression of these genes at the level of idiotypic determinants expressed on lymphocytes allows for the specific expansion of antigen-reactive clones as compared to the nonspecific triggering by IL-1 and IL-2 (33,267).

Feedback loops exist throughout this network, acting to down-regulate the immune response. Specific suppression is mediated by antiidiotype on Lyt 2,3 (Leu 2)-positive T cells, which in turn are induced by Lyt 1,2,3-positive T cells. Nonspecific suppression may be mediated by MHC-linked genes (105).

Because of the complexity of the immunologic network, nutritional factors can affect the immune system at various levels. Specific metabolic requirements for the generation of any of these cell interactions could alter the generation of some or all of these cellular subpopulations in the presence of nutritional deprivation. The cells involved in the immunologic network all develop from precursors derived from yolk sac and fetal liver during embryogenesis and from bone marrow during adult life (96,207). Pluripotential stem cells differentiate into precommitted pre-

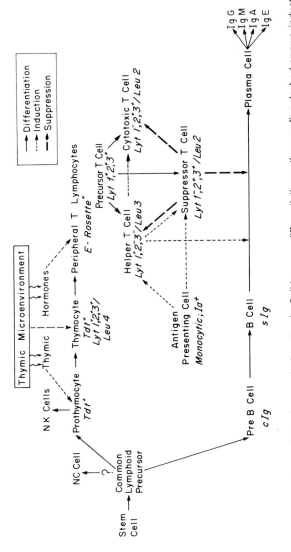

FIG. 1. Major pathways in the immunologic network. *Solid arrows*, differentiation pathways: *fine dashed arrows*, inductive pathways; *heavy dashed arrows*, suppressive effects.

TABLE 1. *Differentiation markers on murine and human T-cell subpopulations*

T-cell subpopulation	Differentiation marker	
	Murine	Human
Prothymocyte	Lyt 1 BAT	OK T 9
Thymocyte (immature)	Lyt 1,2,3 $^+$	OK T 9 Leu 4
Peripheral T cell (mature)	Thy 1	OK T 1 OK T 11 E-rosette $^+$
Helper T cell	Thy 1 Lyt 1 $^+$,2,3 $^-$	OK T 4 Leu 3 E-rosette $^+$
Cytotoxic/suppressor T cell	Thy 1 Lyt 1 $^-$,2,3 $^+$	OK T 5 Leu 2 E-rosette $^+$
Inducers of suppressors	Thy 1 Lyt 1 $^-$,2,3 $^+$	E-rosette $^+$

cursor cells which, under the influence of specific microenvironments and factors produced by these microenvironments, mature into functional cells expressing the markers which we have mentioned.

The lack of protein or specific vitamins and minerals might affect the inducing microenvironment as well as the developing precursor cells. B lymphocytes develop in mammals in the equivalent of the Bursa of Fabricius of birds, although the specific site remains unknown (188). T lymphocytes develop in the thymus, as precursors from the bone marrow enter the epithelial anlage and are induced to differentiate by humoral and/or cellular interactions (70,188) (Fig. 1). Within the thymic microenvironment, multiple subsets of lymphocytes develop. Both Lyt 1 $^+$,2,3 $^-$ (Leu 3) and Lyt 1,2,3 $^+$ (Leu 4) cells mature along separate developmental lineages (126). There is also distinct compartmentalization within the thymus: the outer capsular cortex containing large functionally immature cells, the deep cortex containing medium sized immature cells, and the medullary region containing small functionally competent thymocytes (272). Cells in both the outer and deep cortex are sensitive to cortisone, whereas medullary cells are cortisone resistant. The deficiency of nutrients specifically required for normal thymic epithelial cell growth or secretion of thymic humoral factors would also effect the maturation process for these various cells of the T lymphocyte system.

There are, therefore, multiple sites and varied mechanisms by which nutritional deprivation could mediate an effect on immunologic responses and the development of cells taking part in such responses. We attempt to dissect and discuss these mechanisms so they can be understood with some "specificity."

NUTRITIONAL CONSIDERATIONS

It is no simple task to define malnutrition, in part because it is so difficult to define optimal nutrition. In contrast, specific deficiency diseases, such as the various clinical syndromes due to inadequate intakes of individual vitamins, often are adequately understood. Minimum dietary levels of the nutrient needed to prevent disease manifestations have been determined. At the same time, the biochemical role of most vitamins and the species-specific needs, depending on the metabolic pathways present, have been defined—a major triumph of modern nutritional biochemistry. This model does not work well in other situations, however, such as protein and energy (calorie) intake, and it is precisely these two critical components of the diet that appear to be in limited supply for much of the world's population. Indeed, the term malnutrition as commonly employed refers to combined protein-energy malnutrition (PEM); most of the human studies and much of the animal work on nutrition-immune system interactions have involved PEM.

When protein and/or energy intakes are restricted, the young organism cannot grow normally, and in any age group, weight per unit height will be reduced (176,274). Until there are overt clinical effects, however, the consequences of growth retardation or weight loss may not be obvious. In fact, animal experimentation suggests that underfeeding may prolong lifespan and retard the decline in immune function that accompanies aging (271). In this sense, undernutrition without malnutrition can be beneficial to health. There is a growing recognition that neither undernutrition nor malnutrition can be adequately defined without an examination of effects on the physiologic (functional) state of the host, and efforts to research this area have been initiated.

Since the spectrum of nutritional adequacy or inadequacy relates to some standard, for example, the recommended dietary allowances (RDAs) for various components of the diet, it is worthwhile to consider how these standards are set (197). Let us examine protein, since there has been great concern over the "protein gap" in human nutrition (the concept that diets in many parts of the developing world are increasingly more deficient in utilizable protein than other constituents) and considerable experimental work done with isocaloric-protein-deprived diets in animals. It must be recalled at the outset, however, that protein needs undoubtedly change with age, are influenced by environmental factors, and are subject to complex regulatory metabolic adjustments in the host (adaptation) (277). Protein intake must satisfy the needs for nitrogen and specific amino acids which cannot be biosynthesized within the host (and hence are termed "essential") for tissue repair, tissue maintenance, and, in the young, growth. In addition, dietary protein provides nitrogen for the synthesis of diverse nitrogren-containing compounds and for the balance of obligatory daily losses of nitrogen through turnover and metabolism.

Table 2 lists the essential amino acids for humans and a few selected animal species. Most species require the same basic group of nine amino acids listed for the human, with one or two additional needs in some animals. A few of the "dispensible" (i.e., nonessential) amino acids which can be synthesized in the body

TABLE 2. *Essential amino acids for humans and some animals*

Human	Rat	Mouse	Chick
His (infant, ? adult)	Arg (infant)	Arg (infant)	Arg
Ile	His	His	Gly
Leu	Ile	Ile	His
Lys	Leu	Leu	Ile
Met	Lys	Lys	Leu
Phe	Met	Met	Lys
Thr	Phe	Phe	Met
Trp	Thr	Thr	Phe
Val	Trp	Trp	Thr
	Val	Val	Trp
			Val

are produced only from certain essential amino acids. Thus methionine is required for cysteine production, while phenylalanine can be converted to tyrosine. When cysteine or tyrosine is present in the diet, the requirements for methionine or phenylalanine are reduced. The other nonessential amino acids are made from organic acid intermediates in carbohydrate metabolism, such as α-ketoglutarate or pyruvate, from other amino acids present in excess and from other nitrogen compounds.

How are these needs determined? One important methodology examines the ability of diets depleted in specific amino acids and repleted at varying levels to support maximum growth of a young animal or to maintain nitrogen balance in adults (277). It is more difficult to assess growth potential in humans, because ethical considerations preclude an adequate study design. Nitrogen retention thus becomes the major study tool available. When intact proteins are consumed, additional factors related to digestion and absorption come into play. Moreover, different proteins are not equivalent in satisfying nutritional needs. Animal proteins in general can meet physiologic requirements for amino acids at lower dietary levels of intake than plant proteins. This measure of protein utilization is termed protein quality and is related to the quantities of specific amino acids that become limiting at restricted intake levels (196) (Table 3). However, the apparent biologic value of any given protein also varies with the level of intake; nitrogen retention becomes more efficient (higher biologic value) at low levels of intake. Intake is always less than the amount of protein synthesized each day, indicating extensive reutilization of amino acids. Individual tissues or organs may also respond uniquely. Finally, nitrogen utilization depends on the level of energy intake; at low levels, some protein will be used to meet energy needs through deamination reactions, gluconeogenesis, and excretion of the removed nitrogen.

The complexities in determination of requirements, evident from the foregoing discussion, and methodologic problems inherent in each technique used experimentally (not discussed) make estimates of dietary needs somewhat imprecise.

TABLE 3. *Essential amino acid composition of different dietary proteins*

Amino acid	Amino acid content (mg/g *N*)			
	Egg albumin	Peanut flour	Casein	Wheat gluten
Arg	374	705	244	230
His	151	139	190	124
Ile	403	259	397	284
Leu	548	442	626	450
Lys	450	218	506	126
Met	260	52	203	104
Cys[a]	186	90	25	148
Phe	371	307	338	315
Tyr[b]	208	181	322	174
Thr	305	174	281	175
Trp	72	49	60	48
Val	466	285	460	266
Nutritive value[c]	100	56	77	44

[a]Reduces requirement for Met.
[b]Reduces requirement for Phe.
[c]Relative to egg albumin = 100.

RDAs are recommended levels of intake considered to be adequate "to meet the known nutritional needs of practically all healthy persons" (195,197). They are based on scientific knowledge of requirements for healthy individuals but are not equivalent to requirements. The RDA is set high enough to account for individual variability in utilization and need; for most subjects the RDA represents an excess intake.

Clinical Considerations in Humans

The majority of observations on immune function and nutritional status in the human come from subjects with PEM. Two polar forms occur in patients: (a) marasmus, a balanced reduced intake of protein and energy, or (b) kwashiorkor, a situation in which protein deprivation exceeds the reduction in energy intake. Clinical features that distinguish the two situations include the relative preservation of serum protein levels (e.g., albumin and transferrin) and lack of edema in the former, and dramatic hypoalbuminemia and decreased transferrin levels accompanied by edema in the latter. Intermediate states exist as well, classified marasmic/kwashiorkor in most clinical studies, with more modest reduction in serum protein levels and the presence of traces of edema. In a broad sense, these categories correspond to variations in adaptation of host metabolism to the stress, particularly with respect to the catabolism of body proteins (so-called labile stores) and the apparent priorities for protein synthesis, particularly by the liver.

Unlike experimental animals, humans do not eat formulated diets which attempt to provide a balanced intake of energy, protein, minerals, and vitamins. People eat food according to availability and their ability to grow it or pay for it. The more economically advantaged may consume a varied diet with multiple sources of needed nutrients in great excess; the poor often eat a monotonous diet (in this sense similar to laboratory chow), but not necessarily balanced. Human malnutrition rarely is due to a single nutrient deficiency but rather is a mosaic of deficiency, sufficiency, or excess of multiple nutrients; malnutrition of a single dietary component usually is a luxury of laboratory manipulation. Human PEM, therefore, is probably complicated by other deficiencies which, not looked for, are not considered. Even PEM itself is not necessarily the same in all regions of the world, since the major source of dietary protein is different in various populations; hence different amino acids may be limiting, producing distinct effects on immune function. Genetic differences in assimilation and utilization of proteins can further complicate the problems. These effects probably are magnified by the nature of the protein sources consumed by most of the world's poor, which are generally plant proteins (grains) of relatively low quality. The poor cannot compensate by increasing the amount consumed. In addition, and again unlike animal models, food intake of humans is not constant from day to day in either quantity or quality. Human malnutrition develops over time, during which there is tremendous variability in the availability of individual nutrients. Experimentally manipulated animals experience a smooth or level deprivation according to the protocol and usually for relatively short periods. The consequences of the variable dietary stress in the human for the function of different limbs of the immune system are not necessarily the same as those observed in a controlled model.

Furthermore, the presence of acute, subacute, or chronic infection, so common in the population of developing countries, alters the pattern of utilization, distribution, and retention of nutrients (24,140). Metabolic sequelae of infectious diseases occur in the healthy as well; these alterations are part of the evolved host response to the stress. Major changes occur in the anabolism and catabolism of body proteins, the flow of amino acids within the body, the utilization of energy stores, the biosynthesis of glucose, the distribution of minerals, and the levels of glucoregulatory hormones, including insulin, growth hormone, glucagon, and corticosteroids. These factors can also affect diverse functions, including those of the immune system, which may be activated by the infectious process and modulated by the metabolic and hormonal concomitants of infection or by the infectious agent itself. Since humans are not reared under controlled conditions which guarantee their being specific pathogen free (SPF), as are SPF laboratory animals, and since they are not housed in laminar flow or clean conditions, they may be subject to many stresses in addition to the nutritional insult they have suffered. It is not surprising how difficult it is to exclude the presence of infection when microbiologic examination is limited and histologic examination cannot be conducted at the completion of the experiment. The result, however, is that human subjects in clinical studies can only be divided into groups with either proven infection or no proven infection, each of which is without doubt heterogenous with respect to genetic background, nutritional state, as well as infectious disease history.

The overall conclusion from these considerations is that the human situation is so complex that simplified models of pure deficiencies in controlled animal experiments cannot be directly extrapolated. We can legitimately question whether or not animal models of malnutrition are, in fact, model nonmodels of the human situation. Thus we must always refer back to the observations in the human and attempt to dissect out the multiple variables present which might affect the results. Only rarely has this been done.

Experimental Considerations in Animal Models

The human represents a difficult and delicate system in which to study nutritional-immunologic interactions. For example, access to lymphoid organs for sophisticated immunologic tests is impossible except at autopsy. This is one of the great advantages of working with experimental animal models, as well as the relative ease in producing an animal that is truly deficient in a single nutrient. Only with the inadequacies of parenteral feeding or the occurrence of certain disease states have some single nutrient deficiencies been seen in the human. Even in these instances, the problems of intercurrent infections and endocrinologic changes affecting immunologic parameters still arise. In many human studies, individual variability within a sample group is often more important, when breaking a study down into a multiple analysis of variance, than the variability due to the indice being tested. To get rid of this individual variability, the use of highly inbred strains of mice has become important in immunologic work. Most of the tools used to dissect out immune mechanism have been developed for use in the mouse system and adapted to the human. Most important, the genetic influences on murine immune function are known in considerable detail. Thus in the immunologic sciences, the mouse has become the model of choice. In the nutritional sciences, however, much work has been done in the rat and other animals where nutrient requirements are fairly well established. The nutrient requirements of the different inbred strains of mice have yet to be completely worked out and can be expected to be somewhat different from strain to strain. In the present discussion, we attempt to explain why one model is used over another in order to understand both the drawbacks and the benefits of the model in comparison to the human situation.

In this context, an important consideration when selecting an animal model for nutritional manipulation is whether it is physiologically relevant and what the clinical consequences might be. For instance, the mouse is inappropriate for studying vitamin C deficiency because it synthesizes its own vitamin C *de novo*. Man, primates, and the guinea pig, on the other hand, must consume a source of vitamin C since they are missing a key enzyme in the pathway of ascorbic acid synthesis. Many immunologic changes attributable to nutritional deficiencies probably are the result of enzymatic and cellular subpopulation modulations. Yet the compartmentation of enzymes is not the same in all species. A nutritional deficiency may have selective effects in different animals, depending on the location of the metabolic pathway being affected.

A number of variables can alter the outcome of a study and are relevant to the design of the experiment for optimal results. Factors that must be considered include (a) age in relation to the maturation of the species at the onset of the study, (b) variations in immunologic regulation, such as autoimmune reactivity, (c) differences in growth curves, (d) previous immunologic experience, (e) presence of infection, (f) severity and length of nutritional deficit, and (g) differences between sexes in response to a dietary change. Prohaska and Lukasewycz (218) recently showed that male mice are much more susceptible to dietary copper deficiency than females. Nutrients, such as zinc, that are required for cell division can be expected to cause more profound changes during periods of rapid growth than if deprivation occurs during a steady state. The growth rate of an animal and the half-life of a nutrient within the animal will be important in determining the length of time an animal will need to be on a diet before a deficiency state occurs. For example, it is nearly impossible to deplete a mouse of vitamin A (a fat-soluble vitamin) unless the dam is deprived prior to birth, while a guinea pig shows signs of severe vitamin C deprivation (a water-soluble vitamin) within 3 weeks. It is not clear whether acute severe deficiencies cause effects similar to suboptimal chronic deficiencies.

The question of whether animals should be raised in a germ-free environment often is brought up. Infection causes a redistribution of nutrients within body compartments and can act synergistically with malnutrition to the detriment of the animal (24,140,239). It becomes difficult to distinguish between the changes caused by infection and the nutrient deficiency. Yet a germ-free environment changes the normal colonization of the gut and is physiologically distinct from the situation in humans.

Extrinsic contamination, especially for trace minerals, such as zinc, must be reduced when depriving an animal of such nutrients. This is helped by acid washing cages and equipment and by handling animals with plastic gloves. Deionized distilled water for drinking should be dispensed in acid-washed bottles as well. The diet being fed to the experimental animal, whether it is commercial or self-prepared, must be assayed for the nutrient being studied. For controlled studies, it is best to feed the same diet to the controls and deficient animals and add the deleted nutrient. The level of nutrient addition to pair-fed animals may have to be at a higher level than to *ad lib* controls to assure adequacy. Pair feeding is best done if animals are caged individually in order to measure all the food consumed and lost by a given animal.

As many environmental influences as possible should be controlled in the housing of experimental animals. For rodents, a regulated light-dark cycle (e.g., 12 hr light, 12 hr dark) is necessary: it determines circadian rhythms when food is continuously available. Temperature, humidity, and noise have secondary effects on the cycles and also must be standardized.

One fault with many studies is the absence of a control for the inanition that often coexists with nutrient deprivation. Pair feeding is usually used to account for food consumption differences between experimental groups. However, pair-fed animals consume their food quickly and are in essence on a scheduled feeding pattern rather than the nibbling feeding pattern of those fed *ad lib*. Comparatively, an *ad lib*-fed animal is never in a fasted basal state. For this reason, pair feeding once a day as a control procedure has come under much scrutiny. The concern is justifiable considering the metabolic and biochemical alterations produced by pair feeding.

Although the light-dark cycle is the major synchronizer in circadian rhythms and the pituitary-adrenal system, food restriction can override the influence of the cycle for some variables (146). A single meal in a restricted feeding schedule causes phase shifts in body temperature, liver protein synthesis, corticosterone levels, peak plasma protein and albumin levels, liver glycogen, serum glucose, brain tryptophan and biogenic amines, certain liver enzymes, and behavioral activity (146,199,211,213). The timing of food accessibility in relation to light seems important. If rats are fed a meal early in the light cycle when they are normally resting, these variables are altered, compared to feeding at the beginning of the dark cycle (102,199).

In a study comparing types of pair feeding, rats were subjected to three different restricted feeding schedules: food given 3 hr after the lights came on, 1 hr before the lights went out, or a ⅛ daily ration every 3 hr by an automatic feeder (102). The light-dark cycles were switched at 6 a.m. and 6 p.m. Animals fed by the automatic feeder lost their circadian rhythm and showed no change in their plasma corticosterone levels over time. Animals pair-fed in the morning had a 12 hr shift in their peak corticosterone levels, compared to *ad lib*-fed controls, while animals fed in the evening had normal diurnal rhythms, with peak plasma corticosterone levels occurring 4 hr earlier than controls. A fourth group that was protein restricted (but fed *ad lib*) showed the same corticosterone levels as the controls: the lowest value at 8 a.m., a peak at 8 p.m., and a return to basal level by 4 a.m. The authors suggest that pair feeding in the afternoon just before the lights go out is more appropriate than the customary feeding in the morning hours after the lights go on.

A shift in the circadian rhythm of plasma corticosterone levels has also been observed in animals with restricted water intakes (146). Again, the change is not seen if water is given in the evening. In both food and water restriction, peak corticosterone levels occur just prior to replenishment, and a rapid decline is observed during presentation. It is hypothesized that the postsupplementation decline in corticoids is controlled separately from the presupplementation rise through a process of reinforcement.

Rodents fed a single daily meal also have enhanced lipid formation due to an increase in lipogenic enzymes (158). A number of other enzymes show increased mean activities: examples include the pentose pathway dehydrogenases, citrate cleavage enzymes, and NADP malic dehydrogenases.

Many of these changes are likely to affect basic cellular processes involved in immune system function.

PEM

Human Studies: T Cells

The first link between PEM and altered cell-mediated immunity was the observation of suppressed skin test responses to tuberculin in malnourished children living in a higly endemic area for tuberculosis (114,133), in those with active disease (159), or following Bacillus Calmette-Guérin (BCG) immunization in tuberculin-negative subjects (115). This anergy is well documented in the report of Lloyd in 1968 (159) showing that only 11 of 51 malnourished children with active tuberculosis (TB) had a positive Heaf test response in contrast to positive responses in all of 102 well-nourished children similarly infected. Similarly, Harland and Brown (115) found that growth-retarded children converted the skin test to 2 TU tuberculin less frequently than well-nourished controls. In both studies, however, apparent anergy could be overcome by increasing the dose of skin test antigen. Thus 18 of the 40 nonreactive children with TB responded to 100 TU tuberculin (159), while increasing the dose from 2 to 20 TU eradicated the difference in post-BCG response between well-nourished and undernourished subjects (115).

In the past 15 years, many studies have confirmed the frequency of anergy in PEM and its relationship to decreased numbers of circulating, and presumably central, T cells. The following discussion first presents the evidence for this statement and then addresses the available information which bears on the localization of this defect in the development of the mature T cell, according to current concepts of T lymphocyte biology.

Circulating T Lymphocytes

Until now, the peripheral T lymphocyte has been identified in malnourished subjects by its ability to form nonimmune rosettes with sheep erythrocytes (SRBC) (E-rosettes) (Table 4). Each of these studies in subjects with kwashiorkor has shown a decrease in the percentage of T cells compared to control values, and all document a decrease in the absolute number of circulating E-rosetting cells. In contrast, the few studies performed in marasmic patients often shown normal absolute numbers and percent of E-rosetting cells. Since the percent and number of B lymphocytes are unchanged (see below), there must be an increase in a population of non-T-non-B lymphocytes. Chandra (51) isolated such cells by first removing B cells on an antiimmunoglobulin-coated nylon wool column, subsequently forming E-rosettes with the eluted cells and removing them on a ficoll-hypaque gradient. The non-T-non-B lymphocytes, termed null cells, comprised 51% of the peripheral lymphocyte population, compared to 9% in the control subjects.

In Vitro *Function*

Lymphocytes are induced to proliferate *in vitro* by specific antigens to which they have been previously sensitized or in an immunologically nonspecific fashion to certain mitogenic lectins which bind to carbohydrate moieties on the cell surface and trigger DNA synthesis. The proliferative response serves as a measure of *in vitro* functional integrity of the lymphocyte and is conveniently assessed by measuring the incorporation of tritiated thymidine (^{3}H-Tdr) into acid-insoluble macromolecules. The earliest studies in malnourished children relied on morphologic criteria to detect the mitogenic response, that is, the transformation of small lymphocytes into large blast cells or obvious mitotic figures. Six of seven studies using

TABLE 4. Percentage of peripheral blood E-rosetting lymphocytes in PEM

Author	Year	Ref.	Country	Age range (no.)	Type of malnutrition[a] (no.)	Percentage of E-rosetting cells		
						Time of study		Controls
						Acute	Convalescent	
Bhaskaram	1974	31	India	Infants	M (8)	38	44 (30)[b]	66
					K (14)	38	37 (30)	
Chandra	1974	47	India	Infants	NS[c]	23	60 (42–112)	71
Ferguson	1974	89	Ghana	12–39 mo	M + K (10)	17	63 (7–17)	60
Bang	1975	20	India	4–60 mo	M + K (17)	46	—	63
Bistrian	1975	34	USA	25–72 yr	K (12)	72	—	67
Holm	1976	125	Sweden	25 ± 2 yr	M (10)[d]	67	—	67
Reddy	1976	224	India	12–60 mo	M (11)	38	—	66
					K (14)	38		
Schopfer	1976	237	Ivory Coast	Infants	K (27)	32	—	65
Bistrian	1977	35	USA	23–74 yr	M (12)	65	—	70
Chandra	1977	50	India	6–30 mo	?M (10)	21	—	68
Kulapongs	1977	148	Thailand	12–60 mo	M + K (24)	24	60 (50)	57
Smith	1977	247	Tunisia	3–18 mo	M (23)	42	—	49
					K (28)	43		
Warren	1977	268	England	Adults	M (11)	73	—	62
Kumar	1978	151	India	12–60 mo	M (27)	34	—	66
					K (8)	37		
Chandra	1979	51	India	11–38 mo	M + K (21)	47	—	74
Jackson	1980	131	Bangladesh	14–60 mo	M + K (16)	39	—	54
Lal	1980	154	India	Children	K (10)	24	—	57
Olusi	1980	206	Nigeria	12–60 mo	K (30)	26	—	50

[a]K, kwashiorkor or marasmic kwashiorkor; M, marasmus.
[b]No. of days after admission.
[c]NS, not separated.
[d]10 days of acute starvation in healthy adult volunteers.

this technique reported decreased responses to phytohemagglutinin (PHA) in PEM patients (43,63,103,109,148,249). The exception, a study in marasmic infants, found no difference between patients and controls (234). This apparent distinction in proliferative responses to PHA between kwashiorkor and marasmic patients is supported by several studies in humans (Table 5) and in experimental animals (161) using ^{3}H-Tdr incorporation as the measure of response. We say "apparent distinction" because in some of the reports, either no clinical distinction is made between the polar forms of malnutrition or the data necessary for classification (such as serum albumin or transferrin levels) are not given. Inclusion of both forms of malnutrition might explain the broad range of results obtained. In other reports that do distinguish between kwashiorkor and marasmus, the lymphocyte data are grouped in such a way as to preclude their separation. The concept that the proliferative response is more impaired in patients with limited amino acid supplies certainly makes sense but does not explain the impaired delayed skin test reactivity to recall antigens in marasmus and the failure of sensitization to dinitrochloro (fluoro) benzene (DNCB or DNFB). However, the *in vivo* skin test involves much more than lectin binding or antigen recognition and cellular proliferation (see below).

T Lymphocyte Numbers in Lymphoid Organs

Since the number of total circulating lymphocytes in the malnourished individual is generally either normal (that is, not significantly different from controls) or only mildly depressed, the impressive decrease in E-rosetting cells and apparent increase in non-T-non-B lymphocytes (by the criteria of absence of the E-rosetting marker, surface Ig, or EAC-rosetting cells) could be a consequence of alterations in lymphocyte populations within the central and peripheral lymphoid organs. This is indeed the case. About 125 years before the current resurgence of interest, Simon (244) noted the sensitivity of the thymus gland and other lymphoid collections to nutritional insults, subsequently confirmed in the premodern era of cellular immunology by Trowell et al. (263) in 1954. As noted by Watson and McMurray (269), the extensive review of nutrition and infection interactions by Scrimshaw et al. (239) in 1968 contained no mention of cell-mediated immunity. By 1969, however, the relationship began to be recognized when Watts (270) reported gross thymic atrophy in cases of kwashiorkor coming to autopsy in which the gland was weighed. In 1971, the importance of this finding was clearly registered by Mugerwa (194) in Uganda and Smythe et al. (249) in South Africa. These reports described abnormal histology of the thymus in all kwashiorkor cases and most marasmic patients, consisting of depletion of thymocytes, especially from the cortex, with relative prominence of epithelial and reticular tissue, infiltration with fibroblasts in some, loss of differentiation between cortex and medulla, and a striking decrease in Hassall's corpuscles.

Spleen, tonsil, and lymph node also demonstrate sharp changes from normal (46,200,276). The most dramatic occur in the thymus-dependent areas, such as the paracortical and periarteriolar regions, with relatively better preservation of B lym-

TABLE 5. *Phytohemagglutinin-stimulated proliferative responses in PEM*

Author	Year	Ref.	Country	Age range (no.)	Type of malnutrition[a] (no.)	Autologous plasma	SI ([3H]-thymidine incorporation)		
							Acute	Recovery	Controls
Jose	1970	136	Australia	5–15 yr	NS[b] (20)	NS	2.7	—	3.3
Chandra	1972	46	India	12–36 mo	NS (8)	? Yes	2.8	—	9.6
Sellmeyer	1972	240	S. Africa	14–72 mo	K (11)	No	46	—	220
Law	1973	155	USA	41–97 yr	K (11)	Yes	26	95	103
Work	1973	276	Ghana	Infants	M + K (41)	NS	66	7.9	129
Bhaskaram	1974	31	India	Infants	M (8)	Yes	4.5	18.1	27.3
					K (14)		7.4		
Chandra	1974	47	India	Infants	NS (15)	No	35	97	111
Ferguson	1974	89	Ghana	Infants	M + K (18)	No	30	—	70
Moore	1974	190	Gambia	9–36 mo	M (7)	No	4.4[c]	4.3[c]	4.4[c]
					K (9)		4.3[c]		
Jose	1975	137	Australia	15–69 mo	NS (17)	Yes	38[d]	—	98[d]
Neumann	1975	200	Ghana	6–72 mo	M (7)	NS	60	—	124
					K (18)		65		
Kielmann	1976	143	India	<36 mo	NS (13)	Yes	87[e]	—	118[e]
Reddy	1976	224	India	12–60 mo	M + K (22)	Yes	5	—	17
Bistrian	1977	35	USA	23–74 yr	M (12)	Yes	24	—	34
						No	98		99
Kulapongs	1977	148	Thailand	12–60 mo	NS (24)	Yes	47	139	93
Beatty	1978	22	S. Africa	10–48 mo	NS (12)	Yes	7.8[f]	—	13.7[f]
						No	27.3[f]		32[f]
McMurray	1981	184	Colombia	24 mo	M (8)	No	112	—	162

[a] K, kwashiorkor or marasmic-kwashiorkor; M, marasmus.
[b] NS, not stated.
[c] "Corrected response" = (stimulated cpm − unstimulated cpm) $\log_{10}$.
[d] Percent of simultaneous normal control cpm.
[e] Mean square root of normalized cpm.
[f] Stimulated cpm × 10^{-3}.

phocyte-rich germinal centers and primary follicles, although these, too, are affected (83). Plasma cells are readily found in the tissues; indeed, by electron microscopy, plasmacytoid cells are found in the circulation, characterized by extensively developed rough endoplasmic reticulum typical of antigenic stimulation. Clinical evaluation of acutely malnourished living children shows decreased thymic shadows on X-ray with restoration upon refeeding (106). Similarly, tonsillar and adenoidal tissues assessed by direct observation are decreased in size (46,200,276).

It is clear that the decrease in circulating E-rosetting cells is not due to any failure to release thymocytes to the circulation which might result in a packed thymus gland. Rather, the thymus and T cell regions of other lymphoid organs are underpopulated with lymphocytes. There are two possible explanations for these observations: (a) a defect in the intrathymic environment necessary for the homing of prethymic T cells to the thymus, and/or (b) a defect in the maturation process within the gland.

Thymic Factors in Malnutrition

In the past few years, three groups have found that thymic factors added *in vitro* to lymphocytes from malnourished patients for a short incubation period result in a significant increase in the number of demonstrable E-rosetting lymphocytes. One study employed thymopoeitin, a polypeptide hormone isolated from calf thymus tissue and purified to homogeneity by adsorption and ion exchange column chromatography (131). Sixteen Bangladeshi children from 14 months to 7 years of age were studied, including 10 with marasmus and six with kwashiorkor. All were clinically infected. The group mean percent E-rosettes was 39 without added thymopoeitin and 49 when lymphocytes were preincubated for 2 hr with 1 μg/ml (mean percent increase, $+46\%$). In four subjects, the percentage of E-rosetting cells in the unstimulated incubation was 50% or more. All four patients were classified as marasmic, and the mean percent change in the presence of thymopoeitin was $+6\%$. Data from 11 age-matched controls showed no significant effect of thymopoeitin from the control incubation (54% E-rosettes) to the samples incubated with the thymic factor (52%).

The other two studies used thymosin fraction 5, a partially purified bovine thymic polypeptide mixture containing at least 12 molecular species. One of these studies involved 30 Nigerian children, mean age 2.7 years, with clinical kwashiorkor (206). In no child was the percentage of E-rosettes greater than 40% (mean, 26%) in the absence of thymosin. In the presence of 5 μg of the factor during a 10 min preincubation, a significant increase was observed in 24 subjects (group mean, 50%); and in 15, the percentage of E-rosettes was equal to or greater than 50% (mean, 55%). The second study is our own (G. T. Keusch, B. Torun, and A. Goldstein) and is not yet published in detail. The findings support the above data in a group of 33 Guatemalan children, 3 to 36 months of age, with kwashiorkor. The effect was thymosin dose-dependent; there was a 15% increase in E-rosettes in the presence of 20 μg/ml of the hormone but a 24% increase when the thymosin dose was increased to 200 μg/ml ($p < 0.02$).

Thus *in vitro* studies with thymic factors in children from three different areas of the world support the idea that *in vivo* thymic function may be compromised in the malnourished host. The consequence of this appears to be the circulation of functionally immature lymphocytes which are responsive to thymic hormone action *in vitro* and thus potentially responsive *in vivo*. Conceptually, this would mean that lymphocyte dysfunction in PEM is an endocrine disease, secondary to underproduction of the relevant polypeptide hormone, a situation theoretically amenable to hormone replacement therapy.

These concepts are consistent with the report of Chandra (52) that the level of circulating thymic hormone in children with PEM is decreased from normal. Nine Indian infants, between 9 and 30 months of age, were studied. It is not possible to separate marasmic from kwashiorkor patients, but the report states that two were edematous, two (probably but not necessarily the same patients with edema) had albumin levels less than 3.0 g/dl, and transferrin was below 162 mg/dl in eight. Serum thymic hormone was assessed by the method of Bach and Dardenne (18), in which serial dilutions of patient or age- and sex-matched healthy control serum were incubated with spleeen cells from adult C57BL/6J mice that had been thymectomized 14 days before. The assay measures rosette-forming cells with SRBC. Thymic hormone levels ($\log_2$ reciprocal titer) were between 6 and 8 in the controls and between 3 and 6.5 in patients. Mean values calculated from the scattergram were 6.9 for the controls and 4.7 in the patients ($t = 5.218$; $p < 0.005$).

Immature Lymphocytes in PEM

The enzyme terminal deoxynucleotidyl-transferase (TdT) (nucleosidetriphosphate DNA deoxynucleotidyl-transferase: EC 2.7.7.31) is restricted to immature thymic, bone marrow, and some circulating lymphocytes. It is not found in mature cells and thus is a marker of immature cells, primarily prothymocytes. Chandra (51) has assayed the enzyme activity in peripheral blood lymphocytes in 21 undernourished Indian children, observing a 10-fold increase compared to healthy age-matched controls (11.34 ± 2.42 versus 1.08 ± 0.07 U/10^8 cells). These children were shown to have a decrease in the percent of E-rosetting cells and an increase in the percent of non-T-non-B cells, with no change in B (surface Ig positive) cells. The correlation between TdT activity and non-T-non-B null cells was highly significant ($r = 0.78$; $p < 0.01$), indicating that a population of immature lymphocytes, presumably of the T cell lineage, was in the circulation. Theoretically, this population of cells might be responsive to thymic-inductive influences, such as thymic hormone factors.

Chandra (50) has also reported that the null cells, separated from T and B cells by an antiimmuoglobulin-coated nylon wool column and by sedimentation of E-rosetting cells, were functionally active in a cell-mediated cytotoxicity assay. The target cells were cultured DBA/2 fibroblast monolayers labeled with ^{51}Cr. In four of four subjects studied, significant cell-mediated lysis was produced by the null cells. The cells that produce this toxic activity are classified as natural cytotoxic

(NC) cells. Their origin and lineage are not known at present, but they appear to be immature. To a lesser extent, a C3b receptor-positive cell isolated by EAC rosetting of ficoll-hypaque-purified mononuclear cells was also cytotoxic in this assay. Since phagocytic cells were removed by the use of carbonyl iron magnetism, it is presumed that the active cell population was primarily lymphocytic without a major contribution from monocytes. The exact nature of the $C3b^+$ cytotoxic cell is unclear; however, we cannot exclude the possibility of contamination with an actively cytotoxic but poorly phagocytic $C3b^+$ monocyte which survives the carbonyl iron procedure. For example, M. Dauphineé and N. Talal *(personal communication)* attempted to remove monocytes from ficoll-hypaque mononuclear cell preparation by this technique to study E-rosetting but still found a population of E-rosetting monocytes among the E-positive lymphocytes obtained.

Another circulating immature cell is the natural killer (NK) cell, which is able to recognize and lyse neoplastic cells, such as the K-562 human erythroid leukemia line. The identity of the NK cell is controversial, but we believe it to be an early cell type in T lymphocyte differentiation. It is not controversial, however, that NK activity is regulated *in vivo* by interferon, or that incubation of peripheral blood lymphocytes *in vitro* with interferon will enhance NK activity. In experimental animals, NK activity is increased by thymectomy, and it is high in congenitally athymic nude mice. One might anticipate, therefore, if the same regulatory influences pertain in the human, that nutritional thymectomy would also induce NK activity. Of great interest, then, is the report by Salimonu et al. (231) of NK activity in Nigerian children with kwashiorkor or marasmus. Compared to well-nourished controls, NK activity was similar in both malnourished groups. In contrast to controls, however, incubation *in vitro* with interferon failed to induce NK activity. Indeed, in the kwashiorkor patients, interferon resulted in a statistically significant decrease in NK cytotoxicity. Circulating interferon levels were also measured and, with the exception of three subjects (two controls and one marasmic), was undetectable in all. The three subjects with measurable interferon levels also had the highest level of NK activity, far above that found in the remaining children.

The low to normal NK activity and the failure to induce cytotoxicity by interferon in the malnourished suggest a defect in prethymic precursor lymphocytes in PEM, in addition to the evidence for intrathymic and postthymic abnormalities. One possible mechanism for a prethymic block is defective interferon production in PEM. Two studies in humans have addressed this. Schlesinger et al. (235) examined *in vitro* production of interferon by mixed leukocytes isolated from leukocyte-rich plasma challenged with Newcastle disease virus (NDV). Compared to 31 healthy controls, the marasmic leukocytes produced significantly less interferon activity (58 versus > 220 U/ml; $p < 0.01$). Nichols et al. (201) found decreased interferon production from children with kwashiorkor with serologic evidence of prior exposure to measles virus (natural disease or vaccine virus) when challenged *in vitro* with the Edmonston or Schwartz strains of measles vaccine. Nutritional recovery was associated with an increase in the percent of subjects responding, as well as an increase in the mean titer. If interferon production is limited, regulation of NK activity *in vivo* could be compromised, accounting for the failure of any feedback regulation to induce high levels of cytotoxicity. This could not account for the *in vitro* failure of exogenous interferon to have an effect, however, suggesting a cellular defect as well.

Suppressor Cells and Factors

Immune function abnormalities can be traced at times to the presence of suppressor cells or soluble factors. There is a paucity of data in human malnutrition on immune suppression. Chandra (50) reported that mitomycin-C-treated null cells from four PEM patients (see above) suppressed the response of normal donor T lymphocytes to PHA. The data are presented as the stimulation index (SI) %, which presumably means the SI in the presence of patient cells as a percent of the SI achieved by the normal donor cells alone. Neither the E-rosette nor the EAC rosette-positive cells affected the PHA response of normal lymphocytes, whereas the null cells reduced the SI to 7 to 24%. The nature and origin of this suppressor cell type remains to be explored, as does its role *in vivo* or in the *in vitro* assays of lymphocyte function discussed earlier. For example, would the defect in *in vitro* PHA responsiveness in PEM be corrected by removal of the null cell population?

The presence of humoral suppressor factors was suggested by Heyworth et al. (121), who screened 19 plasma samples from patients with PEM and five normals (four adult and one child) for effects on PHA mitogenesis in lymphocyte cultures from healthy adults. Six samples obtained from malnourished subjects who subsequently died reduced the PHA response of the donor cells to less than one-third of the results obtained in control plasma. Less prominent suppression was found in six additional plasmas, whereas no effect was found in seven. Suppression was more common in kwashiorkor plasma (nine of 11) than in marasmic plasma (three of eight).

Beatty and Dowdle (22) studied 12 children with kwashiorkor and determined the PHA response of their lymphocytes in the presence of autologous serum, pediatric control serum, or normal adult AB serum. Results were equivalent in the two control sera, indicating no intrinsic abnormality in mitogenic response in these patients, but clearly were suppressed in the malnourished patient serum. Kwashiorkor serum also suppressed the response of normal adult lymphocytes. The suppressive effect of patient serum decreased progressively during nutritional therapy over 6 weeks. The effect of AB control or kwashiorkor serum was also tested in a one-way mixed lymphocyte response (MLR) in a crossover design in which the stimulating lymphocytes were either mitomycin-C-treated kwashiorkor or control lymphocytes. In the presence of control serum, the MLR produced by either control or kwashiorkor cells was equivalent; in the presence of kwashiorkor serum, neither malnourished nor normal responder cells demonstrated a proliferative response.

In a subsequent publication, Beatty and Dowdle (23) attempted to characterize the suppressor effect of kwashiorkor serum. In order to evaluate the possibility of a competitive inhibitor of lectin mitogenesis, they studied effects of patient serum on response of normal lymphocytes to three plant proteins with different sugar specificity for binding, PHA, conconavalin A (Con A), and pokeweed mitogen (PWM), and used a range of mitogen dose to determine if there was an end point for inhibition. The suppressive effect was independent of mitogen used or the dose employed. There was no effect on cell viability during the incubation, nor was there an alteration in the kinetics of precursor incorporation but rather only a suppressive effect on the extent of incorporation. The suppressive effect was also detected morphologically by treating 72 hr PHA cultures with pronase and cetrimide to isolate nuclei and then determining size distribution in an electronic particle counter with a multiple channel (size) analyzer. In the presence of AB serum, there was a marked shift to larger nuclei, whereas in the presence of kwashiorkor serum, the distribution of nuclei was intermediate between unstimulated and control (AB serum-stimulated) cells.

Autoradiographs of ^{3}H-thymidine-pulsed cells confirmed the increased proliferation of cells in the absence of patient serum. The mean number of labeled cells was three times greater in the AB serum controls. When serum was switched from AB to kwashiorkor, or vice versa, after 24 or 48 hr and incubation continued, the total incorporation reflected the sum effects of the serum present during the individual segments. Kwashiorkor serum suppressed during both early and late segments and seemed to simply fail to support proliferation. Mixing experiments then were performed to distinguish the presence of an inhibitor from the absence of a required factor. The results suggested the latter to be the case; when increasing amounts of kwashiorkor serum were added to limiting concentrations of AB serum, lymphocyte responses increased with increasing total serum concentration up to 35% serum (v/v). Moreover, addition of a low molecular ultrafiltrate of AB serum (Amicon UM-05 membrane filtrate) in increasing concentration to 5% kwashiorkor serum progressively augmented the proliferative response to control levels. The authors conclude that kwashiorkor serum lacks a low molecular weight factor essential for lymphocyte proliferation and mention, without presenting data, that dialysis of AB serum removes its ability to support lymphocyte transformation.

Delayed Type Hypersensitivity Reactions in Skin

Delayed type skin test reactivity is dependent on intact cell mediated immunity. Specifically reactive lymphocytes first must be sensitized. Most studies have tested this afferent limb of the response by use of the hapten DNCB or DNFB. When sensitized lymphocytes are challenged by introduction of antigen into skin, there is a local proliferation of the sensitized clone with release of various lymphokine mediators, which results in a local inflammatory response. The accumulation of mononuclear and polymorphonuclear phagocytes produces the induration in skin characteristic of the efferent limb of the response.

We have mentioned the failure of skin test responses to tuberculin or purified protein derivative (PPD) in malnourished individuals who would be expected to be reactive because of the frequency of positive responses in controls (114,133). Most individuals have also had contact with other antigens which elicit recall reactions in skin, including *Candida albicans*, and the streptococcal products streptokinase (SK) and streptodornase (SD). Many studies have shown impaired responses to these antigens in the malnourished compared to well-nourished controls. Skin test reactivity is reduced in both marasmic and kwashiorkor patients, perhaps to a greater extent in the latter group, and is observed in both children and adults. Table 6 shows results obtained with recall antigens, including tuberculin.

The delayed skin test also has been investigated by immunization with BCG, DNCB, or DNFB. Failure to respond to these antigens has been observed in the malnourished (Table 6). Two recent studies deserve comment. In the first, McMurray et al. (185) immunized a group of Colombian infants with BCG within the first 24 hr of life. Nutritional status was followed over 2 years, and periodic skin tests were performed with PPD. More than one-half the infants grew poorly during this time and were classified as mildly to moderately malnourished. PPD skin test response rate was lower in the moderately malnourished at 8 and 104 weeks but significantly greater than controls at 52 weeks. At 8 weeks of age, all PPD-negative subjects were sensitized with 10 mg DNCB and then challenged 2 weeks later with 0.5 mg DNCB. Of 18 malnourished children, 89% responded, compared to 58% of 24 well-nourished infants. At 2 years of age, all 71 children remaining in the study were sensitized and challenged with the hapten. Ninety-four percent of 31 normals and 82% of 33 mildly malnourished responded, compared to 57% (four of seven) moderately malnourished. In 48 of the 2 year olds, *in vitro* lymphocyte responses to PHA also were determined. The SI was significantly decreased in the malnourished subjects by 29% ($p < 0.05$). The data could be interpreted to suggest that young children in the process of developing malnutrition transiently pass through a stage during which they exhibit heightened cell-mediated immune responsiveness before suppressed reactivity is observed. However, the small number of subjects in some of the test groups and the lack of temporal concordance between PPD and DNCB results represents a problem in interpretation.

In the second study, by Koster et al. (145), 50 severely malnourished children in Bangladesh, from 1 to 8 years of age, were randomized into four study groups. Slightly more than one-half (27 of 50) were edematous. Four groups were sensitized with 2 mg DNCB at either 2, 8, 15, or 22 days of hospitalization. Nutritional rehabilitation was initiated on admission. A bolus of vitamin A was given at the same time, and folic acid, thiamine, and pyridoxine were administered daily thereafter. Oral iron was begun during the second week of hospitalization. DNCB challenge (0.05 mg) was accomplished 10 days after initial sensitization and at 2 and 4 weeks thereafter. All children developed local erythema within 48 hr of the initial dose. Positive responses to the first challenge dose were obtained in only 29% of those sensitized on the second day of hospitalization (group 1), compared to approximately 75% of those initially sensitized 8, 15, or 22 days after admission (groups 2 to 4) during nutritional recovery. The corresponding figures for the second challenge dose given 24 days after sensitization were 50% for group 1 and 91 to 100% of groups 2 to 4. Evidence of therapeutic response to diet was seen in all

TABLE 6. *DTH reactions in skin in patients with PEM*

Author	Year	Ref.	Country	Age range	Type of malnutrition[a]	DTH reactions (no. positive/no. tested)			
						PPD	Candida	SK/SD	DNCB/DNFB
Harland	1965	114	Uganda	Children	NS[b]	8/16[c] (50)[d]	—	—	—
Harland	1965	115	Uganda	1–36 mo	NS	5/27[c] (19)	—	—	—
Brown	1966	40	Uganda	5–84 mo	K	2/8[e] (25)	—	—	—
Llyod	1968	159	Uganda	<84 mo	K	11/51[e] (20)	—	—	—
Jose	1970	136	Australia	5–15 yr	NS	—	9/43 (21)	—	—
Geefhuysen	1971	103	S. Africa	6–30 mo	NS	—	3/18 (17)	—	—
Smythe	1971	249	S. Africa	Children	NS	—	—	—	0/17 (0)
Chandra	1972	46	India	12–36 mo	NS	9/50[c] (18)	4/30 (13)	5/30 (17)	8/23 (35)
Feldman	1972	88	Argentina	2–68 mo	NS	2/17[f] (12)	2/11 (18)	—	1/6 (17)
Edelman	1973	84	Thailand	12–60 mo	NS	—	2/14 (14)	—	2/10 (20)
Law	1973	155	USA	29–69 yr	K	—	2/16 (13)	—	2/11 (18)
Abbassy	1974	1	Egypt	4–40 mo	M	2/21[c] (10)	—	—	—
					K	4/37[c] (11)	—	—	—
Chandra	1974	47	India	12–36 mo	NS	—	—	—	—
Coovadia	1974	63	S. Africa	8–72 mo	NS	—	—	—	4/23 (17)
Schlesinger	1974	234	Chile	3–18 mo	M	1/12[c] (8)	—	—	4/12 (33)
Jose	1975	137	Australia	15–69 mo	NS	—	4/15 (27)	—	0/18 (0)
Neumann	1975	200	Ghana	6–72 mo	M	—	7/11 (64)	3/11 (27)	—
					K	—	8/22 (36)	5/22 (23)	—
Ziegler	1975	278	India	10–24 mo	M	1/14[c] (7)	—	—	—
Kielmann	1976	143	India	36 mo	NS	27/51[c] (53)	—	—	—
Sinha	1976	245	India	24–78 mo	M	35/73[c] (48)	—	—	—
					K	0/9[c] (0)	—	—	—
Bistrian	1977	35	USA	29–74 yr	M	—	2/11 (18)	—	—
Smith	1977	247	Tunisia	3–18 mo	M	17/40[c] (43)	17/39 (40)	—	2/4 (50)
					K	—	10/29 (37)	—	3/13 (23)
Koster	1981	145	Bangladesh	12–106 mo	K	0/21 (0)	0/21 (0)	—	4/14 (29)
					M				5/20 (0)
McMurray	1981	184	Colombia	18–60 mo	M	1/11 (9)	0/11 (0)	—	3/11 (27)
Pooled controls						399/578 (69)	111/155 (72)	24/42 (57)	79/102 (77)

[a] K, kwashiorkor or marasmic-kwashiorkor; M, marasmus.
[b] NS, not separated.
[c] Documented prior BCG immunization.
[d] Percent positive.
[e] Documented active tuberculosis.
[f] 13/17 with documented prior BCG immunization.

groups by the eighth day of hospitalization in an increase in both weight and total serum proteins.

Group 1, sensitized on hospital day 2, was divided into those subjects with initial serum total protein greater than 5.5 g/dl (mean, 6.4 ± 0.22) and those with protein less than 5.5 g/dl. Four of six of the former but none of eight of the latter responded to challenge 10 days later. This suggests that protein deficits may be the important determinant for the negative skin test in this group. The progressive increase in reactivity observed in these same children when tested on days 24 (50%) and 38 (75%) demonstrates that the afferent limb was intact on admission; the cause of the nonreactivity to challenge must rest in the efferent limb. A similar observation was made by Abbassy et al. (1), who immunized 58 malnourished Egyptian children with BCG. Initially PPD-anergic children ultimately became PPD positive without further immunization during the subsequent 18 months when serum protein levels increased. Harrison et al. (117) were unable to obtain conversion of the PPD response when immunizing children with a serum albumin less than 2.2 g/dl.

Koster et al. (145) suggest that the failure to respond to DNCB challenge may be due to a state of specific immunologic tolerance. In support of this, they describe a child who was initially sensitized before refeeding who not only failed to respond upon challenge but also did not convert with two additional sensitizing doses on days 24 and 70 of nutritional therapy. Bang et al. (20) also reported three children who were sensitized prior to feeding and who failed to demonstrate delayed hypersensitivity after two additional sensitizing doses applied following at least 4 weeks of nutritional therapy.

If the defect is in the efferent limb of the response, there are several possibilities. Production of lymphokines required for the inflammatory response may be restricted by either protein or calorie, or combined, deficiency. The effect of this would be a reduction in the migration and accumulation of monocytes and neutrophils at the skin test site. Only a few studies have attempted to measure lymphokine production as an indicator of the functional integrity of the lymphocyte in the delayed-type hypersensitivity (DTH) response. Selective defects in lymphokines may explain some of the specific patterns of cell-mediated immune responses in malnutrition.

The reported results have been variable, depending on the type of malnutrition in the patients and the stimulus employed to trigger lymphokine release. For example, Lomnitzer et al. (160) observed defective leukocyte inhibitory factor (LIF) production by lymphocytes from children with kwashiorkor. Twenty five children, 6 to 24 months old, with either kwashiorkor or marasmic-kwashiorkor were studied, 14 of whom were overtly infected at the time. Ficoll-hypaque mononuclear cells were stimulated in vitro for 2 hr with 10 μg/ml PHA and then set up in migration chambers. The mean migration index over 72 hr for 12 controls was 0.60 compared to 0.79 in the patients. The migration index was less than 0.80 in 11 of 12 controls but in only 12 of 25 patients (chi square = 6.57; $p < 0.01$). Among the patients, there were no observed correlations between lymphokine activity and age, type or severity of malnutrition, degree of anemia, or presence or type of infection. Ford et al. (97) also found depressed migration inhibition factor (MIF) production by

Australian aboriginal children with moderate PEM but only when *Candida* antigen was employed to stimulate mediator release and not with streptolysin O or a lymphocyte membrane preparation. In contrast, Heresi et al. (120) reported that marasmic children (mean age, 8.3 ± 2.8 months) with a 30 to 40% deficit in weight for age made normal titers of leukocyte inhibitory factor (LIF) when activated by PHA. When cells from BCG-immunized, PPD-positive cases or controls were stimulated *in vitro* with PPD and compared, marasmic patients produced more LIF than did controls (migration inhibition index, 55.7 ± 5.4 versus 38.2 ± 5.0, respectively; $p < 0.05$).

Impaired phagocytic cell function per se could also depress skin test responses by blunting the inflammatory response, the manifestation detected clinically in delayed hypersensitivity reactions. For example, *in vivo* chemotaxis of cells into a Rebuck type skin window is altered in PEM, and impaired neutrophil bactericidal and metabolic activity are often seen *in vitro*. There are few studies of the human monocyte in PEM. A recent review (141) concluded that the monocyte may be functionally intact but that defects in lymphocyte function and depressed complement activity might cause significant abnormalities *in vivo*. More sophisticated studies of monocyte/macrophage functions as antigen-presenting cells have not been carried out. We recently observed that either typhoid vaccine or diphtheria toxoid (DPT) will induce a rise in serum amyloid A protein (SAA) in acute PEM patients (K. P. W. J. McAdam, G. T. Keusch, and B. Torun, *unpublished*), with the peak occurring 36 hr after vaccine administration. Because SAA production is induced by a monokine, the observation suggests that the mononuclear phagocytes retain the ability to respond appropriately to inflammatory stimuli, and that the liver remains responsive to the SAA-stimulating factor. Much work remains to be done.

Corticosteroid Effects

This section addresses the question of cortisol effects on *in vivo* or *in vitro* cell-mediated immunity. Cortisol levels rise in malnourished children when serum albumin drops below 3.0 g/dl (5,63,157,236). Thus marasmic patients have early morning steroid levels in the normal range, whereas kwashiorkor patients show an increase in total cortisol. Because of the normal binding of glucocorticoids to albumin, the percentage of free cortisol rises as well when albumin is depressed. Hence in kwashiorkor, there is a significant rise in biologically active hormone in circulation. The question has been raised many times whether or not this can account for the defects of cell-mediated immunity in malnourished hosts. The first problem with this hypothesis is that cortisol levels in marasmic children are in the normal range; yet some authors describe abnormal skin test responses in such children (1,234,278). However, the latter finding is not as clearly established as is the suppression observed in kwashiorkor, and it may be that marasmic children are a heterogenous group with respect to other nutritional factors that modulate DTH. As noted above, skin test reactivity does seem to be related to serum albumin levels in some studies.

It is now appreciated that glucocorticoid effects on the lymphoid system are species dependent. Rodents are cortisone sensitive, and lympholysis is readily produced. In contrast, the human and the guinea pig are resistant to cortisone-induced lympholysis (214). In these species, the effect of steroid is primarily a cellular redistributional event. Administration of a bolus of hydrocortisone alters the traffic pattern of cells in the circulation and causes a shift from circulation to lymphoid organs, including thymus, spleen, and lymph node (118). T lymphocytes are primarily affected; among the T cells, those with surface receptors for the Fc portion of IgM are preferentially lost from the circulation. This redistribution is more readily attained *in vivo* at lower steroid dosage than is an effect on function *in vitro* (87). Sampling of the blood may lead to unwarranted conclusions *vis-a-vis* lymphocyte function, since the distribution of T cell subsets in circulation will not be normal. Since the Fcμ receptor is thought to be a marker for helper cell functions, and, as a result of the stress, there is a relative enrichment in the number of Fcγ-positive cells, which are markers for suppressor/cytotoxic T cells, *in vitro* correlates of cell-mediated immunity may be altered by the resulting functional imbalance within the immunologic network. The results of these changes could be lymphopenia and/or depressed *in vitro* immune responsiveness of peripheral blood lymphocytes, both of which may be observed in human PEM.

In considering the mechanism of these events, some experiments performed in guinea pigs are relevant since this species, like the human, is quite resistant to steroid lympholysis (59). Adaptive transfer of lymphocytes was performed using lymph node cells from normal or steroid-treated inbred strain animals previously exposed to PPD (273). The cells were then transferred into nonimmune recipients, some of which received cortisol. All were PPD tested 2 days after transfer. Lymphoid cells from normal or cortisol-treated donor animals transferred PPD sensitivity into normal recipients. The response was abrogated by steroid treatment of the recipient, and there was a dramatic decrease noted in the number of macrophages and polymorphonuclear leukocytes in the skin test site. Thus cortisol seems to exert its effect by interfering with the macrophage response to the amplification mechanism of the T cell in the efferent limb. Since infection can alter cortisol levels, the skin test response may be suppressed in infected marasmic infants even if peripheral blood lymphocytes remain responsive to functional tests, such as PHA mitogenesis, as observed in the study of Schlesinger and Stekel (234).

Human Studies: B Lymphocytes

The B lymphocyte has received little attention in malnourished subjects. There are three principal reasons for this "benign" neglect: (a) the relative preservation of B cell regions in spleen and lymph node compared to T-dependent regions, (b) the presence of normal percentage of B lymphocytes in peripheral circulation, and (c) the normal to elevated levels of immunoglobulins in serum (20,49,63,148, 194,236,237). Since immunoglobulin is secreted by differentiated plasma cells rather than B lymphocytes, the maturation pathway is intact in such patients. Indeed, the latter observation is consistent with an immunologic response to the constant antigenic stimulation of repeated infections in the malnourished child and is supported by ultrastructural evidence of plasmacytoid cells or morphologically identifiable plasma cells in the circulation suggestive of B cell activation (Fig. 2). Chandra (51) quantitated the percentage of blood lymphocytes reactive with fluorescein-tagged goat anti-human IgA, IgG, and IgM in a group of Indian children with kwashiorkor and in age-matched healthy children from the same environment. Although the specificity of the reagents was not described, the results demonstrated normal numbers of lymphocytes reactive with anti-IgG and anti-IgM but a significant 125% increase in cells reacting with anti-IgA ($p < 0.01$).

The B cell and humoral specific immunity are not necessarily unaffected by PEM. Many studies have been conducted employing vaccine challenge as a probe of immune responses (49). Antibody titers have been perfectly normal to some antigens and markedly defective with others. The usual probes have been typhoid or tetanus vaccines among the nonviable antigens tested, and polio or measles vaccine among the living vaccines. In general, defects in antibody response are observed with the viruses, in some individuals with typhoid vaccine (especially antipolysaccharide O antigen) and essentially not at all using tetanus toxoid. The presence of clinical infection may be an important conditioner of response; Chandra (49) has observed that infected malnourished children produce much less agglutinating antibody to typhoid O antigen than malnourished noninfected children. The regulatory factors called into play in such circumstances may be complex. Since antibody synthesis depends on antigen presentation by mononuclear phagocytic cells, interaction with T helper cells for most antigens, and, finally, maturation of B lymphocytes into plasma cells, there are many cell-cell interactions that potentially can be affected by malnutrition. Diverse humoral factors may also be involved, including the rise in acute phase proteins, such as C-reactive protein (which can exert immunosuppressive effects on antibody production), the third component of complement (which is frequently depressed in the malnourished and consumed during infection), and hormones, such as cortisol, all of which are altered by the stress of infection. As Mitchell (187) has pointed out, the spatial organization of lymphoid tissue *in vivo* is undoubtedly important in promoting the antigen-B lymphocyte-accessory cell (macrophage, T cell) interaction; therefore, the structural changes in thymus, spleen, and lymph node caused by PEM are probably of importance.

The antigen that seems to be most problematic of those tested is the polysaccharide O antigen of *S. typhi*, which, like other carbohydrates, may be capable of directly engaging the B cell to initiate synthesis of antibody of the IgM class. Such T-independent antigens frequently share several properties, such as polymeric structure, persistence in the host, inability to recruit T cells, and activation of the complement pathway to split C3. Polysaccharide antigens are also the poorest immunogens in the young, the target population most frequently affected by PEM. Some investigators have observed an improved antityphoid O antigen response if the subjects are given additional protein at the time of immunization. The difference is apparent by day 10 after immunization between PEM children given either 30

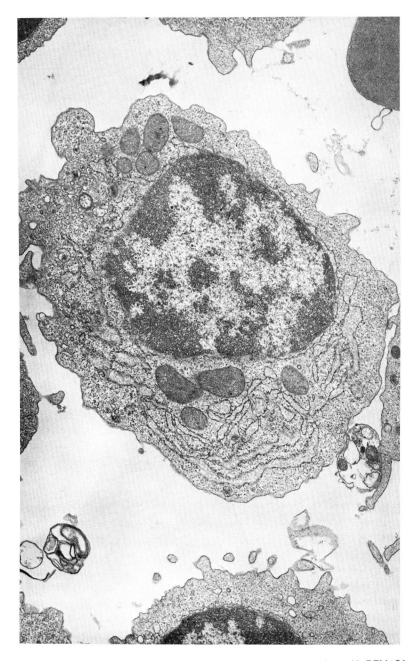

FIG. 2. Electron micrograph of a circulating plasmacytoid cell in a patient with PEM. Of note are the heterochromatic nucleus, prominent nucleolus, prominent Golgi zone, and numerous strands of rough-surfaced endoplasmic reticulum in the cytoplasm. ×14,000. (S. D. Douglas, G. T. Keusch, and J. J. Urrutia, *unpublished.*)

or 50 g protein per day (222,257). The mechanism is unclear but is probably not at the level of plasma cell protein synthesis, since serum immunoglobulin concentrations were not depressed and were, in fact, the same in the two groups. A blunted inflammatory response at the site of infection might be responsible for a failure to deliver antigen to responsive B lymphocytes.

There is an apparent discrepancy in the response to live virus antigens. For example, Ifekwunigwe et al. (128) recently reported the results of immunization of 111 seronegative children in Nigeria with Schwartz strain measles vaccine as well as 193 children lacking a smallpox vaccination scar who were given smallpox vaccine. Independent of nutritional status, 94% seroconverted to measles (titer > 1:20 HI after 6 to 8 weeks), and 97% had a positive take with smallpox. Ninety two percent of 71 moderately malnourished and all of 12 severely malnourished children developed measles antibody, with a geometric mean titer rise equal to the normally nourished group.

In contrast to the variable results discussed above, decreased concentration of secretory IgA (sIgA) in saliva, nasopharyngeal washings, or tears has been a more constant finding in the few studies reported in severe PEM patients (48,183,223,246). Concentration of other proteins in secretions, such as albumin, IgG, lysozyme, and aminopeptidase, may be affected but to a lesser extent. As a result, the ratio of sIgA/IgG in these fluids is reversed from the usual situation in which sIgA predominates. When these subjects are nutritionally rehabilitated, the concentration of sIgA increases proportionally much more than the other proteins; since the parotid flow rate increases as well, this represents a large increment in sIgA production (183).

In one recent study, human small intestinal immunoglobulins were assayed in fluids obtained by peroral intubation (29). The patient groups included malnourished Indonesian children with enteric infection, well-nourished Indonesians with or without infection, Australian aborigines with gastroenteritis, and caucasian Australian children neither malnourished nor infected. Considering the data obtained in the last group as a standard, intestinal juice IgA, G, and M were generally elevated and in no instance depressed in the other patient groups. Interestingly, IgG levels exceeded IgA in the Indonesian children by about twofold, independent of nutritional status or presence of acute enteritis. Since these children all had a history of frequent infection, the implication is that antigenic stimulation, even in the poorly nourished, can stimulate production and transport of immunoglobulins, including sIgA and IgG, into the gut. More than 90% of the IgA was dimeric and the IgG was an intact monomer when molecular size was determined by gel filtration chromatography of iodinated duodenal contents, indicating that rapidly diffusing small molecular weight breakdown fragments were not responsible for the increased size of the precipitin rings used to estimate immunoglobulin content. The increase appears to be real.

However, immunoglobulin levels in mucosal and intestinal secretions are not a measure of the capacity to develop a functional antibody response. Direct measures of antibody activity in response to specific antigen stimulation is required for this assessment. Chandra (48) determined both serum and secretory antibody responses in nasopharyngeal secretions in response to oral immunization with live polio or measles vaccine in malnourished children. Although immunization was successful in that serum antibody responses were obtained, both the percentage responding with sIgA antibody and the titer in the responders were diminished in the malnourished children. This may be significant in the immune response to local enteric pathogens; but in fact, oral immunization with measles is clinically successful even in severely malnourished children (128). At the same time, oral polio vaccine has been reported to fail to even stimulate production of serum antibodies in a proportion of individuals in developing countries (134). However, this may be due to failure of the cold chain in maintenance of vaccine viability in tropical environments or to the presence of interfering enterovirus infection in the gut which precludes establishment of the vaccine strain in the intestine.

Animal Studies: Inbred Mouse Strains

The award of the 1980 Nobel Prize in Medicine to Benaceraf, Snell, and Dousset for their contributions to the understanding of genetic control of immune function was also a recognition of the contribution of countless generations of inbred mouse strains to this work and the beginning application of these principles to the human. Experimental studies in mice eliminate one of the constant variables in human studies: the heterogeneity of the MHC. A second critical aspect of murine studies that must be recognized is the exuberant corticosteroid rise, so readily provoked by stress in mice, and the sensitivity of murine lymphoid cells to steroid lysis (59). While results from murine models may be applicable to the human, it may be restricted to controlled conditions of diet, infection, and treatment not readily obtained in human populations. In fact, the frequent findings of normal or enhanced cell-mediated immune responses and depressed or unaffected antibody responses in mice are at variance with the human studies already described (62). It must be remembered that animals are fed a constant diet deficient in selected nutrients and that *in vitro* immunologic studies are performed with cells obtained from thymus or spleen directly, and not the circulating peripheral lymphocytes in the bloodstream.

T Lymphocytes and Cell-Mediated Immunity

Cooper and colleagues (61,62) have undertaken a sustained effort to understand the effect on immune responses of chronic protein deprivation in mice employing isocaloric diets with a varying content of protein in the form of casein. The model selected compares moderate protein restriction in both dams and their offspring fed 8% casein, with control animals fed a 27% casein diet *ad lib*. Room temperature, humidity, and the lighting cycle (12 hr on, 12 hr off) were controlled, and both *in vivo* and *in vitro* studies of cell-mediated immunity were performed. Graft versus host (GVH) reactivity was assessed by the Simonsen assay, in which normally fed (C3H/Bi X C57BL/6)f$_1$ hybrids were injected with spleen cells from protein insufficient (PI) or pair-fed normal C3H/Bi mice. Ten days later, spleen weight per unit body weight was determined and compared to controls given spleen cells from

(C3H X C57) f_1 mice fed either normal or PI diets. Spleen weight was 131% of control in response to normal C3H spleen cells but significantly increased ($p < 0.02$) to 196% of control when PI C3H cells were given, indicating an enhanced cellular immune reactivity in PI animals. Similarly, skin allograft survival (C57 female donor to C3H female recipient) was significantly shortened in PI mice (16 ± 2 versus 26 ± 2 days, $p < 0.01$). In a separate set of experiments, the influence of protein restricting the donor also was tested in a crossover design grafting C57 skin to SEC/1ReJ mice. There was no influence of diet in the donor when skin was grafted to a normal diet recipient. Regardless of the protein status of the donor, however, allograft survival was shorter in PI recipients (22.2 days) compared to normal recipients (29.9 days) ($p < 0.01$). Neonatal thymectomy of the PI mice at 3 to 12 days of age abolished the differences observed in skin graft rejection when studied at 6 to 10 weeks of age. Thus the accelerated GVH response was dependent on the presence of the thymus during the period of dietary deprivation.

Experiments employing PHA were also performed in C3H and SEC mice. Compared to normal diet controls, the SI of ^{3}H-thymidine incorporation was increased by 68.2 and 50.0% in PI mice of the two strains, respectively ($p < 0.01$). Results were not significantly different in experiments performed in second, third, or fourth generation SEC mice fed the 8% casein diet continuously.

In contrast, a more recent report of long-term protein restriction comparing *ad lib* feeding of 4, 8, and 24% casein diets in male Balb/c mice, initiated at weaning and continued for as long as 717 days, failed to confirm the increase in cell-mediated immunity, measured as proliferative responses to PHA or Con A, or in a one-way MLR to irradiated CBA T_6T_6 spleen cells (255). No significant differences were observed among the diet groups after 125, 373, 567, or 717 days, although age effects were observed. Neither thymus nor spleen weight or serum albumin levels were greatly affected by the 8% casein diet. Body weight, spleen weight, and thymus weight were all decreased in the 4% diet mice at day 125 but not at other times in the study. It is not clear if the difference between these data and the results of Cooper et al. (61,62) are attributable to differences in the strains of mice employed, the time of initiation of diet, or the time of study. Of importance, however, is that neither study found diminished T cell response.

Bell and Hazell (25) also studied protein restriction diets initiated at weaning (17 days) in Balb/c mice using a better quality protein, egg albumin, to formulate the diet. The measure of cell-mediated immunity was the GVH response assessed by the Simonsen assay. In addition, the effect of corticosteroids was controlled by adrenalectomy or sham operation at weaning. Adrenalectomized animals were given 0.9% saline for drinking water. Significant splenomegaly was induced by spleen or mesenteric lymph node cells from control diet donors but not from thymus or Peyer patch. In contrast, cells from all four organs from protein-restricted animals induced the GVH response. The increased response was approximately 4-, 1½-, 2-, and 10-fold in spleen, node, thymus, and Peyer patch, respectively. The enhanced response of protein-restricted spleen cells was apparent as early as 7 days on diet and was unaffected by adrenalectomy. Thus the enhanced reactivity of the cells obtained from the protein-restricted animals cannot be explained by a relative enrichment of spleen cell suspensions by steroid-resistant cells which mediate the GVH. The difference was narrowed by pair feeding but remained significantly higher in the 4% protein animals in both spleen and thymus ($p < 0.005$ and <0.01, respectively). GVH activity was completely removed from both normal and experimental diet spleen suspensions by preincubation with rabbit antimouse thymocyte serum plus complement. Refeeding a normal diet promptly and completely abrogated GVH responses. This depressed reactivity persisted through 16 days of refeeding, returning to normal levels only by day 26. The data suggest that changes in the proportion of T and B cells or T cell subsets in the various organs, particularly the relatively long-lived T cells with GVH reactivity, are responsible for the observed enhancement of cell-mediated immunity in protein-restricted animals. The rapid loss of GVH reactivity upon refeeding could also be due to a change in the proportion of lymphocyte populations, in this case due to a rapid influx of new cells lacking GVH reactivity derived either from the thymus or local proliferation within the spleen itself.

The dietary manipulations employed produced a rapid loss in both thymus and spleen weight due to depletion of cellular content, persisting for the duration of the experiment. The normal pattern of thymus growth is an increase in organ weight through day 28 and subsequent involution. When protein-deficient mice were transferred to a normal diet at day 45, the thymus resumed its growth pattern by increasing in size and cellularity and then regressing, ultimately reaching the adult thymic weight of normal diet controls (26). Thus protein restriction merely held this normal pattern of change in abeyance until adequate protein was supplied.

The functional consequence of these changes was a biphasic proliferative response to PHA (26). Initially decreased at 1 week in both spleen and mesenteric node cell suspensions, the PHA response per cell exceeded control levels by 2 weeks and thereafter was maintained at about twice control. The possibility that these results were due to a loss of suppressor cells was tested. *In vivo* suppression was assayed by intraperitoneal injection of equal numbers of spleen cells from normal or deprived mice which had been given two intraperitoneal injections of KLH prior to cell harvest. These cells were transferred intravenously into recipient mice, which were primed on the same day with an intraperitoneal injection of trinitrophenylated KLH (TNP KLH) adjuvantized in *B. pertussis* vaccine. Four days later, spleen cells were tested in a plaque-forming assay against TNP erythrocytes. Equivalent suppression resulted from transfer of either normal or protein-deprived primed spleen cells into normal recipients. This suggests that reduction in a suppressor cell population was not involved in the enhanced PHA proliferative response. Does this mean that the relative proportion of PHA responsive cells is increased?

Malavé et al. (174) examined the changes in lymphocyte populations in thymus and spleen in C57 BL/6 mice fed 8 or 27% casein diets by determining the "homing" properties of ^{51}Cr-tagged cells and mitogen responsiveness. Various studies have shown that lymph node-seeking cells represent a long-lived, recirculating pool of lymphocytes containing helper T cells, alloreactive killer cells, and specific suppressor T cells. Spleen-seeking cells are more heterogenous, including such recirculating lymphocytes as well as short-lived sessile cells mediating nonspecific suppression and amplification of both help and suppression. Unfortunately, the experimental results in this study are somewhat unusual, in that early changes during the first 4 weeks of diet, even the loss of body weight initially observed, were not sustained during the second 4 weeks. The failure to gain weight during the first 25 days on diet followed by a rapid weight regain and parallel growth to the control diet group is the pattern typically observed in refed PEM subjects, including human children demonstrating catch-up growth. Since other dietary protein restriction studies in mice do not demonstrate this biphasic pattern, we must assume that the deprived mice somehow gained access to control diet in the latter phase of the experiment. Therefore, we consider here only the results obtained in the first 3 week period.

During this interval, the yield of thymus and spleen cells decreased to 27 and 38% of control animal yields, respectively. At the same time, the percentage of cells homing to lymph node in normal syngeneic recipients increased among splenocytes obtained from restricted compared to control diet animals, without a change in homing to the spleen. Thymocytes from the 4% casein diet animals showed the same pattern. When the number of recirculating and nonrecirculating cells was estimated in the spleen and thymus of the protein-deprived animals, there was a decrease in both populations but a proportionately greater decrease in the nonrecirculating cells. Consistent with these changes in cell populations, the response of both thymus and spleen cell suspensions to PHA and Con A progressively increased in relation to the response elicited in cells obtained from the normal diet controls, and the usual inhibition of Con A-induced proliferation by supraoptimal concentrations of the lectin was not observed. However, when 3 week deficient animals were switched to normal diets 96 hr prior to study, body weight rapidly increased, the spleen cell yield improved, and the effects on mitogen response to optimal and supraoptimal doses of PHA and Con A normalized.

In a separate study, Malavé et al. (173) determined the proliferative response to alloantigenic stimulation *in vivo* by transferring lymphoid cells from protein-deprived (8% casein) or control (27% casein) diet animals into lethally irradiated normally fed hemiallogenic f_1 hybrid adult animals. This directly measures the response of the donor cells in the GVH reaction. Donor animals were C57BL/6 mice and recipients were (C57BL/6 X DBA/2)f_1 hybrids. The latter received 770 rads (whole body irradiation) and within 4 hr were given an intravenous injection of donor cell suspensions obtained from animals after 3 to 5 weeks of protein restriction. Response of donor lymphocytes was ascertained by measuring splenic uptake of ^{125}I-IUDR into DNA 96 hr following cell transfer. Precursor uptake was significantly increased when protein-deficient thymus, spleen, or mesenteric node cells were injected, compared to cells obtained from normal diet animals. Furthermore, peak DNA synthesis in the host spleen occurred earlier using deprived compared to normal donor cells. Mixing experiments to detect cellular suppressor responses to the GVH reaction revealed equivalent activity of both protein-deprived and normal diet thymocytes. These data suggest that the former cell population contains a higher proportion of alloantigen reactive cells than does the latter.

Thus the diet-related selective depletion of nonrecirculating lymphocytes leads to a relative enrichment of more mature recirculating cells. This is supported by histologic evidence that the thymic cortex is more severely affected during early protein restriction than is the medullary region wherein the more differentiated T lymphocytes may be found. Thus lymphocyte population changes in lymphoid organs could account for the enhanced GVH and accelerated allogeneic skin graft rejection described by Cooper and colleagues (61,62). Malavé et al. (173) suggest that impaired cell division and/or increased corticosteroid secretion, which might reduce the steroid-sensitive cortical lymphocyte population, could underlie the relative increase in the long-lived medullary cell population.

Both these effects in fact have been shown by Bell et al. (27). In well-designed studies comparing 4 and 28% egg protein diets to standard laboratory chow (18 to 20% protein) initiated at weaning, the authors demonstrated a rapid loss of weight in all lymphoid organs in protein-restricted animals, most marked in the thymus and least so in the mesenteric lymph node. The cell content of each organ was proportional to organ weight, demonstrating that weight loss was due to cellular depletion. Although weight did not decrease in mesenteric nodes, it did remain steady, indicating a lack of cellular proliferation. Adrenalectomized, protein-deprived animals maintained spleen and lymph node weight and showed only a small decrease in thymus weight over 2 weeks. In contrast, the organ weight of sham-operated animals was equivalent to the adrenalectomized animals after 1 week of diet but showed dramatic decreases during the second week, presumably the additive effect of restricted cell division and corticosteroid lympholysis. The limited cell division in the deprived mice was not confined to lymphoid organs alone but included a severe reduction in extramedullary hematopoiesis in spleen and loss of megakaryocytes and cessation of myelopoiesis in the splenic red pulp. The stem cell population was reduced by 90%, and the lack of cell division was further reflected in a sharp decrease in ^{3}H-thymidine suicide reactivity in bone marrow and spleen.

Refeeding normal diets to mice deprived of protein at weaning results in cellular repopulation of thymus, with more or less normal kinetics of growth and involution of the organ beginning at the time of dietary rehabilitation. Increased weight in mesenteric nodes parallels body weight change, whereas spleen rapidly increases in weight during the first week and thymus somewhat later (28). Spleen regrowth is complex, representing a summation of both massive hematopoietic stem cell proliferation and differentiation and repopulation with lymphocytes, including B cells.

The resumption of normal development of thymus after an interval of diet-induced growth retardation raises the dual questions of the nature and source of the repopulating cells. Bell and Hazell (26) report that initiation of a protein-deficient diet 4 weeks after weaning, that is, during the usual thymic involutional phase, does not alter thymus weight, nor is there any effect of reinstituting a normal diet 3 weeks later. The refeeding changes observed after early protein restriction thus appear to be related to normal regulation of the thymus and may represent repopulation of the gland from cells intrinsic to the thymus or by an exogenous source of stem cells. Neither bone marrow nor spleen is required for thymic regrowth, however, since [89]strontium irradiation and splenectomy do not alter the events. Partial restoration of the thymus still occurs after whole body irradiation (400 rads) combined with splenectomy and [89]strontium treatment, whereas lethal irradiation (900 rads) prevents repopulation, even when the spleen is shielded. These data suggest that the thymus itself is the source of the repopulating cells. Treatment with cortisone acetate 3 days before refeeding further reduces thymic weight and results in a disappearance of virtually all remaining cortical lymphocytes but does not affect thymic regrowth, even in the face of [89]strontium therapy, which would remove the bone marrow as a source of stem cells.

The presence of long-lived stem cells in the thymus could be demonstrated experimentally by the Till and McCulloch assay for colony forming units (CFUs). In this assay, the number of CFUs in spleen of irradiated recipient mice is determined histologically 9 days following injection of donor cells. The number of CFUs per 10^6 thymic cells was increased by cortisone treatment of protein-restricted mice, consistent with an enrichment in cortisone-resistant stem cells, even though the total number of CFUs per organ was somewhat lower than observed in nonsteroid-treated animals. These data suggest that the thymic medullary region, wherein relatively radiation-resistant, steroid-resistant stem cells may reside, is the source of the repopulating cells.

B Lymphocytes and Humoral Immunity in Mice

The effects of malnutrition on B cell function and immunoglobulin synthesis is no less complex to dissect than is T cell function and cell-mediated immunity. Antibody production is dependent on far more than the presence of antigen and functioning B cells; it involves macrophages in processing and/or presentation of antigen as well as regulatory effects of T cells in both help and suppression of the response (Fig. 3). Regulatory T cells are also involved in the switch from IgM to IgG production, and even some T-independent antigens, such as pneumococcal capsular polysaccharide or DNP-ficoll, appear to need accessory macrophages to trigger an IgM response or are suppressed by T cell subpopulations. B cell responses in malnutrition, therefore, could be regulated and/or altered up or down by changes in either the APCs or T cell subsets. In fact, experiments in mice have shown decreased, unaltered, or enhanced responses to different antigens and at times to the same antigens in different studies.

We consider the studies reported by Cooper et al. (61) to be the start of a new era in experimental immunology of malnutrition effects in mice. The authors clearly state that their results cannot be directly extrapolated to the human, for the mouse is a controlled model in which experimental manipulation can provide interpretable data concerning immunologic mechanisms. On the basis of these early studies, they reported that protein deficiency of inbred mice leads to enhanced cellular immunity

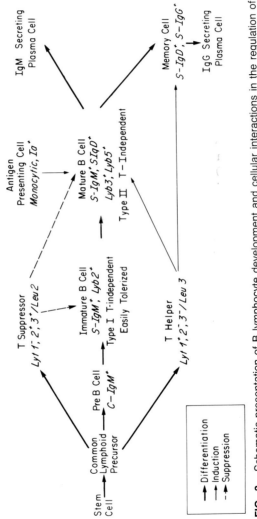

FIG. 3. Schematic presentation of B lymphocyte development and cellular interactions in the regulation of antibody synthesis. *Heavy solid arrows*, differentiation pathways; *fine solid arrows*, inductive (help) interactions; *dashed arrows*, levels of suppression.

Stem Cell → Common Lymphoid Precursor → Pre B Cell *C–IgM*⁺

T Suppressor *Lyt 1⁻, 2⁺, 3⁺/Leu 2*

Immature B Cell *S–IgM⁺, Lyb2⁺* Type I T-independent Easily Tolerized

Antigen Presenting Cell *Monocytic, Ia⁺*

Mature B Cell *S–IgM⁺, SIgD⁺ Lyb3⁺, Lyb5⁺* Type II T–Independent

IgM Secreting Plasma Cell

T Helper *Lyt 1⁺, 2⁻, 3⁻/Leu 3*

Memory Cell *S–IgD⁺, S–IgG⁺*

IgG Secreting Plasma Cell

→ Differentiation
→ Induction
–→ Suppression

and depressed or unaltered humoral immunity. Because of the lack of pair-fed controls in these and other studies, however, one cannot distinguish between protein, energy, or protein-energy malnutrition.

Using the SEC/1 ReJ mouse, Cooper and colleagues (61) demonstrated an equivalent agglutinating antibody response to 10^9 killed *Brucella abortus* cells in animals receiving either 8 or 27% casein diets. This was true of both the primary (1°) response, 8 days after the first injection, and the secondary (2°) response, 18 days following a booster injection. It is important to note that weight of protein-deprived animals was 30% less than controls; therefore, the deficient mice received more antigen per gram body weight than did the normals. Since dose response curves were not done, it is difficult to come to any conclusions about relative responses; different interpretations might become evident from titration experiments. Moreover, the serum albumim dropped by only 15% in the deficient animals, indicative of a mild protein malnutrition; this may also be the key to the normal results obtained. However, the 1° response to injection of SRBC in animals given only slightly less protein (6%) was dramatically depressed. This was shown in two ways. First, the number of PFCs per 10^5 spleen cells was decreased by 92%. Second, the mean agglutinating antibody titer ($\log_2$) was decreased from 9.4 to 6.1. The reduction in PFCs and antibody was proportional, indicating that each PFC produced as much antibody in malnourished as in nourished mice. Since the response to SRBC is highly T cell dependent, and the response to *Brucella* is to the somatic antigens like soluble LPS, "relatively T independent," one explanation for the divergent result would be that protein malnutrition does not directly affect B cell responses but rather may act at the T cell level of help. This is consistent with the fact that the percentage of B cells in spleen and mesenteric node remains constant on a 4% egg protein diet, although the total number of B cells is reduced because of the reduced size of the spleen (27). The mesenteric node retains the capacity for antigen-induced hypertrophy (*B. abortus* or SRBC) but to a lesser extent than normal diet animals, especially for SRBC (27).

Price and Bell (215–217) have attempted to systematically examine the antibody response to several antigens with varying degrees of T cell dependency. The results are complex and depend on the strain of mouse employed, dose and form of the antigen, age of the animal, and duration of the protein deficiency (4% egg albumin diet) before 1° immunization. The data are reported as the total antibody response (the accumulated $\log_2$ titer on days 8, 11, and 14 for the 1° response). For the 2° response, animals were rechallenged 14 days after priming, and the accumulated $\log_2$ titer on days 6, 12, and 18 after boosting was ascertained. At specific antigen dose levels, antibody response was increased to some antigens (polyvinylpyrrolidone 1° and 2°, *B. abortus* 1°, soluble tetanus toxoid 1°) and reduced for others (SRBC 1°, $AlPO_4$ adjuvantized tetanus toxoid, and soluble pneumococcus T-III polysaccharide). The 1° response to $AlPO_4$ tetanus was decreased when animals were primed after 1 week on diet and unaffected when primed after 3 weeks on diet. The increased 1° and decreased 2° response to soluble tetanus toxoid in protein deficiency was accounted for by the enhanced 1° IgM response in the protein-deprived mice and the brisk IgG 2° response to rechallenge in normal mice. In many experiments, the IgM antibody content was assessed by assay in the presence of 2-mercaptoethanol (2-ME). The proportion of total antibody that was sensitive to 2-ME was increased in the deficient mice for *B. abortus* 1° response, SRBC 1° and 2° response, AlPO$_4$ tetanus 2° response, soluble tetanus toxoid 1° and 2° response, and 1° response to soluble tetanus toxoid adjuvantized with *B. pertussis, B. abortus,* or *S. typhimurium* LPS. For pneumoccal T-III capsule, all antibody was 2-ME sensitive, and the 1° response was depressed whether assayed at 5 or 10 days following priming. The increase in the total antibody response to alumtetanus after 3 weeks on the diet was largely accounted for by 2-ME-sensitive antibodies.

Dose response curves were carried out for polyvinylpyrrolidone and pneumococcus T-III polysaccharide (215). Both antigens were tolerizing at high doses and significantly more so in deficient mice.

These data must be put into perspective of our current understanding of the regulation of immunoglobulin production by B cells. B cell development takes place in the mammalian equivalent of the bursa of Fabricius, bone marrow, or fetal liver. Here, stem cells differentiate into committed B cell precursors. These cells then develop into pre-B cells, with cytoplasmic but not surface immunoglobulin (Fig. 3). Maturation then proceeds to a cell which expresses IgM but not IgD on its cell surface, is easily tolerized, expresses no Lyb 3 or Lyb 5 (murine), and responds only to type I T-independent antigens, such as LPS. With further differentiation, both surface IgM and IgD are present, and such cells are functionally more mature and respond to type II T-independent antigens, such as TNP-ficoll, dextran, *Brucella*, and polyvinylpyrrolidone. These cells are also responsive to the action of T cell factors, which induce them to differentiate into IgG-secreting cells. Although such bacterial and synthetic antigens described here as T independent do not require T cell help for the initiation of B cell responses, regulation, which is under T cell control, is nonetheless involved at the level of suppression.

Most B cell responses, however, are under strict T cell control. B cells expressing surface IgD are triggered to produce antibody in response to antigen-specific T cell help. This T cell help is due to both idiotype-specific T cell signals as well as IL-2. This type of T cell help triggers a primary IgM response as well as the switch from IgM to IgG during the 2° response. B cells are also under the influence of regulatory T cells, which affect not only nonspecific suppression at the level of both immature and mature B cells but antigen-specific suppression of mature B cells as well.

Of the antigens used in the studies described above, polyvinylpyrrolidone, pneumococcus T-III polysaccharide, and LPS are relatively T-independent antigens capable of inducing an IgM response in the absence of T cells, whereas SRBC and tetanus toxoid require T cell help for optimal antibody production and for an IgG response. In addition, macrophages probably are involved in the immune response to either T-dependent or type II T-independent antigens. The first general principle to be extracted from the available experimental data demonstrating that the response to polyvinylpyrrolidone and *B. abortus* is enhanced while the response to LPS is normal in protein-deficient mice is that B cell function is largely intact if effective triggering with antigen can be achieved. The reduced response to pneumococcus T-III polysaccharide could mean that an accessory cell required for help is affected by protein deficiency or that a tolerizing as well as an immunizing form of the antigen is present.

Passwell et al. (209) have shown that altering macrophage function by infusion of carbon black into mice prior to immunization with another antigen, highly purified human serum transferrin, qualitatively alters the affinity of the antibody produced and reduces the clearance function for ^{125}I-polyvinylpyrrolidone. Affinity is a measure of the attractive forces between antibody and antigen that causes them to combine. Early antibody of the IgM class is of lower affinity than later antibody of the IgG class. Mononuclear cell blockade prior to immunization with the transferrin proportionally reduces the number of responding mice as well as the affinity of the antibody produced in responding animals. Moderate protein restriction likewise impairs clearance of colloidal particles and results in antibody of reduced affinity. Some of the effects described above may be related to mononuclear phagocyte dysfunction in the malnourished host.

The second principle to emerge is that protein deficiency affects the IgM to IgG switch in antibody response. The switch in immunoglobulin class of antibody that occurs when T-dependent antigens are used for immunization of normal mice does not occur in T cell-deficient animals. In this circumstance, whatever antibody is produced is reduced in amount and limited to the IgM class. Malavé and Layrisse (172) have examined the switch phenomenon in C57BL/6 mice fed 8 or 27% casein diets and immunized with allogeneic DBA/2 cells which differ at the H-2 locus (H-2^b versus H-2^d, respectively). Primary immunization was carried out 1 to 6 weeks after initiation of the experimental diet by intraperitoneal injection of 10^7 donor cells, and the 2° boost was given 14 days later. Antibody production was evaluated by means of a direct (IgM) plaque-forming assay employing the established lymphoma line L51784 (H-2^d) as a target or by hemagglutination assays using DBA/2 (H-2^d) or A/J (H-2^a) erythrocytes, with or without 2-ME to measure IgG and total (IgG plus IgM) antibody. Six weeks of diet reduced spleen weight by 44% and the number of cells per spleen by 55%. At the same time, the total number of PFCs per spleen at day 6 after 1° immunization was only 20% less in the malnourished animals, and the number of PFCs per 10^7 lymphocytes was actually increased by nearly twofold. The increase in the proportion of PFCs became apparent by day 6 after immunization and increased further on successive days. When 1° immunization was carried out after 1, 2, 3, 4, or 6 weeks of diet, the increase in PFCs was found to occur at the earliest time. Comparative antibody titers depended on the day of sampling. Anti-H-2 hemagglutinating antibody, all 2-ME sensitive, was increased in the malnourished animals on day 7 after 1° immunization, while the normal animals had rising titers of 2-ME-resistant antibody from 7 to 11 days after antigen administration. In addition, the antibody titer rose during the 2° response in normal diet animals, especially 2-ME-resistant activity, whereas the malnourished animals failed to show an anamnestic response or develop IgG antibody.

The data demonstrate the following: (a) There is no inhibition of the 1° IgM response to the allogeneic immunization in malnourished mice; indeed, there is enhanced antibody production. (b) There is no anamnestic response in the malnourished animals. (c) These mice fail to switch IgM to IgG antibody production. These observations are consistent with prior reports by Jose and Good (135) on the failure of C3Hf/Umc mice to develop IgG-blocking antibody to DBA/2 mammary adenocarcinoma when protein or specific amino acid (phenylalanine plus tryosine, valine, threonine, methionine plus cystine, isoleucine, or tryptophan)-deficient diets are fed to the animals.

One mechanism to account for the observations would be preferential reduction during malnutrition of splenic lymphocyte populations not involved in the IgM alloantibody response. Selective sensitivity of lymphocyte T cell subsets to protein deprivation is described above. Relative preservation of cells capable of the IgM allogenic response, however, would not account for the observed enhanced IgM response, and it is necessary to postulate a nutritionally induced disruption of regulatory responses, such as a reduction in supressor cells. This mechanism would be consistent with the increased antibody response to polyvinylpyrrolidone, but not with the results obtained following immunization with pneumococcal T III polysaccharide in which the total antibody response is significantly reduced.

Bongiorni-Malavé and Pocino (38) determined the suppressor cell response in C57B1/6 mice fed 8 or 26% casein diets. Spleen cell suspensions prepared from normal or malnourished mice were injected into lethally irradiated syngeneic mice which were immediately sensitized with 10^8 SRBC. The number of direct PFCs per recipient spleen was determined 5 days later. The response was significantly greater (1.9-fold; $p < 0.01$) in recipients reconstituted with malnourished splenocytes.

To eliminate the possibility that differences in homing of transferred cells accounted for these results, normal or malnourished spleen cells were stimulated *in vitro* in the presence of 5×10^{-5} M 2-ME with varying numbers of SRBC (5×10^5 to 10^8) and the PFC response measured 5 days later. At all levels of stimulation, the malnourished cells produced a greater PFC response. The increased response at suboptimal antigen dose suggests that helper cell activity was not affected by the dietary manipulations. The level of suppressor activity then was tested by isolating spleen cells from experimental or control diet mice 2 weeks after a single intraperitoneal injection of 2×10^9 SRBC; 3×10^7 primed spleen cells were transferred intravenously into syngeneic recipients, and an immunizing dose of 2×10^8 SRBC was given immediately after cell transfer. Control groups received nonimmune spleen cells or SRBC alone, and the PFC response was assessed 5 days later. Transferred nonimmune spleen cells did not change the PFCs of recipient cells. Normal primed cells significantly suppressed the response by 61% ($p < 0.05$). The level of suppression by the malnourished primed cells (27%) was not significantly different from nonprimed normal spleen cells ($p > 0.05$).

In five of six additional experiments performed after priming donor mice following 1, 2, or 3 weeks on diet, the normal donor cells resulted in a significant suppression (40 to 80%; $p < 0.05$ to <0.001), whereas malnourished cells caused statistically significant suppression only once. The suppressor effect was antigen specific and not expressed when recipient animals were challenged with pigeon erythrocytes. The suppressor cell population was present in the effluent of nylon wool column fractionated lymphocytes and rapidly appeared when deficient animals were refed normal diet beginning 3 days prior to immunization. When nutritional rehabilitation was delayed until 3 days prior to harvesting donor cells, there was no significant suppressor activity; the low level observed was similar to the results in animals maintained on 8% casein throughout the experiment.

The suppressor activity of normal donor primed cells was abrogated when transferred into a recipient on the low protein diet for 3 weeks as well as in normal recipient mice treated with 10 mg/kg cyclophosphamide 24 hr prior to cell transfer. The data suggest that feedback-induced suppression, mediated by a short-lived cyclophosphamide-sensitive cell, does not occur in the malnourished recipient host. This may be explained if an Ly $1,2,3^+$ precursor suppressor cell has been depleted from the malnourished spleen cell population, so that normal antigen-specific Ly $1^-,2,3^+$ suppressor cells cannot induce and amplify the generation of such feedback-induced suppressor T cells. Phenotypic characterization of lymphocyte populations from malnourished mice have not yet been reported, however, and the explanation remains to be proved.

Animal Studies: Rats

Considerable work has employed the rat as a model for protein-energy deprivation. Histologic changes in central and peripheral lymphoid organs (primarily loss of cellularity in T-dependent regions) and lymphopenia, more marked in intact compared with adrenalectomized animals, and elevated plasma corticosterone levels have been reported (7–12,73,81,139,142,177,178,181,189,195). B cells and B cell regions are better preserved. Antibody responses to tetanus toxoid (195) and SRBC (8) are decreased, as is the proportion of PFCs to the latter, without change in antibody production per PFC. In one study, reduced dietary protein (8%) impaired the development of serum cytotoxic antibody responses against xenogeneic tumor cells (135). In these manifestations, the rat responds in similar fashion to the mouse.

Species differences have been reported in the studies of cell-mediated immunity. In contrast to the mouse data, PHA responsiveness and GVH reactivity of spleen cells from protein-deprived animals are both impaired (9,181). The differences may be due, at least in part, to the model of malnutrition employed in the rat, an unrealistic total deprivation of protein.

Heresi and Chandra (119) have studied the effects of dietary restriction (at a level of 30% of intake of a laboratory chow diet by *ad lib*-fed controls) on PHA-stimulated mitogenesis of spleen cells. After 8 weeks of restricted diet, the body, spleen, and thymus weights were all severely reduced. The lymphocyte content per gram organ was also depressed by 40 to 50% in the restricted group. The SI to PHA in malnourished animals was significantly reduced from 35.7 ± 8.5 in the controls to 10.4 ± 3.8. This was entirely due to an increase in the basal (unstimulated) thymidine incorporation in the latter. The authors postulate that either subclinical infection or a reduction in suppressive influences could be responsible. The observed normal stimulated response would not be consistent with the latter ideas, however, and is similar to the results reported in marasmic human patients.

Thymic hormone activity in serum was also determined in these animals by the method of Bach and Dardenne (18). Activity was significantly depressed in the diet-restricted group. The functional importance of this observation is unclear, since the spleen cell population did respond well to PHA, but might be an important defect leading to the lymphocyte depletion noted in the lymphoid organs.

Another observation has been made in protein-deprived rats that has not been reported in other animal studies, namely, a depletion in mucosal lymphocytes in the gut. Keusch et al. (142) found a marked reduction in lymphoid aggregates and single gut lymphocytes in animals severely restricted in protein in the diet (0.5 to 2.0% lactalbumin). In a later study, Maffei et al. (171) reported that total protein deprivation resulted in a quantitative decrease in mucosal lymphoid cells in the jejunum. Morphometric techniques were used to count the number of intraepithelial lymphocytes (IEL) per 100 villus epithelial cells, the absolute number of cells per millimeter muscularis mucosa, and, in PAS-stained sections, the percentage of lymphocytes crossing the basement membrane. In protein-deprived rats, IEL per 100 villus cells and per millimeter were each reduced by 37%, while the percentage of lymphocytes crossing the basement membrane increased from 1.6% in controls to 7.0% in malnourished animals. These alterations undoubtedly are a reflection of the general change in number and distribution of lymphocyte populations in the protein-deprived host and may offer a mechanism in explanation of the impaired IgA response in humans with PEM.

ZINC

Human Studies

Zinc deficiency occurs in patients with PEM (106), acrodermatitis enteropathica (53), Down syndrome (36,100), and hospitalized patients receiving zinc-free total parenteral nutrition (4). Common features of all these instances of documented zinc deficiency are thymic atrophy, decrease in thymic hormone levels, and an associated decrease in certain T cell populations. The observation that the thymus undergoes involution in zinc deficiency may be related to the fact that more than 70 metallo enzymes are zinc dependent. Among these enzymes are thymidine kinase and both DNA polymerase and DNA-dependent RNA polymerase. In addition, thymic hormone is a zinc-containing metallopeptide produced by the epithelial cells of the thymus. The thymic atrophy, therefore, could be attributable to multiple defects, such as depressed epithelial function resulting in the decreased secretion of thymic hormones or the inability of immature T cells and prothymocytes to differentiate properly, because of either a decrease in epithelial function or the fact that both these populations contain terminal deoxynucleotidyl transferase, a zinc-containing DNA polymerase. Impaired thymic function can account for reduced T cell numbers in the periphery, as well as specific defects which result in the loss of functional subpopulations dependent on the presence of recirculating thymic hormone.

Golden and co-workers (106) studied malnourished children who exhibited thymic atrophy. In order to assess whether zinc supplementation could reverse the effects seen on the thymus, the patients received oral zinc sulfate. This intervention induced a rapid increase in thymic size as well as an increased response in DTH to *Candida* antigens. In eight malnourished children who were supplemented with zinc sulfate, the observed increase in thymic size, as assessed by chest autoradiography, correlated with the increase in plasma zinc levels.

Franceschi et al. (100) investigated 28 noninstitutionalized zinc-deficient Down syndrome subjects and observed a significant reduction of circulating T lymphocytes when compared to cells obtained from normal controls. No significant differences were reported in the ability to respond in an allogeneic MLR; however, there was a significant decrease in the autologous MLR ($15,716 \pm 826$ cpm in controls compared to $8,406 \pm 1,778$ cpm in the Down subjects), a test for a regulatory subset of T cells which is defective in various autoimmune disorders.

Thymic hormone activity was also measured in Down syndrome by assessing *facteur thymique serique* (FTS) levels using the azathioprine-sensitive, rosette-forming cell assay (100). Induction of rosetting in this assay takes place only in the presence of active FTS. FTS activity was reduced in Down subjects as compared to controls in every age group studied.

Björkstén et al. (36) also assessed the effects of zinc supplementation in 12 patients with Down syndrome. Initial zinc levels, determined by atomic absorption spectrophotometry, were dramatically reduced (16 μg/dl) as compared to healthy controls (180 μg/dl). After 2 months of zinc therapy, serum zinc levels increased to the normal range (158 μg/dl). This correlated with an increase in neutrophil chemotactic activity and lymphocyte reactivity. Ten of 11 patients showed an increase in DTH responses to DNCB and an increase in PHA responsiveness after correction of zinc levels.

Acrodermatitis enteropathica, inherited as an autosomal recessive trait, is characterized by diarrhea, skin lesions, neurologic symptoms, frequent infection, and zinc malabsorption. Chandra (53) studied lymphocyte responses to PHA in a group of these patients. In the majority of the children (eight of 10) with low serum zinc levels, there was a depressed proliferative response of lymphocytes to the mitogen. DTH responses were also assayed using a battery of recall antigens, with total anergy exhibited by seven of 10 patients. The patients not displaying anergic responses had normal serum zinc levels. When zinc sulfate was administered for a 2 week period, these patients showed rapid improvement, with plasma zinc levels rising to a normal level. Eight patients subsequently developed a positive response to one or more of the recall antigen panel. Oleske et al. (205) reported a child with observed hypergammaglobulinemia and an immune deficiency involving both T and B cell functions. The patient's lymphocytes showed weak responses to the T cell mitogens, PHA and Con A, as well as to the polyclonal T-dependent activator of B cells, PWM. After initiation of zinc therapy, T cell numbers returned to normal. Lymphocytes also began to respond to the mitogens, and skin test reactivity returned as well.

Allen et al. (4) studied patients who had developed a severe zinc deficiency during parenteral hyperalimentation. Circulating T lymphocyte counts in these patients were decreased compared to normal levels. One of the two patients studied for PHA mitogen response had a significantly reduced proliferation, approximately 30% below control. After intravenous zinc supplementation, both patients showed exaggerated proliferative responses to PHA above control levels.

Animal Studies

Danish cattle with lethal trait A46 have been shown to have a characteristic hypoplastic thymus, deficient cell-mediated immunity, and associated zinc deficiency due to intestinal malabsorption of zinc, a syndrome equivalent to human acrodermatitis enteropathica (41). Like acrodermatitis, this trait is inherited as an autosomal recessive. Affected animals display not only marked depletion of cortical thymic lymphocytes, but also hypoplasia in the peripheral lymphoid organs, such as spleen, regional nodes, and Peyer patches. Brummerstedt et al. (41) have shown that these cows have a decreased humoral response to tetanus toxoid and reduced cell-mediated immunity in skin responses. Supplementation of the diet with zinc sulfate restores thymic morphology as well as peripheral lymphoid function. This restoration continues as long as zinc treatment is maintained; however, discontinuation of treatment results in a relapse of immunologic defects.

Recently, a number of experimental studies have been performed in zinc-deficient rat and murine models. Fernandes and associates (92) produced zinc-deficient mice and demonstrated the occurrence of thymic atrophy with cortical depletion, as well as a reduction in peripheral lymphoid T cells. Mice were divided into groups that were pair-fed either zinc-deficient, zinc-supplemented, or *ad lib* Purina lab chow diets. There was an appropriate rapid drop in serum zinc levels in the zinc-deficient diet group. FTS activity was then measured by the azathioprine-sensitive rosette assay. The zinc-deficient group showed a drop of FTS after only 3 weeks on the diet; by 5 weeks, no detectable FTS activity was found (129).

Fraker and colleagues (76,77,98,99,167,168) performed a series of studies on the effect of varying dietary zinc levels on the immune response of different mouse strains. Thymus weight in the zinc-deficient mice was reduced by approximately 85% as compared to mice fed with marginal or adequate dietary zinc (98). Antibody responses in zinc-deficient mice to T-dependent antigens, such as SRBC and KLH, were significantly decreased in both IgM and IgG PFCs. Primary antibody responses (IgM) to SRBC were reduced from approximately 4,000 PFCs in controls to 2,000 PFCs in zinc-deficient mice. Indirect plaques (IgG) showed a more dramatic decrease, from approximately 22,000 PFCs in controls to 4,000 PFCs in zinc-deficient mice. When zinc-deficient mice were reconstituted with 6×10^6 normal thymocytes, there was an increase from about 6,000 to 37,000 IgG PFCs per spleen.

In subsequent studies, Fraker and co-workers (99) used pair-fed controls. Their data demonstrate that thymic atrophy and the impairment of T cell helper function are the result of zinc deficiency rather than reduced daily food intake. Luecke et al. (168) also determined the effects of zinc deficiency on different mouse strains. A comparison of outbred Swiss mice and inbred mice showed no significant differences in the effect of dietary zinc deficiency on either growth, diet consumption, or immunologic responses.

Since corticosteroids can dramatically alter cell-mediated immune responses, DePasquale-Jardieu and Fraker (76) determined whether or not stress secondary to the zinc deficiency induced in A/J mice led to an elevation of glucocorticoid hormone levels. Indeed, steroid levels were markedly increased in zinc-deficient mice. Both zinc-deficient and control mice then were divided into adrenalectomized and sham-operated groups (77). Adrenalectomy did not reverse the depletion of cortical thymic lymphocytes or thymic atrophy. When zinc-deficient mice were fed a zinc-adequate diet for 1 week, the indirect (IgG) PFC response to SRBC returned to about 70% of control levels (15,260 versus 22,410 PFCs), and thymic weight increased (99). By 2 weeks after initiation of the zinc supplementation, the PFC response was slightly higher in treated animals (27,720 PFCs) as compared to controls (20,270 PFCs). By 4 weeks, the response was equivalent in control and supplemented animals.

In a series of studies by Fernandes et al. (92) in mice fed a zinc-deficient diet, serum zinc was reduced to 35 to 60 μg/dl after 4 weeks, compared to 110 to 125 μg/dl in pair-fed and *ad lib*-fed mice. Deficient mice showed a dramatic decrease in indirect PFCs to SRBC when assessed 4 weeks after the initiation of the deficient diet. IgG responses in depleted animals were about 50% of pair-fed control values (14,913 compared to 31,934 PFCs). By 6 weeks, the response in zinc-deficient mice was decreased to 5,128 PFCs, whereas in pair-fed controls, there were approximately 70,000 PFCs.

The generation of cytotoxic effector cells (CTLs) after *in vivo* immunization with EL-4 tumor cells was also studied. After 2 weeks on the diet, there was a 50% reduction in CTL activity of lymphocytes isolated from zinc-deficient mice. By 8 weeks, deficient mice showed 14.7% killing against allogeneic cells compared to 78% killing in pair-fed controls at the same 100:1 effector to target ratio. NK cell activity was determined by measuring the ability of spleen cells to lyse ^{51}Cr-labeled RL-1 lymphoma cells. NK cell activity was significantly reduced after 2 weeks on the diet. After 8 weeks, spleen cells derived from zinc-deficient mice were also assayed for their ability to mediate antibody-dependent cell-mediated cytotoxicity (ADCC) against ^{51}Cr-labeled chicken erythrocyte targets. ADCC is thought to be mediated by Fc receptor (FcR)-positive lymphoid cells, and no significant reduction was observed during the 8 weeks on the zinc-deficient diet. These data are consistent with the decreasing numbers of Thy 1-positive spleen and lymph node cells, while the percentage of FcR-positive cells remained normal or elevated in zinc-deficient mice.

Chandra and Au (54) also studied NK cell activity, ADCC, and the generation of CTLs in zinc-deficient mice. There was a reduction in the ability of spleen cells derived from zinc-deficient mice to generate CTLs against allogeneic targets. However, in contrast to the findings of Fernandes et al., Chandra observed an increase in both NK cell activity and ADCC in splenocytes from zinc-deficient animals.

Gross et al. (111) reported that the effects of zinc deficiency in rats could be reversed by treatment with levamisole. PHA stimulation of spleen cells derived from zinc-deprived rats was significantly reduced (SI of 87.9 as compared with 143.3 in control rats). However, levamisole treatment markedly improved the PHA response of spleen cells from the zinc-deprived group (SI = 135) without changing the SI of the control group (SI = 143). Similar effects were seen in the PHA response of peripheral blood lymphocytes derived from control and zinc-deprived rats. The SI of 146 in zinc-deprived rats increased to control values (SI = 317) after levamisole treatment. Since levamisole acts in some fashion on precursor cells, these studies suggest that the stem cells in zinc-deficient animals are normal and, therefore, the effects of zinc deficiency are at the thymus and/or peripheral T cell level.

Studies on zinc deficiency in both humans and animal models thus have shown a consistent impairment of cell-mediated immunity. Data also indicate a role for zinc *in vitro* in lymphocyte responses of normal cells. It appears that there is an absolute requirement for zinc during *in vitro* proliferation responses of lymphocytes to PHA and Con A in both animal and human cells. Studies by Rao et al. (221) have shown that zinc can act alone or in combination with mitogens to induce the proliferation of T lymphocytes. In these studies, zinc appears to affect the cell membrane to both induce proliferation in the absence of any mitogen and to cause a redistribution of receptors so that there is increased sensitivity of the response of lymphoid cells to PHA and Con A.

These studies indicate that zinc has a central effect on the development of the cell-mediated limb of the immune response. The atrophy and associated loss of thymic humoral function may inhibit the development of thymic precursors into mature thymus-derived lymphocytes. The reversal of zinc deficiency effects with levamisole further supports this hypothesis, since its proposed mechanism of action is to mimic thymic factors in the induction of prothymocyte to thymocyte differentiation.

IRON

Human Studies

Studies on the role of iron and iron-binding proteins on immune functions have been conducted primarily in humans. There is a clinical suggestion, by no means conclusively supported by evidence from well-designed epidemiologic studies, that individuals with moderate to severe iron deficiency anemia have depressed resistance mechanisms to infection and increased infection morbidity. Iron deficiency in humans is a result of inadequate iron intake, inadequate iron absorption, or blood loss. Etiology becomes important in order to properly understand associated immunologic defects, since parasitic or other infection, tumors, or gut lesions that lead to blood loss can potentially affect the immune system directly, while intestinal malabsorption is probably not specific for iron and can affect other nutrients that influence immune function.

In addition to their critical role in oxygen transport, iron and iron-binding proteins have diverse biologic functions, among which may be a direct effect on the development and function of the immune system. Iron is a required element in many enzymes and metabolic cofactors, including cytochrome c, cytochrome c reductase, cytochrome oxidase, succinic dehydrogenase, aconitase, peroxidase, and xanthine oxidase. However, there are no clues at present about the specific role of iron in the immune response.

Srikantia et al. (252) reported the immunologic status of 88 children divided into four groups based on hemoglobin levels. In the groups with severe to moderate iron deficiency (<8.0 and 8.1 to 10.0 g/dl hemoglobin), there was a significant depression in E-rosette formation and PHA responsiveness of peripheral blood lymphocytes, compared to mild anemia or nonanemic controls. In the group with severe iron deficiency, E-rosettes were reduced from 58.7 to 37.9%, while the PHA SI decreased from 19.4 to 5.9. In the group with moderate deficiency, 47.3% of the lymphocytes formed E-rosettes, and the SI was 13.3. The data in the group with mild iron deficiency (10.1 to 12.0 g dl^{-1}) did not differ from those in the normal control group ($\geq$12 g dl^{-1}). Unfortunately, no biochemical parameters were reported to rule out other, concomitant nutrient abnormalities of potential importance in the severely anemic, such as folic acid or vitamin B$_{12}$. The subjects were also separated into two groups with low (<10.0 g dl^{-1}) or high ($\geq$10 g dl^{-1}) hemoglobin and further subdivided according to percent transferrin saturation. In the group with low hemoglobin levels, those with transferrin saturation of greater than 15% had 34% E-rosetting cells and a PHA SI of 3.6, whereas children with transferrin saturation of less than 15% had 44% T cells in the peripheral blood and a SI of 10.4. Thus transferrin saturation may be a more sensitive indicator of depressed T lymphocyte functions than is the degree of anemia.

Bhaskaram and Reddy (32) found the same changes in nine iron-deficient children and also determined the effect of iron supplementation. There was a significant reduction in the percentage of circulating T cells in these subjects (42 versus 65% in 11 controls) and in the proliferative response to PHA (4.5 versus 27.3). With iron supplementation, however, the T cells increased to 52% by the fourth week of treatment, although the PHA proliferative response continued to be depressed (SI = 5.0). The data are difficult to fully evaluate because methods are not well described and there is an enormous and overlapping range of values for each parameter tested. The controls are not age or sex matched, and the presence of infection is not considered.

Similar studies by Chandra and Saraya (56) also showed a depression in immunologic responsiveness associated with iron deficiency. Twenty children were classified as iron deficient based on several criteria, including hemoglobin levels, serum iron, transferrin saturation, and the presence of hypochromia. PEM was excluded by anthropometry and serum albumin levels. As in previous studies, there was a reduction in rosette-forming T cells and PHA response, which was reversible by iron supplementation. Compared to 20 healthy matched controls, there was a depression of DTH skin responses to recall antigens in the iron-deficient children. Fewer of the latter responded to *Candida*, tricophyton, SK/SD, or mumps. Unfortunately, the statistical significance of the differences in the data is not presented.

MacDougall et al. (170) studied 27 iron-deficient children, 20 with hemoglobin less than 10 g dl^{-1} (mean, 8.1 $\pm$ 1.7) and seven termed "latent iron deficient" who had hemoglobin values greater than 10.0 g dl^{-1} (mean, 10.8 $\pm$ 0.5). However, serum iron was similarly reduced to 34 μg dl^{-1} in both these groups. Total lymphocyte and white blood cell counts were slightly but not significantly elevated in the subjects with iron deficiency, possibly related to recent infections reported in 75% of the group. Immunologic status was examined by assessing *in vitro* responses to PHA and *Candida* and DTH skin responses to DPT and *Candida in vivo*. Compared to 14 controls (mean hemoglobin, 12.8 $\pm$ 1.2 g dl^{-1}; serum iron, 76 $\pm$ 26 μg dl^{-1}), DTH responses to DPT were reduced from 86 to 18% positive, although a similar response rate to *Candida* was observed in the controls and iron-deficient groups (79 versus 64%). Interestingly, there were fewer positive reactions in the group with latent iron deficiency (0 for diphtheria and 43% for *Candida*), but there were only seven subjects in this category. A significant decrease in PHA responsiveness was measured by mitotic index in both iron-deficient groups as compared to control levels (13.4 $\pm$ 4.0). Again, the value was lowest in the latent group (6.6 $\pm$ 1.5) compared to the severely anemic subjects (9.7 $\pm$ 4.6). The initiation of iron therapy by the administration of intramuscular iron dextran in 11 anemic and four latent iron-deficient children reversed the hematologic abnormalities and corrected the immunologic responses to near normal levels when tested 2 to 3 months later. At that time, 82% responded to diptheria and 100% to *Candida*, while the PHA mitotic index rose to 16.2 $\pm$ 3.5 in the anemic and to 17.2 $\pm$ 3.0 in the latent group. The separation of anemic and latent iron-deficient subjects seems somewhat arbitrary, since these infants all had similar biochemical indices of iron deficiency. The greater degree of anemia in the former may be related to the high incidence of recent infection in these subjects.

The studies by Wakabayashi and Takaku (266) examined the ability of peripheral blood lymphocytes derived from patients with iron deficiency anemia to respond to PHA. The proliferative response was significantly lower in the iron-deficient group as compared with normal controls. Ferrous sulfate added *in vitro* to the culture medium of both iron-deficient and control cells resulted in an increase in proliferation in all groups tested, with the greatest increase in the iron-deficient cells cultured with 2 μg ferrous sulfate. These data suggest that iron must be present in sufficient quantity at the time of stimulation, since the defect is corrected so rapidly *in vitro*. This brings up the general problems of demonstration of altered cellular function due to nutritional deficiencies which may be corrected by the medium employed for *in vitro* cell culture and in the process obscure *in vivo* defects. By 3 months of treatment, proliferative responses were back to control levels.

These various studies reveal similar immunologic defects in subjects with either severe iron deficiency anemia or iron deficiency with lesser degrees of anemia, that is, suppression of cell-mediated immune responses at the level of T cell proliferation to mitogens, reduced responses to PPD *in vitro*, and depressed DTH to recall antigens. No careful studies have been done to explore the effects of iron on B cell responses or humoral immunity in the human.

Animal Studies

Nalder et al. (195) employed several protocols to create iron deficiency in weanling Sprague-Dawley rats. In one such study, a 20% casein stock diet was progressively diluted with sucrose. As the percentage of dietary sucrose increased from 0 to 75% and the iron and protein content decreased, body weight, hemoglobin, and serum protein content all diminished in the animals when assessed after 6 weeks on the diet. At week 3 and 4, these animals were immunized with a killed *Salmonella pullorum* vaccine, and the resulting agglutinating antibody response was measured at week 6. Even in the minimal 10% sucrose dilution diet group, antisalmonella antibody titers were decreased. This effect was more marked with higher sucrose content in the diet. However, the regimen not only altered iron content but dramatically changed the overall nutritional quality of the diet as the protein/calorie ratio was altered. Thus, while hemoglobin levels did not change in the 10% sucrose group, total serum protein dropped from 8.5 to 7.1 g dl^{-1}.

To focus on iron per se, another group of rats, obtained from iron-deficient dams, were fed with diets containing either 20 or 0 mg ferrous sulfate/kg of diet. Eight to 10 weeks after birth, the animals were immunized with 6 weekly tetanus toxoid injections, using a proportional dose based on body weight. At week 15, hemoglobin was significantly reduced (from 12.9 to 4.7 g/dl) as was serum protein (7.5 to 3.4 g/dl). A qualitative precipitin reaction was employed to measure antibody and demonstrated a reduction in the mean titer from 310 in controls to 19 in the iron-deprived rats.

In a similar protocol, male weanling rats were fed diets adequate in all nutrients but iron, which was added in a range of concentrations from 20 to 5 mg/kg diet. Each rat was immunized twice with tetanus toxoid as above after 7 weeks on diet. Antibody titers at week 13 were determined and were found to be significantly decreased, even in animals with minimal reductions in iron intake from 20 to 18, 16, or 14 mg/kg diet. These diets had no effect on body weight or serum and liver iron levels and caused only a slight reduction in hemoglobin, suggesting an effect of mild or tissue-selective iron depletion on the antibody response.

Additional studies on the effects of iron deficiency on immune functions have employed a model helminth infection, *Nippostrongylus brasiliensis*, in the rat (37,68,82). When rats are infected with larval stages of this worm, the adults develop in the small intestine; but after a few weeks, they are expelled in an immunologically specific fashion. Such immune rats are resistant to rechallenge. The mechanism of the immune rejection of worms is complex and involves antibody, sensitized T cells, and an essential bone marrow constituent. The first attack on the adult worm is via antibody, rendering the worms susceptible to a T cell-mediated expulsion, which may be related to release of pharmacologic mediators. Antibody damage alone is ineffective in producing worm expulsion, however, since this does not occur in irradiated or T cell-deficient animals.

Worm expulsion is also defective (delayed) in combined iron and protein deficiency induced by dietary deprivation. Cummins et al. (68) determined the effect of transfer of syngeneic mesenteric lymph node cells from normal or iron/protein deprived *N. brasiliensis*-infected inbred DA rat donors on worm expulsion by normal or deprived DA recipients. Weanling donors were placed on diet for 5 weeks and then infected twice at a 3 week interval with 1,000 larvae. Cells were obtained 7 days later, and 1.25×10^8 pooled mesenteric node cells were transferred intravenously on the day of infection of recipients. Worm counts in the latter were determined 10 days later. Body weight, serum albumin, and hemoglobin were significantly reduced in the experimental diet groups. When cells from normal controls were transferred to normal recipients, there were only 5 ± 1.1 worms recovered after rechallenge, compared to 275 ± 44.4 from normal rats which were not given sensitized lymphocytes. Cells transferred from deficient donors to normal recipients were also effective; there were only 17 ± 7.9 worms remaining at day 10 compared to 320 ± 50 in untransfused deficient infected controls. However, sensitized cells from either nutrient-sufficient or -deficient donors were ineffective when given to deficient recipients (269 ± 43.7 and 298 ± 52.6 worms present at 10 days in animals receiving dietary-sufficient or -deficient donor cells, respectively). This demonstrates that delayed expulsion is not due to any permanent intrinsic defect in deficient donor cells, which are able to function normally in the milieu of the normally nourished animal. The locus of the defect is uncertain from these studies, and it is impossible to separate the effects of protein deficiency from iron deficiency.

Duncombe et al. (82) studied a single deficiency of iron or protein as well as a combined deficiency on the acquired resistance to reinfection with *N. brasiliensis*. Groups of 3-week-old Wistar rats were placed on the three diets. Seven weeks later, all were infected with 1,000 *N. brasiliensis* larvae. On day 9 of $1°$ infection, some animals were treated with a high dose (50 mg/kg) of mebendazole to kill and expel the worms present. These rats were rechallenged with 1,000 larvae 7 days later, and worm survival was determined 11 days later. Hemoglobin levels in iron-deficient, protein-deficient, iron/protein-deficient, and control groups were 5.4, 11.9, 7.3, and 13.2 g dl^{-1}, respectively, while corresponding body weight was 242, 190, 111, and 269 g. In the control diet group, 26 worms remained from primary infection on the day of rechallenge (day 16). When these animals received mebendazole on day 9, however, the infection was virtually eliminated by day 16 (0.2 worms present per animal). The strong rejection of worms on $2°$ challenge is obvious from the count of 8 ± 4 obtained on day 27 in mebendazole-treated, reinfected controls. In contrast, the worm count on day 27 of similarly manipulated rats on the iron-, protein-, or iron/protein-deficient diets was 66 ± 12, 48 ± 8, and 140 ± 23, respectively. Thus either iron or protein deficiency significantly reduced the 2° immune expulsion of *N. brasiliensis*, and combined deficiency further impaired rejection.

Nutritional rehabilitation (normal diet plus intramuscular iron-dextran) begun 2 days before either 1° infection or rechallenge successfully reversed the abnormal (delayed) expulsion, assessed again on day 27 of the protocol. This result in animals repleted only after 1° infection demonstrates that the afferent limb of sensitization to *N. brasiliensis* is intact in iron- and protein-deficient animals. The data suggest that an effector mechanism, such as production or release of lymphokines or pharmacologic mediators (possibly bioactive mast cells products), may be at fault. The affected mechanism remains uncertain.

In an abstract, Kuvibidila et al. (153) reported impaired lymphocyte function in mice made iron deficient. Details of mouse strain, diets employed, or the effect on iron metabolism are not stated. Splenic lymphocytes were isolated from iron-deficient, pair-fed, and *ad lib*-fed control mice and were stimulated *in vitro* with Con A, PHA, PWM, and LPS. Proliferative responses in the iron-deficient anemic groups were said to be less than 50% of control levels. Although the decreased responsiveness to PHA did not correlate with the degree of anemia, lymphocyte proliferation was restored *in vitro* by the addition of ferric chloride ($FeCl_3$) or transferrin. Con A responses did correlate with the degree of iron deficiency, but the abnormality was not reversible *in vitro*. Unfortunately, the data are not presented for careful examination. This study is important, however, because most other animal studies examine only the effects of iron deficiency on resistance to infection or determine effects on growth of microoganisms *in vivo* or *in vitro*.

In Vitro Iron Supplementation

Recent studies have explored the role of iron and iron-binding proteins in regulation of immune responses *in vitro*. Receptors on the surface of human and murine lymphocytes and murine lymphoma cells for ferritin, lactoferrin, and transferrin have been described as well.

De Sousa, Nishiya, and co-workers (78,202,203) have studied the effect of addition of $FeCl_3$ or iron citrate on the E-rosetting of human peripheral blood lymphocytes. Addition of the iron salts, but not sodium citrate or zinc chloride, reduced the percentage of E-rosetting cells by 30 to 90% at concentrations of 10^{-5} to 10^{-4} M. A significant but less marked inhibition of EAC rosettes was also found. Maximum inhibition was 60% at 10^{-4} M iron citrate concentration. In contrast, there was no effect on EA rosette formation. Inhibitory effects were reversed by addition of iron chelators, and the iron salts were, in themselves, nontoxic. Native purified human transferrin was inactive in the above studies unless it was fully saturated with iron, whereas lactoferrin had no observable influence regardless of the degree of iron saturation.

Bryan et al. (42) studied effects of iron in the MLR. At a concentration of 10^{-2} M, $FeCl_3$ totally depressed the proliferation of human peripheral blood lymphocytes in the MLR, while 10^{-4} M $FeCl_3$ reduced the response by 40%. Treating the stimulating and responding cell populations individually with iron, washing the treated cells, and mixing demonstrated that the inhibition is mediated by iron binding to the responding T cell population. These treatments did not affect cell viability. HLA typing of donors demonstrated that responding cells expressing the HLA-A2 phenotype were significantly less affected by iron than non-A-2 donors.

These studies grew out of the observation that Hodgkin disease patients show abnormal accumulation of E-rosetting cells in spleen and other tissues containing high iron concentrations. The suggestion is that iron may also alter the migration of T cells *in vivo*. In this context, the effect of iron and iron-binding proteins on regulation of surface markers and function of T cells as well as traffic suggests that these effects take place at the T cell surface membrane via specific receptors and may be responsible for impaired cell-mediated immunity in iron deficiency.

MAGNESIUM

The mineral magnesium is an important constituent of bone and soft tissues and is present in the intracellular milieu and in serum. Of the 20 to 25 g body magnesium in the human adult, more than 70% is combined with calcium and phosphorus in bone. In trace concentrations, Mg^{2+} is a critical activating ion for many biologic reactions, as diverse as the activation of the complement pathway or specific enzymes in the glycolytic pathway of metabolism. Indeed, oxidative phosphorylation and the transfer of high energy phosphate would be impossible in the absence of Mg^{2+}.

It has been difficult to define clinical syndromes of magnesium deficiency, in part because of the large reserves in bone. It is clear, however, that magnesium deficiency causes tetany, muscular weakness, and seizures in the human. Acute deprivation of dietary magnesium in the growing rat leads to a rapidly developing deficiency disease characterized by vasodilation, neuromuscular abnormalities, and hyperkinesia. The usual and concomitant changes in serum calcium do not occur in the rat, however, and in this sense the model is unlike the human counterpart. Although there is little in the literature on immune function in magnesium deficiency, it has virtually all been done in the rat model.

Cichocki (58) reported on lymphocyte numbers, distribution, and mitogen responsiveness during magnesium deficiency in Wistar rats. Changes in thymus as well as peripheral lymphoid organs were observed. Degeneration of both epithelial and lymphoid elements of the thymus, disappearance of paracortical areas of lymph nodes, and stimulation of germinal centers were found. At the same time, there was peripheral blood lymphocytosis, attributed to the escape of lymphocytes from the nodes to the circulation. Significant lymphocytosis occurred from day 19 through day 26 of the deficient diet. When the counts returned to normal levels, animals were killed, submandibular lymph node cells were isolated, and the proliferative response to PHA was measured. Using ^{14}C-leucine incorporation as the measure of stimulation, Cichocki (58) observed no difference between Mg^{2+}-deficient and control groups. The significance of this is unclear, however, since the protocol employed a short incubation of only 8 hr, which may be insufficient to detect differences even in the mitogen-stimulated burst of protein synthesis that occurs in the first 24 hr of culture, inasmuch as the SI in the controls was only 1.2. This study was not well designed. Eighteen experimental and three control rats were used. Rats of different ages and probably with different degrees of Mg^{2+} deficiency were pooled for analysis; levels of magnesium in the diets were not measured; nor was the degree of deficiency assessed in the experimental animals. The author makes no mention of body weight due to the deficient diet, and pair-fed controls were not used to estimate the effect of concomitant inanition on the histologic changes observed.

Alcock and Shils (3) reported a 50% decrease in IgG levels in deficient Sprague-Dawley rats after 10 to 14 weeks of diet, compared to normal controls. The decrease in IgG correlated with the serum Mg^{2+} level; when Mg^{2+} was repleted in pair-fed controls, there was a rapid normalization of both serum Mg^{2+} and IgG levels. In fact, subcutaneous injection of Mg^{2+} resulted in an increase in IgG significantly above control within a week and completely restored the depressed serum protein level to normal. It should be noted, however, that no specific probe of antibody synthesis was employed in these experiments. McCoy and Kenney (179) examined both IgM and IgG levels and antibody response to SRBC in magnesium-deficient Wistar rats. Although body weight diminished, spleen weight as a precentage of body weight increased in the Mg^{2+}-deficient animals. The authors found little or no change in immunoglobulin levels, although there was a significant decrease in both agglutinin and hemolysin titers to SRBC 5 to 9 days after immunization.

Two papers report magnesium deficiency in mice produced with diets of reduced magnesium content (4 to 6 mg Mg^{2+} per 100 g diet, compared to 40 mg/100 g). Guenounou et al. (113) used *ad lib*, pair-fed, and deficient diet groups to compare the anti-SRBC response to immunization on day 15 and again on day 29 of the experiment. There were no changes in the pair-fed group; but in the deficient animals, the primary IgM PFC response was significantly reduced (335 ± 351), compared to *ad lib* controls (1,585 ± 161/10^6 spleen cells). The indirect IgG PFC response on day 33 was also diminished in the Mg^{2+}-deprived animals (35 ± 24 versus 308 ± 133; $p = 0.009$). Similarly, Elin (86) found a decrease in body weight in acutely deprived male Swiss albino mice and in the anti-SRBC response in spleen measured 4 days after immunization on either day 2 or day 8 of diet. With either protocol, there was a significant suppression of the PFC response in the deficient animals (254 ± 24 versus 816 ± 43 on day 6, or 106 ± 18 versus 1,071 ± 48 on day 12; $p = 0.001$ for both). Serum immunoglobulin levels were also measured on days 3, 6, 9, and 12 of diet. There was a consistent and significant decrease in IgG_2 and IgM and a less constant decrease in IgA, with little or no effect on IgG_1 in the deficient mice.

Each of these studies demonstrates some effect of magnesium deficiency on immunolgobulin or antibody levels. It is unclear, however, whether the effect is primarily on the B cell, indirect through a T cell or macrophage effect, or simply related to a metabolic effect on protein synthesis in general. We are not aware of any studies that examine cell-mediated immunity in magnesium deficiency states.

COPPER

Recent investigations of copper deficiency in mouse models clearly show effects on several distinct immunologic responses. In 1981, Prohaska and Lukasewycz (218) reported that antibody production in hypocupric C58 mice in response to immunization with SRBC measured by the PFC assay in splenic lymphocytes was variable from animal to animal but correlated directly with biochemical evidence of copper deficiency, assessed as serum ceruloplasmin enzymatic activity. Indeed, the antibody response was virtually absent in those animals with undetectable ceruloplasmin activity. The variability in the response to copper deprivation was attributed, in part, to differences in the individual growth pattern of the animals. Male mice in general showed greater evidence of mineral depletion in terms of weight loss, anemia, decreased liver copper, increased liver iron, and hypoceruloplasminemia.

In a subsequent study (presented at present only in abstract form), the ability to generate a cytotoxic T lymphocyte response *in vivo* to I_b syngeneic lymphocytic leukemia cells was found to be impaired in copper-deficient male mice (219). This was evidenced by the death of 20 of 22 deficient animals, compared to zero mortality in copper-sufficient control animals. Proliferative responses to *in vitro* Con A stimulation also were reduced by 90%, suggesting a defect in T cell function.

Further supportive evidence of a copper-induced T cell defect derives from *in vitro* models of copper deficiency (95). RPMI medium and fetal calf serum were depleted of divalent cations by chelation, and calcium, magnesium, and zinc were added back to create a specific copper-depleted system. Controls included untreated RPMI and medium supplemented with all trace elements, amino acids, sodium, and potassium. Mineral levels were determined by direct measurements. Lymphocyte survival was not affected in this medium; however, the ability to generate antibody, CTLs, or helper factors produced by Lyt 1^+ T cells was impaired. T cell replacement factors produced by normal helper T cells during an MLR between Balb/c and C57 BL/6 splenocytes permitted normal generation of immunologic effector cells when added to lymphocytes in copper-depleted medium. The effects of copper deficiency, therefore, appear to be at a peripheral rather than central level and are in contrast to the effects of PEM, in which the thymus and spleen are severely affected.

Copper deficiency in humans is rare, and only recently has it been conclusively demonstrated. One example is Menkes syndrome, a sex-linked genetic disease of copper absorption, with varied manifestations, including physical and mental retardation, hypothermia, skin depigmentation, peculiar white stubby hair, and frequent infections. Two patients with Menkes syndrome have been studied immunologically and reported in brief, with conflicting results on the functional integrity of the T lymphocyte system (210,256). Thus it is not possible to draw any conclusions on the immunologic effects of copper deficiency in humans. On the basis of the experimental work in animals, however, we can suggest that copper deficiency affects the ability of Lyt 1 + helper cells to interact with B lymphoctes in the antibody response to T-dependent antigens and to function in the generation of cytotoxic T cells, perhaps through impaired production of T cell factors, such as IL-2.

VITAMIN A

Animal Studies: Supplementation

Vitamin A and the retinoids are essential for the differentiation and function of secretory epithelial cells. When vitamin A is depleted in animals, there is a marked metaplasia of secretory epithelium in tissues such as prostate and pancreas, which become multilayered and keratinized. These effects can be reversed by supplementation with retinoids. Recent work has suggested that vitamin A might function to inhibit certain types of neoplastic cell growth, such as carcinoma of the skin (85). Reports, more anecdotal than scientific, have suggested a lower incidence of lung cancer in heavy smokers who have supplemental vitamin A in their diet over those smokers who do not (186). These types of suggestive observations have prompted many interesting studies on the effect of retinoids on immunologic defense mechanisms.

The best designed *in vitro* studies on the effects of added vitamin A on immune responsiveness were reported by Dennert and co-workers (74,75), who studied the role of retinoic acid (RA) on T cell function both *in vivo* and *in vitro*. C57BL/6 mice were treated daily for 6 days with various dose schedules of RA. On day 8, the mice were injected with allogeneic S 194 tumor cells at suboptimal doses. Seven days later, spleen cells from mice receiving only corn oil failed to show significant killing against ^{51}Cr-labeled tumor cells. However, animals receiving 25 or 100 μg RA/day were able to generate killer cells with marked lytic capability. There was no significant difference with increased amounts of RA or with injections given three times weekly for up to 3 months. Experiments also were performed on spleen cells obtained from RA-injected or corn oil-treated control mice which were stimulated with antigen *in vitro*. There was a significant increase in the ability to generate specific cytotoxic effectors *in vitro* in cells from RA-treated animals. Elimination of effectors using anti-Thy 1 sera plus complement proved that the killing was caused by T cells.

The ability of RA to influence recognition and killing of syngeneic tumor cells was also tested using Balb/c (H-2^d) mice and syngeneic S 194 tumor cells or C57BL/6 (H-2^b) and syngeneic EL-4 lymphoma targets. RA, in doses of 5 to 300 μg, was injected for 1 to 5 days, and spleen cells then were isolated and sensitized *in vitro* for 5 days. Both Balb/c anti-S 194 and C57BL/6 anti-EL-4 responses were significantly enhanced at doses of 10, 25, and 100 μg RA, and neither stimulated nor suppressed at doses of 5 and 300 μg per mouse. These experiments show that both strong (allogeneic) and weak (syngeneic) T cell killing can be stimulated with RA. The mechanism of action is unclear, but RA may act on helper cells to induce IL-2 production, on killer cell precursors to activate cytotoxic mechanism, or on suppressor T cells to eliminate down-regulation.

In vitro effects of RA, which were investigated by Dennert, demonstrate similar enhancement or suppression of CML activity, depending on the dose of RA injected as well as the number of stimulator cells present in the culture; 10^{-7} M RA and 10^4 stimulating cells were optimal for maximum killing in the culture conditions reported. Stimulating cells also were treated with RA; these results suggest that they were rendered more immunogenic than untreated control tumor cells (67 versus 51% killing). The adjuvant effect of RA depended on addition during the induction phase; RA had no effect when added during the CML assay itself.

C57BL/6 mice, pretreated with RA, were primed with an intravenous dose of SRBC. DTH responses, measured by footpad swelling following a challenge injection of 10^8 SRBC into the footpad 4 days after priming, were either not altered or suppressed by supplemental RA, depending on the dose; 500 μg/day for 7 days completely abrogated the DTH responses. Similar effects were seen on the MLR, with no effect at doses of 10^{-6} or 10^{-7} M RA but a 50% suppression at a concentration of 10^{-5} M. Since the DTH response is mediated by Lyt 1,2,3$^+$ cells and the MLR by Lyt 1$^+$ cells, the data suggest that RA may act specifically on Lyt 2,3$^+$ killer and/or suppressor T cells.

RA exerted no effect on Con A or PHA proliferative responses by murine spleen cells. There was a significant dose-dependent effect of RA on the LPS response, however, with 80% inhibition at concentrations of 10^{-6} M. This effect on B cell proliferation prompted experiments on the humoral limb of the immune response to SRBC. RA pretreatment *in vivo* did not affect PFC responses to SRBC, whereas pretreatment *in vitro* and subsequent *in vitro* immunization with SRBC dramatically suppressed the PFC response.

In a small number of animals, the effect of RA on T helper populations was assessed. TNP SRBC were used for immunization, and immune splenocytes from control or RA-treated animals were mixed *in vitro* with normal splenocytes and 10^6 SRBC. Carrier priming was assessed by a plaque assay against TNP burro erythrocytes 5 days later. Since the results were negative, there is no evidence for an action of RA on T help.

In earlier studies, Floersheim and Bollag (94) examined the adjuvant effects of vitamin A on cell-mediated immunity as measured by homograft rejection in mice. In this study, male C3H or CBA/H mice were given vitamin A derivatives orally rather than parenterally. Vitamin A therapy was begun 2 weeks prior to grafting or on day 1 or 10 after grafting skin from one strain to the other. Vitamin A treatment decreased the median survival time from 40–42 to 19–29 days, depending on the dose and schedule of administration. Vitamin A started on either day 1 or 10 after grafting was equally effective. The results were more pronounced in the weak rejection of CBA/H skin to C3H recipients, compared to the stronger reverse protocol, suggesting an adjuvant effect for vitamin A that is antigen specific. These studies also showed a decrease in graft survival in mice immunosuppressed with ALS, with mean survival time changing from 90 to 64 days and a toxic effect of high doses (200 mg/kg twice weekly) on both grafts and recipient animals.

Jurin and Tannock (138) assessed the effects of vitamin A on both the anti-SRBC hemagglutinating antibody response and rejection of male to female skin grafts in the C57BL/6 mouse model. The antibody response increased dramatically when 250 IU vitamin A was injected intraperitoneally for 5 days before or immediately after antigen administration. Ten days after sensitization, the titer was 1,024, compared to 64 in saline-injected controls. Injection of vitamin A beginning 5 days after sensitization had no effect on the anti-SRBC titer. C57BL/6 female mice were grafted with isogenic male skin in order to investigate the effects of vitamin A on rejection of weak antigens. Mean total rejection time was reduced to 23 to 24 days for the vitamin A-injected group as compared to 35.3 days in saline-injected controls. These experiments, however, lacked a control given the vehicle alone.

Cohen and Cohen (60) used vitamin A to reverse corticosteroid suppression of the anti-SRBC response in C57BL/6J mice. Pretreatment of animals with 1,000 to 30,000 IU vitamin A palmitate increased the anti-SRBC PFC response, whether or not the mice also received hydrocortisone. A single dose of 1 mg hydrocortisone acetate injected intraperitoneally 2 days prior to immunization with SRBC decreased the subsequent response from 21,983 to 725 PFCs. If, in addition, 5,000 IU vitamin A were given 1 day before and on the day of immunization, the PFC response increased to 3,563 PFCs. Administration of steroid at the same time as immunization with SRBC had a definite but less dramatic effect on PFC response (14,800). However, 2 days of vitamin A prior to SRBC immunization restored and slightly increased the response to 25,433 PFCs, whereas this dose of vitamin A without hydrocortisone clearly enhanced the PFC response still further to 33,938.

All these reports corroborate the classic studies of Dresser (80) in 1968, reporting that retinol could substitute for *B. pertussis* as an adjuvant in the immune response of CBA mice to soluble bovine gammaglobulin. In the absence of adjuvant, immune paralysis resulted, whereas a strong antibody response occurred when either *B. pertussis* vaccine in saline or retinol in liquid paraffin was injected 1 day prior to immunization. Dresser suggested that the retinol might alter the integrity of lysosomal membranes and stimulate cell division.

More recently, Rhodes and Oliver (225) presented evidence that trans-RA can alter functional aspects of the human monocyte membrane. Culture of peripheral blood monocytes results in spreading of the glass-adherent cells, normally accompanied by an increase in the number of FcRs, assessed as the percentage of rosette-forming cells using antibody-coated erythrocytes for detection. However, in the presence of RA in a concentration of 10^{-6} to 10^{-7} M, there is significant inhibition of this change in receptor number during a 24 hr culture of human monocytes. In contrast, 10^{-6} M arachidonic acid has no effect.

Animal Studies: Experimental Vitamin A Deficiency

Rats fed a vitamin A-deficient diet develop clinical manifestations of eye lesions and xerophthalmia, along with anorexia and suboptimal weight gain. Serum vitamin A levels reflect this deficiency, dropping to 1.9 μg/dl^{-1} in experimental groups compared to 33.8 μg/dl^{-1} in controls. Nauss et al. (198) studied vitamin A deficiency in Lewis rats, comparing deficient diet to vitamin A-supplemented deficient diet pair-fed controls. There were no significant differences in body weight or thymus, spleen, or liver weights per 100 g body weight due to vitamin A deficiency. Mitogen-proliferative responses were assessed in thymic and splenic lymphocyte populations. No effect on Con A responses of thymic cells was found. In contrast, the splenic lymphocyte response to PHA, Con A, or LPS was significantly suppressed in the deficient animals. Mitogen responsiveness was restored 3 days after repletion of experimental animals with 500 μg retinyl acetate.

Histologic observations by Krishnan et al. (147) are consistent with these observations. Although many experimental details are not presented, vitamin A deficiency produced in albino Holtzman rats resulted in a decrease in spleen and thymus weight per unit body weight that was significantly more profound than observed in pair-fed, vitamin A-supplemented animals. There was virtual ablation of the thymic cortex in the deficient rats, with relative sparing of the medullary regions. In the spleen, a decrease in the number of germinal centers and loss of cellularity of the germinal centers and mantle zone was found. When the splenic 1° PFC response to SRBC was assayed, however, there were no differences between vitamin A-deficient and pair-fed animals, although the response in both these groups was significantly depressed compared to *ad lib*-fed controls. When DPT was used for immunization, somewhat reduced titers to diphtheria and tetanus were found in the deficient compared to pair-fed rats.

In a study by Bang et al. (19), White Leghorn chicks were put on various vitamin A-deficient diets from the time of hatching. By 30 days, there was premature involution of the bursa of Fabricius, with irregular maturation of the follicles and interfollicular and medullary fibrosis. When normal and deficient chicks were challenged intranasally with NDV, there were striking alterations in the bursa of deficient birds. These included rapid attrition of lymphocytes, vascular atrophy, involution and progressive surface epithelial metaplasia, and marked keratinization. The epithelium was disorganized and pseudostratified, in contrast to the normal single row of regularly aligned secretory cells. There were no pair-fed controls in these experiments, however, and it is clear that the diets were deficient in nutrients other than vitamin A, since the changes observed were not reversed by simply replacing vitamin A. Nevertheless, the data suggest that vitamin A deficiency may have a direct effect on B cell maturation, in addition to any effects on humoral immunity via induced T cell defects.

Human Studies

Vitamin A deficiency is not an uncommon problem in the developing world; data on the effect of vitamin A on immune function, however, are exceedingly uncommon. We have found three publications worthy of comment. In 1958, Jayalakshmi and Gopalan (133), investigating the tuberculin response in malnourished children, found an association between vitamin A deficiency and negative skin tests. Because of concomitant PEM in these subjects, it is difficult to interpret the data. Bhaskaram and Reddy (32), therefore, studied nine Indian children, 2 to 10 years old, in whom PEM could be excluded by anthropometry (weight for age > 80% of standard). All had clinical and biochemical evidence of vitamin A deficiency, including conjunctival xerosis, Bitot spots, and low serum levels of vitamin A. The percentage of circulating T cells was decreased (47.0 versus 65.7% in controls; $p < 0.01$), and the proliferative response to PHA was reduced (SI = 13.1 versus 27.3), although the latter was not statistically significant because of the wide range of values obtained in patients and controls. Unfortunately, the methods used are not clearly described, other nutrient deficiencies or the presence of infection are not ruled out, and the controls are not age or sex matched, making it difficult to interpret the importance of vitamin A depletion in these subjects.

In a different type of study, Brown et al. (39) attempted to determine if vitamin A could play an adjuvant role in humans as defined in animal experiments. One hundred and four Bangladeshi village children, 1 to 6 years of age, with no history or antibody evidence of prior tetanus immunization were studied. Complete physical examination, nutritional assessment, anthropometry, hematocrit, serum protein, carotene, and vitamin A levels were done, and skin tests with PPD and *Candida* were performed. Skin tests were read 2 days later, and children were paired by age and sex. All study subjects received 0.3 ml unadjuvantized tetanus toxoid, and one of each pair was randomly selected to receive 200,000 IU water-miscible vitamin A palmitate. The tests were repeated 4 weeks later, and the antitoxin level was determined. There was no positive titer in any child, consistent with a primary immunization response to this antigen, and controls and vitamin A-supplemented children did not differ with respect to weight, serum protein, and hematocrit, or in the reactivity to the two skin test antigens. A second injection of tetanus toxoid was given and, 8 weeks later, the antibody response was again measured. At this time, the geometric mean titer was similar in the two groups (0.016 in the vitamin A-treated children and 0.011 in the controls). There were no significant correlations between antibody titer and age, weight for age, or serum vitamin A levels. To further validate the results, the same toxoid preparation was given to groups of mice that received varying doses of 3,000 to 30,000 IU vitamin A. There was a significant increase in antibody titer when 3,000 to 15,000 IU vitamin A were simultaneously administered with the vaccine, confirming previous experimental results. It is not clear whether the discrepancy in the murine and human data is related to the relatively high dose of vitamin A in the animal, since a comparable dose per kilogram weight in the human would likely cause toxicity, or if this is a species-related response.

B VITAMINS

Animal Studies

Some of the earliest studies in nutrition and immunologic responses involved the family of B vitamins. This complex group of essential nutrients affects multiple biochemical pathways in cellular function. Most of the experimental work has focused on pyridoxine, with limited studies of riboflavin, thiamine, pantothenic acid, folic acid, and vitamin B_{12}. The majority of the work has been performed in animal models, since it is difficult to produce mononutrient deficiency in human subjects.

Work began in the 1940s with a well-designed study on pyridoxine deficiency in rats by Stoerk and Eisen (253). In this experiment, both normal (*ad lib*-fed) controls and pair weighed controls were used to compare with the deficient group. Furthermore, control diets were identical to deficient diets, with the missing vitamin added back as a supplement. Both these features make this and many of the other early studies in vitamin B deficiency remarkable for the time, or, indeed, for the present. Given the level of understanding of immunity 30 to 40 years ago, the experimental questions were directed to determine whether or not antibody could be produced against antigens such as SRBC. Pyridoxine-deficient rats demonstrated a decrease in agglutinin and hemolysin titers as compared to pair weighed and *ad lib*-fed controls. In a subsequent comparative study of pyridoxine, thiamine, riboflavin, and pantothenic acid, only pyridoxine-deficient rats showed a significant depression of antibody titers against SRBC (254). Antibody activity was actually slightly enhanced in pair weighed inanition controls. It is interesting to note that in 1947, Stoerk reported decreased lymphocyte numbers in pyridoxine deficiency as well as such developmental changes as thymic cortical atrophy with replacement of lymphocytes by epithelial cells and stroma.

It was during this period that Axelrod and colleagues (15) began a series of experiments on the effects of B vitamins on antibody responses. Using human erythrocytes as the antigen, the authors confirmed the observation that pyridoxine-deficient rats had a striking and highly significant reduction in hemagglutination titers. In contrast to the prior work, however, they found that pantothenic acid or riboflavin deficiency resulted in a profound or modest depression in antibody responsiveness, respectively. The discrepancy may be attributable to differences in the strain of animal, the antigen used, and/or the immunization schedule. Several subsequent reports have confirmed the suppressive effects of both pantothenic acid and pyridoxine deficiency on the antibody response against T-dependent antigens (164–166).

Ludovici and Axelrod (163) compared a dietary deficiency of folate, niacin, and vitamins A, B_{12}, and D in rats in terms of the hemagglutinating antibody response to human erythrocytes. Only folate deficiency resulted in severe depression in antibody titers. It can be difficult to make animals deficient in some nutrients, however, and the effects of the diets were not assessed. Pruzansky and Axelrod

(220) repeated these experiments in rats, using alum-precipitated DPT as the antigenic probe. Folic acid deficiency again completely abrogated both the 1° and 2° responses. In addition, pantothenic acid, pyridoxine, riboflavin, biotin, vitamin D, and vitamin A all depressed diphtheria antitoxin production to a greater or lesser extent.

Gershoff et al. (104) produced dietary pyridoxine deficiency in Charles River rats and found a modest decrease in antibody response to either SRBC or the synthetic antigen poly Glu^{52} Lys^{33} Tyr^{15} (GLT). Virtually complete suppression was obtained with addition of the antivitamin deoxypyridoxine to the diet (5 to 10 mg/kg diet). Partial restoration of the antibody response in the deoxypyridoxine-treated rats was obtained by supplementing the diet with 2.1% L-serine in the case of SRBC and with 3% glycine for GLT. While this can be explained by an effect of the antivitamin on glycine and serine availability, the significant decrease in antibody production in the face of amino acid supplementation is evidence of the requirement for pyridoxine per se. Axelrod et al. (14) extended the studies on pyridoxine deficiency to the guinea pig; using DPT for immunization, they demonstrated a decrease not only in the antibody response but in the Arthus type reaction to intradermal toxoid as well. Harmon et al. (116) used swine to demonstrate the depressive effect of pyridoxine deficiency on antibody titers to either human erythrocytes or *S. pullorum* and restoration of the immune response with dietary repletion of the vitamin.

Lederer, Kumar, and Axelrod (149,156) later used the Jerne plaque assay to evaluate the splenic PFC response to SRBC in pyridoxine, pantothenic acid, riboflavin, thiamine, folic acid, and biotin deficiency in Holtzman rats. Pyridoxine deficiency reduced the 1° PFC response from $232/10^6$ splenic cells to $4/10^6$ splenocytes (149). Vitamin B_6 repletion, beginning 3 days before immunization and continuing until the antibody response was measured, completely restored the PFC response, despite the severe reduction in body weight. In contrast, there was a relative increase in PFC to $1,012/10^6$ splenocytes in the pair-fed (inanition) controls. Antigenic delivery, assessed as the accumulation of ^{51}Cr-tagged SRBC in spleen over 96 hr, was not affected by pyridoxine deficiency, even though spleen weights were reduced by about 60%. The kinetics of the PFC response over a 7 day period was similar in the control and deficient animals, and increasing the antigen load by 200-fold also was without effect. These data are consistent with a restricted proliferative response, since pyridoxine is required for nucleic acid synthesis in 1 carbon transfers from serine.

Results in pantothenic acid deficiency were essentially identical to those for pyridoxine, except for a slight decrease in labeled SRBC uptake in spleen in the first 5.5 hr after injection in pantothenic acid-deficient animals (156). The studies with the other vitamins are not as well designed, involve different time periods of diet, and do not clarify a number of methodologic questions, such as the dose used for the rehabilitation studies (151). All the deficiencies reduced the PFC response, least so in the case of thiamine, and, except for biotin and folic acid, were corrected with 7 days of repletion. In a different study, Koros et al. (144) showed that pyridoxine, pantothenic acid, or riboflavin deficiency increased the background PFC response to sheep, human, or rat erythrocytes by three- to fourfold in unimmunized rats, suggesting a possible alteration in regulatory influences or a shift in cellular populations within the spleen.

Axelrod, Trakatellis, and co-workers (16,262) examined the effect of pyridoxine deficiency on cell-mediated immune responses in BCG-immunized guinea pigs. Animals were loaded with 1 mg i.p. vitamin daily for 4 days before initiating the diet and administering BCG. The PPD responsiveness, measured at 6 weeks, was markedly reduced in the deficient compared to control animals receiving either the vitamin-supplemented purified diet or lab chow. Within 1 week of rehabilitation with the complete (vitamin-sufficient) diet, the PPD response was normal. When deoxypyridoxine was later administered to these same PPD-responsive animals, the DTH reaction was sharply curtailed within 1 week of treatment. These data indicate that acute or chronic pyridoxine deficiency can impair the expression of skin sensitivity. That this is not a nonspecific effect on skin reactivity was shown by the normal response elicited by histamine in the deoxypyridoxine-treated animals and the minimal blunting of the histamine reaction after 48 days of continuous deficient diet.

Passive transfer of sensitized peritoneal cells from control or pyridoxine-deficient animals successfully transferred PPD sensitivity to unimmunized normal diet recipients. Equivalent reactivity of normal or deficient splenocytes to PPD *in vitro* also could be shown, employing an assay for the lymphokine MIF. Since sufficient pyridoxine was probably available in the *in vitro* as well as *in vivo* studies, these experiments suggest that the effect of the vitamin deficiency is localized to the effector limb of the DTH response. Antigen recognition by sensitized lymphocytes and/or the ability of these cells to respond and to recruit other mononuclear cells by proliferation and production of lymphokines may be impaired. Interestingly, there appears to be some specificity to the altered responses of the deficient animal. Since the BCG vaccine contained BSA, anaphylactic responses to intraperitoneal PPD or intravenous BSA were determined on day 82 of the experiment. Anaphylactic death due to PPD correlated with skin reactivity to this antigen, and both were suppressed in the pyridoxine-deficient animals. In contrast, all immunized animals, regardless of pyridoxine nutrient status, succumbed to intravenous albumin. The systemic response to PPD was restored after transfer to a complete diet and was normal in inanition controls or scorbutic guinea pigs used as a nutrient specificity control.

Akpom and Warren (2) employed a different system, the lung granuloma model of *Schistosoma mansoni* in female Swiss white mice, to evaluate the effects of thiamine, riboflavin, pantothenic acid, or pyridoxine deficiency on DTH responses. Intravenous injection of *S. mansoni* eggs into microvasculature of the lungs results in the formation of an immunologically specific granuloma around the egg. Neither pantothenic acid- nor riboflavin-deficient diets affected the granulomatous reaction. A significant decrease in granuloma volume was observed in mice fed the thiamine-deficient diet; however, there was severe anorexia and weight loss in these mice.

While the pyridoxine-deficient diet alone was without effect, addition of deoxy-pyridoxine in doses as low as 0.005 mg/mouse/day, which did not affect body weight, sharply reduced granuloma size.

Homograft and autograft rejection in pyridoxine-deficient Wistar or Long-Evans rats were assessed by Axelrod et al. (17). Graft survival was improved when donor skin was obtained from or grafted to deficient animals. The results were even more striking in animals maintained in normal pyridoxine status until immediately after skin transfer.

Axelrod and Trakatellis (13) also found that tolerance to skin grafts could be induced by administering donor splenocytes to pyridoxine-deficient mice if the deficiency was present at the time of cell transfer. C3H/HeJ skin was grafted to CBA/J recipients that had previously received C3H/HeJ, A/HeJ, or no spleen cells. All animals had been receiving complete diet for 10 days when the skin graft was performed. Prolonged survival of the graft was observed in recipients given syn-geneic donor spleen cells in the presence of pyridoxine deficiency but not when allogeneic splenocytes were used. When male to female skin isografts in C57B1/6J mice were studied in an identical protocol, tolerance was observed much more readily when mice were vitamin deficient at the time of spleen cell transfer, requiring only a fraction of the cells needed for induction of immune tolerance in nondeficient recipients (261).

This result was not confirmed by Fisher and Schewe (93), who studied skin grafts from Sprague-Dawley to Long-Evans recipients. The only protocol that suc-cessfully prolonged graft survival was to perform the skin graft within 3 to 5 days of detecting the first signs of pyridoxine deficiency. Prior transfer of splenocytes to normal or deficient recipients had no effect on survival of skin grafts performed at a later time. A second graft from the same donor to recipient was performed in 27 rats with prolonged (42 to 63 days) survival of the first graft. Eighty one percent of the second set were rejected by 2 weeks, and in only 1 of 27 animals did the graft persist for 6 months. In contrast, 56% of the first grafts remained intact during that period of time. Lymph node cells from normal recipients rejecting grafts from the same donors supplying skin to tolerant recipients adversely altered graft viability in 8 of 13 animals so treated, with some suggestion of a dose response curve.

Surviving grafts in the pyridoxine-manipulated recipients were successfully trans-ferred back to the original Sprague-Dawley donors but promptly rejected when they were placed on Long-Evans recipients 4 months later. Grafts transferred back to Sprague-Dawley rats other than the original donor did not take. Thus it is not likely that the antigenicity of the grafted skin was changed in the environment of the recipient animal.

The generalized depression of these various cell-mediated immune responses by B group vitamin deficiencies, and especially pyridoxine, suggests an effect on T lymphocytes, including Lyt 1,2,3$^+$ DTH-responding cells and Lyt 2,3$^+$ killer cells. This could be at the level of the Lyt 1,2,3$^+$ precursor cell or perhaps earlier within a pyridoxine-requiring population of pre-T cells. This would be consistent with the suppression of B cell responses to T-dependent antigens such as SRBC. To the extent that the various B vitamins have similar effects on cell-mediated or antibody-dependent immune reactions, it is reasonable to look for a common mechanistic pathway for their actions. This is not easy, however, given the diverse physiologic roles of these various factors. For example, thiamine is a coenzyme for oxidative decarboxylation of pyruvate or α-ketoglutarate in energy metabolism; riboflavin in the form of FAD is a critical constituent of a number of intermediary metabolism reactions involving hydrogen transfer; pyridoxine is essential for amino acid metabolism in decarboxylation, deamination, transamination, transulfuration, desulfuration, and transfer of amino acids into cells; pantothenic acid is a constituent of coenzyme A and therefore required for the activation of acetate for 2 carbon transfer reactions in intermediary metabolism, for activation of succinate to succinyl-Co A in heme synthesis, and for the oxidation and biosynthesis of fatty acids; and folic acid serves in 1 carbon transfer reactions in nucleic acid synthesis. It is possible, however, that the distinct metabolic effects of these vitamins could, in common, limit the proliferative responses essential to either T or B cell-mediated immune reactions. It is ironic that proliferative responses to T or B cell mitogens were not determined in these studies; in the case of the B vitamins, such nonspecific stimuli could provide meaningful insights.

Several recent studies on pyridoxine deficiency serve to clarify some of the mechanisms of immunodepression involved. Davis (71) induced pyridoxine deficiency in pregnant Sprague-Dawley rats and determined the effects on the fetus. The protocol utilized a B_6-deficient diet, deoxypyridoxine in the drinking water, with pyridoxine supplements provided to the controls. In addition to an alarming incidence of fetal congenital anomalies in the deficient offspring, there was significant splenic hypoplasia and a slight decrease in thymic weight in these animals. Congenitally pyridoxine-deficient nonrunted Sprague-Dawley or Lewis rats did not convert the tuberculin test following immunization with BCG or *M. tuberculosis* in complete Freund's adjuvant, respectively, although there was no difference in the response of another group of similarly treated animals to $1°$ or $2°$ immunization with SRBC as compared to controls (72). Robson and Schwarz (226,227) were unable to confirm the splenic atrophy in the progeny of vitamin B_6-deficient dams but did find a 48% decrease in the MLR of Lewis strain thoracic duct lymphocytes (TDL) to Lewis X Brown Norway f_1 hybrid stimulator cells and a significantly depressed GVH reaction in skin. Similar observations were made in dietary pyridoxine deficiency in weanling rats.

Willis-Carr and St. Pierre (275) evaluated the ability of thymic epithelium (TE) from pyridoxine-deficient or normal Lewis rats to induce functional differentiation of T cell precursors *in vitro*. This was assessed by means of a one-way MLR to mitomycin-treated Wistar splenocytes and proliferative responses to PHA and Con A. TE monolayers were prepared from control, pyridoxine-deficient, and deficient/pyridoxine-repleted animals. Spleen, bone marrow, and mesenteric lymph node cells were obtained from control, deficient, and neonatally thymectomized rats. Normal TE or TE from vitamin B_6-repleted deficient animals was capable of significantly improving responses of all donor lymphocyte populations from thymectomized animals in the MLR and mitogen stimulation assays, whereas TE from pyridoxine-deficient animals failed to induce functional responses in these same cell populations. *In vitro* responses of spleen or lymph node cells from pyridoxine-deficient animals were similar to these results, except that the bone marrow cells from the deficient animals gave MLR and mitogen responses equivalent to normal cells, with or without TE induction. The main flaw in these studies is the failure to include pair-fed controls for the pyridoxine-deficient TE induction studies. Histologic examination of thymus from the deficient animals showed a severe depletion of lymphocytes and loss of corticomedullary differentiation, all of which was reversed by pyridoxine repletion. No defects in TE were discernible in the deficient group at the light or electron microscope level. The defect in cell-mediated immunity in pyridoxine, therefore, is in part localizable to the TE cell in its role in T cell differentiation and not at the level of the T cell precursor, since normal *in vitro* differentiation of pyridoxine-deficient precursors occurred during coculture with normal TE.

Chandra et al. (57) measured serum thymic hormone activity by the Bach and Dardenne method in pyridoxine-deficient and pair-fed control Sprague-Dawley rats. Depletion of thymic and splenic lymphocyte populations, depression of PHA responsiveness, an increase in the background, and a decrease in the direct PFC response to SRBC were documented in these animals. Serum thymic hormone activity was reduced in both pair fed and deficient animals compared to *ad lib*-fed normals but much more depressed in the B_6-deficient animals. Unfortunately, the controls were fed a lab chow diet different in composition from the deficient diet; with the exception of the thymic hormone assay, *ad lib* diet controls were not used. The latter is important in order to be certain that the responses of the deficient group are suppressed rather than a situation in which the responses of the pair-fed group are enhanced. At any rate, the data are consistent with a defect in TE function, expressed as a decrease in circulating thymic factors.

Human Studies

Hodges et al. (124) produced experimental combined pyridoxine and pantothenic acid deficiency in a small number of human volunteers by means of a deficient diet formulation and administration of deoxypyridoxine and omega-methyl-pantothenic acid. Without the addition of the antagonists, diet alone caused no effect on antibody response to tetanus toxoid or typhoid vaccine. Diet plus antivitamin resulted in a complete lack of antibody to tetanus or typhoid O antigen, a reduced antityphoid H titer, and a good response to polio vaccine. Nutritional rehabilitation restored the tetanus and typhoid antibody responses in these subjects.

By the same methods, pyridoxine or pantothenic acid deficiency alone was induced in six subjects each (122,123). With only two individuals per group and the variability in the antibody responses to the vaccine probes, it is impossible to draw conclusions, but there is a suggestive reduction in the antitetanus titers in the deficient subjects. These studies are mentioned primarily because they are unlikely to be repeated, and no other human data are available.

Effects of both vitamin B_{12} and folate deficiency have been examined in a small number of patients with pernicious anemia receiving maintenance vitamin B_{12} therapy or folate deficiency megaloblastic anemia due to dietary deprivation or pregnancy (169). There were no alterations in the percentage of T or B cells in circulation in the pernicious anemia patients and no change in morphologic assessment of blast transformation to PHA. However, ^{3}H-Tdr incorporation, assessed by either autoradiography or scintillation counting, was significantly depressed in these patients, even though they were receiving adequate vitamin B_{12} supplementation.

Gross et al. (112) also found significantly depressed PHA-stimulated ^{3}H-Tdr incorporation in patients with clinical folate deficiency. This defect correlated well with a failure to induce sensitization to DNCB. With therapy, however, DNCB responsiveness returned in 10 of 13 patients within 6 to 23 days, and the mitogen response improved to well above normal in 7 to 14 days, returning to normal by day 24 of treatment. Because of the essential role of folate and vitamin B_{12} in nucleic acid metabolism, it is not surprising that abnormal proliferative responses occur in deficiency states. The limited studies available at this time do not permit further assessment of any specific defects that these deficiencies may also cause.

ASCORBIC ACID

Animal Studies

Vitamin C has become a popular entity in any discussion on host resistance and immunity. Studies on vitamin C deficiencies have been done primarily in the guinea pig model because, like primates and humans, they cannot convert L-gulonolactone to L-ascorbic acid, whereas other species biosynthesize their requirements. On a deficient diet, however, guinea pigs become severely vitamin C deficient within a 14 day period. This is accounted for by the rapid half-life of ascorbate (4 days) in this species. Ascorbic-deficient diets also result in diminished food intake, however, and the animals dramatically lose body weight, far in excess of the weight loss of pair-fed animals. The degree of inanition due to continuing anabolic events in the scorbutic animal is a major problem in such investigations and in the interpretation of the specificity of the immunologic changes observed. Hartley strain guinea pigs also have a particularly high requirement for folic acid, and care must be exercised to be certain that sufficient folate is administered.

There have been many studies to ascertain the effects of ascorbic acid deficiency on T and B lymphocytes. For example, Fraser et al. (101) used vitamin C-free diets in the guinea pig model, with daily parenteral supplementation of 25 mg sodium ascorbate for the controls, including pair-fed animals. All animals were placed on the ascorbic-free diet with parenteral supplementation for 10 days, at which time BSA in complete Freund's adjuvant was injected. At this time, pair feeding was initiated and groups were given either 25 or 250 mg ascorbate daily. Fourteen days later, a booster dose of BSA in saline was administered. The ascorbate-free diet resulted in marked depletion of tissue vitamin C. For example, spleen levels were

0.3 ± 0.0 versus 32.2 ± 9.6 in controls, while comparable adrenal levels were 1.0 ± 0.5 versus 68.0 ± 10.4. Although there were no changes in total peripheral blood leukocyte counts, there was a significant decrease in T cell numbers using the E-rosette assay in the scorbutic animal from 50.0 to 34.8%. There was a concomitant increase in the percentage of B cells (surface IgG positive) from 43.0 to 62.6%. In the supplemented animals, T cells increased and B cells decreased over the 28 days of observation. There was little difference between modest (25 mg) or megadose (250 mg) sodium ascorbate supplements. In animals receiving the high or low sodium ascorbate treatment, the percentage of T lymphocytes increased from 47.6 to 62.0% and from 48.9 to 57.8%, respectively. However, only three to five animals per group were examined at 0, 14, and 28 days.

Frazer et al. (101) also analyzed peripheral blood lymphocyte responses to T and B cell mitogens in these same animals. However, baseline (no mitogen) proliferative responses were increased following the initial immunization with BSA in complete Freund's adjuvant, especially in the megadose supplemented group. Therefore, it is appropriate to analyze only the difference in stimulated-unstimulated ^{3}H-TdR incorporation between groups. There was little difference in PHA or Con A responses after 14 days; at 28 days, however, the deficient animals showed an impaired Con A response, while the high ascorbate supplemented animals had an increased response to PHA. Unfortunately, only one dose of each mitogen was employed, the standard error of the mean was broad, and there were only three to five animals per group. The response to LPS was generally suppressed compared to baseline proliferation. This was least so in the scorbutic animals. At 28 days, this group had a mean ^{3}H-TdR incorporation of $+23,322$ cpm compared to $-7,925$ and $-13,800$ cpm in the low and high supplemented animals, respectively.

Anthony et al. (6) used a different protocol for supplementing ascorbic acid. Control animals received 4 g/kg ascorbic acid in their diets instead of parenteral sodium ascorbate. In these studies, the percentage of E-rosetting peripheral blood cells was similar in all the groups tested at 2 and 4 weeks of diet (for example, after 4 weeks, $37 \pm 3\%$ in controls, $33 \pm 5\%$ in pair-fed groups, and $32 \pm 4\%$ in ascorbic acid-deficient animals). Agglutinating antibody responses to intradermal injection of chicken erythrocytes in Freund's complete adjuvant was no different between experimental and control groups, although the range of titers was somewhat lower in the former. The authors then examined the ability of T cells derived from the spleens of control and experimental guinea pigs to generate CTLs. Cytotoxicity was assayed on target cells at 10:1 and 50:1 effector/target cell ratios. In these studies, there was no significant change in the percentage of E-rosette-forming spleen cells in the ascorbic acid-deficient guinea pigs as compared to both control and pair-fed mice. Even in the presence of normal numbers of E-rosette-forming cells from immunized animals, however, there was a significant decrease in cytotoxicity at low (10:1) target/effector ratio in scorbutic animals ($13 \pm 3\%$ compared to $32 \pm 4\%$ and $27 \pm 3\%$ in the pair-fed and control immunized groups, respectively). At a 50:1 target/effector ratio, there was a 50% reduction in the activity in the deficient animals, while in the pair-fed group consuming less diet, and therefore less ascorbic acid, a 25% decrease was observed.

Kumar and Axelrod (150) examined the ability of guinea pigs to make an antibody response after immunization with alum-precipitated DPT given 1 week after initiation of the diet. These studies also used groups of control *ad lib*-fed, control pair-fed, and ascorbic acid-deficient animals. There was no discernible difference between serum antibody titers 3 weeks after primary immunization in the various groups tested. Skin responses to formol DPT (Arthus type hypersensitivity) were reduced; however, there was also a reduction in the response to a histamine control injection.

Studies by Mueller et al. (193) explored the effect of vitamin C deprivation in the guinea pig model of experimental allergic encephalomyelitis (EAE), which has been shown to be a T cell-mediated disease. The experimental group was put on a vitamin C-deficient diet and daily intraperitoneal saline injections, while control groups were given 50 μg ascorbic acid in saline. There were no pair-fed controls. One week after the initiation of ascorbic acid-deficient diets, the animals were injected with 4 mg bovine spinal cord and *M. butyricum* complete adjuvant. Severity of disease was then assessed by neurologic symptomatology and histologic changes, such as the inflammatory (mononuclear) response. Eight of 12 controls showed limb paralysis characteristic of EAE; in 11 of the 12, mononuclear infiltrates were present on histologic examination. In contrast, guinea pigs on the scorbutic diet failed to develop clinical changes, and only 1 of 11 exhibited histologic changes. Since EAE-induced damage is attributable to cytotoxic T lymphocytes, these studies demonstrate an impairment of cytotoxic T cell function *in vivo* in ascorbic acid deficiency, which correlates well with the demonstrated depression of T cell killing *in vitro*. The specificity of the effect on the cytotoxic and not the helper T cell is suggested by the observed normal antibody responses against T-dependent antigens. Plasma 17-hydroxycorticosteroid levels were elevated three- to fourfold in scorbutic or calorie-deprived controls. Although the scorbutics were protected from EAE and could not be sensitized to tuberculin, the calorie-deprived animals, which had even higher steroid levels, were susceptible to EAE and were easily sensitized.

Zweiman et al. (279) further analyzed the ability of ascorbic acid-deficient guinea pigs to mount a DTH response against tuberculin. After 1 week on ascorbic acid-deficient diets, experimental and control animals were given injections of complete Freund's adjuvant containing 1.0 mg/ml heat-killed *M. tuberculosis* in the footpads and multiple subcutaneous sites on the back. They were challenged with PPD 14 days later, and skin reactivity was observed 24 hr later. The mean reaction size to first strength PPD in scorbutic animals was 0.3 mm, compared to 9.0 mm in the normal diet animals. There was an absence of the normal heavy infiltration of mononuclear cells at the reaction site in the deficient guinea pigs as compared to the response observed in guinea pigs supplemented with vitamin C. The defect in the delayed type response to PPD is interesting, because it is also mediated by a class of helper T lymphocytes. The discrepancy in the help function in antibody versus DTH may reflect an inability of proper production of lymphokines and recruitment of other mononuclear cells into the site of induration. Despite the negative skin response, transfer of lymph node and/or peritoneal cells from sensitized scorbutic animals to normal unsensitized recipients transferred responsiveness to PPD. The reverse experiment was unsuccessful and is consistent with the explanation offered above. Both the yield of peritoneal cells in response to intraperitoneal Bayol oil and the nonspecific skin inflammatory response to intradermal 1% benzyl alcohol were depressed in the ascorbic-deficient animals.

Dieter (79) examined the effects of ascorbic acid deficiency on the production and activity of thymic humoral factors. Extracts of thymus or spleen were prepared from guinea pigs which were ascorbic acid deficient or supplemented. Extracts were injected into 300 rads irradiated Sprague-Dawley rats, and the effect on the increase in organ weight and the ability to induce lymphopoiesis and organ regeneration in irradiated rats were determined. Only the thymic extracts from control guinea pigs had a significant positive effect, most marked on the regenerated thymus.

Studies by Siegel and Morton (243) in the Balb/c mouse (which cannot be used as a model of vitamin C deficiency) examined the effect of ascorbic acid supplementation in drinking water (250 mg/100 ml) on the antibody response to SRBC, a T-dependent antigen, as well as the proliferative response to lipopolysaccharide, a T-independent antigen. There was no effect on the *in vivo* response of Balb/c mice to immunization with either antigen, although *in vitro* Con A stimulation of spleen cells was increased after ascorbic acid supplementation. Although there was a dramatic increase in background proliferation in vitamin C-supplemented animals as compared to control groups, there was a significant increase in the stimulated-unstimulated ^{3}H-TdR incorporation in the vitamin C-supplemented animals. The treatment did not alter the splenic stem cell population, however, since no differences were observed between supplemented and control animals in the generation of CFUs in the spleen following 400 to 600 rads.

Balb/c mice were given ascorbic acid in drinking water over a period of 3 months and challenged with Raucher leukemia virus (241). Siegel (241) also determined the circulating immune interferon response and found a 62 to 145% increase in *in vivo* circulating interferon levels in ascorbate-supplemented mice, depending on the dose of challenge virus. Further studies were performed *in vitro* using mouse L-cell monolayers challenged with VSV virus or poly I/poly C (242). Again there was an increase in the ability of these cells to make interferon in the presence of vitamin C. Dahl and Degré (69) determined the effects of vitamin C on human embryonic lung fibroblasts or human embryonic skin cells stimulated with NDV or poly I/poly C. There was a small reproducible increase in interferon titers assayed as VSV protection in human embryonic lung cell monolayers. In addition, activity of a standard leukocyte interferon was enhanced by 0.2 to 0.4 $\log_{10}$ units in the presence of 5 to 100 μg/ml ascorbic acid.

VITAMIN E AND SELENIUM

Vitamin E functions as an intracellular antioxidant and stabilizes polyunsaturated fatty acids as well as the intermediate metabolites involved in the biosynthesis of lipids. Some of the most recent work on nutrition and immune responsiveness concerns the role of vitamin E and selenium. The role of vitamin E as an antioxidant is the basis for investigating its effects on biologic regulatory mechanisms and is the reason for the association of selenium in such studies, since the latter appears to be important in the glutathione peroxidase system. In addition, vitamin E has been shown to be important in the maintenance of the stability of biologic membranes.

Initially, studies on vitamin E were done in chickens and examined the effects of high dose supplementation on the humoral limb of the immune response. Tengerdy (259) reported that chickens given five times the usual dietary intake of vitamin E significantly increased the generation of anti-SRBC PFCs. In subsequent studies, supplementation with 60 to 180 mg/kg diets in mice significantly increased the humoral immune response, as measured by increased PFC responses to SRBC and increased antibody to tetanus toxoid (260). When CDF 1 mice were placed on a vitamin E-deficient diet for 30 days, there was a decrease from $1,225$ PFCs/10^6 cells in control groups to $419/10^6$ cells in the deficient animals. The antioxidant N,N-diphenyl-p-phenylenediamine (DPPD) was unable to significantly replete the PFC response, whereas vitamin E supplementation increased the PFCs by nearly 10-fold. There was a greater response to the vitamin of direct (IgM) compared to indirect (IgG) PFCs.

Experiments by Campbell et al. (44) examined *in vitro* effects of vitamin E on antibody responses to SRBC. In these studies, *in vitro* addition of α-tocopherol or its acetate form at the initiation of the Mishell Dutton cultures enhanced the anti-SRBC PFC response compared to control cultures. In a separate series of experiments, spleen cells were depleted of adherent cells by passage over a polystyrene column. The effluent cells were considered macrophage depleted since subsequent stimulation with SRBC *in vitro* produced low numbers of responding cells. When tocopherol or 2-ME were added to the adherent cell-depleted cultures, normal antibody responsiveness was restored, suggesting that vitamin E was either acting directly on helper T cells in a manner similar to 2-ME or was stimulating the release of lymphocyte-activating factors (LAF) from remaining adherent cells. It is known that even multiple passages over Sephadex G 10 columns will not completely remove the splenic adherent cell population.

Corwin and Shloss (65,66) have examined the mitogenic effects of tocopherol on murine lymphocytes. Vitamin E and 2-ME both were found to have mitogenic properties. While the addition of vitamin E had no effect on lymphocyte proliferation in the presence of optimal concentrations of Con A, dietary supplementation with 5 mg/kg diet increased responses 2.5-fold, and 50 mg/kg increased the response eightfold. These studies also suggest that vitamin E induces a shift in the relative response of spleen and lymph node cells to PHA and Con A, which might be due to the release of factors affecting maturation of T cells. Vitamin E has also been shown to affect antibody synthesis in the absence of T lymphocyte help. The authors found that vitamin E stimulates the response to DNP-ficoll, a type II T-independent antigen. Since anti-DNP-ficoll is a macrophage-dependent response, the effect of vitamin E could be at the level of stimulating factors from the adherent cell population which nonspecifically trigger lymphocyte responses. This argument is supported by the observation that the response to the macrophage-independent type I antigen TNP LPS is not affected by vitamin E. Although vitamin E may act via a macrophage effect, it appears to be a mitogen for B cells as well as T cells, since it is able to induce proliferation of sIg-positive cells.

Corwin and co-workers (64,67) selected T cell subpopulations to ascertain the nature of the cell affected by vitamin E. They showed that vitamin E enhances the proliferation of more mature T cells which are resistant to hydrocortisone and respond to PHA. Vitamin E appears to specifically affect the Ia-negative, PHA-responsive population, since treatment of spleen cells with anti-Ia plus complement enriches for the responsive cell, which is, in addition, responsive to suboptimal but not optimal doses of Con A and is hydrocortisone resistant. Although vitamin E may affect the immune response at many different levels, for example, via helper T cells, B cells, or macrophages, the studies to date most strongly point to an action on the macrophage membrane to induce the release of regulatory molecules, such as IL-1, which would trigger T cell help, or other molecules which might directly affect B cell responses.

Because of its association with vitamin E in the glutathione peroxidase system, selenium is also being studied for possible immunoadjuvant effects. There have been few well-controlled studies in this area, however. In a series of studies, Spallholz et al. (250,251) found that addition of sodium selenate to the diet at 2.8 ppm increased the antibody responses to SRBC. The suggestion that this is a significant increase does not seem to be supported by statistical evaluation. The paucity of studies at present does not permit a conclusion as to the site of action, if any. The data do suggest, however, that the IgM to IgG switch may be affected, since there was little enhancement of IgG plaques.

SUMMARY AND CONCLUSIONS

The influences of various nutritional factors involved in biologic regulatory mechanisms are complex, exerting their effects at multiple levels. We have attempted to analyze the role of specific nutrients on the distinctive subpopulations of interacting cell types in the immunologic network. This has been a difficult undertaking because so many biologic pathways are potentially affected by nutritional factors that it is not always clear whether the observed effects on the immunologic system are primary or secondary in nature. It is certain, however, that nutritional status plays a critical role in immunologic defense mechanisms at a number of important levels.

First, nutrition profoundly affects multiple organ systems during the differentiation and maturation of many cell types. For example, in both PEM and vitamin B_6 deficiency, there is a central effect on the thymus microenvironment, which in turn inhibits the ability of this organ to properly maintain the development of differentiating lymphocytes. This event has secondary repercussions on the peripheral lymphoid component over time because no lymphocyte renewal can take place.

Second, nutritional status can also affect mature peripheral lymphoid cells, either via cell membrane changes or by altering the production or release of regulatory molecules which control certain immune functions and cellular interactions. The effects of vitamin E and selenium on the integrity of membrane lipids or the effects of iron and iron-binding proteins on surface receptors of lymphocyte subpopulations are examples of the former. The apparent influence of copper on the production or release of IL-2 by T helper cells is an example of the latter.

Third, nutritional status may induce changes in antigen processing of bacteria or viruses by macrophage-like cells. This could result in the subsequent suppression of the immunologic system by bacteremia or viremia. In addition, direct effects on tissues by retinoids, which might induce neoplastic growth, could cause a secondary suppression of the immune system.

The nutritional factors discussed in this review exert an influence on immune function by varied mechanisms but at apparently specific loci. For example, PEM acts in this way to affect multiple areas of immune function both centrally and in the periphery. In many of these situations, more conclusive results can now be obtained by use of monoclonal antibodies directed against individual subpopulations of lymphocytes. Future studies in PEM will also need to rule out the influence of individual minerals or vitamins through mechanisms associated with but not directly due to PEM.

Until this is accomplished, any conclusions remain speculative. On the basis of current evidence, we suggest that the vitamins exert their influences at either central (e.g., pyridoxine and thymus epithelium) or peripheral (vitamin A and cytotoxic T cells) limbs of the network. Minerals, such as zinc, iron, magnesium, or copper, appear to affect different peripheral lymphocyte subpopulations (e.g., effects of copper on T cell help, magnesium on B cell production of antibody, or iron on peripheral T cell functions) or have central effects on development and function of T lymphocytes (e.g., zinc effects on thymus epithelium and/or factors). These studies on nutritional status and immune functions are far from complete, and much more work needs to be done. It is evident, however, that this is an exciting area of research, encompassing many disciplines. We have attempted to summarize and illustrate the specificity of nutritional influences on the immune system in Fig. 4. Future work to elaborate on and refine this scheme will also accomplish the goals set by our colleagues from the nutritional sciences, succinctly expressed by Whitehead et al. (274): "A state of malnutrition must be characterized in terms of malfunction; malnutrition is not just a synonym for dietary deprivation."

In closing, it is interesting to note that the specificity of some of the described effects of nutrients on the immune system may be useful in the therapeutic intervention in autoimmune diseases or in the enhancement of immune responsiveness in malignant diseases. One model for such an approach is described in the studies by Mueller et al. (193) on vitamin C deficiency and experimental autoimmune encephalomyelitis, which revealed an inhibition in the ability to induce neurologic damage by an effect of the deficiency state on the cytotoxic T cell responsible for

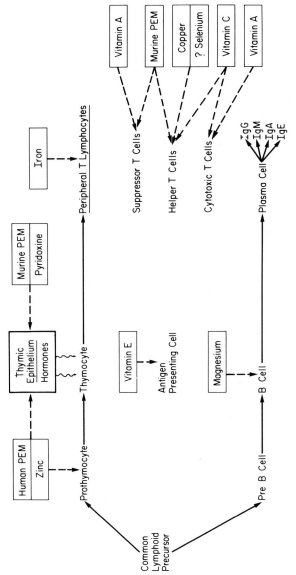

FIG. 4. Localization of the specific effects of nutrients on the immunologic network. *Dashed arrows*, site or specific cell type affected by the various nutrients listed for effects elicited by nutrient deprivation or supplementation.

the central nervous system lesions. Unfortunately, vitamin C deprivation also causes major immune defects at many other levels as well.

Dietary factors have been shown to play an important modulating role in murine models of systemic lupus erythematosis. PEM and restriction of polyunsaturated fatty acids have decreased the severity of autoimmune manifestations in NZB/W mice. Recent studies by Beach and co-workers (21) on zinc restriction in these mice demonstrate both a decrease in autoantibody formation (anti-DNA) and a dramatic increase in survival. The zinc deprivation exerted a significantly greater effect on disease pathology than did the PEM produced in the pair-fed controls. In the problem of malignant disease, since the addition of either vitamin A or C increases cytotoxic T cell reactivity, these nutrients are being actively investigated as immunoadjuvants in the host response to autologous neoplastic cells. In both autoimmune disease and enhancement of immunologic responses against neoplasia, specific application of nutritional therapy may ultimately be used to alter disease pathology without affecting other peripheral events. This is the challenge for the future.

ACKNOWLEDGMENTS

This work was supported by the Rockefeller Foundation, grant 77088, to the Division of Geographic Medicine under the direction of Dr. Gerald T. Keusch and by grants CA 29282 (S. D. Waksal, principal investigator) and HD 11844 (G. T. Keusch, principal investigator) from the National Institutes of Health.

Dr. S. D. Waksal is a Scholar of the Leukemia Society of America.

REFERENCES

1. Abbassy, A. S., Badr El-Din, M. K., Hassan, A. I., Aref, G. H., Hammad, S. A., El-Araby, I. I., Badr El-Din, A. A., Soliman, M. H., and Hussein, M. (1974): Studies of cell-mediated immunity and allergy in protein-energy malnutrition. I. Cell-mediated delayed hypersensitivity. *J. Trop. Med. Hyg.*, 77:13–17.
2. Akpom, C. A., and Warren, K. S. (1975): The inhibition of granuloma formation around *Schistosoma mansoni* eggs. VI. Protein, calorie, vitamin deficiency. *Am. J. Pathol.*, 79:435–450.
3. Alcock, N. W., and Shils, M. E. (1974): Serum immunoglobulin G in the magnesium-depleted rat. *Proc. Soc. Exp. Biol. Med.*, 145:855–858.
4. Allen, J. I., Kay, N. E., and McClain, C. J. (1981): Severe zinc deficiency in humans: Association with a reversible T-lymphocyte dysfunction. *Ann. Intern. Med.*, 95(2):154–157.
5. Alleyne, G. A. O., and Young, V. H. (1966): Adrenal function in malnutrition. *Lancet*, 1:911–912.
6. Anthony, L. E., Kurahara, C. G., and Taylor, K. B. (1979): Cell-mediated cytotoxicity and humoral immune response in ascorbic acid-deficient guinea pigs. *Am. J. Clin. Nutr.*, 32(8):1691–1698.
7. Aschkenasy, A. (1965): Influence of alimentary proteins on the size of blood lymphocytes in the rat. The role of the thymus in this effect. *Isr. J. Med. Sci.*, 1:552–562.
8. Aschkenasy, A. (1973): Differing effects of dietary protein deprivation on the production of rosette-forming cells in the lymph nodes and the spleen and on the levels of serum haemagglutinins in rats immunized to sheep red cells. *Immunology*, 24:617–632.
9. Aschkenasy, A. (1974): Effect of a protein-free diet on mitotic activity of transplanted splenic lymphocytes. *Nature*, 250:325–326.
10. Aschkenasy, A. (1975): Effect of a protein-free diet on lymph node and spleen cell response in vivo to blastogenic stimulants. *Nature*, 254:63–65.

11. Aschkenasy, A. (1978): Protein deprivation induces a premitotic block on the lymphocytes of rats and primarily suppresses cortisone-sensitive T cells. *Nutr. Rep. Int.*, 18(2):177–185.
12. Aschkenasy, A., Adam, Y., and Joly, P. (1966): Quelques données sur l'efat fonctionnel des corticosurrénales chez le rat carencé en protéines ou en certains acides aminés. *Ann. Endocrinol.*, 27:21–36.
13. Axelrod, A. E., and Trakatellis, A. C. (1964): Induction of tolerance to skin homografts by administering splenic cells to pyridoxine-deficient mice. *Proc. Soc. Exp. Biol. Med.*, 116:206–210.
14. Axelrod, A. E., Hopper, S., and Long, D. A. (1961): Effects of pyridoxine deficiency upon circulating antibody formation and skin hypersensitivity reactions to diphtheria toxoid in guinea pigs. *J. Nutr.*, 74:58–64.
15. Axelrod, A. E., Carter, B. B., McCoy, R. H., and Geisinger, R. (1947): Circulating antibodies in vitamin deficient states: 1. Pyridoxine, riboflavin, and pantothenic acid deficiencies. *Proc. Soc. Exp. Biol. Med.*, 6:137–140.
16. Axelrod, A. E., Trakatellis, A. C., Block, H., and Stinebring, W. R. (1963): Effects of pyridoxine deficiency upon delayed hypersensitivity in guinea pigs. *J. Nutr.*, 79:161–167.
17. Axelrod, A. E., Fisher, B., Fisher, E., Chiung Puh Lee, Y., and Walsh, P. (1958): Effect of pyridoxine deficiency on skin grafts in the rat. *Science*, 127:1388–1389.
18. Bach, J. F., and Dardenne, M. (1972): Thymus dependency of rosette-forming cells. Evidence for a circulating thymic hormone. *Transplant Proc.*, 4:345–350.
19. Bang, B. G., Bang, F. B., and Foard, M. A. (1972): Lymphocyte depression induced in chickens on diets deficient in vitamin A and other components. *Am. J. Pathol.*, 68:147–162.
20. Bang, B. G., Mahalanabis, D., Mukherjee, K. L., and Bang, F. B. (1975): T and B lymphocyte rosetting in undernourished children. *Proc. Soc. Exp. Biol. Med.*, 149:199–202.
21. Beach, R. S., Gershwin, M. E., and Hurley, L. S. (1982): Nutritional factors and autoimmunity. II. Prolongation of survival in zinc-deprived NZB/W mice. *J. Immunol.*, 128:308–313.
22. Beatty, D. W., and Dowdle, E. B. (1978): The effects of kwashiorkor serum on lymphocyte transformation *in vitro*. *Clin. Exp. Immunol.*, 32:134–143.
23. Beatty, D. W., and Dowdle, E. B. (1979): Deficiency in kwashiorkor serum of factors required for optimal lymphocyte transformation *in vitro*. *Clin. Exp. Immunol.*, 35:433–442.
24. Beisel, W. R. (1980): Effects of infection on nutritional status and immunity. *Fed. Proc.*, 39(13):3105–3108.
25. Bell, R. G., and Hazell, L. A. (1975): Influence of dietary protein restriction on immune competence. 1. Effect on the capacity of cells from various lymphoid organs to induce graft-vs-host reactions. *J. Exp. Med.*, 141:127–137.
26. Bell, R. G., and Hazell, L. A. (1977): The influence of dietary protein insufficiency on the murine thymus. Evidence for an intrathymic pool of progenitor cells capable of thymus regeneration after severe atrophy. *Aust. J. Exp. Biol. Med. Sci.*, 55(5):571–584.
27. Bell, R. G., Hazell, L. A., and Price, P. (1976): Influence of dietary protein restriction on immune competence. II. Effect on lymphoid tissue. *Clin. Exp. Immunol.*, 26:314–326.
28. Bell, R. G., Hazell, L. A., and Sheridan, J. W. (1976): The influence of dietary protein deficiency on haemopoietic cells in the mouse. *Cell Tissue Kinet.*, 9:305–311.
29. Bell, R. G., Turner, K. J., Gracey, M. J., Suharjono, and Sunoto (1976): Serum and small intestinal immunoglobulin levels in malnourished children. *Am. J. Clin. Nutr.*, 29:392–397.
30. Benaceraf, B., and McDevitt, H. O. (1972): The histocompatibility-linked immune response genes. *Science*, 175:273–279.
31. Bhaskaram, C., and Reddy, V. (1974): Cell mediated immunity in protein calorie malnutrition. *J. Trop. Pediatr. Environ. Child Health*, 20:284–286.
32. Bhaskaram, C., and Reddy, V. (1975): Cell-mediated immunity in iron and vitamin-deficient children. *Br. Med. J.*, 3:522.
33. Binz, H., and Wigzell, H. (1978): Induction of specific immune responsiveness with purified mixed leukocyte culture-activated T lymphoblasts as autoimmunogen. II. An analysis of the effects measured at the cellular and serological levels. *J. Exp. Med.*, 147(1):63–76.
34. Bistrian, B. R., Blackburn, G. L., and Scrimshaw, N. S. (1975): Cellular immunity in semi-starved stages in hospitalized adults. *Am. J. Clin. Nutr.*, 28:1148–1155.
35. Bistrian, B. R., Sherman, M., Blackburn, G. L., Marshall, R., and Shaw, C. (1977): Cellular immunity in adult marasmus. *Arch. Intern. Med.*, 137:1408–1411.

36. Björkstén, B., Bäck, O., Gustavson, K. H., Hallmans, G., Hägglöf, B., and Tärnvik, A. (1980): Zinc and immune function in Down's syndrome. *Acta Paediatr. Scand.*, 69(2):183–187.

37. Bolin, T. D., Davis, A. E., Cummins, A. G., Duncombe, V. M., and Kelly, L. D. (1977): Effect of iron and protein deficiency on the expulsion of Nippostrongylus brasiliensis from the small intestine of the rat. *Gut*, 18:182–186.

38. Bongiorni-Malavé, I., and Pocino, M. (1980): Abnormal regulatory control of the antibody response to heterologous erythrocytes in protein-calorie malnutrition. *Clin. Immunol. Immunopathol.*, 16:19–29.

39. Brown, K. H., Rajan, M. M., Chakraborty, J., Aziz, K. M. A., and Phil, M. (1980): Failure of a large dose of vitamin A to enhance the antibody response to tetanus toxoid in children. *Am. J. Clin. Nutr.*, 33:212–217.

40. Brown, R. E., and Opio, E. A. (1966): Associated factors in kwashiorkor in Uganda. *Trop. Geogr. Med.*, 18:119–124.

41. Brummerstedt, E., Basse, A., Flagsted, T., and Andresen, E. (1977): Acrodermatitis enteropathica, zinc malabsorption. Animal model: Lethal trait A46 in cattle (hereditary parakeratosis, hereditary thymic hypoplasia, hereditary zinc deficiency). *Am. J. Pathol.*, 87(3):725–728.

42. Bryan, C. F., Nishiya, K., Pollack, M. S., Dupont, B., and De Sousa, M. (1981): Differential inhibition of the MLR by iron: Association with HLA phenotype. *Immunogenetics*, 12:129–140.

43. Burgess, B. J., Vos, G. H., Coovadia, H. M., Smythe, P. M., Parent, M. A., and Loening, W. E. L. (1974): Radio-isotopic assessment of phytohaemagglutinin-stimulated lymphocytes from patients with protein calorie malnutrition. *S. Afr. Med. J.*, 48:1870–1872.

44. Campbell, P. A., Cooper, H. R., Heinzerling, R. H., and Tengerdy, R. P. (1974): Vitamin E enhances *in vitro* immune responses by normal and nonadherent spleen cells. *Proc. Soc. Exp. Biol. Med.*, 146:465–469.

45. Cantor, H., and Boyse, E. A. (1975): Functional subclasses of T lymphocytes bearing different Ly antigens. II. Cooperation between subclasses of Ly$^+$ cells in the generation of killer activity. *J. Exp. Med.*, 141:1390–1399.

46. Chandra, R. K. (1972): Immunocompetence in undernutrition. *J. Pediatr.*, 81:1194–1200.

47. Chandra, R. K. (1974): Rosette forming T lymphocytes and cell mediated immunity in malnutrition. *Br. Med. J.*, 3:608–609.

48. Chandra, R. K. (1975): Reduced secretory antibody response to live attenuated measles and poliovirus vaccines in malnourished children. *Br. Med. J.*, 2:583–585.

49. Chandra, R. K. (1977): Immunoglobulins and antibody response in protein-calorie malnutrition— a review. In: *Malnutrition and the Immune Response*, edited by R. M. Suskind, pp. 155–168. Raven Press, New York.

50. Chandra, R. K. (1977): Lymphocyte subpopulations in human malnutrition: Cytotoxic and suppressor cells. *Pediatrics*, 59(3):423–427.

51. Chandra, R. K. (1979): T and B lymphocyte subpopulations and leukocyte terminal deoxynucleotidyl transferase in energy-protein undernutrition. *Acta Paediatr. Scand.*, 68(6):841–845.

52. Chandra, R. K. (1979): Serum thymic hormone activity in protein-energy malnutrition. *Clin. Exp. Immunol.*, 38:228–230.

53. Chandra, R. K. (1980): Acrodermatitis enteropathica: Zinc levels and cell-mediated immunity. *Pediatrics*, 66(5):789–791.

54. Chandra, R. K., and Au, B. (1980): Single nutrient deficiency and cell-mediated immune responses. 1. Zinc. *Am. J. Clin. Nutr.*, 33:736–738.

55. Chandra, R. K. (1977): *Nutrition, Immunity and Infection. Mechanism of Interactions*. Plenum, New York.

56. Chandra, R. K., and Saraya, A. K. (1975): Impaired immunocompetence associated with iron deficiency. *J. Pediatr.*, 86(6):899–902.

57. Chandra, R. K., Heresi, G., and Au, B. (1980): Serum thymic factor activity in deficiencies of calories, zinc, vitamin A and pyridoxine. *Clin. Exp. Immunol.*, 42:332–335.

58. Cichocki, T., Stachura, J., Komorowska, Z., and Bigaj, M. (1977): Cytoenzymatic studies on the lymphocytes of peripheral blood and lymphocyte nodes of rats in an experimental magnesium deficiency. *Acta Vitaminol. Enzymol.*, 31:187–193.

59. Claiman, H. N., Moorehead, J. W., and Benner, W. H. (1971): Corticosteroids and lymphoid cells *in vitro*. I. Hydrocortisone lysis of human, guinea pig and mouse thymus cells. *J. Lab. Clin. Med.*, 78:499–507.

60. Cohen, B. E., and Cohen, I. K. (1973): Vitamin A: Adjuvant and steroid antagonist in the immune response. *J. Immunol.*, 111(5):1376–1380.
61. Cooper, W. C., Good, R. A., and Mariani, T. (1974): Effects of protein insufficiency on immune responsiveness. *Am. J. Clin. Nutr.*, 27:647–664.
62. Cooper, W. C., Mariani, T. N., and Good, R. A. (1975): The effects of protein deprivation on cell-mediated immunity. *Birth Defects*, 11(1):223–228.
63. Coovadia, H. M., Parent, M. A., Loening, W. E. K., Wesley, A., Burgess, B., Hallet, F., Brain, P., Grace, J., Naidoo, J., Smythe, P. M., and Vos, G. H. (1974): An evaluation of factors associated with the depression of immunity in malnutrition and measles. *Am. J. Clin. Nutr.*, 27:665–669.
64. Corwin, L. M., and Gordon, R. K. (1982): Vitamin E and immune regulation. *Ann. NY Acad. Sci. (in press)*.
65. Corwin, L. M., and Shloss, J. (1980): Influence of vitamin E on the mitogenic response of murine lymphoid cells. *J. Nutr.*, 110(5):916–923.
66. Corwin, L. M., and Shloss, J. (1980): Role of antioxidants on the stimulation of the mitogenic response. *J. Nutr.*, 110:2497–2505.
67. Corwin, L. M., Gordon, R. K., and Schloss, J. (1982): Studies of the mode of action on vitamin E in stimulating T-cell mitogenesis. *Scand. J. Immunol.*, 14: *(in press)*.
68. Cummins, A. G., Duncombe, V. M., Bolin, T. D., Davis, A. E., and Kelly, J. D. (1978): Suppression of rejection of Nippostrongylus brasiliensis in iron and protein deficient rats: Effect of syngeneic lymphocyte transfer. *Gut*, 19:823–826.
69. Dahl, H., and Degré, M. (1976): The effect of ascorbic acid on production of human interferon and the antiviral activity *in vitro*. *Acta Pathol. Microbiol. Scand. [B]*, 84:280–284.
70. Davies, A. J. S. (1969): The thymus and the cellular basis for immunity. *Transplant. Rev.*, 1:43–91.
71. Davis, S. D. (1970): Teratogenicity of vitamin B6 deficiency: Omphalocele, skeletal and neural defects, and splenic hypoplasia. *Science*, 169:1329–1330.
72. Davis, S. D. (1974): Immunodeficiency and runting syndrome in rats from congenital pyridoxine deficiency. *Nature*, 251:548–550.
73. Delmonte, L., Eyquem, A., and Aschkenasy, A. (1962): Recherches sur le compartement immunologique du rat carencé eu protéines. *Ann. Inst. Pasteur*, 102:420–436.
74. Dennert, G., and Lotan, R. (1978): Effect of retinoic acid on the immune system: Stimulation of T killer cell induction. *Eur. J. Immunol.*, 8:23–29.
75. Dennert, G., Crowley, C., Kouba, J., and Lotan, R. (1979): Retinoic acid stimulation of the induction of mouse killer T-cells in allogeneic and syngeneic systems. *J. Natl. Cancer Inst.*, 62(1):89–94.
76. DePasquale-Jardieu, P., and Fraker, P. J. (1979): The role of corticosterone in the loss in immune function in the zinc-deficient A/J mouse. *J. Nutr.*, 109(11):1847–1855.
77. DePasquale-Jardieu, P., and Fraker, P. J. (1980): Further characterization of the role of corticosterone in the loss of humoral immunity in zinc-deficient A/J mice as determined by adrenalectomy. *J. Immunol.*, 124(6):2650–2656.
78. De Sousa, M., and Nishiya, K. (1978): Inhibition of E-rosette formation by two iron salts. *Cell. Immunol.*, 38:203–208.
79. Dieter, M. P. (1969): Studies on thymic humoral factor prepared from guinea pigs: The influence of dietary vitamin C. *Proc. Soc. Exp. Biol. Med.*, 132:1147–1152.
80. Dresser, D. W. (1968): Adjuvanticity of vitamin A. *Nature*, 217:527–529.
81. Duffus, W. P. H., and Allan, D. (1971): The kinetics and morphology of the rosette-forming cell response in the popliteal lymph node of rats. *Immunology*, 20:345–361.
82. Duncombe, V. M., Bolin, T. D., and Davis, A. (1979): The effect of iron and protein deficiency on the development of acquired resistance to reinfection with Nippostrongylus brasiliensis in rats. *Am. J. Clin. Nutr.*, 32:553–558.
83. Edelman, R. (1977): Cell-mediated immune response in protein-calorie malnutrition—A review. In: *Malnutrition and the Immune Response*, edited by R. M. Suskind, pp. 47–74. Raven Press, New York.
84. Edelman, R., Suskind, R., Olson, R. E., and Sirisinha, S. (1973): Mechanisms of defective delayed cutaneous hypersensitivity in children with protein-calorie malnutrition. *Lancet*, 1:506–508.

85. Elias, P. M., and Williams, M. L. (1981): Retinoids, cancer, and the skin. *Arch. Dermatol.*, 117:160–180.
86. Elin, R. J. (1975): The effect of magnesium deficiency in mice on serum immunoglobulin concentrations and antibody plaque-forming cells. *Proc. Soc. Exp. Biol. Med.*, 148:620–623.
87. Fauci, A. S. (1979): Glucocorticoid effects on circulating human mononuclear cells. *J. Reticuloendothel. Soc.*, 26:727–738.
88. Feldman, G., and Gianantonio, C. A. (1972): Aspectos immunologicos de la desnutricion en el niño. *Medicina (B. Aires)*, 32:1–9.
89. Ferguson, A. C., Lawler, G. J., and Neumann, C. G. (1974): Decreased rosette-forming lymphocytes in malnutrition and intrauterine growth retardation. *J. Pediatr.*, 85:717–723.
90. Fernandes, G., Yunis, E. J., and Good, R. A. (1976): Influence of protein restriction on immune functions in NZB mice. *J. Immunol.*, 116(3):782–790.
91. Fernandes, G., Friend, P., Yunis, E. J., and Good, R. A. (1978): Influence of dietary restriction on immunological function and renal disease in (NZB × NZW)F$_1$ mice. *Proc. Natl. Acad. Sci. USA*, 75(3):1500–1504.
92. Fernandes, G., Nair, M., Onoe, K., Tanaka, T., Floyd, R., and Good, R. (1979): Impairment of cell-mediated immunity functions by dietary zinc deficiency in mice. *Proc. Natl. Acad. Sci. USA*, 76(1):457–461.
93. Fisher, B., and Schewe, E. (1962): Further observations on skin homografts in pyridoxine deficient animals. *Ann. Surg.*, 155:457–463.
94. Floersheim, G. L., and Bollag, W. (1972): Accelerated rejection of skin homografts by vitamin A acid. *Transplantation*, 15(4):564–567.
95. Flynn, A., and Yen, B. R. (1981): Mineral deficiency effects on the generation of cytotoxic T-cells and T-helper cell factors *in vitro*. *J. Nutr.*, 111:907–913.
96. Ford, C. E., Micklem, H. S., Evans, E. P., Cray, J. G., and Ogden, D. A. (1966): The inflow of bone marrow cells to the thymus: Studies with part body irradiated mice injected with chromosome marked bone marrow and subjected to antigenic stimulation. *Ann. NY Acad. Sci.*, 129:283–296.
97. Ford, G. W., Jakeman, M., José, D. G., Vorbach, E. A., and Kirke, D. K. (1975): Migration inhibitory factor production by lymphoid cells of Australian aboriginal children with moderate protein calorie malnutrition. *Austr. Paediatr. J.*, 11:160–164.
98. Fraker, P. J., Haas, S. M., and Luecke, R. W. (1977): Effect of zinc deficiency on the immune response of the young adult A/J mouse. *J. Nutr.*, 107:1889–1895.
99. Fraker, P. J., DePasquale-Jardieu, P., Zwickl, C. M., and Luecke, R. W. (1978): Regeneration of T-cell helper function in zinc-deficient adult mice. *Proc. Natl. Acad. Sci. USA*, 75(11):5660–5664.
100. Franceschi, C., Licastro, F., Chiricolo, M., Bonetti, F., Zannotti, M., Fabris, N., Mocchegiani, E., Fantini, M. P., Paolucci, P., and Masi, M. (1981): Deficiency of autologous mixed lymphocyte reactions and serum thymic factor level in Down's syndrome. *J. Immunol.*, 126(6):2161–2164.
101. Fraser, R. L., Pavlović, S., Kurahara, C. G., Murata, A., Peterson, N. S., Taylor, K. B., and Feigen, G. (1980): The effect of variations in vitamin C intake on the cellular immune response of guinea pigs. *Am. J. Clin. Nutr.*, 33(4):839–847.
102. Gallo, P. V., and Weinberg, J. (1981): Corticosterone rhythmicity in the rat: Interactive effects of dietary restrictions and schedule of feeding. *J. Nutr.*, 111:208–218.
103. Geefhuysen, J., Rosen, E. U., Katz, J., Ipp, T., and Metz, J. (1971): Impaired cellular immunity in kwashiorkor with improvement after therapy. *Br. Med. J.*, 4:527–529.
104. Gershoff, S. N., Gill, T. J., Simonian, S. J., and Steinberg, A. I. (1968): Some effects of amino acid deficiencies on antibody formation in the rat. *J. Nutr.*, 95:184–189.
105. Gershon, R. K., Lance, E. M., and Kondo, K. (1974): Immuno-regulatory role of spleen localizing thymocytes. *J. Immunol.*, 112:546–554.
106. Golden, M. H. N., Jackson, A. A., and Golden, B. E. (1977): Effect of zinc on thymus of recently malnourished children. *Lancet*, 2:1057–1059.
107. Gordon, J. E., Jansen, A. A. J., and Ascoli, W. (1965): Measles in rural Guatemala. *J. Pediatr.*, 67:779–786.
108. Gordon, J. E., Wyon, J. B., and Ascoli, W. (1967): The second year death rates in less developed countries. *Am. J. Med. Sci.*, 254:357–380.
109. Grace, H. J., Armstrong, D., and Smythe, P. M. (1972): Reduced lymphocyte transformation in protein calorie malnutrition. *S. Afr. Med. J.*, 46:402–403.

110. Gross, R. L., and Newberne, P. M. (1980): Role of nutrition in immunologic function. *Physiol. Rev.*, 60:188–302.
111. Gross, R. L., Osdin, N., Fong, L., and Newberne, P. M. (1979): *In vitro* restoration by levamisole of mitogen responsiveness in zinc-deprived rats. *Am. J. Clin. Nutr.*, 32:1267–1271.
112. Gross, R. L., Reid, J., Newberne, P. M., Burgess, G., Marston, R., and Hift, W. (1975): Depressed cell-mediated immunity in megaloblastic anemia due to folic acid deficiency. *Am. J. Clin. Nutr.*, 28:225–232.
113. Guenounou, M., Armier, J., and Gaudin-Harding, F. (1978): Effect of magnesium deficiency and food restriction on the immune response in young mice. *Int. J. Vitam. Nutr. Res.*, 48(3):290–295.
114. Harland, P. S. (1965): Tuberculin reactions in malnourished children. *Lancet*, 2:719–721.
115. Harland, P. S., and Brown, R. E. (1965): Tuberculin sensitivity following B.C.G. vaccination in undernourished children. *East Afr. Med. J.*, 42:233–238.
116. Harmon, B. G., Miller, E. R., Hoefer, J. A., Ullrey, D. E., and Luecke, R. W. (1963): Relationship of specific nutrient deficiencies to antibody production in swine. II. Pantothenic acid, pyridoxine, or riboflavin. *J. Nutr.*, 79:269–275.
117. Harrison, B. W. D., Tugwell, P., and Fawcett, I. W. (1975): Tuberculin reaction in adult Nigerians with sputum positive pulmonary tuberculosis. *Lancet*, 1:421–424.
118. Haynes, B. F., Katz, P., and Fauci, A. S. (1979): Effect of hydrocortisone on the kinetics and function of peripheral blood immunoregulatory cells in man. In: *Antibody Production in Man. In Vitro Synthesis and Clinical Implications*, edited by A. S. Fauci and R. Ballieux, pp. 291–302. Academic Press, New York.
119. Heresi, G., and Chandra, R. K. (1980): Effects of severe calorie restriction on thymic factor activity and lymphocyte stimulation response in rats. *J. Nutr.*, 110(9):1888–1893.
120. Heresi, G. P., Saitra, M. T., and Schlesinger, L. (1981): Leukocyte migration inhibitory factor production in marasmic infants. *Am. J. Clin. Nutr.*, 34:909–913.
121. Heyworth, B., Moore, D. L., and Brown, J. (1975): Depression of lymphocyte response to phytohaemagglutinin in the presence of plasma from children with acute protein energy malnutrition. *Clin. Exp. Immunol.*, 22:72–77.
122. Hodges, R. E., Bean, W. B., Ohlson, M. A., and Bleiler, R. E. (1962): Factors affecting human antibody response. III. Immunologic responses of men deficient in pyridoxine acid. *Am. J. Clin. Nutr.* 11(2):85–93.
123. Hodges, R. E., Bean, W. B., Ohlson, M. A., and Bleiler, R. E. (1962): Factors affecting human antibody response. IV. Pyridoxine deficiency. *Am. J. Clin. Nutr.*, 11:180–186.
124. Hodges, R. E., Bean, W. B., Ohlson, M. A., and Bleiler, R. E. (1962): Factors affecting human antibody response. V. Combined deficiencies of pantothenic acid and pyridoxine. *Am. J. Clin. Nutr.*, 11:187–199.
125. Holm, G., and Palmblad, J. (1976): Acute energy deprivation in man: Effect on cell-mediated immunological reactions. *Clin. Exp. Immunol.*, 25:207–211.
126. Huber, B., Cantor, H., Shen, F. W., and Boyse, E. A. (1976): Independent differentiative pathways of Ly 1 and Ly 2,3 subclasses of T cells. *J. Exp. Med.*, 144:1128–1133.
127. Hughes, W. T., Price, R. A., Sisko, F., Havion, W. S., Kafatos, A. G., Schonland, M., and Smythe, P. M. (1974): Protein-calorie malnutrition. A host determinant for *Pneumocystis carinii* infections. *Am. J. Dis. Child.*, 128:44–52.
128. Ifekwunigwe, A. E., Grasset, N., Glass, R., and Foster, S. (1980): Immune response to measles and smallpox vaccinations in malnourished children. *Am. J. Clin. Nutr.*, 33:621–624.
129. Iwata, T., Incefy, G. S., Tanaka, T., Fernandes, G., Menendez-Botet, C. J., Pih, K., and Good, R. A. (1979): Circulating thymic hormone levels in zinc deficiency. *Cell. Immunol.*, 47:100–105.
130. Jackson, C. M., editor (1925): *The Effects of Inanition and Malnutrition Upon Growth and Structure*. P. Blakiston's Son, Philadelphia.
131. Jackson, T. M., and Zaman, S. N. (1980): The *in vitro* effect of the thymic factor thymopoietin on a subpopulation of lymphocytes from severely malnourished children. *Clin. Exp. Immunol.*, 39(3):717–721.
132. Jandinski, J., Cantor, H., Tadakuma, T., Peavy, D. L., and Pierce, C. W. (1976): Separation of helper T cells from suppressor T cells expressing different Ly components. I. Polyclonal activation: Suppressor and helper activities are inherent properties of distinct T-cell subclasses. *J. Exp. Med.*, 143:1382–1390.

133. Jayalakshmi, V. T., and Gopalan, C. (1958): Nutrition and tuberculosis. I. An epidemiologic study. *Indian J. Med. Res.*, 46:87–92.

134. John, T. J., and Jabal, P. (1972): Oral polio vaccination of children in the tropics. I. The poor seroconversion rates and the absence of viral interference. *Am. J. Epidemiol.*, 96:263–269.

135. Jose, D. G., and Good, R. A. (1973): Quantitative effects of nutritional essential amino acid deficiency upon immune responses to tumors in mice. *J. Exp. Med.*, 137:1–9.

136. Jose, D. G., Welch, J. S., and Doherty, R. L. (1970): Humoral and cellular immune responses to streptococci, influenza and other antigens in Australian aboriginal school children. *Aust. Paediatr. J.*, 6:192–202.

137. Jose, D. G., Shelton, M., Tauro, G. P., Belbin, R., and Hosking, C. S. (1975): Deficiency of immunological and phagocytic function in aboriginal children with protein calorie malnutrition. *Med. J. Aust.*, 2:699–705.

138. Jurin, M., and Tannock, I. F. (1972): Influence of vitamin A on immunological response. *Immunology*, 23:283–287.

139. Kenney, M. A., Roderbuck, C. E., Arnrich, L., and Piedad, F. (1968): Effects of protein deficiency on the spleen and antibody function in rats. *J. Nutr.*, 95:173–178.

140. Keusch, G. T. (1979): Nutrition as a determinant of host response to infection and the metabolic sequellae of infectious diseases. *Sem. Infect. Dis.*, 2:265–303.

141. Keusch, G. T. (1981): Effect of nutritional factors on macrophage production and function. In: *CRC Handbook of Nutritional Requirements in a Functional Context*, edited by M. Rechcigl, pp. 115–125. CRC Press, Boca Raton.

142. Keusch, G. T., Douglas, S. D., Braden, K., and Geller, S. A. (1978): Antibacterial functions of macrophages in experimental protein-calorie malnutrition. 1. Description of the model, morphological observations and macrophage surface IgG receptors. *J. Infect. Dis.*, 138(2):125–133.

143. Keilmann, A. A., Uberoi, L. S., Chandra, R. K., and Mehra, V. L. (1976): The effect of nutritional status on immune capacity and immune responses in preschool children in a rural community in India. *Bull. WHO*, 54:477–483.

144. Koros, A. M. C., Axelrod, A. E., Hamill, E. C., and South, D. J. (1976): Immunoregulatory consequences of vitamin deficiencies on background plaque-forming cells in rats. *Proc. Soc. Exp. Biol. Med.*, 152:322–326.

145. Koster, F., Gaffar, A., and Jackson, T. M. (1981): Recovery of cellular immune competence during treatment of protein-calorie malnutrition. *Am. J. Clin. Nutr.*, 34:887–891.

146. Krieger, D. T. (1974): Food and water restriction shifts corticosterone, temperature, activity and brain amine periodicity. *Endocrinology*, 95:1195–1201.

147. Krishnan, S., Bhuyan, U. N., Talwar, G. P., and Ramalingaswami, V. (1974): Effect of vitamin A and protein-calorie undernutrition on immune response. *Immunology*, 27:383–392.

148. Kulapongs, P., Suskind, R. M., Vithayasai, V., and Olson, R. E. (1977): *In vitro* cell mediated immune response in Thai children with protein calorie malnutrition. In: *Malnutrition and the Immune Response*, edited by R. M. Suskind, pp. 99–109. Raven Press, New York.

149. Kumar, M., and Axelrod, A. E. (1968): Cellular antibody synthesis in vitamin B6-deficient rats. *J. Nutr.*, 96:53–59.

150. Kumar, M., and Axelrod, A. E. (1969): Circulating antibody formation in scorbutic guinea pigs. *J. Nutr.*, 98:41–44.

151. Kumar, M., and Axelrod, A. E. (1978): Cellular antibody synthesis in thiamin, riboflavin, biotin, and folic acid-deficient rats. *Proc. Soc. Exp. Biol. Med.*, 157:421–423.

152. Kumar, K. K., Agrawal, T., Yadav, S. K., and Dhamija, J. P. (1978): A study of cell mediated immune response in protein calorie malnutrition. *Indian Pediatr.*, 15(10):803–808.

153. Kuvibidila, S., Nauss, K. M., Suskind, R. M., and Baliga, B. S. (1979): Impairment of mitogenic response by splenic lymphocytes isolated from iron deficient anemic mice. *Fed. Proc.*, 38:763.

154. Lal, N., Bazaz-Malik, G., and Sehgal, H. (1980): Profile of T and B lymphocytes in malnourished children. *Indian J. Med. Res.*, 71:576–580.

155. Law, D. K., Dudrick, S. J., and Abdou, N. I. (1973): Immunocompetence of patients with protein-calorie malnutrition. The effects of nutritional repletion. *Ann. Intern. Med.*, 79:545–550.

156. Lederer, W. H., Kumar, M., and Axelrod, A. E. (1975): Effects of pantothenic acid deficiency on cellular antibody synthesis in rats. *J. Nutr.*, 105:17–25.

157. Leonard, P. J. (1973): Cortisol-binding in serum in kwashiorkor: East African studies. In: *Endocrine Aspects of Malnutrition, Marasmus, Kwashiorkor and Psychosocial Deprivation*, edited by L. I. Gardner and P. Amacher, pp. 355–362. Kroc Foundation, Santa Ynez.

158. Leveille, G. A., and Hanson, R. W. (1966): Adaptive changes in enzyme activity and metabolic pathways in adipose tissue from meal-fed rats. *J. Lipid Res.*, 7:46–55.

159. Lloyd, A. V. C. (1968): Tuberculin test in children with malnutrition. *Br. Med. J.*, 3:529–531.

160. Lomnitzer, R., Rosen, E. U., Geefhuysen, J., and Rabson, A. R. (1976): Defective leukocyte inhibitory factor (LIF) production by lymphocytes in children with kwashiorkor. *S. Afr. Med. J.*, 50:1820–1822.

161. López, V., Davis, S. D., and Smith, N. J. (1972): Studies in infantile marasmus. IV. Impairment of immunologic responses in the marasmatic pig. *Pediatar. Res.*, 6:779–788.

162. Lotan, R., Mokady, S., and Horenstein, L. (1980): The effect of lysine and threonine supplementation on the immune response of growing rats fed wheat gluten diets. *Nutr. Rep. Int.*, 22:313–318.

163. Ludovici, P. P., and Axelrod, A. E. (1951): Circulating antibodies in vitamin-deficiency states. Pteroylglutamic acid, niacin-tryptophan, vitamin B_{12}, A and D deficiencies. *Proc. Soc. Exp. Biol. Med.*, 77:526–530.

164. Ludovici, P. P., Axelrod, A. E., and Carter, B. B. (1949): Circulating antibodies in vitamin deficiency states. Pantothenic acid deficiency. *Proc. Soc. Exp. Biol. Med.*, 72:81–83.

165. Ludovici, P. P., Axelrod, A. E., and Carter, B. B. (1951): Circulating antibodies in vitamin-deficient states. Pantothenic acid and pyridoxine deficiencies. *Proc. Soc. Exp. Biol. Med.*, 76:665–670.

166. Ludovici, P. P., Axelrod, A. E., and Carter, B. B. (1951): Circulating antibodies in vitamin deficiency states. Pantothenic acid-sparing action of DL-methionine. *Proc. Soc. Exp. Biol. Med.*, 76:670–672.

167. Luecke, R. W., and Fraker, P. J. (1979): The effect of varying dietary zinc levels on growth and antibody-mediated response in two strains of mice. *J. Nutr.*, 109:1373–1376.

168. Luecke, R. W., Simonal, C. E., and Fraker, P. J. (1978): The effect of restricted dietary intake on the antibody mediated response of the zinc deficient A/J mouse. *J. Nutr.*, 108:881–887.

169. MacCuish, A. C., Urbaniak, S. J., Goldstone, A. H., and Irvine, W. J. (1974): PHA responsiveness and subpopulations of circulating lymphocytes in pernicious anemia. *Blood*, 44(6):849–855.

170. MacDougall, L. G., Anderson, R., McNab, G. M., and Katz, J. (1975): The immune response in iron-deficient children: Impaired cellular defense mechanisms with altered humoral components. *J. Pediatr.*, 86:833–843.

171. Maffei, H. V. L., Rodriques, M. A. M., DeCamargo, J. L. V., and Campana, A. O. (1980): Intraepithelial lymphocytes in the jejunal mucosa of malnourished rats. *Gut*, 21(1):32–36.

172. Malavé, I., and Layrisse, M. (1976): Immune response in malnutrition. Differential effect of dietary protein restriction on the IgM and IgG response to alloantigens. *Cell. Immunol.*, 21:337–343.

173. Malavé, I., Németh, A., and Blanca, I. (1978): Immune response in malnutrition. Effect of protein deficiency on the DNA synthetic response to alloantigens. *Int. Arch. Allergy Appl. Immunol.*, 56:128–135.

174. Malavé, I., Németh, A., and Pocino, M. (1980): Changes in lymphocyte populations in protein-calorie-deficient mice. *Cell. Immunol.*, 49:235–249.

175. Martinez, C., and Chaves, A. (1979): Nutrition and development of children from poor rural areas. VII. The effect of nutritional status on the frequency and severity of infections. *Nutr. Rep. Int.*, 19:307–314.

176. Mata, L. J. (1977): *The Children of Santa Maria Cauqué: A Prospective Field Study of Health and Growth*. The MIT Press, Cambridge.

177. Mathur, M., Ramalingaswami, V., and Deo, M. G. (1972): Influence of protein deficiency on 19S antibody-forming cells in rats and mice. *J. Nutr.*, 102:841–846.

178. McAnulty, P. A., and Duckerson, J. W. (1973): The cellular response of the weanling rat thymus gland to undernutrition and rehabilitation. *Pediatr. Res.*, 9:778–785.

179. McCoy, J. H., and Kenney, M. A. (1975): Depressed immune response in the magnesium-deficient rat. *J. Nutr.*, 105:791–797.

180. McEndy, D. P., Boon, M. A., and Furth, J. (1944): On the role of thymus, spleen and gonads in the development of leukemia in a high-leukemia strain of mice. *Cancer Res.*, 4:377–383.

181. McFarlane, H., and Hamid, J. (1973): Cell mediated responses in malnutrition. *Clin. Exp. Immunol.*, 13:153–164.

182. McKenzie, D., Hansen, J. D. L., and Becker, W. (1959): Herpes simplex virus infections: Dissemination in association with malnutrition. *Arch. Dis. Child.*, 34:250–256.

183. McMurray, D. N., Rey, H., Casazza, L. J., and Watson, R. R. (1948): Effect of moderate malnutrition on concentrations of immunoglobulins and enzymes in tears and saliva of young Columbian children. *Am. J. Clin. Nutr.*, 30:1944–1948.

184. McMurray, D. N., Watson, R. R., and Reyes, M. A. (1981): Effect of renutrition on humoral and cell-mediated immunity in severely malnourished children. *Am. J. Clin. Nutr.*, 34(10):2117–2126.

185. McMurray, D. N., Loomis, S. A., Casazza, L. J., Rey, H., and Miranda, R. (1981): Development of impaired cell-mediated immunity in mild and moderate malnutrition. *Am. J. Clin. Nutr.*, 34:68–77.

186. Micksche, M., Cerni, C., Kokron, O., Titscher, R., and Wrba, H. (1977): Stimulation of immune response in lung cancer patients by vitamin A therapy. *Oncology*, 34:234–238.

187. Mitchell, G. F. (1977): Observations and speculations on the influence of T cells in the cellular events of induction of antibody formation and tolerance in vivo. In: *The Lymphocyte. Structure and Function. Part I*, edited by J. J. Marchalonis, pp. 227–256. Marcel Dekker, New York.

188. Mitchell, G. F., and Miller, J. F. A. P. (1969): The thymus and antigen reactions. *Transplant. Rev.*, 1:3–42.

189. Mokady, S., Lotan, R., and Horenstein, L. (1979): The effect of dietary wheat gluten in protein malnutrition on the immune response of growing rats. *Nutr. Rep. Int.*, 20:615–624.

190. Moore, D. L., Heyworth, B., and Brown, J. (1974): PHA-induced lymphocyte transformations in leukocyte cultures from malarious, malnourished and control Gamerian children. *Clin. Exp. Immunol.*, 17:647–656.

191. Morley, D. (1969): Severe measles in the tropics. *Br. Med. J.*, 1:297–300.

192. Morley, D., Woodland, M., and Martin, W. J. (1963): Measles in Nigerian children. A study of the disease in West Africa and its manifestations in England and other countries during different epochs. *J. Hyg.*, 61:115–134.

193. Mueller, P. S., Kies, M. S., Alvord, E. C., and Shaw, C. M. (1962): Prevention of experimental allergic encephalomyelitis (EAE) by vitamin C deprivation. *J. Exp. Med.*, 115:329–338.

194. Mugerwa, J. W. (1971): The lymphoreticular system in kwashiorkor. *J. Pathol.*, 105:105–109.

195. Nalder, B. N., Mahoney, A. W., Ramakrishnan, R., and Hendricks, D. G. (1972): Sensitivity of the immunological response to the nutritional status of rats. *J. Nutr.*, 102(4):535–542.

196. National Academy of Science-National Research Council (1963): *Evaluation of Protein Quality*, publication 1100. National Academy of Sciences, Washington, D.C.

197. National Research Council (1980): *Recommended Dietary Allowances*, ninth edition. National Academy of Sciences, Washington, D.C.

198. Nauss, K. M., Mark, D. A., and Suskind, R. M. (1979): The effects of vitamin A deficiency on the *in vtiro* cellular immune response of rats. *J. Nutr.*, 109(10):1815–1823.

199. Nelson, W., Scheving, L. E., and Halberg, F. (1975): Circadian rhythms in mice fed a single daily meal at different stages of lighting regimen. *J. Nutr.*, 105:171–184.

200. Neumann, C. G., Lawler, G. J., and Stiehm, E. R. (1975): Immunologic responses in malnourished children. *Am. J. Clin. Nutr.*, 28:89–104.

201. Nichols, K. E., Solomons, N., Waner, J., Cruz, J. R., Urrutia, J. J., and Toru, B. (1980): Interaction of protein-energy nutrition and *in vitro* production of interferon in lymphocyte cultures: Studies in Guatemalan infants and children. *Western Hemisphere Nutrition Congress VI*, Los Angeles, pp. 74–75.

202. Nishiya, K., Gupta, S., and De Sousa, M. (1979): Differential inhibitory effect of iron on E, EA, and EAC rosette formation. *Cell. Immunol.*, 46(2):405–408.

203. Nishiya, K., De Sousa, M., Tsoi, E., Bognacki, J., and De Harven, E. (1980): Regulation of expression of human lymphoid cell surface marker by iron. *Cell. Immunol.*, 53:71–83.

204. Ogbeide, M. I. (1967): Measles in Nigerian children. *J. Pediatr.*, 71:737–741.

205. Oleske, J. M., Westphal, M. L., Shore, S., Gorden, D., Bogden, J. D., and Nahmias, A. (1979): Zinc therapy of depressed cellular immunity in acrodermatitis enteropathica. *Am. J. Dis. Child.*, 133:915–918.

206. Olusi, S. O., Thurman, G. B., and Goldstein, A. L. (1980): Effect of thymosin on T-lymphocyte rosette formation in children with kwashiorkor. *Clin. Immunol. Immunopathol.*, 15:687–691.

207. Owen, J. J. T., and Ritter, M. A. (1969): Tissue interaction in the development of thymus lymphocytes. *J. Exp. Med.*, 29:431–437.

208. Parent, M. A., Loening, W. E. K., Coovadia, H. M., and Smythe, P. M. (1974): Pattern of biochemical and immune recovery in protein calorie malnutrition. *S. Afr. Med. J.*, 48:1375–1378.

209. Passwell, J. H., Steward, M. W., and Soothill, J. F. (1974): The effects of protein malnutrition on macrophage function and the amount and affinity of antibody response. *Clin. Exp. Immunol.*, 17:491–495.

210. Pedroni, E., Bianchi, E., Ugazio, A. G., and Burgio, G. R. (1975): Immunodeficiency and steely hair. *Lancet*, 1:1303–1304.

211. Philippens, K. M. H., Von Mayersbach, H., and Scheving, L. E. (1977): Effects of the scheduling of meal-feeding of different phases of the circadian system in rats. *J. Nutr.*, 107:176–193.

212. Philips, I., and Wharton, B. (1968): Acute bacterial infection in kwashiorkor. *Br. Med. J.*, 1:407–408.

213. Pocknee, R. C., and Heaton, F. W. (1978): Changes in organ growth with feeding pattern. The influence of feeding frequency on the circadian rhythm of protein synthesis in the rat. *J. Nutr.*, 108:1266–1273.

214. Prendergast, R. A., and Henney, C. S. (1977): Cellular immune reactions. In: *The Lymphocyte. Structures and Functions. Part I*, edited by J. J. Marchalonis, pp. 257–277. Marcel Dekker, New York.

215. Price, P. (1978): Responses to polyvinyl pyrrolidone and pneumococcal polysaccharide in protein-deficient mice. *Immunology*, 34:87–96.

216. Price, P., and Bell, R. G. (1976): The effects of nutritional rehabilitation on antibody production in protein-deficient mice. *Immunology*, 31:953–960.

217. Price, P., and Bell, R. G. (1977): The response of protein-deficient mice to tetanus toxoid. Effects of antigen dose, adjuvants, period of deprivation and age on antibody production. *Immunology*, 32:65–74.

218. Prohaska, J. R., and Lukasewycz, O. A. (1981): Copper deficiency suppresses the immune response of mice. *Science*, 213:559–561.

219. Prohaska, J. R., and Lukasewycz, O. A. (1982): Immunological consequences of copper deficiency in mice. Proceeding on the *Role of Copper and Other Essential Metals in Inflammatory Diseases*. Human Press, Clifton *(in press)*.

220. Pruzansky, J., and Axelrod, A. E. (1955): Antibody production to diphtheria toxoid in vitamin deficiency states. *Proc. Soc. Exp. Biol. Med.*, 89:323–325.

221. Rao, K. M., Schwartz, S. A., and Good, R. A. (1979): Age-dependent effects of zinc on the transformation response of human lymphocytes to mitogens. *Cell. Immunol.*, 42:270–278.

222. Reddy, V., and Srikantia, S. G. (1964): Antibody response in kwashiorkor. *Indian J. Med. Res.*, 52:1154–1158.

223. Reddy, V., Raghuramulu, N., and Bhaskaram, C. (1976): Secretory IgA in protein calorie malnutrition. *Arch. Dis. Child.*, 51:871–874.

224. Reddy, V., Jagadeesan, V., Ragharamula, N., Bhaskaram, C., and Srikantia, S. G. (1976): Functional significance of growth retardation. *Am. J. Clin. Nutr.*, 29:3–7.

225. Rhodes, J., and Oliver, S. (1980): Retinoids as regulators of macrophage function. *Immunology*, 40:467–472.

226. Robson, L. C., and Schwarz, M. R. (1975): Vitamin B6 deficiency and the lymphoid system. 1. Effects on cellular immunity and *in vitro* incorporation of ³H-uridine by small lymphocytes. *Cell. Immunol.*, 16:135–144.

227. Robson, L. C., and Schwarz, M. R. (1975): Vitamin B6 deficiency and the lymphoid system. II. Effects of vitamin B6 deficiency in utero on the immunological competence of the offspring. *Cell. Immunol.*, 16:145–152.

228. Rosenstreich, D. L., and Mizel, S. B. (1978): The participation of macrophages and macrophage cell lines in the activation of T lymphocytes by mitogens. *Immunol. Rev.*, 40:102–135.

229. Rosenthal, A. S. (1978): Determinant selection and macrophage function in genetic control of the immune response. *Immunol. Rev.*, 40:136–152.

230. Rous, P. (1914): The influence of diet on transplanted and spontaneous mouse tumors. *J. Exp. Med.*, 20:443–451.

231. Salimonu, L. S., Ojo-Amaize, E., Williams, A. I. O., Johnson, A. O. K., Cooke, A. R., Adekunle, F. A., Alm, G. V., and Wigzell, H. (1982): Depressed natural killer cell activity in children with protein-calorie malnutrition. *Clin. Immunol. Immunopathol. (in press)*.

232. Salomon, J. B., Mata, L. J., and Gordon, J. E. (1968): Malnutrition and the common communicable diseases of childhood in rural Guatemala. *Am. J. Public Health*, 58:505–516.

233. Saxton, J. A., Jr., Boon, M. A., and Furth, J. (1944): Observations on the inhibition of development of spontaneous leukemia in mice by underfeeding. *Cancer Res.*, 4:401–409.

234. Schlesinger, L., and Stekel, A. (1974): Impaired cellular immunity in marasmic infants. *Am. J. Clin. Nutr.*, 27:615–620.

235. Schlesinger, L., Ohlbaum, A., Grey, L., and Stekel, A. (1976): Decreased interferon production by leukocytes in marasmus. *Am. J. Clin. Nutr.*, 29:758–761.

236. Schonland, M. M., Shanley, B. C., Loening, W. E. K., Parent, M. A., and Coovadia, H. M. (1972): Plasma cortisol and immunosuppression in protein-calorie malnutrition. *Lancet*, 2:435–436.

237. Schopfer, K., and Douglas, S. D. (1976): *In vitro* studies of lymphocytes from children with kwashiorkor. *Clin. Immunopathol.*, 5:21–30.

238. Scragg, J. N., and Applebaum, P. C. (1978): Septicemia in kwashiorkor. *S. Afr. Med. J.*, 53:358–360.

239. Scrimshaw, N. S., Taylor, C. E., and Gordon, J. E. (1968): *Interactions of Nutrition and Infection*. WHO Monograph Series no. 57. WHO, Geneva.

240. Sellmeyer, E., Bhettay, E., Truswell, A. S., Meyers, O. L., and Hansen, J. D. L. (1972): Lymphocyte transformation in malnourished children. *Arch. Dis. Child.*, 47:429–435.

241. Siegel, B. V. (1974): Enhanced interferon response to murine leukemia virus by ascorbic acid. *Infect. Immun.*, 10(2):409–410.

242. Siegel, B. V. (1975): Enhancement of interferon production by poly(rI) · poly(rC) in mouse cell cultures by ascorbic acid. *Nature*, 254:531–532.

243. Siegel, B. V., and Morton, J. I. (1977): Vitamin C and the immune response. *Experientia*, 33:393–395.

244. Simon, J. (1845): *Physiological Essay on the Thymus Gland*. Renshaw, London.

245. Sinha, D. P., and Bang, F. B. (1976): Protein and calorie malnutrition, cell mediated immunity, and BCG vaccination in children from rural West Bengal. *Lancet*, 2:531–534.

246. Sirisinha, S., Suskind, R., Edelman, R., Asvapaka, C., and Olson, R. E. (1975): Secretory and serum IgA in children with protein-calorie malnutrition. *Pediatrics*, 55:166–170.

247. Smith, N. J., Khadroui, S., Lopez, V., and Hamza, B. (1977): Cellular immune response in Tunisian children with severe infantile malnutrition. In: *Malnutrition and the Immune Response*, edited by R. M. Suskind, pp. 105–109. Raven Press, New York.

248. Smythe, P. M. (1968): Changes in intestinal bacterial flora and role of infection in kwashiorkor. *Lancet*, 2:724–727.

249. Smythe, P. M., Schonland, M., Brereton-Stiles, G. G., Coovadia, H. M., Grace, H. J., Loening, W. E. K., Mafoyane, A., Parent, M. A., and Vos, G. H. (1971): Thymolymphatic deficiency and depression of cell-mediated immunity in protein-calorie malnutrition. *Lancet*, 2:939–943.

250. Spallholz, J. E., Martin, J. L., Gerlach, M. L., and Heinzerling, R. H. (1973): Immunologic responses of mice fed diets supplemented with selenite selenium. *Proc. Soc. Exp. Biol. Med.*, 143:685–689.

251. Spallholz, J. E., Martin, J. L., Gerlach, M. L., and Heinzerling, R. H. (1973): Enhanced immunoglobulin M and immunoglobulin G antibody titers in mice fed selenium. *Infect. Immun.*, 8(5):841–842.

252. Srikantia, S. G., Bhaskaram, C., Prasad, J. S., and Krishnanchari, K. A. V. R. (1976): Anaemia and immune response. *Lancet*, 1:1307–1309.

253. Stoerk, H. C., and Eisen, H. N. (1946): Suppression of circulating antibodies in pyridoxine deficiency. *Proc. Soc. Exp. Biol. Med.*, 62:88–89.

254. Stoerk, H. C., Eisen, H. N., and John, H. M. (1947): Impairment of antibody response in pyridoxine-deficient rats. *J. Exp. Med.*, 85:365–371.

255. Stoltzner, G. H., and Dorsey, B. A. (1980): Life-long dietary protein restriction and immune function: Responses to mitogens and sheep erythrocytes in BALB/c mice. *Am. J. Clin. Nutr.*, 33:1264–1271.

256. Sullivan, J. L., and Ochs, H. D. (1978): Copper deficiency and the immune system. *Lancet*, 2:686.

257. Suskind, R., Sirishinha, S., Vithayasai, V., Edelman, R., Damrongsak, D., Charupatana, C., and Olson, R. E. (1976): Immunoglobulins and antibody response in children with protein-calorie malnutrition. *Am. J. Clin. Nutr.*, 29:836–841.

258. Templeton, A. C. (1970): Generalized herpes simplex in malnourished children. *J. Clin. Pathol.*, 23:24–30.

259. Tengerdy, R. P., Heinzerling, R. H., and Nockles, C. F. (1972): Effect of vitamin E on the immune response of hypoxic and normal chickens. *Infect. Immun.*, 5(6):987–989.

260. Tengerdy, R. P., Heinzerling, R. H., Brown, G. L., and Mathias, M. M. (1973): Enhancement of the humoral immune response by vitamin E. *Int. Arch. Allergy*, 44:221–232.
261. Trakatellis, A. C., and Axelrod, A. E. (1969): Effect of pyridoxine deficiency on the induction of immune tolerance in mice. *Proc. Soc. Exp. Biol. Med.*, 132:46–49.
262. Trakatellis, A. C., Stinebring, W. R., and Axelrod, A. E. (1963): Studies on systemic reactivity to purified protein derivative (PPD) and endotoxin. I. Systemic reactivity to PPD in pyridoxine-deficient guinea pigs. *J. Immunol.*, 91:39–45.
263. Trowell, H. C., Davies, J. N. P., and Dean, R. F. A. (1954): *Kwashiorkor.* Edward Arnold, London.
264. Vint, F. W. (1937): Post-mortem findings in natives in Kenya. *East Afr. Med. J.*, 13:332–340.
265. Wagner, H., Hardt, C., Heeg, K., Pfizenmaier, K., Solbach, W., Bartlett, R., Stockinger, H., and Röllinghoff (1980): T-T cell interactions during cytotoxic T lymphocyte (CTL) responses: T cell derived helper factor (Interleukin 2) as a probe to analyze CTL responsiveness and thymic maturation of CTL progenitors. *Immunol. Rev.*, 51:215–255.
266. Wakabayashi, Y., and Takaku, F. (1978): Effect of iron on the DNA synthesis in peripheral lymphocytes from patients with iron deficiency anemia. *Acta Haematol. Jpn.*, 41(5):846–851.
267. Ward, K., Cantor, H., and Nisonoff, A. (1978): Analysis of the cellular basis of idiotype-specific suppression. *J. Immunol.*, 120(6):2016–2019.
268. Warren, J. V., and Hill, G. L. (1977): T cells and protein nutrition in hospitalized surgical patients. *Br. J. Surg.*, 64:897–899.
269. Watson, R. R., and McMurray, D. N. (1979): The effects of malnutrition on secretory and cellular immune processes. *CRC Crit. Rev. Food Sci. Nutr.*, 12(2):113–159.
270. Watts, T. (1969): Thymus weights in malnourished children. *J. Trop. Pediatr.*, 15:155–158.
271. Weindruch, R. H., Kristie, J. A., Cheney, K. E., and Walfold, R. L. (1979): Influence of controlled dietary restriction on immunological function and aging. *Fed. Proc.*, 38(6):2007–2016.
272. Weissman, I. L., Small, M., Fathman, C. G., and Herzenberg, L. A. (1975): Differentiation of thymus cells. *Fed. Proc.*, 34:141–144.
273. Weston, W. L., Mandel, M. J., Yeckley, J. A., Krueger, G. G., and Claman, H. N. (1973): Mechanism of cortisol inhibition of adoptive transfer of tuberculin sensitivity. *J. Lab. Clin. Med.*, 82:366–371.
274. Whitehead, R. G., Coward, W. A., and Lunn, P. G. (1973): Serum-albumin concentration and the onset of kwashiorkor. *Lancet*, 1:63–66.
275. Willis-Carr, J. I., and St. Pierre, R. L. (1978): Effects of vitamin B6 deficiency on thymic epithelium cells and T lymphocyte differentiation. *J. Immunol.*, 120(4):1153–1159.
276. Work, T. H., Ifekwunigwe, A., Jelliffe, D., and Jelliffe, P. (1973): Tropical problems in nutrition. *Ann. Intern. Med.*, 79:701–711.
277. Young, V. R., Rand, W. M., and Scrimshaw, N. S. (1977): Measuring protein quality in humans: A review and proposed method. *Cereal Chem.*, 54(4):929–948.
278. Ziegler, H. D., and Ziegler, P. B. (1975): Depression of tuberculin reaction in mild and moderate protein calorie malnourished children following BCG vaccination. *Johns Hopkins Med. J.*, 137:59–64.
279. Zweiman, B., Schoenwetter, W. F., and Hildreth, E. A. (1966): The effect of the scorbutic state on tuberculin hypersensitivity in the guinea pig. 1. Passive transfer of tuberculin hypersensitivity. *J. Immunol.*, 96:296–300.

Subject Index

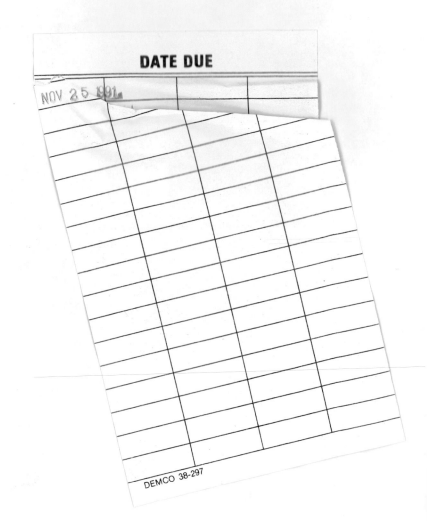

DATE DUE

NOV 25 1991

DEMCO 38-297